Y0-AFX-008

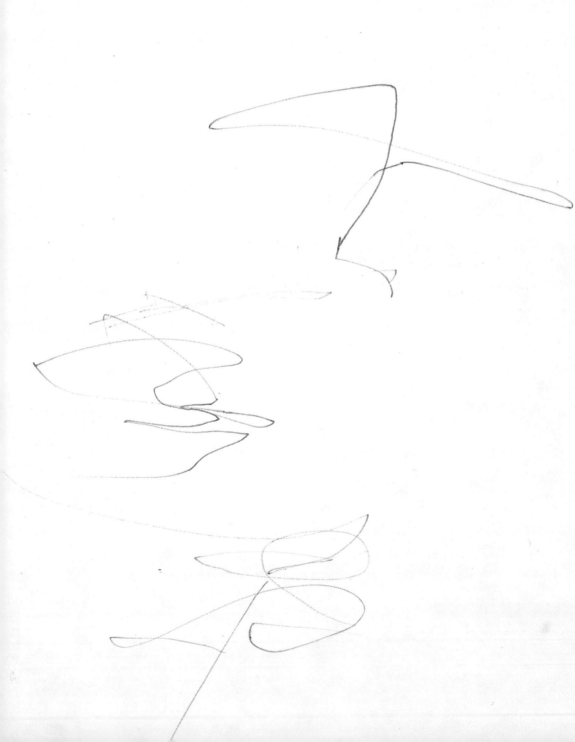

Human
Communication
Disorders

Human Communication Disorders

An Introduction

edited by

George H. Shames
University of Pittsburgh

and

Elisabeth H. Wiig
Boston University

Charles E. Merrill Publishing Company
A Bell & Howell Company
Columbus   Toronto   London   Sydney

Published by
Charles E. Merrill Publishing Co.
A Bell & Howell Company
Columbus, Ohio 43216

This book was set in Korinna.
Cover Design Coordination: Will Chenoweth.
Text Designer: Francie Margolin
Production Coordination: Martha Morss

Cover photographs by Robert L. Goodman, courtesy of Columbus Speech and
Hearing Center, Columbus, Ohio.

Excerpts on page 428 from Howard Gardner, *The Shattered Mind,* copyright
1975 by Alfred A. Knopf, Inc. Reprinted by permission. Selection on page 447
from *Wings* by Arthur Kopit. Copyright © 1978 by Arthur Kopit. Reprinted by
permission of Hill and Wang, a division of Farrar, Straus and Giroux, Inc.

Copyright © 1982, by Bell & Howell Company. All rights reserved.
No part of this book may be reproduced in any form, electronic or mechanical,
including photocopy, recording, or any information storage and retrieval system,
without permission in writing from the publisher.

Library of Congress Catalog Card Number: 81–84346
International Standard Book Number: 0–675–09837–8

Printed in the United States of America

2 3 4 5 6 7 8 9 10—86 85 84 83 82

Contents

Foreword

This book provides an introduction to the profession of speech-language pathology and audiology. It also introduces a rapidly growing, instrumental academic field. The authors attend closely to the ground rules of the American Speech-Language and Hearing Association and clearly describe both its humanistic and its scientific philosophy. The scope of the book is impressive. More importantly, it defines the boundaries of the expanding field; while standing upon the foundations of speech and hearing, it authoritatively addresses language and its related interpersonal usage systems.

Because of the rapid changes that science has brought to the speech-language and hearing field, the planners of *Human Communication Disorders* were faced with difficult choices in content selection. This text builds upon an accepted knowledge base with treatments of the many recent advances derived from research and clinical experience. The material is organized into a readable, comprehensive statement that students with limited backgrounds can understand with the help of competent teachers. Also, the material meets the tests imposed by knowledgeable scholars in the several areas covered.

The planners and contributors have produced a book of remarkable cogency. The content is distinguished by its scope and perspective, by its informativeness, and by its readability. Each of these features deserves a brief explanation.

This is a *perspective* book. The reader can use the book to gain an overview of human communication and the many hazards and impairing conditions that children and adults experience on their way to personal development. The book is especially valuable because it explains the various categories of disorder in terms of both process (speech, voice, and language) and etiology (cleft palate, cerebral palsy, aphasia, and so on). The orienting value of this approach is apparent to all who seek to gain an understanding of communicative disorders and who wish to build subsequent competencies upon a sound base of scholarship.

It is an *informative* book. It covers new developments and synthesizes them with the main knowledge base of a distinguished field. For instance, the book discusses early language development, language differences, learning disabilities, and nonvocal language, all new and exciting areas that have emerged in recent years. Also considered are cerebral palsy, cleft palate, adult aphasia, auditory disorders, and functional articulation disorders, all areas that have long been a traditional part of the field. However, I do not intend to imply that any part of the book is "traditional" in presenting information that is standardized or outdated. Each of the chapters provides recent, updated information that helps us project our thinking well into the future and that will make this book a useful text for many years to come.

It is a *readable* book. The writing style is lucid, and numerous examples, case descriptions, and editorial inserts guide the reader. The case studies are especially apt and illustrative. They help the reader to extend the principles and the multidimensional information into human experience. Also, accompanying audio examples bring to life different speech, language, and communication variations. The strategy followed throughout is to present the information in a vivid, interesting, and meaningful way.

My comments would be incomplete if I did not call attention to the list of competent authors. Noted scholars, they are also successful clinicians and researchers. Their demonstrated effectiveness in these important respects gives validity to the subject matter and provides an authoritative stamp to each chapter of the book.

Richard L. Schiefelbusch
University of Kansas

Preface

The purpose of *Human Communication Disorders: An Introduction* is to lead you gradually into the world of the person who has problems communicating with other people. As guides for this journey, leading authorities in the fields of speech and hearing science, speech pathology, language pathology, and audiology have contributed chapters which focus on individual facets of this multidimensional topic. While each author presents his or her own personal perspective, we have tried to blend the parts into a cohesive picture of a complex profession. A common thread is our interest in *serving people* with communication problems. This book is for the beginner, for whom it may well be the first venture into a rewarding career as a speech-language pathologist, audiologist, special educator, classroom teacher, concerned and informed citizen.

The book is divided into three major parts. Part I, *Bases of Human Communication,* provides basic information that underlies our understanding of problems of communication and how they are studied and managed. One chapter develops a view of the profession—its history, philosophy, and ethics. In addition, this section discusses the theoretical and scientific principles that help us understand human communication problems. Separate chapters describe the communication process and what language is, language differences, and the physical basis of the act of speaking.

Part II, *Disorders of Speech, Voice, and Language* considers each of the major categories of disordered communication. For each disorder, the author discusses basic theories of causation, characteristics, and special procedures of assessment and therapy.

In Part III, titled *Communication Disorders of Special Populations,* we turn to populations of children and adults that have certain unique physical characteristics that are associated with or contribute to a specific type of communication problem. This section ends with a view of those systems and events which can facilitate your task of helping the communication handicapped. You are introduced to the world of the clinician, including feelings, reactions, values, and philosophies, and how they mesh with the problems of the clients.

Each disorder chapter in Parts II and III opens with a concrete, real-life case history so that you can readily understand some of the human, social, and emotional aspects of these problems. To augment your understanding, we have included audio disc recordings so that you can hear samples of various problems. In addition, marginal notes in each chapter define key terms to help you clearly understand material; many of these definitions also appear in a glossary at the end of the book, for ready reference. Because speech and language problems in real people cannot be as easily categorized as chapters in a book, we have also included numerous cross-references from chapter to chapter.

Human communication and its disorders are a part of the overall human condition. Each of us lives and exists as a uniquely synthesized unit. We express ourselves to one another and relate to one another, not as a mouth or a tongue or an ear, but as individual thoughtful, caring, feeling people. The momentary focus on separate aspects of human communication in separate chapters reflects our own attempts to analyze a complex process in order to try to understand it. But when we communicate, the body and mind respond together as a unit; and it is with this synthesis that we are concerned in this book.

Acknowledgments

Writing projects like this one requires significant contributions at strategic times by many people. Each contribution has its own unique impact on the final result.

From its inception, this book had the dedication of Ms. Marianne Taflinger and Ms. Vicki Knight of Charles E. Merrill. Marianne brought us together to begin this project. As our tireless developmental editor, Vicki handled the logistics of manuscript preparation and transmission in a firm yet sensitive manner. Hers was the responsibility for meeting deadlines, for permission forms, for manuscript preparation, and, perhaps above all else, for maintaining warm, productive communication among the authors.

All of the chapter authors deserve special commendations for their ability to come down from their highly sophisticated level of thought to put together their ideas at an introductory and basic level for the beginning student. In addition, the authors were able to translate their special areas of interest and research into concepts involving the "whole person" and "total rehabilitation," to show their personal commitment to helping people with communication disorders. A special thank you goes to Bill and Therese Zemlin, who created all the excellent illustrations in his chapter (except as noted).

Wayne Secord receives our gratitude for his in-depth review of the entire manuscript, including multiple drafts of individual chapters. Based on his experience teaching the course, Wayne's constructive comments helped shape the final book.

Joel Kahane, Nancy Creaghead, Kennon Shank, Ron Tikofsky, William Melnick, Betty Webster, Richard Culatta and Laura W. Kretschmer, as the reviewers of these many chapters, brought their critical observations of the field of Speech Pathology to the mission of this book. Their evaluations of each chapter and of the total volume as an integrated whole greatly influenced the final product.

We would also like to thank Marc E. Fey for providing tape-recorded material for chapter 8 and Martha Selvik Lansing for her tireless assistance on this project.

In the later stages of preparation, Francie Margolin, as the rewrite editor, worked on the manuscript. With her view of grammar and syntax, her facile vocabulary, and her sense of dramatic composition, she pulled the separate chapters into smooth sections of a well-integrated volume.

We sincerely thank G. Paul Moore and Leonard L. LaPointe for their contributions to the editorial comments for Parts II and III.

Finally, the two editors (Shames and Wiig) would like to acknowledge each other for the mutual joy and support that this collaboration has brought to them as they shared in this editorship.

*When we are children we learn to
understand the nature of the world we live
in and to accept love and caring from
those who are around us.*

*When we are adults we learn to share
those understandings and to care for those
who are in need.*

*The mission of this book is to promote a
special kind of understanding and caring
for those children and adults and their
families who live with communication
problems.*

*It is to the achievement of this mission that
the editors humbly dedicate this book.*

Human
Communication
Disorders

part I

Bases of
Human
Communication

THE PROFESSIONS OF SPEECH-LANGUAGE PATHOLOGY AND AUDIOLOGY

Jack Matthews

This book is about people—people with communication disorders, the people speech-language pathologists and audiologists work with and try to help. Some of their problems stem from physical causes, such as cleft palate, brain damage, hearing loss. Some have roots in the environment in which a child grows up, lack of language stimulation for example. Some grow out of the way people feel about themselves. Some may stem from some unmeasurable combination of these factors. Regardless of the cause or causes, speech-language pathologists and audiologists try to help the *whole person* who is experiencing a communication problem.

As you get to know more about some of these people, you will realize that speech-language pathologists and audiologists have to know a good deal about people, how they communicate, and what breakdowns can occur in their communication. You will soon become acutely aware that becoming a professional involves much more than learning about communication disorders and how to alleviate them. In fact, sometimes we cannot restore certain lost or impaired functions, but instead must modify and train residual or retained abilities. And you will see that speech-language pathologists and audiologists often work with other professionals in education, medicine, social work, psychology, rehabilitation, and dentistry to provide the necessary help for the person who has a communication disorder. To begin, let us look at three people whose lives were changed by speech-language pathologists.

Let me start by telling you about Annabelle. Until she was about 5, she lived almost like a caged animal. The adults in her world hid her from society because she was illegitimate. Her grandparents, with whom she and her mother lived, believed that the family's "disgrace" would be concealed by keeping Annabelle out of sight. The little room she grew up in was more a closet than a child's nursery. She saw no sunshine. She had no friends. She was fed much like an animal. At the time that the juvenile court authorities found her (early 1940s), Annabelle was malnourished, was not able to walk, and had no language or speech, even though she was almost 5 years old. In many ways she was more a little beast than a little girl. Because Annabelle's mother was thought to be mentally retarded and because Annabelle could not talk, some juvenile court workers assumed that Annabelle, too, was retarded and should be placed in the state institution, which in those days was known as the State School for the Feebleminded.

Annabelle was brought to Children's Hospital in Columbus, Ohio. While she was there, she was seen by a speech-language pathologist, and several graduate students played with Annabelle. They bounced and tossed a ball to each other; and as they played with it, kept saying, "ball, ball, ball." After a few minutes of patient stimulation of this kind, Annabelle responded to the ball by uttering the sounds "ba-ba," as she, too, tossed the ball.

Annabelle smiled broadly when a wristwatch was held to her ear. She could hear. It was clear she could see the ball and other people and objects in her environment. While she was in Children's Hospital, physicians, psychologists, and speech-language pathologists carried out a series of diagnostic examinations. They concluded that Annabelle had the necessary "equipment" to speak. What she needed was appropriate stimulation and training, in addition to general health care.

Because I subsequently married one of the graduate students who helped train Annabelle, I had an especially good opportunity to watch her develop. To me it was almost a miracle to observe Annabelle as she grew from a near animal into a youngster who showed promise of leading a normal life.

Annabelle has not proved to be a genius. She has not won a Nobel Prize. But she did grow into a healthy, attractive child and was adopted by a warm, loving family. When last I heard, she had completed high school and was about to enter nursing school. Annabelle did not have to spend the rest of her life in a state institution. She was given a chance to develop her potential. Both Annabelle and our society have profited from the efforts of a team of professionals, which included several knowledgeable and concerned speech-language pathologists.

Next I want to describe Roger, a young man for whom speaking was unpleasant. When he spoke, he had severe blocks and many repetitions. People called him a stutterer. He finished college and, without a personal interview, was somehow hired as a teacher in a remote rural school. During the first few minutes of his first day of teaching, he avoided talking by writing the names of texts, assignments, and everything else on the blackboard. Shortly after class began, the superintendent stopped by. He came into the classroom by the rear door. Roger immediately fled through the front door. A number of hours later, he was found near death from carbon monoxide poisoning. He had started the motor of his car and closed the garage doors. Fortunately, Roger was revived. He was encouraged to seek professional help for his speech problem at a clinic affiliated with a large university. Here he was given an opportunity to talk through his problem with a speech pathologist. He learned some techniques for handling it and was helped to change his attitude toward his speech and himself. While he was doing all of this, Roger decided to enter graduate school to learn more about the nature of stuttering, communication disorders, and psychology. At the same time, he continued working on his own speech in the speech clinic. In a few years he completed his doctorate. His speech improved, and I am pleased to report that today he is successfully engaged in the profession of his choice. Speech-language pathology gave Roger an opportunity to develop many fine capabilities that he had never used—instead of becoming nothing more than a suicide statistic. Society is richer today because Roger was given a chance to develop his potential. Speech-language pathologists played an important role in Roger's development, a role which involved much more than simply correcting a stutter.

Finally, let's look at Jerry, another example of the kind of person speech-language pathologists try to help. He came to the clinic where I was working to get some vocational guidance. He told me he wanted to study sheet metal work. Everything he communicated to me was written on a slip of paper. The few times he tried to speak, he was very difficult to understand. The tests Jerry took indicated that he had very little aptitude for sheet metal work. I told him the test results, and he was very upset. I finally succeeded in getting him to tell me his story. Jerry's speech had been a problem for as long as he was able to remember. He had managed to finish high school and begin college. Shortly after entering college, however, he dropped out and decided to get a job that would not require him to speak. Very naively, he thought that as a sheet metal worker he would not have to talk to people. He thought he would be able to take an order for a furnace, deliver it, and install it. He hoped he might be able to do all of this without having to speak at all.

As Jerry returned for subsequent visits to the clinic, we helped him realize that sheet metal workers, like most people, have to communicate. With the aid of the clinic audiologist, we discovered that he had a hearing loss that contributed to his speech problem. He began a program in our clinic which helped him manage his hearing problem and which also helped him speak more intelligibly. While we could not cure his hearing loss, Jerry was able to profit from the use of a hearing aid. As his speech began to improve, Jerry revealed many things about his earlier life and about some of his real ambitions. He told me that he had spent many rewarding hours coaching youth groups. That was what he really enjoyed doing best. As his speech continued to improve, we encouraged him to return to college, where he majored in physical education. Shortly before I saw Jerry for the last time, he had received a letter from the superintendent of a nearby school offering him a teaching and coaching job.

The three people I have just described were not geniuses; none of them made the cover of *Time* magazine. But Annabelle was saved from a useless existence as an inmate in an institution and instead became a successful nurse. Roger eventually earned a PhD and has made an outstanding contribution to his profession. Jerry did not become the number one athletic coach in the United States, but he did not become a failure in work he was not suited for. Instead, he became a happy and useful teacher and greatly admired athletic coach. All three of these people share one thing in common—each was helped to develop unrealized potential which had been blocked because of communication problems.

These examples are obviously dramatic, and all have happy endings. Of course, not all of the people speech-language pathologists and audiologists work with have such dramatic appeal and provide us with such happy endings. I can assure you, however, having been in this field for almost 40 years, that the kinds of stories I just reported are not at all unusual. Anyone who begins a career in this field can expect to experience some similar satisfactions.

HOW MANY PEOPLE HAVE COMMUNICATION DISORDERS?

The information we have about the exact number of people with communication disorders is not as accurate as I would like. While there have been many studies to determine the number of people with communication disorders, reliable figures are hard to come by. One problem is comparing a study done by one investigator with that carried out by another. Not all studies employ exactly the same definition of *communication disorder.* Another problem is sampling. One report may be based on a population that is very different from the population another researcher studies. There are so many variables to consider that the best we can do is to make some estimates about the incidence and prevalence of communication disorders.

Incidence *refers to the number of new cases of a condition identified within a group over a specific period of time;* prevalence, *to the total number of cases existing at a particular place or time.*

One of the early large-scale efforts to determine the prevalence of communication disorders was the 1950 White House Conference (ASHA Committee, 1952). The committee which studied the problem at the time estimated that 5% of the population between ages 5 and 21 had defective speech. Let me present a brief quotation from the White House Conference report.

> It is to be stressed that the figures are presented as the lowest defensible estimate; they would be regarded as serious underestimates in certain respects by some authorities. They leave out of account an estimated additional 5% or 2,000,000 children who have minor speech and voice defects, unimportant for the most practical purposes but serious in their effects on personal and social adjustment in some cases, and obviously significant for children destined for fields of work, such as teaching, requiring good speech. (p. 129)

This report concentrated on children, but not all individuals with communication disorders are between ages 5 and 21. In fact, some communication disorders are found more frequently in an older population. Robert Milisen, in *Handbook of Speech Pathology and Audiology* (1971, pp. 621–622), summarized the studies of the incidence and prevalence of communication disorders. Later in this book, the authors writing about various types of communication disorders will provide more specific information about the incidence and prevalence of particular communication disorders. For the time being, it is safe for us to say that communication disorders affect millions of people of all ages.

SCOPE OF THIS BOOK

This book is only an introduction to communication disorders. Because it is an introduction, it cannot include everything that is known about communication disorders. Indeed, we do not deal with all communication disorders but, instead, concentrate on the oral-verbal part of communication. Other books and other professions are concerned with communication disorders related to reading, writing, spelling, and so on. In this chapter, we will focus on the professions of speech-language pathology and audiology, which specialize in the oral-verbal aspects of communication.

Throughout this book you will find discussions of many elements of disordered oral-verbal communication. Some specialists will tell you about children and adults who have difficulty producing certain sounds, that is, with articulation. In many instances, it's hard to understand what a person is saying. Sometimes you can understand what is being said, but the "defective" sound production is so noticeable that you concentrate on the unfamiliar sounds. In so doing, you can miss much that the person is trying to say. Other specialists will describe speakers whose voices are not appropriate for their age and sex or who are not pleasant to listen to. You will learn about cases in which the problem is neither voice nor sound production, but the rhythm with which the speech is produced. You will learn that in some instances the disorder of communication is related to how a speaker feels about the way he talks. You will learn about children who do not talk, or who at age 8 sound like a child of 3. We will discuss communication disorders associated with special problems such as hearing impairment, brain damage, cleft palate, and mental retardation. You will learn about communication problems in which sound production, voice, and rhythm are not involved, but where the individual has trouble associating the appropriate word or sound with the object or the concept he wishes to talk about.

In addition to learning about problems, you will read about the processes used to help. You will learn about the diagnostic procedures speech-language pathologists and audiologists carry out, and how the information obtained by other professional workers can help you understand the nature and causes of the communication disorder. You will learn about remedial procedures employed directly by speech-language pathologists, as well as procedures which are developed by speech-language pathologists and carried out by parents, teachers, and a variety of others who are in contact with the person with a communication disorder. You will learn that, in some instances, it is possible to restore a lost or impaired function, as is the case of plastic surgery for a child with a cleft palate; in other cases, the most that can be done is to modify a residual function, as might be true with someone who has paralysis following a stroke. In still other cases, we prescribe adaptive equipment, such as a hearing aid, to help perform the function of a damaged or even missing body part.

OTHER PROFESSIONS CONCERNED WITH COMMUNICATION DISORDERS

It is important to realize that there are many professions which are concerned with certain communication disorders. Almost 30 years ago, Dorothea McCarthy (1954) noted that increasingly large numbers of individuals with normal intelligence and intact senses have difficulty in acquiring facility in the various essential forms of communication.

> This phenomenon has in turn given rise to the several professions concerned with remediation, such as speech therapists and remedial reading teachers who together with clinical psychologists and psychiatrists are concerned with alleviating the various language disorders. . . . Whether a child is referred to a speech therapist, to a psychologist, or to a remedial reading teacher is largely a matter of timing. It is a question of when a particular symptom becomes intolerable to someone in the environment and what facilities are available in the community. (p. 514)

If McCarthy were writing today, she might add several additional specialists who are concerned with communication disorders: pediatricians, otolaryngologists, audiologists, neurologists, classroom teachers, and specialists in learning disabilities.

In a text directed to otolaryngologists and pediatricians, Matthews (1982) points out that the variety of specialists concerned with communication disorders can be a source of confusion to parents.

> It can be confusing to the parents of a 3-year-old child who is not speaking to receive different and often conflicting opinions concerning the etiology of delayed language. The otolaryngologist may stress the role of hearing loss. The psychologist may attribute the problem to mental retardation. The psychiatrist may give major importance to emotional problems in the home. Other specialists may blame an environment lacking adequate language stimulation or confusion growing out of a bilingual background. The presence of one of these factors does not rule out the possible influences that may be exerted by the others. The incidence of hearing loss is, indeed, higher in the mentally retarded than in the nonretarded population (Birch & Matthews, 1951), and hearing loss can result in frustration and emotional prob-

lems. A physical disability can result in parents overly protecting a child so the child finds little need to learn to talk. The task of differential diagnosis in the child with a language disorder is difficult and goes beyond the scope of training of most pediatricians and otolaryngologists, even though the contributions of these physicians are important in the diagnosis and treatment of the disorders.

In both diagnosing and treating a communication disorder, it is often desirable to involve specialists from speech-language pathology, audiology, special education, psychology, social work, neurology, psychiatry, pediatrics, otolaryngology, and other medical and dental specialties. But of all these professions, only speech-language pathology has communication disorders as its *central* concern. For this reason, we will begin our text on communication disorders with a discussion of the profession of speech-language pathology.

WHAT DO SPECIALISTS IN COMMUNICATION DISORDERS CALL THEMSELVES?

In this book, we use the term *speech-language pathologist* as the title for specialists who diagnose and treat individuals with communication disorders. In a recent survey (Taylor, 1980), there were 19 professional titles applied by state departments of education to the speech-language pathologist working in the school setting. These titles included speech and language clinician, speech correctionist, communication disorders specialist, speech and hearing therapist, speech clinician, teacher of speech handicapped, and speech therapist. Some state departments of education do not use any of the 19 professional titles for the *specialists* in communication disorders, but instead designate the *specialty area* by employing one of 14 different terms, including speech correction, speech pathology, speech disorders, speech and hearing therapy, and speech and language pathology. To work as a speech-language pathologist in a school system, you must have a certificate issued by the state department of education. At the present, eight states employ the professional title of speech pathologist or speech and language pathologist. None of the other titles is employed by more than three states.

In contrast, *audiologists* are concerned with identification, measurement, and study of hearing and hearing impairments. The audiologist is usually the professional who prescribes the hearing aid, if necessary. Because hearing problems are often related to communication disorders, audiologists and speech-language pathologists work together to determine both the sources of a problem and a coordinated program of rehabilitation.

WHERE DO SPEECH-LANGUAGE PATHOLOGISTS AND AUDIOLOGISTS WORK?

The profession of speech-language pathology is made up only in part of specialists who work in school systems. Many speech-language pathologists work in hospitals, rehabilitation centers, university speech clinics, and community speech and hearing centers. Thirty-one states now issue licenses for individuals to carry on the practice of speech pathology.

An estimated 50% of the working speech-language pathologists in the United States are members of the American Speech-Language-Hearing Association (ASHA). Using the results of a recent ASHA membership analysis (ASHA, 1980b), we estimate that about 45% of speech-language pathologists and audiologists are employed in elementary or secondary schools. About 12% work in universities, and about 19% are employed in nonuniversity clinics in hospitals, rehabilitation centers, community speech and hearing centers, and so on. About 20% are employed in other settings. Nearly 5% at any one time are voluntarily unemployed.

Although the majority of speech-language pathologists and audiologists work as clinicians in schools, hospitals, and rehabilitation centers, more and more speech-language pathologists are working as private practitioners who serve their clients in much the same way as doctors or lawyers who are in private practice. Still others are employed by a clinical facility, but devote some "after hours" time to private practice.

WHAT ARE THE MAJOR WORK ACTIVITIES OF SPEECH-LANGUAGE PATHOLOGISTS AND AUDIOLOGISTS?

Although over 70% of the speech-language pathologists and audiologists spend most of their time as clinicians helping people with communication disorders, some (about 6%) devote much of their time carrying out research to learn about the causes of communication disorders and the improvement of procedures to help people with communication disorders. An increasing number (almost 9%) devote the major part of their work activity to administration as directors of clinics, supervisors of clinical staffs, coordinators of research, and so on. Another 2.6% teach handicapped children in classroom settings. Speech-language pathologists and audiologists have the opportunity of working in a variety of job settings and engaging in a wide variety of work activities.

These figures also come from the 1980(b) ASHA survey.

ESTABLISHING THE COMPETENCE OF SPEECH-LANGUAGE PATHOLOGISTS AND AUDIOLOGISTS

As we have mentioned, approximately 50% of the specialists working in the field of communication disorders are members of ASHA. This association has approximately 35,000 members and maintains a national headquarters. ASHA sets standards for colleges and universities which train speech-language pathologists and audiologists as well as for facilities which provide services for people with communication disorders. ASHA issues a certificate of clinical competence (CCC) for individuals who have successfully completed a program of graduate study in speech-language pathology or speech-language and hearing science, have passed a national written examination, and have completed a year of full-time clinical experience under the supervision of someone holding a certificate of clinical competence. An equivalent certificate is available for audiologists. Although most holders of the certificate of clinical competence are members of ASHA, membership in the association is not required for certification. The certificate is not a membership card, but instead is proof of having completed both the graduate academic and the clinical experience to demonstrate competence in performing professional

The address of ASHA national headquarters is 10801 Rockville Pike, Rockville, MD 20852.

duties. The requirements for the ASHA certificates of clinical competence are considerably higher than those of any of the 31 states which issue a license for speech-language pathologists or audiologists. ASHA certification has become the best way for members of the general public as well as for other professional workers to identify a professional who has been adequately trained either as a speech-language pathologist, an audiologist, or both.

If you plan a career as a speech-language pathologist or an audiologist, you should be aware of the requirements for the certificates of competence issued by the American Speech-Language-Hearing Association. These requirements are revised periodically. The January 1, 1981, revision is presented in Appendix A. Future revisions may be obtained by writing to the ASHA headquarters.

By writing to ASHA, you can also obtain a list of colleges and universities which offer accredited master's degree programs in speech-language pathology or audiology. The list includes programs which have applied for, but not yet received, accreditation. The most recent list (ASHA, 1982) includes more than 125 colleges and universities throughout the United States and Canada.

Taking a certain number of courses at "approved" training centers does not guarantee that you will be an effective professional, nor does the possession of a license to practice. The truly effective professional in the helping professions should have not only a certain level of information, knowledge, and skills, but also a desire to help others and an ability to relate to people seeking help. These traits, concerns, and sensitivities are difficult to build into an examination for license or the requirements for certification by a professional society. In spite of such limitations, the certificates of clinical competence issued by ASHA are the best protection the public has today in selecting an ethical and competent speech-language pathologist or audiologist.

As a further protection to the public, ASHA is encouraging the development of continuing education programs, which will help certified speech-language pathologists and audiologists to update their training continuously to keep up with new research findings and clinical procedures—not only in their own field but in other areas which relate directly to communication disorders. As you begin your training, you should be prepared to continue to improve your skills and your understanding of communication disorders throughout all of your professional career. Important though the certificate of clinical competence may be, it does not mean that your learning stops with the receipt of the certificate. Nor are the knowledge and skills associated with the certificate a substitute for your commitment to helping people with communication problems develop to the maximum of their capabilities.

AMERICAN SPEECH-LANGUAGE-HEARING ASSOCIATION

A more detailed account of this history can be found in Elaine Paden's (1970) A History of the American Speech and Hearing Association, 1925–1958.

Because the American Speech-Language-Hearing Association is such an important part of our profession, you may be interested in looking back a few years to see how this organization came into being. In a sense this will give us a general picture of the history of speech-language pathology as a profession in the United States.

Of course, before ASHA was founded, there were people in the United States who were helping other people with hearing and communication disorders. Workers relied heavily on information available in writings which appeared in Germany, Austria, France, and England. In fact, throughout Europe until World

War II, most communication disorders were treated by members of the medical profession.

Actually, references to speech disorders go back to biblical times. Greek writers several centuries before the birth of Christ mentioned a variety of communication disorders. Perhaps the best known legend regarding speech disorders deals with a description of Demosthenes going down to the ocean and shouting over the waves as he attempted to talk with a mouth full of pebbles. Legend has it that this technique was recommended to cure his stuttering. Although our records of this story are not reliable, it has been suggested that the person who advised this treatment for Demosthenes was an actor named Satyrus.

Unfortunately, wherever you encounter people with problems, you often discover a few unscrupulous individuals who are willing to exploit the person with a problem. This has been true in the field of communication disorders. Over the years, certain people have made wild claims about their ability to cure communication disorders, often claiming secret techniques and charging exorbitant fees. These wild claims have not proved to be true. Equally unfortunate is the fact that many of these people have been permitted to practice their unethical procedures without any regulation or monitoring. In the United States, some of the worst offenders were those who promised cures for stuttering, often founding schools for "the cure" of stuttering and stammering. They held out false hope to those with problems and often extracted large sums of money from people who could ill afford their exorbitant fees.

While all of this was going on, a number of concerned and ethical practitioners from a variety of fields were trying to apply the knowledge available in the field of communication disorders. These individuals did not make any wild claims. Their fees were reasonable—in fact, in many instances these professional workers were affiliated with universities and did not even charge fees for the services they rendered.

By the early 1900s, a number of ethical practitioners were actively engaged in the treatment of communication disorders. At that time there were no formal training programs in the United States for the individual who wished to concentrate in this field. Clinicians practicing in the United States in the early 1900s often went to Germany and Austria to learn from the workers there. It was not until well into the second decade of the 20th century that a number of Americans began to contribute to the literature in the field of communication disorders. Although Alexander Graham Bell is best known for his work in the development of the telephone, he must also be credited as one of the first people in the United States to write in the field of hearing and communication disorders. Among other early American writers in the field were Elmer Kenyon, Edward Scripture, Charles Blumel, and Knight Dunlap. Often these American writers repeated the theories which were prevalent in Europe. More often than not, their writing consisted of highly subjective reports and descriptions of observations of clients and treatment procedures.

Early in this century, American school systems began to employ specialists to work with children with communication disorders. Paden (1970) reports that, as early as 1910, the Chicago public schools employed 10 speech correction teachers. At that same time, the city of Detroit had two speech correctionists in the school system. Boston's schools began a program of speech correction in 1913, and New York and San Francisco had established programs by 1916. In the state of Wisconsin eight cities had speech correction teachers in the public schools by 1916. This trend for school systems to establish programs of therapy for children with communication disorders developed to such an extent that in 1918 Dr. Walter B. Swift published a paper entitled "How to Begin Speech Correction in the Public Schools" (Paden, 1970).

By the early 1920s there was a considerable increase in the publication of scientifically based studies in the field of communication disorders. Along with this increase of scientific studies came the development of university courses concerned with the nature and treatment of communication disorders. Somewhere around 1915 the University of Wisconsin established what is probably the first speech clinic in any American university. The same university granted the first PhD in the field of communication disorders to Sarah M. Stinchfield in 1921.

The University of Wisconsin was followed by other universities in establishing programs for training specialists in communication disorders. Included among these pioneer programs were Columbia University, University of Pennsylvania, and the University of Iowa. There was continued development of university-level training programs dealing with communication disorders. This growth proved to be particularly strong throughout universities in the Midwest.

Although many clinicians working in the field of communication disorders came from university departments in the broad field of speech and communication, many of those contributing to the field of speech pathology in its early years in the United States were not academic teachers of speech but came from such fields as otolaryngology, psychology, neurology, and psychiatry. From the very beginning of speech-language pathology in the United States, the field has profited from the contributions of experts from a variety of disciplines.

During the first quarter of the 20th century, the National Association of Teachers of Speech (NATS) provided the opportunity for workers in the field of communication disorders to present papers and to publish papers in the official journals of that association. By 1920 enough members of the National Association of Teachers of Speech were interested in communication disorders to form a small interest group. This group met with NATS to hold meetings concerned entirely with communication disorders. Of the 84 articles published from 1921 to 1923 in the *Quarterly Journal of Speech Education,* 10 dealt with speech correction and 7 were concerned with phonology and phonetics. During the 1920s, the *Quarterly Journal of Speech Education* showed a good deal of interest in the field of communication disorders. This can be seen in reviews of new books of concern to speech-language pathologists. It can also be seen by an examination of various reports of research in progress.

The increasing interest in the field of communication disorders grew to the point where, in 1925, a small group met in Iowa City and proposed the creation of an organization devoted entirely to the study and treatment of communication disorders. Credit for bringing this small group together is often given to Dean Carl E. Seashore of the University of Iowa Graduate School. By training, Seashore was a psychologist, and many of the early organizers of the group which eventually became ASHA came out of a strong background in psychology. December 29, 1925, is considered to be the date of the formal action which established an association devoted to the study of the field of communication disorders. Eleven individuals are mentioned in the official minutes of that first meeting. The group chose as a name the American

Academy of Speech Correction and stated as its purpose "the promotion of scientific, organized work in the field of speech correction" (Paden, 1970). The membership of the new organization was limited to members of the National Association of Teachers of Speech who met certain requirements, which included actually working in the field of communication disorders, teaching others to become specialists in communication disorders, and conducting research dealing with the causes and treatment of communication disorders. In those early days, membership in the American Academy of Speech Correction required individuals to be involved not only in clinical activities but also in teaching and research as well. For almost 25 years, the American Academy of Speech Correction continued to meet each year with the National Association of Teachers of Speech.

In 1935 the organization changed its name to American Speech Correction Association. It now had 87 members, who decided to begin a publication titled *Journal of Speech Disorders*. The first editor of the *Journal of Speech Disorders* was G. Oscar Russell, who served in this capacity for 7 years. Some indication of the rapid growth of the profession can be seen from the fact that, within my own professional lifetime, the membership in the professional association devoted to communication disorders has grown from about 100 members to nearly 35,000. The increase in the number of association publications has increased in an equally dramatic fashion.

At the December 31, 1947, business meeting of the American Speech Correction Association held in Salt Lake City, a motion was passed to amend the constitution to change the name of the association to include reference to hearing rehabilitation. The new name became the American Speech and Hearing Association. This name continued until 1978, when the present name, American Speech-Language-Hearing Association, was adopted.

The inclusion of the term *hearing* in the name of the association recognized the rapid growth of interest in aural rehabilitation during World War II. Four retraining centers had been established during the war to serve the needs of military and navy personnel with hearing impairments. With the end of the war in 1945, the staff of the programs established for the hearing casualties of the war began applying their knowledge and skills to the needs of the civilian population. A new profession, audiology, began. Today audiologists are one of several specialists serving the needs of those with communication disorders.

From the beginning, the members of the American Academy of Speech Correction had a deep commitment to a strong code of ethics. As early as 1926, one of the five qualifications for membership listed in the original constitution was:

> Possession of a professional reputation untainted by a past record (or present record) of unethical practices such as latent commercialization of professional services or guaranteeing of "cures" for stated sums of money. (Paden, 1970)

As early as 1930, a section of the constitution was devoted to a statement of principles of ethics. Section III was devoted to a list of unethical practices. These unethical practices included:

(1) To guarantee to cure any disorder of speech.
(2) To offer in advance to refund any part of a person's tuition if his disorder of speech is not arrested.
(3) To make "rash promises" difficult of fulfillment, in order to secure pupils or patients.

(4) To employ blatant or untruthful methods of self-advertising.

(5) To advertise to correct disorders of speech entirely by correspondence.

(6) To seek self-advancement by attacking the work of other members of the society in such a way as might injure their standing and reputation. Reproaches or criticisms should be sympathetically discussed with the member involved.

(7) For persons who do not hold a medical degree to attempt to deal exclusively with speech patients requiring medical treatment without the advice or the authority of a physician.

(8) To extend the time of treatment beyond the time when one should recognize his inability to affect further improvement.

(9) To charge exorbitant fees for treatment. (Paden, 1970)

These same ethical concerns are incorporated in ASHA's present code of ethics. Additional statements have been incorporated into the present-day code of ethics to provide further protection to the clients whom members of the profession serve. Upholding the code of ethics is one of the most valuable functions of ASHA. As Paden (1970) stated in concluding her chapter dealing with ethics in the history of the American Speech and Hearing Association,

> The stature which ASHA has held, however, is due in no small degree to its early and continued concerns for the high ethical principles which it has insisted be upheld in the relations to all members, to the public, and which has, in turn, brought substantial reward to the members themselves.

YOU AND THE CODE OF ETHICS

As someone who is considering a career in speech-language pathology or audiology, you need to be aware of the ethical concerns which led to the formation of the professional society which eventually became the American Speech-Language-Hearing Association. You should also be aware of the ethical responsibilities you would be asked to assume as a practicing member of the profession today. For this reason, you should carefully read the most recent statement of the code of ethics of ASHA (Appendix B). The ASHA code of ethics includes the following six major principles, each of which involves certain ethical proscriptions or matters of professional propriety.

(1) Individuals shall hold paramount the welfare of persons served professionally.

(2) Individuals shall maintain high standards of professional competence.

(3) Individuals' statements to persons served professionally and to the public shall provide accurate information about the nature and management of communicative disorders, and about the profession and services rendered by its practitioners.

(4) Individuals shall maintain objectivity in all matters concerning the welfare of persons served professionally.

(5) Individuals shall honor their responsibilities to the public, their profession, and their relationships with colleagues and members of allied professions.

(6) Individuals shall uphold the dignity of the profession and freely accept the profession's self-imposed standards.

Responsibility to Client

A code of ethics is more than a statement of "Thou shalt nots." The real basis of a code of ethics is giving highest priority to the welfare of the clients a profession is to serve. What is ethical or not ethical in your behavior as a professional boils down to the kinds of choices you make. You will very frequently be confronted with making choices which could be based on your answers to three questions:

(1) What is the appropriate decision as far as the best interest of my client?
(2) What is the best decision in terms of the organization I work for? and
(3) What is the best decision for me personally?

It is safe to say that any time you make a decision on the basis of "what is best for my organization" or "what is best for me personally" rather than *"what is best for my client,"* there is a real chance that the answer may be unethical. Speech-language pathologists and audiologists have an overriding responsibility for the welfare of people who have communication disorders. Part of the responsibility we believe speech-language pathologists should take is the responsibility to serve as advocates for the communicatively handicapped who are not receiving the services they should have and to which they are entitled under legislation.

P.L. 94–142, one federal law affecting the rights of children with communication handicaps, will be discussed later in this chapter.

In trying to bring needed help to an individual with a communication disorder, you may occasionally encounter a situation where you seem to be in competition with a professional from another discipline who is also trying to help. This can lead to such differences of opinion as to whether a child with a language problem should receive therapy from a speech-language pathologist, from a specialist in learning disabilities, or from a classroom teacher. There is no one right approach. In each instance you—as an ethical professional—will have to decide which type of service delivery will be best for the person with the communication disorder. Your decision cannot ethically be made on the basis of the status of your profession, income to the agency you work for, or your own financial or prestige enhancement.

There is also the possibility of a "jurisdictional dispute" between a speech-language pathologist and the physician who has the overall responsibility for the health of a child or adult who has a communication disorder. In this situation, the physician may become involved in decisions relating to speech-language therapy for which he or she has no training, or the speech-language pathologist may become involved in aspects of care which are clearly outside the realm of speech-language pathology. Again, ethics demands that decisions be made on the basis of what is best for the person with the communication problem.

Because it is difficult to completely separate and isolate a communication disorder from the health, educational, social, and psychological characteristics of the person with the disorder, speech-language pathologists and audiologists frequently work very closely with teachers, physicians, dentists, psychologists, social workers, and other professionals equally committed to human service. As a speech-language pathologist, you will be trained to work with representatives of many professions so that you will be able to best treat the *person* with a problem rather than the communication disorder.

Responsibility to Society

The profession also has a responsibility to society in general. As more and more questions are being raised about how our tax dollars are being spent, our profession will be subjected to public demands for accountability. We can point to Annabelle, to Jerry, and to Roger and say, "Look what speech-language pathology has accomplished by making it possible for these individuals to develop their potential." We can point to happier lives resulting from the correction of communication disorders. We can also show that the treatment of people with communication disorders results in economic benefits to the larger society, which in a very real sense pays the cost of our treatment efforts. We will need to point out that spending a few hundred dollars for speech-language treatment for Annabelle helped her to develop into a normal, happy person who now earns a living and pays taxes. Without the help of speech-language pathology, Annabelle would have been supported in a state institution at tax payers' expense for the rest of her life. We have ample evidence to show that, in the long run, our services contribute to the economic well-being of society by helping people with communication disorders become productive, tax-paying citizens. As more and more competition develops for the tax dollar that supports education and rehabilitation programs, our profession will have to inform the public of how providing help for those with communication disorders not only enriches their individual lives, but also enriches society in general in economic as well as human terms.

Another part of our responsibility to society is to continuously evaluate our procedures. Do our treatment techniques accomplish their purposes? Is the system we use to deliver services the most effective? Does it reach the people who need our services? Is there a less costly way to provide the needed services? All of these questions will be raised by the general public as well as those responsible for allocating funds for education, health, and "the general welfare."

As we try to answer some of these questions of accountability, we may come to realize that certain of the traditional activities of speech-language pathologists need to be modified or can be carried out more economically by other workers. This has already happened in some other professions. For example, prior to World War II, most shots were given by physicians. Now the majority of shots are administered by other members of the health professions who have had less training than MDs. X-ray technicians and a host of medical technicians carry out other procedures which once were exclusively handled by physicians. Today the cleaning of teeth is frequently done by dental hygienists rather than by graduate dentists. In contrast, the profession of speech-language pathology has not accepted the concept of the paraprofessional or trained technician to the extent that it has been adopted by providers of health care. Part of our responsibility as professionals is to find the most effective ways of helping those with communication disorders, which could quite possibly involve using paraprofessionals. You, as a new member of the profession, will have the opportunity and responsibility to guide the development of our profession in the forthcoming years. You face the challenge of taking the information and the skills presented in this book and evaluating their effectiveness in the settings in which you will be working. For this reason, we will not try to give you cookbook recipes for diagnosis and treatment, but instead will give you general principles. Where possible, we will explain the extent to which these principles are based on research findings or on clinical observations or impressions. As practicing speech-language pathologists, we will try to tell you what we know, what we don't know, and how we have decided what we think we know. As the speech-language pathologist or audiologist of tomorrow, you will be called upon to assume more responsibility and to be more directly accountable to the public than has been true for most of us in our careers. As a professional, you will need to know not only the procedures to follow in helping your students or clients but also how to evaluate your own effectiveness and that of your profession as a whole. It is not enough to understand evaluation procedures; you must be honest and open to self-evaluation in the best interests of the individuals you are committed to help and of the society which pays for a large portion of that help.

Prevention and Research

As we assume greater responsibility for accountability as speech-language pathologists, we also have a responsibility to try to prevent communication disorders, which requires us to learn more about their causes. This knowledge will come from the research efforts of speech-language pathologists and of other professionals as well. In speech-language pathology research, we try to better understand normal communication in order to better understand disordered communication. In turn, our increasing knowledge of the disordered will contribute to our understanding of the normal.

Some research projects are carried out by speech-language pathologists working in university and hospital laboratories; others, in schools and clinics. As we seek better treatment procedures for individuals with communication disorders, we will try new approaches and compare them with the old in an effort to find the most effective therapies—effective both in terms of results and costs. A person about to embark on a career in speech-language pathology can look forward to stimulating work in research as well as clinical service.

For those with an interest in the teaching of a new generation of speech-language pathologists, there will also be opportunities as college and university teachers and supervisors of clinic practice in the many training programs.

A LOOK AT THE FUTURE OF SPEECH-LANGUAGE PATHOLOGY

It is difficult to predict how speech-language pathology in 5 years will differ from the profession as we know it today, but we can make a few educated guesses, based in part on some current federal legislation. One piece of legislation that already is beginning to affect speech-language pathology is Public Law 94–142, the Education for All Handicapped Children Act. In addition to providing more federal money to identify and treat children with communication disorders, this legislation requires that services to handicapped students be provided in "the least restrictive environment." This mandate is often referred to as "mainstreaming"; it means that, as much as possible, a child is not segregated from nonhandicapped peers but instead receives as much therapy and education as possible in the regular classroom. This suggests that many of the remedial procedures speech-language pathologists have historically carried out in special speech rooms will in the future be carried out in the regular classroom—often by the classroom teacher with advice and consultation from the speech-language pathologist. To be effective in working in the classroom, the speech-language pathologist will have to learn about classroom procedures, about curriculum, about how reading and spelling are taught, and so on. The speech-language pathologist working in a school setting in the future will have to be able to work as part of a team concerned with more than the problem of a communication disorder. The speech-language pathologist in tomorrow's schools will be more involved with the overall education of children with communication disorders.

For a discussion of trends in audiology, refer to chapter 10.

With the current trend to cut back federal government spending and regulations, it is hard to predict what will happen to P.L. 94–142.

Chapter 9 covers the school-age person with language/learning disabilities.

Another effect of P.L. 94–142 will be an increase in attention directed to identifying children with learning disabilities and designing programs of remediation for them. Speech-language pathologists will be particularly well-qualified to work with those students whose primary learning disability is manifested by disorders of language acquisition, comprehension, and production. Speech-language pathologists will be called upon to help assess children suspected of having learning disabilities in order to determine if there is a language disorder. Speech-language pathologists on their own, and in cooperation with special educators, will plan programs to assist children with language disorders and language-based learning disabilities (Gruenewald, 1980). Speech-language pathologists in some instances will carry out remedial procedures themselves. In other instances, they may design programs to be carried out by teachers or other specialists. Thus, speech-language pathologists will be providing consulting services as well as direct services to individuals. In keeping with the long-standing tradition of the profession as well as ASHA's code of ethics, any jurisdictional problems should again be resolved by making decisions which are in the best interest of the individual student. P.L. 94–142 requires that all placement and program decisions be made by a team comprised of at least the classroom and special teacher, the parents, an administrator, and all relevant specialists, which would include the speech-language pathologist. Thus, the school speech-language pathologist of the future will need to be able to participate effectively both as a team member and as an expert in the field.

Another effect of P.L. 94–142 will be the extension of services to previously unserved populations. The law mandates services to handicapped children between the ages of 3 and 21, which means that more preschoolers will be evaluated and, presumably, treated. Children with more severe handicaps, including the hearing impaired, the mentally retarded, and the physically handicapped, will be moving into regular classrooms and regular schools—in some cases, from institutions. The public school speech-language pathologist is likely to see students with a broader range of communication disorders than used to appear in that setting. It is also likely that audiologists will evaluate more children referred by the public schools.

See chapter 8 for more on language development and problems in early childhood; chapter 10, on hearing and auditory disorders; chapter 12, on cerebral palsy.

For 1980, $35,000,000 was allocated to implement P.L. 95–561. This amount was increased to $41,000,-000 for 1981. However, at the time of this writing, the effects of the Reagan budget cutbacks on this funding were not yet known.

Another piece of federal legislation likely to affect the profession of speech-language pathology is the Education Amendments of 1978, Public Law 95-561, which expanded the definition of *basic skills* to include listening and speaking skills. Under this legislation, federal support will be available to develop programs to serve all children, youth, and adults needing to improve their listening and speaking skills. This support will not be limited to those who are communicatively handicapped. Thus, in the future, speech-language pathologists will have opportunities to develop oral communication programs for people who are not handicapped but who need to improve basic skills in listening and speaking. This overall concern with developing programs designed to improve communication skills—reading, writing, listening, and speaking—is likely to continue. This new emphasis may very well result in our questioning the arbitrary separation between spoken and written language as well as between "normal" and "disordered" communication. Tomorrow's speech-language pathologist may be more involved in the reading and writing aspects of both normal and disordered communication. This broader concern with the entire communication process (oral and written) and its disorders is similar to that which I observed several years ago in the training of speech-language pathologists in the Soviet Union (Matthews, 1974).

Certain other shifts in emphasis are also likely. We will be called upon to serve more senior citizens as well as more preschoolers. We will be called upon to provide more services to the multiply and severely handicapped. Caseloads will probably shift from an emphasis on problems of articulation to language and learning disabilities. As speech-language and audiology services are integrated into student's total educational programs, we can expect to be more involved with team teaching and other cooperative activities with special education and classroom teachers.

This team participation will make it desirable for some speech-language pathologists and audiologists to supplement their ASHA membership with membership in other professional associations which have overlapping interests. Speech-language pathologists in public schools may become more active in the Council for Exceptional Children (CEC). Those who see many cleft palate patients will find value in affiliation with the American Cleft Palate Association (ACPA). The American Association for Mental Deficiency (AAMD) may be attractive to those working with retarded children and adults; The Association for the Severely Handicapped (TASH), to those working with the multiply handicapped.

Along with these developments, we can expect to see increasing opportunities for private practice. Donna R. Fox, President of the Academy of Private Practice, pointed out that "in the past 25 years, private practice has grown from a few isolated practitioners to thousands of practitioners in both full- and part-time practice" (1980, p. 383). She concludes a recent guest editorial in *Asha* with the following statement about the challenges and rewards of private practice.

> Clinicians in private practice understand the dilemma of serving two masters: the need to provide quality service at a reasonable price and the need to actively contribute to their profession through research and organizational affiliation. This dedication to serving both makes private practice an exciting and rewarding professional setting. (p. 384)

CONCLUSION

Speech-language pathology and audiology have been satisfying careers for many. Some of us have experienced satisfaction as clinicians; some as researchers; some as teachers and administrators. We have in our lifetime seen our professional association, ASHA, grow from less than 100 members to nearly 35,000. We have been able to observe the results of our efforts as we see people with communication disorders helped to become happy and productive citizens. The future is equally bright for someone about to embark on a career in this field. We only hope that the balance of this book will lead many of you to that rewarding career.

SELECTED READINGS

Matthews, J. Communicology and individual responsibility. *Asha,* 1964, *6* (1).

Matthews, J. Personal and professional responsibilities related to current social problems. *Asha,* 1971, *13* (6).

Matthews, J. Disorders of language. In C. Bluestone & S. Stool (Eds.), *Pediatric Otolaryngology*. Philadelphia: W. B. Saunders, 1982.

Nicolosi, L., Harryman, E., & Kresheck, J., *Terminology of communication disorders.* Baltimore: Williams and Wilkins, 1978.

Paden, E. P. *A history of the American Speech and Hearing Association, 1925–1958.* Washington, D.C.: American Speech and Hearing Association, 1970.

Perkins, W. H. *Human perspectives in speech and language disorders.* St. Louis: C. V. Mosby, 1978.

Van Riper, C. *A career in speech pathology.* Englewood Cliffs, N.J.: Prentice-Hall, 1979.

Wiig, E. H., & Semel, E. M., *Language disabilities in children and adolescents.* Columbus, Ohio: Charles E. Merrill, 1976.

REFERENCES

American Speech-Language-Hearing Association. Accredited education and training programs and those in the accreditation process. *Asha,* 1980, *22*(7), 487–490. (a)

American Speech-Language-Hearing Association. ASHA is 35,000 strong. *Asha,* 1980, *22*(10), 867. (b)

American Speech-Language-Hearing Association. Requirements for certificates of clinical competence. *Asha,* 1980, *22*(6), 433–437. (c)

American Speech and Hearing Association, Committee on the Mid-Century White House Conference. *Journal of Speech and Hearing Disorders,* 1952, *17*(1), 129–137.

Birch, J., & Matthews, J. The hearing of mental defectives: Its measurement and characteristics. *American Journal of Mental Deficiency,* 1951, *55*, 384–393.

Fox, D. R. Competency and commitment. *Asha,* 1980, *22*(5), 383–384.

Gruenewald, L. Language and learning disabilities ad hoc develops position statement. *Asha,* 1980, *22*, 628–636.

Matthews, J. Speech and language development. In J. J. Gallagher (Ed.), *Windows on Russia.* Washington, D.C.: U.S. Government Printing Office, 1974.

Matthews, J. Disorders of language. In C. Bluestone & S. Stool (Eds.), *Pediatric otolaryngology.* Philadelphia: W. B. Saunders, 1982.

McCarthy, D. Language disorders and parent-child relationships. *Journal of Speech and Hearing Disorders,* 1954, *19*(4), 514–523.

Milisen, R. The incidence of speech disorders. In L. E. Travis (Ed.), *Handbook of speech pathology.* New York: Appleton-Century-Crofts, 1971.

Paden, E. P. *A history of the American Speech and Hearing Association, 1925–1958.* Washington, D.C.: American Speech and Hearing Association, 1970.

Taylor, J. S. Public school speech-language certification standards: Are they standard? *Asha,* 1980, *22*(3), 159–165.

HUMAN LANGUAGE AND COMMUNICATION 2

John Irwin

Before we can look at disorders of communication and language, we must understand what *communication* is and what *language* is. In a general sense, developed through years of experience, we all know what we mean when we use these words. But when we try to define them precisely and completely, we run into trouble. For example, think about these questions. If I write this chapter and no one reads it (!), have I "communicated"? Does communication depend upon language? If the answer to that is yes, is an infant who is crying because he's hungry communicating? What about a nod of the head—does that communicate? And is it language? Does a two-year-old speak English (or French or Swahili or whatever) or a different kind of language? Do animals communicate, or only people? (After all, my dog lets me know when she wants to go outside—most of the time.) Is written communication simply a formal transcription of speech, or is it a different "thing" altogether?

It would be wonderful to be able to present clear-cut answers to these questions. Unfortunately, we cannot; scholars in the field have not been able to come up with pat definitions and simple conclusions. In fact, their answers to these and other similar questions are often contradictory. The difficulty here reflects the complexity of the communication process—a complexity which extends into the realm of defining and identifying disordered communication. In this chapter, we will take a look at the elements of the communication process and, more specifically, at one critical tool for communication, language. Our ultimate goal is to develop a functional understanding that will help you deal with individual people with communication and language problems.

WHAT IS COMMUNICATION?

In the broadest sense, *communication* is the transmission of information (Moerk, 1977). With this interpretation, communicative events can range from the gestures of a primate to the flight of a heat-seeking missile. Further, human communication would encompass almost all interpersonal interactions, including those which involve verbal symbolism and those which are entirely nonverbal. We can even include *intra*personal communication—when you plan "in your head" what you will say in a job interview, for example.

Elements of Communication

In intrapersonal communication, the sender and the receiver would be the same person in two different roles.

The different types of communication we have mentioned have at least three elements in common: a sender, a message, and a receiver. We can even draw a simple diagram of the process.

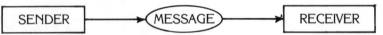

We can now identify these elements in a specific communication event. When I see you on the street and say "Hello!" I am the sender, the message is "Hello!" and you are the receiver. But we can go into much more detail in describing this event. First, I have an idea—to greet you. After choosing a word to accomplish my purpose, I send a message from my brain to my breathing and speech muscles. They cooperate to produce a sound wave that travels through the air and reaches your ears. Your auditory tract picks up the sound wave pattern and sends a signal to your brain, which transmits the message "Hello!" to you. And even more, it calls back a lifetime of your accumulated experience—with the sound pattern "hello," with being greeted on the street, with me. It's easy to see that this is a tremendously complex event that could be interrupted at any stage by a physical disorder (in you or in me), by a language difference or deficiency, by a feeling or reaction.

Various chapters in this book examine what happens when the process is interrupted.

Our simple model is obviously a flat statement of a miraculous process. It fails to show that the sender can use many channels other than speech, or that the receiver may react to other elements in the situation—fatigue, another message being sent by a second sender—that are not perceived by the sender. That communication is ever effective is a tribute both to the intelligence of the communicators and the adequacy of the system.

Levels of Communication

Besides describing elements of communication, we can describe levels. Weaver (1964) has described three levels of communication: the technical level—how precisely symbols can be exchanged; the semantic level—how precisely the symbols used reflect the intended meaning; and the effectiveness level—how precisely the response in the receiver reflects the intent of the sender. We are concerned about all levels. Speech-language pathologists, audiologists, and telephone engineers are concerned with the accurate transmission of the sounds of speech; teachers and airline pilots are concerned with precision of meaning; politicians and preachers are concerned with the effect of the message. Again, each of these levels relates to both verbal and nonverbal messages. We'll look at **nonverbal communication** first, and then move on to verbal communication. This, in turn, will take us directly to an examination of language.

*Words in **boldface** in the text are defined in the glossary, beginning on page 491.*

NONVERBAL COMMUNICATION

Categories of Nonverbal Communication

It is difficult to define nonverbal messages by example, for the range is great. Facial expression and gesture come to mind at once, but less obvious examples like the distance between speaker and listener are also important. Because the list of specific nonverbal techniques is so large, complete definition by example is almost impossible. Yet a definition by description may fail to convey either the variation in or importance of this type of communication. If we accept the point of view that a **symbol** is any stimulus that represents something other than itself, then a nonverbal symbol is any symbol other than those of spoken or written language. In general, these nonverbal signs will have meaning to both senders and receivers, although the range of subject matter and the precision of language are probably more restricted than with verbal signs. Only rarely do we use any single method of communicating (Moerk, 1977). Many nonverbal techniques tend to be complementary and unconscious; they tend to supplement rather than replace the verbal part of the message.

Eisenberg and Smith (1971) have divided nonverbal communication techniques into three basic categories: **paralanguage,** variables of voice and voice use; **kinesics,** body movements; and **proxemics,** body positions and spatial relationships.

Paralanguage refers to sounds produced in speaking that are not part of the phonemic code, that is, the recognized speech sounds, of a particular language. Perhaps the most obvious of these, as noted by Trager (1958), is voice quality, but changes in vocal pitch and loudness are also important. In addition, noises such as yawns, crying and laughing, the style of articulation, fluency, and rhythm are all paralinguistic elements.

Paralanguage

We will delve into phonology, the study of the speech code, later in this chapter.

Crystal (1969) has reviewed the literature with respect to both the concepts of and the vocabulary of vocal changes. He recognizes pitch, loudness, duration, and timbre (quality) as paralinguistic elements. To Crystal, voice quality is a single impression of a voice existing throughout the whole of a normal utterance. Crystal distinguishes between prosodic and paralinguistic features. He defines **prosodic features** as vocal effects related to variations of pitch, loudness, duration, and silence, thus excluding effects which do not result primarily from the direct working of the vocal bands. These prosodic effects are often used intentionally, and can be controlled. He defines *paralinguistic effects* as those which result from the direct workings of the pharyngeal, oral, or nasal cavities, recognizing always that these cavities may have some effect on pitch, loudness, and duration. When used, these paralinguistic effects are noticeable and call attention to themselves; in contrast, prosodic effects are *always* present. Prosodic effects can reinforce the verbal message, or contradict it. A good example of this kind of contradiction is found in sarcasm, where the voice quality very deliberately belies the words.

See chapter 4 for a description of these body parts and how they work in the speech process.

Kinesics

Where paralanguage deals with auditory nonverbal signals, *kinesics* involves visual signals, the signals we send with body movements. Gesture, facial expression, and posture are all included. In his study of bodily movements—particularly gestures—Birdwhistell (1970) notes a striking parallel between movement and language. He conceives of movement as being almost an extension of the sound. Birdwhistell is convinced that visible bodily activity can predictably influence the behavior of listeners. These movements, however, may not have a common significance across different cultures. That is, the group must learn the full meaning of these movements as it must learn the full meaning of the sounds and words of the shared language.

We can classify nonverbal bodily communication activities into three groups: arbitrary, iconic, and intrinsic. **Arbitrary** movements are interpreted on the basis of convention rather than resemblance to what they refer to. For instance, in our culture, we interpret a side-to-side head shake as negative, and up-and-down movement as affirmative. **Iconic** movements bear some resemblance to what they refer to, as when you use your hands to direct the parking of a car. Churchill's famous "V" for victory sign may be interpreted as either iconic or arbitrary. It is iconic in that it resembles the letter *V*, which is the first letter of the written word *victory;* it is arbitrary in that it has no connection to the concept of victory itself. **Intrinsic** movements are part of the condition signified, as in the body movements made in crying or laughing.

Nierenberg and Calero (1971) have tried to make the art of reading gestures and postures practical. Among the many attitudes that these authors describe are openness, defensiveness, suspicion, confidence, boredom, and acceptance. For example, a defensive attitude can be revealed by what Nierenberg and Calero call a *crossed arm defensive position.* Variations in this position can reveal variations in attitude—hands made into fists indicate some degree of willingness to fight; hands wrapped tightly around the biceps indicate a greater degree of apprehension.

Proxemics

Proxemics is concerned with the use of space in the communication process—most importantly the use of interpersonal space. Interpersonal space affects the act of communication in at least two ways (Hall, 1959). First, the space between speaker and listener has communicative significance; that is, it affects how a message is interpreted. Within the American culture, Hall recognizes four spatial categories, ranging from the intimate (0 to 18 inches) to public (over 12 feet). Second, different cultures have different interpersonal spatial codes. For example, Arabs and Latins tend to stand closer together when talking face to face than do North Americans.

Violations of interpersonal spatial codes are often interpreted negatively. For instance, you may not like a stranger who stands too close while talking to you. A violation of the spatial code may be very innocent, especially in intercultural communication, for two speakers with different sets of interpersonal spatial values may violate each other's standards. For instance, imagine a young American woman talking to a South American at a party. As he steps forward, she steps back, perhaps thinking that he is being fresh. And he, in turn, is offended, perhaps thinking that she is not interested in what he is saying. In these instances, neither party is aware of what is disturbing the interaction.

*The term **metacommunication** is sometimes used to denote any or all of the nonverbal aspects of communication.*

Effectiveness of Nonverbal Communication

Nonverbal messages between people may vary in specificity, in degree of awareness, and in degree of control. Moreover, people show great individual variations in their awareness of nonverbal signs and their intent to use them. Although verbal communication can be used to send almost any message, the functional range of nonverbal behavior is relatively limited. It is particularly effective in the affective realm; that is, in interactions in which the feelings of the sender are made known to the receiver.

Affective communication may be verbal or nonverbal. If nonverbal, it may be used intentionally or unintentionally either to reinforce or to contradict the verbal message. If used to reinforce, the voice quality and pitch, the bodily posture and gestures, and the interpersonal space must all be in harmony. For sincere speakers from the same cultural background, this kind of harmony is probable, although the degree of reinforcement may vary in kind and amount from person to person. For insincere speakers, this harmony may be absent.

Not only can there be a lack of harmony between verbal and nonverbal behaviors but between different types of nonverbal behaviors themselves (Nierenberg & Calero, 1971). For example, a nervous laugh is a prime illustration of nonverbal incongruence. A laugh is usually an intrinsic indicator of happiness. A nervous laugh, on the other hand, occurs only when the rest of the nonverbal signals indicate nervousness and strain. Like other workers in this field, Nierenberg and Calero feel that lack of fit between either verbal and nonverbal behavior or between nonverbal behaviors should serve as a warning to the receiver. Given a lack of harmony between verbal and nonverbal communication, they prefer to rely upon nonverbal clues.

Lowen (1958), in his preface to *The Language of the Body,* explores the relationship between expression and emotion. He believes that the human organism expresses itself in movement, in posture, in pose, and in gesture more clearly than in words. He also addresses the theoretical question of whether the character of an individual can be changed without also affecting some change in bodily structure and mobility. He concludes that the therapist must analyze not only the psychological problems of the client, but also the physical expression of the problem.

Can nonverbal techniques of communication be used intentionally? Can they be taught? Or can they only be interpreted? Evidence is accumulating that these behaviors cannot only be read but that they can be taught and can be used intentionally. Nierenberg and Calero attempt to teach position and gesture. Elocutionists sought to standardize the entire realm of nonverbal behavior: the nasal voice indicated sarcasm; a stooped body, depression; hands above the head, a noble impulse. The skill of the actor is, at least in part, in the use of these nonverbal reinforcers and contradictions. But while improvement seems possible, complete mastery seems unlikely. We are just beginning to understand how nonverbal messages affect interpersonal interactions, and we still have much to learn. For the most part, speech-language pathologists do not deal directly with possible contradictions between nonverbal and verbal messages, or with other difficulties with nonverbal communication. However, it is important for them to try to keep their own nonverbal messages in harmony with their words.

Speech-language pathologists do help people learn to control their voice quality; see chapter 6.

Nonspeech Communication

Many populations do not have adequate speech for communication (Silverman, 1980). These may include people with profound hearing losses, motor problems such as cerebral palsy, and/or profound mental retardation. For some of these people, nonspeech communication modes may be helpful. Procedures for coding and transmitting messages without directly using the vocal tract are currently being developed and refined. A good example is sign language. Although many of the skills involved in the use of these procedures are nonverbal, the final output tends to be verbal, in that specific symbols are used in a regulated sequence to communicate specific meanings.

See the discussions of these problems in individual chapters.

VERBAL COMMUNICATION

As we have implied already in this chapter, verbal communication tends to be much more intentional and specific than nonverbal communication. Adult users of a language translate their ideas into specific words and arrange those words into (we hope) orderly sequences which they use to transmit their messages. The message can be transmitted either in written or oral form. This whole process is called **encoding.** When the receiver perceives the message (either by reading or listening) and translates it into an understood meaning, the process is called **decoding.** Clearly, for the receiver to have any chance of receiving the meaning the sender intended to send, the two parties must be using the same or very similar systems of sounds, word meanings, and word and phrase order. These systems used to encode and decode messages are called **languages.** We now amplify our earlier diagram.

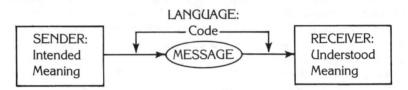

LANGUAGE

Impact of Specific Languages

If a language is a system that two people (or a group of people) use to encode and decode meanings, we might ask how the common meanings people have affect the language that they use and how the language system affects the meanings. That is, does a specific language that a young child learns affect or even control how that child perceives the world around him? Again, we have found another question that we cannot answer with certainty. Some linguists feel that we are bound hand and foot by our language, that we learn only those concepts for which we have words. That is, our language controls our reality. This hypothesis, known as the *Sapir-Whorf hypothesis,* has been rejected by many theorists, but it continues to be studied.

Today, the consensus is that languages do differ both in labels and in grammar with respect to how cultural groups organize reality. But these differences may reflect differences between the ways groups of people perceive reality rather than control that reality. That is, a language may influence perception but can scarcely control it (Slobin, 1971). A language may be a guide to how a culture organizes its world, but it is not a formula that determines all behavior.

Components of Languages

We have seen that nonverbal communication techniques can be arbitrary, iconic, or intrinsic. Verbal communication, in contrast, is almost completely arbitrary. That is, there is usually no correspondence between the sound or sounds we use and the objects or ideas they represent. (An exception would be words like *bow-wow* or *hiss* that name sounds.) Further, word order is also arbitrary. Clearly, for a language to be functional, members of a group must use the same rules to choose their sounds and words and compose utterances. That is, when I see you on the street, I have my choice of sounds, words, and word order in speaking to you. But if I want you to understand and even respond, I'd better use the same rules you do in making some basic word and word order selections.

We can identify three types of language rules: rules of **phonology,** of **morphology** and **syntax,** and of **semantics.** These rules can be extended with rules of **pragmatics.** Phonological rules deal with the sound segments used in speech. Morphology is concerned with the arrangements of sounds into words or other units which carry meaning. It is a part of syntax, which is the system which governs how we arrange units of meaning in an utterance, both at the level of individual words and the larger level of phrases, clauses, and sentences. Semantics relates phonology and syntax to meaning. The fourth component of language, pragmatics, relates to how the situational context or the speaker's intent can affect our choice of utterances.

As a speaker, my intended meaning, the context, and the phonological, morphological, and syntactical structure of my language ultimately determine what I say and how I say it. I do not have completely free choice of sounds, words, or structures. For example, if you want to describe a beautiful scene to your friend, you may choose the word *green* from your vocabulary. This choice reflects your meaning; it is an appropriate selection from the thousands of words in your vocabulary. But the form of the word is controlled by the constraints of English on sound order. The form /grin/ is permissible; the form /grni/ is not. At the syntactic level, the sequence of words *the green meadow* or *the meadow is green* are permissible and statistically probable; the sequence *the meadow green* is permissible but not probable and would tend to be reserved for poetic contexts; the sequence *meadow the green* would not be permissible.

Let us now look at each of these kinds of rules in more detail.

PHONOLOGY

Phonology is primarily concerned with the rules of combining sound segments into morphemes and longer linguistic units; phonetics, then, is the study of the actual spoken signal. Phonology may be concerned with three different aspects: (*a*) physical properties, (*b*) perceptual properties, and (*c*) production properties. Physical properties include the organization of the sounds, the insertion of sounds, the deletion of segments, and changes in the identity of segments. Perceptual properties include length, stress, tone, effects of neighboring sounds, pitch, loudness, and frequency. Production properties include duration of sound, place and manner of articulation, and the role of segments at junctures. Both in practice and in theory, the distinction between phonetics and phonology may sometimes be obscure.

Problems with phonology are called articulation problems; they are discussed in depth in chapter 5.

The Sound System of English

The sounds of English are typically classified as vowels and consonants. This distinction is largely based on production characteristics. For the vowels, the vocal tract is relatively open or unconstricted; at no point is a friction noise produced by the outgoing air stream. English vowels are **voiced.** For the consonants, the vocal tract is either completely closed or relatively tightly constricted. A friction noise is usually produced at the point of constriction for most English consonants. English consonants can be either voiced or **unvoiced.**

The number of separate sounds recognized in English varies somewhat with the classification system, with dialectal variations, and with the system of transcription. For example, Leutenegger (1963) recognizes a total of 20 vowels and 28 consonants. Thomas (1958) recognizes 17 vowels and 25 consonants. Gleason (1955) recognizes 22 vowels and 24 consonants. In this

*A **voiced** sound requires the vocal folds to vibrate; an **unvoiced** sound does not require vibration. The physiology of the vocal tract and how sounds are produced are described in detail in chapter 4.*

TABLE 2.1
The Sounds of English.

Vowels, Phonemic Diphthongs, and Syllabics		Consonants	
Phonetic Symbol	Key Word	Phonetic Symbol	Key Word
i	peat	m	sum
ɪ	pit	n	sun
e	pate	ŋ	sung
ɛ	pet	p	pot
ɚ	pat	b	bob
ɑ	pot	t	tot
ɔ	pall	d	dot
o	poll	g	got
u	pool	k	cot
ʊ	pull	f	fine
ɝ ɜ	purr	v	vine
ɚ ə	putter	θ	ether
ʌ	putt	ð	either
ɔɪ	coy	s	seal
au	cow	z	zeal
aɪ	my	ʃ	bash
ɪu	mew	ʒ	beige
ṇ	button	h	hump
ḷ	saddle	tʃ	chump
m̩	chasm	dʒ	jump
		l	led
		r	red
		w	wet
		j	yet

book, we use a system of 46 sounds—22 vowels and 24 consonants. They are presented in Table 2.1, using International Phonetic Alphabet transcription (IPA).

Three terms that require careful definition are **phone**, **allophone**, and **phoneme**. Phones are the actual sounds produced by speakers. Because they are produced by a fallible mechanism, no two productions—whether by the same or by different speakers—are ever completely identical. Phones are typically enclosed in brackets. Allophones are groupings of phones that in any one language are interpreted as belonging to one phoneme. Yet the various allophones of a phoneme may differ perceptibly to any reasonably attentive listener. A frequently cited example of allophonic variation involves the phoneme /p/. At the end of a word, as in *stop,* /p/ is *aspirated.* That is, it involves a little puff of air that can be heard quite clearly. In phonetic transcription, the final segment would be written as [pʰ]. (Allophones also are written in brackets.) But in the production of the phoneme /p/ in *speak,* the phoneme is not aspirated. In phonetic transcription it would be written as [p]. Although the sounds differ at the phonetic level, and although we can hear the difference, in English we do not differentiate between any two words by this difference. So the two variants are classified in English as allophones of the phoneme /p/.

The phoneme is an abstraction. It may be defined as the smallest sound unit that, although meaningless in itself, makes a semantic difference when

Note that other languages may have sounds that are not used in English and vice versa. For example, German has a gutteral sound often represented by "ch" that is not used in English.

combined with other phonemes. Phonemes of a given language are identified by the technique of the minimal pairs constrast. For example, in English the two phonetic sequences /kɪt/ and /kot/ differ by one phone. In English, this difference identifies two separate words: *kit* and *coat*. Thus /ɪ/ and /o/ are called phonemes of English, because in at least one instance the resulting minimal pairs contrast makes a difference in the meaning of at least two forms. (Transcription of phonemes is placed within slashes.) Consider the two phonetic sequences /kot/ and /kout/. Although we can hear a difference in these sound patterns, English does not differentiate any words on this basis. Thus, by this test, [o] and [ou] are allophones of the same phoneme. However, this test is not infallible because of differences in dialects and the pronunciations of different speakers.

You may wish to refer to Table 2.1 for the IPA notation used throughout this book.

A relatively new movement in the field is to recognize a higher level of abstraction than the traditional phonemes (Schane, 1973). The new level recognizes, for example, that in words such as *pirate* the final consonant is realized as /t/ in *piratical* and as /s/ in *piracy*. This new level, which seeks to systematically explain such changes, is called the **systematic phonemic,** whereas the traditional phonemic level is called the **autonomous phonemic**.

The distinction between the phone and the phoneme is particularly important in attempts to transcribe the speech of infants and young children. It is quite possible that an adult listener who is a native speaker of a language may impose the phonemic structure of the adult upon the phonetic output of the infant. This same difficulty may arise when a speaker of one language tries to describe the phonemes used by a speaker of a different language.

The Classification of English Phonemes

As we have stated, the two basic groups of English phonemes are vowels and consonants, traditionally described in terms of presumed differences in the basic modes of production. These classification systems assume that there is essentially uniform production across all sounds and all speakers of a language. Almost certainly, this uniformity does not exist. Yet, because evidence from direct observation and certain physical tests tends to support a common pattern of position and sound, the traditional descriptions have survived with only slight variations. They are accepted as having at least limited validity. Primarily because of the greater degree of constriction in the consonants, the oral positions of these sounds can be described with more precision than can those of the vowels.

The descriptions that follow are relatively conventional for their type, but particularly reflect the works of Gleason (1955), Wise (1958), and Thomas (1958).

A recent trend is to describe phonemes not as units but as bundles of distinctive production features. In this approach, each phoneme is described in terms of the feature scale being used. This kind of description is known as a *distinctive feature matrix*. Table 2.2 presents a simplified distinctive feature matrix for three phonemes and three features. The symbols "+" or "−" in-

TABLE 2.2

Example of a Simplified Distinctive Feature System for Three English Consonants.

	Phonome Specification		
Feature	**b**	**p**	**m**
Nasalty	−	−	+
Voicing	+	−	+
Continuancy	−	−	+

+ = feature is present in phoneme; − = feature is not present.

dicate the presence or absence of the feature. Thus, the phoneme /m/ is nasal, voiced, and continuant.

At present opinions are somewhat divided as to the relative merits of the traditional and the distinctive feature approaches to the description of English phonemes. Both methods are being used. The traditional system places the emphasis on the phoneme as the unit of analysis; the distinctive feature approach emphasizes the constituents of the phoneme rather than the phoneme itself. For instance, in describing how young children develop speech, the traditional approach might describe which phonemes usually develop by age 24 months, which by age 30 months, and so on. The distinctive feature approach would look at which *distinctive features* develop first. The same approach would be used to describe an articulation problem. We will first present traditional classification for both vowels and consonants. Then we will discuss the distinctive feature classification of the consonants of English.

Chapter 5 discusses how these approaches affect the speech-language pathologist in assessing and remediating articulation processes.

Traditional Linguistic Approach

Table 2.3 presents the traditional classification of the vowels of English. The major elements in traditional vowel descriptions are tongue position—its height and front-to-back position—and lip rounding. These positions are shown in Figure 2.1. In addition, the distinction between tense and lax is sometimes introduced, although it is more difficult to perceive and describe. Let us look at each of these descriptions.

TABLE 2.3
Traditional Vowel Classification.

Tongue Height	Front T+	Front L+	Central T	Central L	Back T	Back L
High	i	ɪ			u*	ʊ*
Medium	e	ɛ	ɝ*ɜ	ɚ*ə	o*	ʌ
Low		ɚ			ɑ	ɔ*

*Some degree of lip rounding.
+T = tense; L = lax

As Schane (1973) has stated, it is possible to recognize different patterns of tongue height and front-to-back positions. The classification of height presented here is based on a three-position scale—high, mid, and low. It is important to recognize that height, as used in this classification scheme, refers to the highest arched portion of the tongue. As shown in Table 2.3, the vowel /i/ is high; the vowel /ɛ/, mid; the vowel /a/, low.

The three front-to-back positions are front, central, and back. Again, the terminology refers to the position within the mouth of the highest arched portion of the tongue. The vowel /i/ is front; the vowel /ɜ/, central; and the vowel /u/, back.

Refer to Table 2.1 for words using each of these vowel sounds and the consonant sounds described below.

The position of the lips in producing vowels is described in terms of relative closure or rounding. In the rounded or somewhat closed position, the lips protrude slightly in an "O" shape. The degree of lip rounding is more marked in some speakers than in others. In English, lip rounding is a characteristic only of certain back vowels. Thus the back vowel /u/ is rounded, but the back vowel /ʌ/ is not.

Vowels may also be described as lax or tense. Tense vowels, as the designation suggests, are produced with greater muscular tension than are lax vowels. But tense vowels are also held longer, and their articulation is more

FIGURE 2.1

Relative Positions for Articulation of the Cardinal Vowels. The range of articulation is shown as a solid line; high back and front tongue shapes are shown as dashed lines. At the bottom is a vowel quadrilateral, showing the tongue positions for the English vowels, within the limits of articulation for the cardinal vowels. (Drawing courtesy of W. R. Zemlin.)

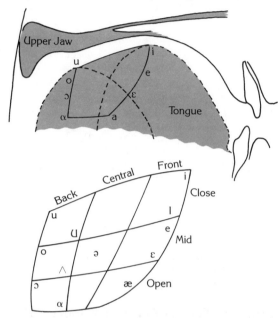

definite. One way to recognize this distinction is to place your forefinger on the midline of your throat while pronouncing the vowels /i/ and /ɪ/ alternately. You will note that as you say /i/, as in the word *seat,* you will feel a forward pressure on your finger. But as you pronounce /ɪ/ as in the word *sit* you will find that this forward pressure is lacking. As you can see from Table 2.3, this is a major production difference in these two vowels.

The traditional classification of English consonants is shown in Table 2.4. The major elements in consonant classification in the traditional system are (*a*) manner, (*b*) place of constriction, and (*c*) voicing. It is difficult to compare these three elements with those of the traditional vowel classification. Manner, which refers to mode of production, really has no equivalent category in the vowel classification system. Place is somewhat analogous to tongue position in the vowel system. Voicing, which refers to the presence or absence of vibration of the larynx, is not specified in the vowel classification because all English vowels are voiced.

Manner   Manner refers to some general characteristic in the production of a consonant, particularly with respect to the release of the sound. As shown in Table 2.4, manner is superimposed across place and voicing. There are six categories of manner in the traditional approach: nasals, plosives, fricatives, affricates, liquids, and glides.

The three nasals of English (/m, n, ŋ/) are made with the oral passageway completely occluded (closed) at one of the constriction points indicated, but with the velopharyngeal valve open so that the air-sound stream escapes through the nose. The acoustic differences among the three nasals results

More detail on sound production is presented in chapter 4.

TABLE 2.4
Traditional Classification of the Consonants of English, with Examples.

Place of Constriction*	Nasals		Plosives		Fricatives		Affricates		Liquids		Glides	
	U⁺	V⁺	U	V	U	V	U	V	U	V	U	V
Front												
Bilabial	m (su<u>m</u>)		p (<u>p</u>ot)	b (<u>bob</u>)								w (<u>w</u>et)
Labiodental					f (<u>f</u>ine)	v (<u>v</u>ine)						
Middle												
Linguadental					θ (e<u>th</u>er)	ð (ei<u>th</u>er)						
Alveolar	n (su<u>n</u>)		t (<u>t</u>ot)	d (<u>d</u>ot)	s (<u>s</u>eal)	z (<u>z</u>eal)			l,r (<u>l</u>ed) (<u>r</u>ed)			
Palatal					ʃ (ba<u>sh</u>)	ʒ (bei<u>g</u>e)	tʃ (<u>ch</u>ump)	dʒ (<u>j</u>ump)				j (<u>j</u>et)
Back												
Velar			k (<u>c</u>ot)	g (<u>g</u>ot)								
Glottal	ŋ (su<u>ng</u>)				h (<u>h</u>ump)							

*Place of constriction is arranged from external or front (lips) to internal or back (glottis).
⁺U = unvoiced; V = voiced.

from variation in the size and shape of the oral cavity and not from variation in the nasal passageway. The nasals of English are all voiced.

The plosives (/p, b, t, d, k, g/) are characterized by a complete obstruction of the air-sound stream. In a complete plosive, the pressure is built up and then abruptly released with an audible aspiration or puff of air. In many phonetic contexts, however, as in the word *speak* /spik/, the /p/ is not aspirated but the /k/ may be. These differences are allophones of the various plosives and are usually not consciously noticed by American listeners. The six plosives of English are found in three pairs, or **cognates**.

Cognates *are two sounds that differ only by voicing.*

The fricatives will be (/f, v, θ, ð, s, z, ʃ, ʒ, h/) are characterized by a light contact between the opposed constrictors so that, as the air-sound stream passes through the relatively constricted aperture, a friction noise or hiss is produced. In voiced fricatives, the friction noise is superimposed upon the laryngeal vibration; in the unvoiced fricatives, the friction noise constitutes the phoneme. The different kinds of constriction produce different noises, so that it is possible to differentiate an /f/ from an /s/. Except for /h/, the one glottal fricative, each of the remaining eight fricatives occur as voiced and unvoiced cognates.

The affricates (/tʃ, dʒ/) represent a blend of plosive and fricative. The two affricates of English are described as beginning with a complete closure at the lingua-alveolar region and as being released as linguapalatal fricatives. The two English affricates are cognates. The IPA symbolism, as shown in Table 2.4, reflects the blend of the two separate elements.

Although /l/ and /r/ are grouped as liquids, they are best described separately. The allophones of /l/ are laterals; that is, the tongue makes a midline closure in the alveolar region, but the air-sound stream is permitted to escape around one or both sides of the tongue. The release is accomplished without perceptible turbulence, so that /l/ has an acoustic quality somewhat similar to that of the vowels. Indeed, as a syllabic in a word such as *saddle,* /l/ may perform a vowel function. The /r/ of English has no complete closure. The sound is produced by elevating either the front or the rear of the tongue in the mouth. Like /l/, /r/ also has a vowel-like quality. In their consonant variations in particular, both liquids are characterized by movement. For this reason writers such as Kantner and West (1941) have categorized /l, r/ as glides.

As classified in this chapter, the true glides are /w/ and /j/. A glide may be defined as a sound produced during the movement of the articulators from one vowel position to another. The /w/ and /j/ are produced by glides from the /u/ and /i/ positions, respectively. Because little friction noise is produced, these sounds are sometimes called **semivowels**. In our terminology, we call glides to the /u/ or /i/ positions **diphthongs**.

Place　Place refers to that point along a continuum from the lips to the glottis at which the greatest degree of constriction occurs. The constriction may be partial, as in the fricatives, or complete, as in the plosives. In the nasals, the oral passageway is completely blocked, but the nasal passageways are open. The sites of maximum constriction may be specified as follows (Irwin & Wong, 1981):

- *Bilabial*—The essential articulatory posture is between the upper and lower lips. Examples are /b, p, m/.
- *Labiodental*—The essential articulatory posture is between the lower lip and the upper incisors. Examples are /f, v/.
- *Linguadental*—The essential articulatory posture is between the front tongue and the upper incisors. Examples are /θ, ð/.
- *Lingua-alveolar*—The essential articulatory posture is between the front tongue and the upper alveolar ridge. Examples are /s, z/.
- *Linguapalatal*—The essential articulatory posture is between the tongue and hard palate. Examples are /ʃ, ʒ/.
- *Linguavelar*—The essential articulatory posture is between the back tongue and the velum or soft palate. Examples are /k, g, ŋ/.
- *Glottal*—The essential articulatory posture is at the glottis. An example is /h/.

See chapter 4 for complete descriptions of how each of these physical structures functions in speech. The structures are shown in Figure 2.2.

Voicing　The three nasals of English are all voiced. But in the plosives, fricatives, and affricatives, as can be seen in Table 2.4, the sounds are arranged in voiced and unvoiced pairs. The one exception is /h/, which has no voiced equivalent. Finally, the liquids and glides are all voiced. In our system, the nasals, liquids, and glides are all sonorants. That is, as Schane (1973) has stated, they have a vowel-like quality. The plosives, fricatives, and affricates, even when voiced, lack this quality.

We have just described the sounds of English. As Whatmough (1957) has reported, other languages use some other sounds with other production characteristics, such as the palatization of Russian, the pitch of Chinese, and the clicks of some African languages. But, as Whatmough affirms, these exceptions may be viewed as rather trivial limitations to the finding that the number of classes is quite small and that most of them are represented in most languages. Or, to rephrase, languages differ primarily not in their sounds but in the way they permit the patterning of sounds and sentences.

FIGURE 2.2

The Articulators and Places of Articulation for Consonant Production. (Drawing courtesy of W. R. Zemlin.)

1. *Lips (Labial)*
2. *Teeth (Dental)*
3. *Alveolar Ridge (Alveolar)*
4. *Hard Palate (Palatal)*
5. *Pharynx (Pharyngeal)*
6. *Soft Palate (Velar)*
7. *Uvula (Uvular)*
8. *Tongue (Tip)*
9. *Tongue (Blade)*
10. *Tongue (Front)*
11. *Tongue (Back)*

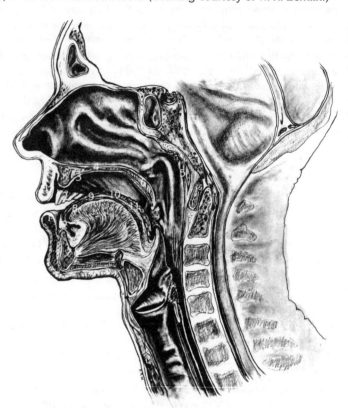

In this discussion, we have treated the phonemes as if they were discrete units in speech. Bear in mind, however, that the physical speech signal is essentially continuous, so continuous that the identification of the boundaries of individual segments or phonemes is virtually impossible. Nevertheless, speakers of a language intuitively feel that not only sounds but also words and sentences are discrete units. However, while we physically could stop speaking in the middle of a word or a sentence, we typically do not.

Generative Phonology

A key event in the development of interest in distinctive feature analysis of speech sounds was the publication of Preliminaries to Speech Analysis *by Jakobson, Fant, and Halle in 1951.*

In contrast to the traditional linguistic approach, the distinctive feature approach of the generative phonologists assumes that phonemes may be broken down into smaller units, the distinctive features. Singh (1976), in reviewing distinctive feature analysis, notes that the features may be (a) acoustical, as in the system of Jakobson, Fant, and Halle (1951); (b) perceptual, as in the systems of Singh, Woods, and Becker (1972); or (c) articulatory, as in the system of Chomsky and Halle (1968). Systems may be either binary or scaled. In a binary system, the feature is either present or absent; in a scaled system, a feature is treated as a continuum on which usually three or more points are located. The Chomsky and Halle (1968) system is binary; the Singh and Black (1966) system is scaled. A single system may combine one or more theoretical bases of classification; that is, it may be perceptual in one feature and articulatory in another or scaled in one feature and binary in a second. Many of the features used in these systems are similar to or the same as the characteristics used to describe sounds in traditional phonology (for example, voicing, tenseness).

Distinctive features have been used in studies of the way most children develop language, in the study of deviant phonology, and in the study of the validity of the distinctive feature concept. Research on "normal" children to date has been relatively scarce, but two comprehensive studies stand out. In one, Olmsted (1971) described the spontaneous utterances of 100 children in the age range from 15 to 30 months. Irwin and Wong (1981) studied the spontaneous development of 100 children with 20 each at ages 18, 24, 36, 48, and 72 months. These two studies differ in the type of sample, the age and language of the children, and in the distinctive feature systems used. But the studies have shown at least partial agreement on these findings: (*a*) within any one system, some features seem to emerge earlier than do others; (*b*) within any one system, some pattern of emergence may be described; and (*c*) regardless of system, the features seem to be generally available at relatively early ages.

See the studies of Menyuk (1968), Prather, Hendrick, and Kern (1975), and Hodson and Paden (1978).

Distinctive feature systems differ obviously in the number of phonemes they seek to describe and in the number of features they use in the analysis. But systems also differ with respect to degree of abstraction. Both Walsh (1974) and Ingram (1976) have referred to this problem. The system of Chomsky and Halle (1968) is relatively abstract; the systems of Singh, Woods, and Becker (1972) and of Irwin and Wong (1981) are more concrete. But such differences are only relative. Inevitably, any distinctive feature approach is an abstraction.

An interesting concept in distinctive feature theory is that the degree of difference between two phonemes can be assessed by counting the number of features by which they differ. Thus two phonemes that differ by only one feature may be assumed to be more like each other than two phonemes that differ by several features. Thus /p, b/ would be considered more like each other than /t, g/, for in most systems the feature difference count would be greater for the second pair.

Despite the intuitive validity of these notions, Singh (1976) notes that, of necessity, the theory assumes that each theory has the same value and, in a scaled system, with each feature each degree has the same value. Singh concludes that, although the concept does have some value in quantifying differences in phonemes, the quantification cannot be taken literally. Moreover, the appropriateness of such a difference may depend upon whether the effect is studied, for example, by production or by perception. Greenberg and Jenkins (1964) studied perceptual differences in selected English consonants. They found that, if the two consonants compared were both voiced, other features of manner and place made little difference. But if the paired consonants were unvoiced, manner and place were much more important. These data do not support the hypothesis of an equal count and an equal difference. Miller and Nicely (1955) found that consonants within phonetic groups were easily confused with each other, but that comparisons of consonants across groups were much less confused.

Postal (1968), incidentally, has noted that such perceptual studies involve coarticulatory effects and thus go somewhat beyond the confines of distinctive feature theory.

Research on the application of distinctive feature theory to the study of deviant phonology is again somewhat limited. Ingram (1976) effectively reviewed the current status of applications of distinctive feature techniques to phonological problems. He concludes that, although distinctive features may be a useful descriptive device and would at times be helpful, use of the tech-

These questions are explored in depth in chapter 5.

nique is not essential and frequently does not add any new information. He looks also at the problem of using distinctive features to predict the emergence of speech sounds. The argument of proponents of the approach, again, is that children develop phonemes by feature rather than by phoneme. But Ingram, using studies of fricatives as examples, concludes that each segment seems to have its own development. Finally, Ingram reviews the generalization process, that is, whether the teaching of a feature in one segment will result in or facilitate its spread to other segments. He cautiously concludes that the generalization hypothesis has not been supported conclusively and that it should be studied further.

In conclusion, distinctive features are a convenient way to describe natural classes of sounds. The fewer features needed to describe a class, the larger the class. Thus vowels and consonants—large natural classes—can be differentiated by relatively few features.

Irwin and Wong (1981), in order to use the Chomsky and Halle (1968) system with a full set of English vowels and consonants, arbitrarily and perhaps inappropriately extended the system in two ways: they included the features voice, continuant, nasal, and strident in vowel summaries and the features round and tense in consonant summaries. A summary description of each feature follows. The Chomsky and Halle feature matrix, as extended for consonants, appears as Table 2.5.

TABLE 2.5
English Consonants Including the Glottal Stop by Chomsky-Halle Extended Features.

Feature	k	q	t	d	p	l	f	v	θ	ð	s	z	ʃ	ʒ	tʃ	dʒ	m	n	ŋ	l	r	h	w	j	ʔ
Vocalic	−	−	−	−	−	−	−	−	−	−	−	−	−	−	−	−	−	−	−	+	+	−	−	−	−
Consonantal	+	+	+	+	+	+	+	+	+	+	+	+	+	+	+	+	+	+	+	+	+	−	−	−	−
High	+	+	−	−	−	−	−	−	−	−	−	−	+	+	+	+	−	−	+	−	−	−	+	+	−
Back	+	+	−	−	−	−	−	−	−	−	−	−	−	−	−	−	−	−	+	−	−	−	+	−	−
Low	−	−	−	−	−	−	−	−	−	−	−	−	−	−	−	−	−	−	−	−	−	+	−	−	+
Anterior	−	−	+	+	+	+	+	+	+	+	+	+	−	−	−	−	+	+	−	+	−	−	−	−	−
Coronal	−	−	+	+	−	−	−	−	+	+	+	+	+	+	+	+	−	+	−	+	+	−	−	−	−
Round																							+	−	−
Tense																								−	−
Voice	−	+	−	+	−	+	−	+	−	+	−	+	−	+	−	+	+	+	+	+	+	−	+	+	−
Continuant	−	−	−	−	−	−	+	+	+	+	+	+	+	+	−	−	−	−	−	+	+	+	+	+	+
Nasal	−	−	−	−	−	−	−	−	−	−	−	−	−	−	−	−	+	+	+	−	−	−	−	−	−
Strident	−	−	−	−	−	−	+	+	−	−	+	+	+	+	+	+	−	−	−	−	−	−	−	−	−

Blank = not relevant.
− = binary feature not present.
+ = binary feature present.

- *Vocalic*—Constriction in the oral cavity is not greater than required for the high vowels /i, u/.
- *Consonantal*—The sound is made with a radical constriction in the mid-sagittal region of the oral cavity.
- *High*—The body of the tongue is elevated above the neutral position.
- *Back*—The body of the tongue retracts from the neutral position.
- *Low*—The body of the tongue is lowered below the neutral position.
- *Anterior*—The sound is produced further forward in the mouth than /ʃ/.
- *Coronal*—The sound is produced with the blade of the tongue raised from the neutral position.
- *Round*—The lip orifice is narrowed.
- *Tense*—The sound is produced deliberately, accurately, and distinctly.

- *Voice*—During the production of the sound, the larynx vibrates periodically.
- *Continuant*—The vocal tract is partially constricted during the production of the sound.
- *Nasal*—The velopharyngeal valve is sufficiently open during the production of the sound to permit the air-sound stream to be directed through the nose.
- *Strident*—The air stream is directed over a rough surface in such a way as to produce an audible noise.

Suprasegmental Systems

The phonology of a language defines more than the sounds of that language, which are frequently treated as the segments of a language. The **supraseg-mental** features are those phonological characteristics that typically cut across more than one segment or sound. Known also as the prosodic features, they primarily include variations in the laryngeal tone such as pitch, quality, loudness, and duration.

Although voice pitch is a suprasegmental feature in English, in some languages, such as Chinese, pitch is used to identify units of meaning (morphemes). According to Langacker (1968), the largest number of different pitches used in any one language to differentiate morphemes seems to be about five.

Coarticulation

The sounds of a language are also affected by **coarticulation**. *Coarticulation* has been defined by Daniloff and Hammarburg (1973) as the influence of one speech segment on another, that is, as the effect of phonetic context on a sound or sounds. Thus coarticulation is concerned with the effects of adjacent sounds on each other so far as production is concerned.

Current writers recognize two major types of coarticulation. If one segment exerts an influence on a following segment, the coarticulation effect is described as left-to-right or carry-over. If one segment influences a preceding segment, the coarticulatory effect is described as right-to-left or anticipatory. Thomas (1958) describes anticipatory coarticulation as the more common of the two types in English. Coarticulatory effects are not limited to immediately adjacent segments. They have been shown to cut across not only two or more segments, but also across the boundaries of syllables, morphemes, and words.

The acceptability of coarticulatory changes seems to be a function of many factors. Among them are the conspicuousness of the perceptual effect, possible semantic confusion, the degree of simplification in the production process, and the status of the people who use the effect. But, whether accepted as "standard" or not, coarticulatory effects continue to be part of the natural history of a language. The rendering of *captain* /kɚptn̩/ as /kɚpn̩/ seems as natural as the production of vision /vɪzjən/ as /vɪʒən/, but only the latter change is well enough established in this country as not to attract attention.

MORPHOLOGY AND SYNTAX

Morphology: The Forms of English

Morphemes may be defined as the smallest grammatical units in a language that have meaning. Smallest simply means that the unit cannot be subdivided without either destroying the morpheme or changing its meaning so as to make it function as a different morpheme. Morphemes contribute to meaning in several ways. First, and most obvious, as independent words such as *car* or *giraffe*, morphemes carry referential meaning or make subject matter meaning possible. Second, as modifications of such content words as nouns, verbs, and adjectives, morphemes simplify the expression of such grammatical relationships as plurals (cats), past tense (sang), and adverbs (swift*ly*).

The forms of morphemes vary. A morpheme may be a phoneme, as the plural /s/, or a sequence of phonemes, as the superlative -*est*. A morpheme may be a syllable, as the *un-* of *unclean*, or a word, as *boy, girl*, or *phone*. But not all phonemes are morphemes; indeed, not all /s/ phonemes are morphemes. Consider the /s/ of *sister*. Not all syllables are morphemes; consider the *la* of *latex*. And not even all words are morphemes; consider *railroad*, which can be subdivided into two morphemes *rail* and *road*.

Langacker (1968) has recognized three contrasting forms or pairs of morphemes.

(1) Free vs. bound
  (a) Free morphemes can stand alone; they are words. An example is *walk*.
  (b) Bound morphemes cannot stand alone. An example is -*ing*, as *walking*.
(2) Full vs. empty
  (a) Full morphemes carry independent meaning. They can be nouns, such as *boy*.
  (b) Empty morphemes do not carry independent meaning. They can be articles and prepositions, such as *into*.
(3) Root vs. affix
  (a) A root is the core of a word, such as *intent*.
  (b) Affixes—prefixes, infixes, and suffixes—are added to roots. For example, in the word *unintentionally*, *un-* is a prefix, -*ion* and -*al* are infixes, and -*ly* is a suffix.

In addition, we can make a useful distinction between lexical morphemes, such as nouns and verbs, and grammatical morphemes, such as the indicators of plural, superlative, or third person singular.

Certain characteristics hold generally for morphemes. For example:

(1) The meaning of a morpheme is usually consistent.
(2) Certain morphemes are essentially meaningless, as for example the morpheme *to*.
(3) The phonological presentation of a morpheme may change. The plural morpheme takes the phonemic form /s/ following a grammatical morpheme that terminates in /p, t, k/ or /f/. But if the plural morpheme is added to a lexical morpheme that terminates in /s, z, ʒ, ʃ, tʃ, dʒ/, it takes the phonemic form /ɪz/. In all other contexts, the plural morpheme takes the phonemic form /z/.
(4) A given sound sequence may be a morpheme in one context but not in another. The *un-* of *unclean* in a morpheme; the *un* of *under* is not.
(5) A given sound may act as one morpheme in one context and another morpheme in a different context. The /s/ of *cats* expresses plurality; the /s/ of the verb *hits*, third person singular.
(6) Two morphemes may be spelled alike and pronounced differently. Consider the verb *read* in its present and in its past tense.

(7) Two morphemes may be pronounced alike but spelled differently, as in the nouns *route* and *root* in the dialects of many speakers.

The skilled speaker of English uses morphological rules to:

(1) Modify the meaning of root words and produce distinctions in meaning, by the addition of number, case, and tense markers and suffixes.
(2) Derive certain words, such as nouns from verbs (teach*er*), adjectives from nouns (spott*y*), adverbs from adjectives (quick*ly*), and specify their syntactic roles in sentences.
(3) Extend or modify the meaning of root words by the addition of prefixes (Wiig & Semel, 1980).

While these rules are common to speakers of a language, they may be varied in certain dialects.

See chapter 3.

Syntax

The words of a language—the morphemes in a general sense—are combined into sentences. The sentence is probably the most vital unit in the understanding of a language. It is a string of morphemes derived from a base formulation through **transformations** and rewrite rules. Sentences can be characterized in terms of (*a*) the sequential arrangements of words in what is said or spoken, (*b*) the type of units included, and (*c*) hierarchical arrangements as demonstrated at the performance level by pauses in either speech or writing.

We use rules of syntax to form sentences from words; like the rules of morphology, these rules are mastered and used automatically by skilled speakers of a language. The term used for a system of describing the syntactic rules of a language is a *grammar.*

Just as the morpheme sequence within words is controlled, so is the sequence of words in a sentence. *Horse the ran* is not an English sentence; *The horse ran* is. If we were to create a grammar for English, it should not permit the first sequence but should permit any acceptable sequence. A grammar should generate not only an infinite number of sentences, but it must generate any conceivable sentence and permit its interpretation. In some respects, this is the most challenging task requirement and test of a grammar. It must permit the speaker to generate any sentence, perhaps one that has never been spoken before. And it must permit the listener to interpret this sentence or any other sentence, whether he or she has ever heard it before. This creativity of generation and interpretation is indeed wondrous.

However, although the allowable sentences must be infinite, the number of rules must be finite. Created rules would not predictably have uniform application and interpretation. In English, we have a finite and stable number of phonemes. At the morpheme level, the number is finite but tremendous and is increasing (that is, it is finite at a given point in time). But new morphemes will—in any given language—take a predictable form, with the potential exception of morphemes borrowed from other languages.

At a practical level, the length of sentences is restricted. The human brain can process only within limits; these limits may vary, but they are always present and cannot be exceeded. Nevertheless, grammars that permit embedding and conjoining provide mechanisms for grammatical sentences of infinite length.

The users of a language must be able to differentiate **ambiguous** sentences and recognize **homonymous** sentences. A typical ambiguous sentence is:

Counseling parents can be fun.

Embedding involves placing a word, phrase, or clause within an existing sentence; conjoining involves joining two syntactically equal elements.

Homonymous sen-
tences have the same
meaning.

Does this sentence describe the act of counseling parents as fun, or does it say that parents who counsel are fun? Native speakers recognize both possibilities, although without any context they may not be able to choose the intended meaning.

In contrast, these sentences mean approximately the same thing:

> The boy mowed the grass.
> The grass was mowed by the boy.

Native speakers—despite the many differences in the word order of the sentence—will recognize the similarity of meaning.

Whatmough (1957) puts these matters much more simply. Each language, he says, has a small number of speech sounds as compared with the number of formative elements that it uses, and these are fewer than the total number of words, and these are less than the total number of meanings. Arrangement and rearrangement of sequence permits endless variety.

In summary, syntax can be described as a finite set of rules which determine both the order of components in an utterance and the relationship of those components within an utterance. The morpheme is the smallest unit of syntax; the sentence is the largest.

SEMANTICS

Semantics is the study of meaning in language. It is concerned with the meaningful relationships between words, groups of words, sentences, and other linguistic entities. It is concerned with the linguistic elements and what they are signs of. Leonard (1976) has identifed three concepts of meaning as it relates to language and language use. These are *referential* meaning, the **referent**(s) of the sign or signs; *pragmatics,* the response to a context; and the *rational,* which can be defined as that which is meant.

A referent is the object,
action, or idea a word
refers to.

The study of semantics is closely related to human psychology. Our unanswered question here is whether our descriptions of language, our grammars, if you will, describe the way people use language. A language may express how an individual thinks, a grammar may give the rules for his expression, but neither reveals how the person thinks. To date, the psychological reality of theoretical grammars has not been established.

PRAGMATICS

Our choice of utterances is often affected by the context of the interaction and the social roles of the sender and receiver. For instance, most children quickly learn to use somewhat different vocabulary and even syntax with their parents, their peers, and their teachers—even if they wish to express the same idea. Furthermore, certain utterances become a part of social rituals and lose their original meanings. A good example is "How are you?" which is used as a common American greeting rather than a request for a medical report. Like the other rules of a language, pragmatic rules are used unconsciously by adults.

THE ORGANIZATION OF LANGUAGE

The presentation in this chapter thus far has reflected a classical or structural linguistic concept of the organization of a language. This type of grammar system breaks the sentence down into hierarchical levels. In descending order, these levels are the sentence, phrases, morphemes, and phonemes. This model implies that speakers actually construct sentences from the lower levels up.

Unfortunately, this approach provides little real information either as to how individuals use language or as to how they acquire it. Many theories have been developed to account for these processes. These theories have largely come from two groups of investigators: psychologists and psycholinguists.

One early theory was referred to as the *finite state* model. Although now largely discredited, it has been described in some detail by McNeill (1970). This model, espoused by early psychologists, held that any element of a sentence was generated on a probability basis from the preceding element. Viewed literally, the model held that a sentence was generated in the exact same order as its final form or surface structure. It has been easy to demonstrate the weaknesses of this model of serial sentence generation. One of its greatest problems is that it does not account for embedding. Another is that, although it was expressed in probabilities, it allowed no real opportunities for choice.

The theory can perhaps be better understood if the term *word* is substituted for the word *state*. A finite word machine produces sentences in a left to right order. Each word is treated as if it could be chosen at random from the user's entire vocabulary. But a string of words generated in this fashion will not necessarily be coherent. Also, in a complex sentence, particularly one with embedding, the effect of a word may be remote rather than immediate. Thus the constraints of actual meaning may be lost completely in the process. In practice, the functional constraints between two words are semantic as well as syntactic. That is, we can say "a *young* girl," "a *blond* girl," or even "a *plastic* girl," but not "a *three* girl."

Various psychologists have proposed other language models based primarily upon stimulus-response psychology. They say that a response made in the presence of a stimulus comes under the control of that stimulus if the response is consistently reinforced. This kind of learning theory becomes more reasonable if it takes into account meaning and total environmental context. Skinner (1957) has identified six kinds of language-related responses and, consistent with his beliefs, feels that the use of each is controlled by its reinforcement. Although relatively straightforward, the theory leaves unexplained much of the detail of language, particularly in the acquisition of syntax.

This theory, as advanced by B.F. Skinner in Verbal Behavior *(1957), has not had wide critical acceptance.*

More sophisticated learning theories have retained the notions of reinforcement and of probability but tie the final structure to context. Osgood (1963), although retaining the idea of serial sentence generation, introduced the concepts of phrase structure grammar and thus made some provision for the effects of remote elements. But, in general, we may conclude that learning theory approaches account well for the acquisition of word meaning and poorly for the acquisition of syntax.

A phrase structure grammar can be used to describe the structure of a language as pictured by the structural linguists.

To a group of linguists called the *generative grammarians,* none of the traditional approaches is satisfactory. These approaches deal only with the surface structure of the sentence. Transformational generative grammarians conceive of a two-level grammar: a deep-structure level and a surface-structure level (Chomsky, 1957, 1965). The deep-structure level embodies the semantic intent of the message. Indeed, it is possible that deep level formulations are constant across all languages. The deep-structure level formulation is converted to the surface-structure level by rewrite and transformation processes, as needed.

We often use pragmatic rules to decide what transformations to make. For example, the context of needing information leads to the transformation from affirmative to interrogative.

A transformation is an operation in which base elements are substituted, deleted, or rearranged, thereby transforming the original base structure into an appropriate surface structure. A transformation is always dependent on structure and restricted by context. Examples of transformations include the negative, the passive, subject-postponement, formal interrogative, echo question, and the imperative. Here are some examples.

> Rearrangement: The weather is nice today.
>   Today the weather is nice.
> Addition: John went to the movies.
>   John and Bill went to the movies.
> Active to passive: John hit the ball.
>   The ball was hit by John.

The transformational approach accounts for ambiguous sentences. It suggests that the different meanings of one single surface structure account for two different deep structures. The same mechanism in reverse accounts for homonymous sentences.

Transformational grammar has greatly influenced the study of language and its acquisition. As of today, these views have not been completely accepted either as describing language or as describing how the human brain functions in thinking and in talking. In the meantime, we will continue to use language to study language.

CONCLUSION

To put all this together, let us return to our early description of the communication event. A sender has a message which he wishes to communicate. From his vocabulary, he chooses a word to symbolize each concept in the message. He uses rules of morphology to form some of these words and to choose other words, and arranges the words in a sequence that conforms to the syntax of his language. The words are related to the concepts they symbolize by semantics. The choice of both the words and word sequences may be affected by pragmatic rules that relate to the current situation.

In written language, a different set of physiological mechanisms produces a message that is interpreted through a different channel in the receiver.

Having constructed a sentence (we could say "encoded an idea"), the sender transforms a mental image of the message into an acoustical pattern. That is, he applies appropriate phonological rules to the words and pronounces each one in turn. (Again, this requires a complex act of a variety of physiological mechanisms.) At the same time, he may intentionally or unintentionally reinforce the verbal message with nonverbal messages. The receiver, in turn, uses the same systems to decode or interpret the perceived message.

Of course, skilled users of a language perform all of these steps at virtually the same moment. And again, the process can fail at any point. It falls to the speech-language pathologist and audiologist to find the point of interruption, (often) its cause, and the best way to overcome it.

SELECTED READINGS

Bolinger, D. *Aspects of language.* New York: Harcourt Brace Jovanovich, 1975.

Clark, H., & Clark, E. *Psychology and language.* New York: Harcourt Brace Jovanovich, 1977.

Howell, R., & Vetter, H. *Language in behavior.* New York: Human Sciences Press, 1976.

Lock, A. (Ed.). *Action, gesture and symbol: The emergence of language.* New York: Academic Press, 1978.

Pollio, H. *The psychology of symbolic behavior.* Reading, Mass.: Addison-Wesley, 1974.

REFERENCES

Birdwhistell, R. *Kinesics and context.* Philadelphia: University of Pennsylvania Press, 1970.

Chomsky, N. *Syntactic structures.* The Hague: Mouton, 1957.

Chomsky, N. *Aspects of the theory of syntax.* Cambridge, Mass.: MIT Press, 1965.

Chomsky, N., & Halle, M. *The sound pattern of English.* New York: Harper & Row, 1968.

Crystal, D. *Prosodic systems and intonation in English.* Cambridge: Cambridge University Press, 1969.

Daniloff, R. G., & Hammarburg, R. E. On defining coarticulation. *Journal of Phonetics,* 1973, *1,* 185–194.

Eisenberg, A. M., & Smith, R. R. *Nonverbal communication.* Indianapolis: Bobbs-Merrill, 1971.

Gleason, H. A. *An introduction to descriptive linguistics.* New York: Henry Holt, 1955.

Greenberg, J. J., & Jenkins, J. J. Studies in the psychological correlates to the sound system of American English. *Word,* 1964, *20,* 157–177.

Hall, E. *The silent language.* Greenwich, Conn.: Fawcett, 1959.

Hodson, B., & Paden, E. Phonological feature competencies of normal four-year-olds. *Acta Symbolica,* 1978, *9,* 37–49.

Ingram, D. *Phonological disability in children.* New York: Elsevier, 1976.

Irwin, J., & Wong, S. *Phonological development: 18 to 72 months.* Carbondale; University of Southern Illinois Press, 1981.

Jakobson, R., Fant, C. G., & Halle, M. *Preliminaries to speech analysis.* Cambridge, Mass.: MIT Press, 1951.

Kantner, C. E., & West, R. *Phonetics.* New York: Harper & Row, 1941.

Langacker, R. W. *Language and its structure.* New York: Harcourt, Brace & World, 1968.

Leonard, L. *Meaning in child language.* New York: Grune & Stratton, 1976.

Leutenegger, R. R. *The sounds of American English.* Chicago: Scott, Foresman, 1963.

Lowen, A. *The language of the body.* New York: Collier Books, 1958.

McNeill, D. *The acquisition of language.* New York: Harper & Row, 1970.

Menyuk, P. The role of distinctive features in children's acquisition of phonology. *Journal of Speech and Hearing Research,* 1968, *11,* 138–146.

Miller, G. A., & Nicely, P. E. An analysis of perceptual confusion among some English consonants. *Journal of the Acoustical Society of America,* 1955, *27,* 338–352.

Moerk, E. L. *Pragmatic and semantic aspects of early language development.* Baltimore: University Park Press, 1977.

Nierenberg, G. I., & Calero, H. H. *How to read a person like a book.* New York: Hawthorne Books, 1971.

Olmsted, D. L. *Out of the mouth of babes.* The Hague: Mouton, 1971.

Osgood, C. On understanding and creating sentences. *American Psychologist,* 1963, *18,* 735–751.

Postal, P. *Aspects of phonological theory.* New York: Harper & Row, 1968.

Prather, E., Hendrick, D., & Kern, C. Articulation development in children aged two to four years. *Journal of Speech and Hearing Disorders,* 1975, *40,* 179–191.

Schane, S. A. *Generative phonology.* Englewood Cliffs; N.J.: Prentice-Hall, 1973.

Silverman, F. H. *Communication for the speechless.* Englewood Cliffs; N.J.: Prentice-Hall, 1980.

Singh, S. *Distinctive features theory and validation.* Baltimore: University Park Press, 1976.

Singh, S., & Black, J. W. Study of twenty-six intervocalic consonants as spoken and recognized by four language groups. *Journal of the Acoustical Society of America,* 1966, *39,* 372–387.

Singh, S., Woods, D. R., & Becker, G. M. Perceptual structure of 22 prevocalic English consonants. *Journal of the Acoustical Society of America,* 1972, *52,* 1698–1713.

Skinner, B. F. *Verbal behavior.* New York: Appleton-Century-Crofts, 1957.

Slobin, D. I. *Psycholinguistics.* Glenview, Ill.: Scott, Foresman, 1971.

Thomas, C. K. *An introduction to the phonetics of American English* (2nd ed.). New York: Ronald Press, 1958.

Trager, G. L. Paralanguage: A first approximation. *Studies in Linguistics,* 1958, *13,* 1–12.

Walsh, H. On certain practical inadequacies of distinctive feature systems. *Journal of Speech and Hearing Disorders,* 1974, *39,* 32–43.

Weaver, W. Recent contributions to the mathematical theory of communication. In C. E. Shannon & W. Weaver, *The mathematical theory of communication.* Urbana: University of Illinios Press, 1964.

Whatmough, J. *Language.* New York: The New American Library of World Literature, 1957.

Wiig, E. H., & Semel, E. M. *Language assessment and intervention for the learning disabled.* Columbus, Ohio: Charles E. Merrill, 1980.

Wise, C. *Introduction to phonetics.* Englewood Cliffs, N.J.: Prentice-Hall, 1958.

LANGUAGE
DIFFERENCES

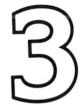

Orlando L. Taylor

James M. is a 7-year-old, Black male who attends a recently integrated elementary school in Prince Georges County, Maryland. James was referred by his teacher, who reported that he was inattentive, disruptive, and receiving failing grades in reading and language arts.

James was seen by the school psychologist who administered the WISC-R test of intelligence on which James scored in the 40th percentile. His mother reports that James is one of six children within the home. James moved to Maryland from Mayfield, North Carolina, at age 5. He is reported to have had a normal childbirth and normal development. His mother, a single, working parent, reports that she has little time to read to James or to assist him with his assignments.

James was given the Peabody Picture Vocabulary Test and the North-western Syntax Screening Test. Test scores revealed that James possessed a disorder of expressive language.

Most experts in the field of communication disorders would agree that communication is disordered when it deviates from the community standards clearly enough that it: (*a*) interferes with the transmission of messages, (*b*) stands out as being unusually different, or (*c*) produces negative feelings within the communicator. Central to this notion is the idea that a communication disorder can only be determined in the context of a community, more specifically a **speech community.** We can say that a speech community is any group of people who routinely and frequently use a shared language to interact with each other (Hymes, 1974; Gumperz & Hymes, 1972). Before we can look carefully at communication disorders, we need to have some understanding of the distinction between a *difference* and a *disorder.*

In a specified geographical area or political unit—the United States, for example—there might be several speech communities, although a common national language (in this case, English) is spoken. From community to community, use of one or all of the major components of language—phonology, morphology, syntax, or semantics or the rules of the language use and interaction—might differ in varying degrees. These varieties of the national language are called *dialects* of that language. Despite their differences, speakers of varying dialects of a language can generally communicate across speech communities. For example, a New Englander like Teddy Kennedy could converse with a Southerner like Jimmy Carter, if he wanted to. (Obviously, the

Remember, we saw in chapter 2 that a language is a set of verbal symbols and rules for their use in transmitting messages.

boundaries of political units and speech communities are not always the same. One country might have more than one language: for example, Quebec contains both French and English communities.)

Because of the intrinsic differences among the dialects of a single language, a dialect speaker often *seems* to meet our criteria for having a communication disorder. You can probably remember, for instance, having trouble understanding the pronunciation of certain words or the meaning of certain idioms used by people or cultural groups different from your own background. Clearly, it would be absurd to say that every person with a different dialect of the national language has a communication disorder, even if those differences result in breakdowns of communication, excessive audience attention, or (because of ridicule) emotional problems for the speaker. Your job as a speech-language pathologist is to understand this interplay between *difference* and *disorder* so you can accurately determine which people can profit from your professional services versus those who may need instruction in a second dialect (or language). In dealing with children or adults who appear to have communication problems, you must consider not only the communication behavior, but its context—the cultural community from which the speaker comes. That is, the speech-language pathologist must take a descriptive rather than a prescriptive posture. Dialects should be viewed in terms of their intrinsic rules and characteristics, and in terms of value judgments made by society or, indeed, the profession. As you will see later in this chapter, this may involve the interactional aspects of communication, as well as the phonology and syntax of the native language.

To evaluate a person's language relative to his or her speech community, you will need to understand some basic concepts pertaining to the interplay of language and culture, as well as to be familiar with some of the major dialects of American English. You will also need to be aware of the many ways cultural considerations can be a part of the practice of speech-language pathology. We will look at each of these topics in turn.

BASIC CONCEPTS RELATED TO LANGUAGE AND CULTURE

No matter how you define it, language is a universal human phenomenon. Some form of language is used by every group of people known on the planet, regardless of its race, region, education, or economic and technical development. But despite the existence of thousands of languages in the world, they all share a common set of "universal" rules (Greenberg, 1966). Even their patterns of acquisition are universal in some ways. And it is also true that social and cultural factors universally affect the nature and use of language within human groups. The study of social and cultural influences on language structure falls within the domain of **sociolinguistics.** Similarly, the study of language use in communication interactions, which by definition involves

See chapter 2.   social and cultural considerations, falls within the domain of pragmatics.

Since the 1960s and early 1970s, with the rise of interest in sociolinguistics and pragmatics, authorities in communication disorders have increasingly recognized that disordered speech and language structure and use can only be evaluated in the context of a specific culture.

The notions of language **dialects** and language standards are central to the understanding of sociolinguistics and its role in the study and practice of communication disorders. A dialect is a variety of a language which has developed through a complex interplay of historical, social, political, educational, and linguistic forces. In the technical sense, the term *dialect* is never used negatively, as is frequently the case with the lay public. In other words, we cannot assume that a dialect is an inferior variety of a language; it is merely a variety. In this context, *all dialects are considered to be linguistically legitimate and valid.* No dialect is intrinsically a "better" way of speaking the language.

But despite the linguistic legitimacy of dialects, people often have social attitudes toward the various dialects within a language. The people who use the **standard dialect** may look down on people who use nonstandard variations. Standard dialects are those spoken by politically, socially, economically, and educationally powerful and prestigious people. These standard dialects become the *de facto* official versions of the national language, and are used in business, education, and mass media. There may be several standard dialects within a national language.

In the United States, several varieties (dialects) of standard English do, in fact, exist. Virtually all of these varieties are identified with specific regions of the country or with certain racial, ethnic, or language groups. While the dialects of standard English—or General American English—may contain differences in dimensions of language like phonology, semantics, and pragmatics (particularly in informal situations), they share a common set of grammatical rules. It is, indeed, in syntax and morphology where social attitudes regarding dialect prestige are strongest (Wolfram, 1969).

Within the dialects of a language, there may be structural, stylistic, or social variations. For example, a **vernacular** or colloquial variation may be used in informal, casual, or intimate situations, but not in writing or in school. A social variation occurs when people communicate with each other. Thus, a specific linguistic structure may have various functions or values depending on the intent of the speaker. For instance, an interrogative sentence such as "Do you have the time?" is not always intended as a question, but may also be used to request the time or to command someone to tell you the time. The selection of a specific linguistic structure, then, depends upon the speaker's perception of the social situation as well as his or her communication intention. Finally, certain **sociolinguistic variables** such as the speaker, listener, audience, topic, or setting, identify the nonlinguistic dimensions of the social context which influence the selection of a particular language variety.

Vernacular is the common, informal language used among members of the same speech community.

That is, when you talk to your boss, you may use different words or sentence structures than when you talk to your best friend.

Seven major factors typically influence language behavior and acquisition throughout the world.

(1) Race and ethnicity
(2) Social class, education, and occupation
(3) Region
(4) Gender
(5) Situation or context
(6) Peer group association or identification
(7) First language community or culture

Race and Ethnicity

Racial and ethnic influences on language and communication are neither biological nor genetic in nature. Instead, they are related to the cultural attitudes and values associated with a particular racial or ethnic group. Some linguistic forms are so characteristic of certain racial or ethnic groups that, when they are used, they immediately mark the speaker as either being from that group, or as having had a great deal of interaction with the group.

We must be careful, however, not to assume that racial or ethnic group membership automatically predicts language behavior or prevents an individual from using language codes usually associated with other groups. To do so would be prejudicial stereotyping. In fact, many people learn to use the language of several different racial and ethnic groups effectively.

Social Class, Education, and Occupation

Like race and ethnicity, linguistic behavior tends to reflect social class, education, and occupation. In some societies, it is considered highly inappropriate for members of the servant classes to speak the language of the aristocracy (Edwards, 1976). Even in these societies, however, it is not unusual for language behavior to be further restricted by factors such as segregation or geographical isolation. In addition to these factors, educational achievement and occupation may have a major role in determining language function (Hollingshead, 1965).

Researchers have attributed many dimensions of language variation to a number of social class influences. The chief social factors listed include: (*a*) poverty and home environment (Anastasiow & Hanes, 1976; Lawton, 1968; Williams, 1970); (*b*) child-rearing practices and maternal teaching styles (Bee, Van Egeren, Strissguth, Nyman, & Leckie, 1969; Brandis & Henderson, 1970; Lawton, 1968; Snow, Arlman-Rupp, Hassing, Jobse, Jootsen, & Vorster, 1976); (*c*) family interaction patterns (Adlam, 1977; Lawton, 1968; Rosch, 1977); and (*d*) travel and experience (Lawton, 1968).

Bernstein (1971) has been at the forefront of those scholars who claim that social class determines a person's access to certain communication codes. He suggests that lower-class groups use a more restricted, context-dependent code with particularistic meanings and that the upper classes use a more elaborated, context-independent code with universalistic meanings. The argument against Bernstein's theory is that it has a built-in bias toward middle-class communicating styles, because it implicitly assumes that it, and not the style of the lower class, is "normal." This type of bias is seen in such measures as mean length of utterance (MLU) to assess level of language acquisition. Furthermore, it may be that many children who have access to so-called elaborated codes choose not to use them in certain situations.

Region

Regional dialects are closely tied to social dialects, but are generally defined by geographic boundaries. There are at least 10 regional dialects recognized in the United States, including Southern, Eastern New England, Western Pennsylvania, Appalachian, Central Midland, Middle Atlantic, and New York City (Nist, 1966). Figure 3.1 shows a map delineating these dialect regions.

The distribution of linguistic forms as a function of geography is typically related to such factors as (*a*) geographical features (climate, topography, water supply), (*b*) trade routes, (*c*) cultural and ethnic backgrounds of settlers, (*d*) religion, and (*e*) power relationships in the region (Wardhaugh, 1976).

In general, regional dialects are marked by specific linguistic patterns. Few native-born Americans, for example, would have difficulty recognizing a stereotyped Appalachian, New York City, or Boston dialect. The speech of people from these geographical regions is unusually marked by sounds, word choices, idioms, syntax, and prosodic or pragmatic features.

FIGURE 3.1

Major American English Speech Varieties. (From J. Nist, *A Structural History of English.*
New York: St. Martin's Press, 1966, p. 371. Used by permission.)

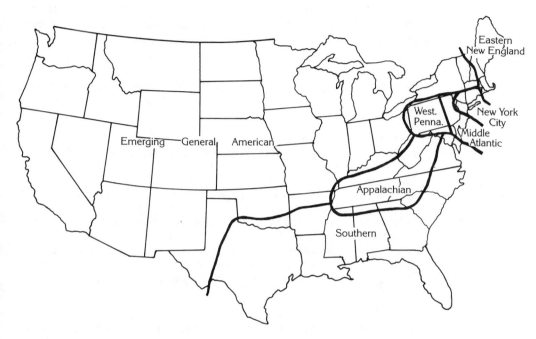

A particular speaker may choose to use a regional dialect for a variety of reasons, including local pride, local activities, or a deliberate rejection of wider affiliations. Other people may give up regionalisms because of their occupational, political, or social aspirations. Some regional dialects are viewed negatively by outsiders or by members of the upper class from the same region. Some speakers compromise by using regional dialects locally or in intimate situations, and more nonregionalized dialects away from home or in formal situations. But since regional standards within a given language tend to be close to the general standard, many speakers do not find it necessary to abandon their regional dialects.

Gender

Few would argue that it is difficult to distinguish between male or female speakers. We usually identify gender by pitch and intonation differences. The male voice is generally thought to be lower than the female voice because males have longer, thinner vocal cords. However, there is good reason to believe that social programming greatly influences men to use "masculine" voices. Women are also influenced by social definitions of voice usage. Wardhaugh (1976) argues, for instance, that women typically vary their intonation patterns more extensively than men to signal endearment, excitement, "mothering," pleasure, and so on. The key point to be kept in mind when discussing gender and voice usage is that culture may be as important, if not more so, than biology in determining voice use. We need only observe different voice patterns of men (or women) in various cultures around the world, even when race is kept constant.

Vocabulary and pragmatics may be even greater markers of gender than voice. For instance, in the United States there are certain taboo words (such as curse words) and topics (such as off-color jokes) that are often considered inappropriate for women to use in middle-class mixed company. These same words and topics, when used by men, are signs of masculinity and toughness. Trudgill (1974) even notes that men tend to use more nonstandard forms than women, as women tend to place more value on the status of standard language usage.

Speaking more explicitly, Wardhaugh (1976) makes the following observations concerning the difference between the "characteristic language uses of men and women":

> Women tend to be more precise and "careful" in speaking: for example, they are more likely than men to pronounce the final -*ing* forms with a *g*, to say *fighting* rather than *fightin'*. In general, they take more "care" in articulation. This behavior accords with other findings that women tend to be less innovative than men in their use of language and to be more conscious of preferred usages. They are also more likely than men to use "appeal tags" such as "isn't it?" or "don't you think?" . . . Women use more different names for colors than men: mauve, lavender, turquoise, lilac, and beige are good examples. Men either do not use such color words or, if they do, tend to use them with great caution. Intensifiers such as *so, such,* and *quite,* as in "He's so cute," "He's such a dear," and "We had a quite marvelous time" comprise a set of words used in a way that most men avoid; emotive adjectives such as *adorable, lovely,* and *divine* are hardly used at all by men. (p. 128)

In the Western world, where traditional sex roles are coming under attack, it is likely we will see fewer surface differences between male and female speech in the future. Indeed, many modes of communication previously restricted to men are beginning to be used by women without penalty.

Situation or Context

Language may vary according to the situation and context in which it is spoken. Several important situational and contextual variables may influence all dimensions of language behavior, the most important being:

(1) Setting
(2) Location
(3) Occasion
(4) Participants
(5) Topic
(6) Purpose
(7) Spatial positions of participants
(8) Speaker's role in two-person interactions

See Ferguson, 1964; Newport, 1976; Snow, 1972.

For example, several researchers have identified a special form of address used by parents to children, often called baby-talk or "motherese." They claim that parents, particularly mothers, tend to vary their pitch, intonation patterns, speed, sentence length, structure, and vocabulary to meet the needs of their children. Both Moerk (1974) and Bruner (1978) claim the mother's language gradually becomes more complex as the child's language becomes more complex.

Some researchers have also suggested that children, like adults, vary their speech as a function of the listener (Ervin-Tripp, 1977; Gleason, 1973;

Mitchell-Kernan & Kernan, 1977; Shatz & Gelman, 1973). For instance, children may use a more "restricted" linguistic code when talking to strangers, especially if the strangers belong to an "outside" group. This point is of extreme importance for the speech-language pathologist who is attempting to obtain a valid linguistic sample from a child.

Peer Group Association/Identification

It is widely believed that linguistic behavior, particularly during childhood, is under the control of the speech community and the parents. There is also strong research evidence to support the claim that the role of peers, including brothers and sisters, is of equal importance. Thus, a child with strong associations or identification with children from other speech communities might learn forms of language which are different from the home community or family. In these cases, the child may use the "nonhome" language or dialect only for communicating with people outside the home or home community.

Wolfram and Fasold (1974) are among several researchers who stress the importance of peer influence on language during adolescence. They report that adolescents typically learn an "in-group" dialect that is primarily used by their immediate peers. Sometimes peer pressure prevails over parental standards during this period. This point often shows up in parents' complaints that they "don't understand their teenaged children."

Finally, language is a fairly good indicator of a person's age. Language patterns of the elderly, for instance, are different from those of younger adults, which, in turn, vary from those of teenagers, and so on. Violations of linguistic age constraints tend to draw attention to the speaker. Thus, it is not unusual to hear pronouncements like "That boy talks like a man" or "That man sounds like a teenager."

First Language Community/Culture

People whose native language or culture is different from the official language and culture of a society typically learn the official language but retain distinct vestiges of their first language. These persons are considered bilingual, in that they presumably control parts or all of two languages.

In recent years, the term bidialectal *has been coined to refer to persons who control parts or all of two languages.*

Bilingual persons typically **code-switch** from one language to another, depending on the social situation (Bell, 1976). In the process of code-switching, the first language may interfere with the use of linguistic structures from the second language. A Chicano, for example, might mix English and Spanish words in the same sentence: "May I have coffee con leche?" Some speakers make morphological errors, such as deleting the plural or possessive morphenes. Phonology and syntax in the second language may also be affected by the first language. For example, English sounds such as /b/, /c/, and /l/ do not occur in Spanish, and adjectives follow nouns rather than preceding them. The Spanish rules may be followed by Spanish speakers who learn English as a second language.

Code-switching *is an individual's ability to move effectively from one language or dialect to another, as a function of the social situation (Gleason, 1973; McCormack & Wurm, 1976).*

Social factors such as age, education, and situation influence an individual's efficiency in code-switching. Also, the frequency with which a person hears and interacts within the second language code and the nature of instruction in the second language code and the nature of instruction in the second language also determine his or her skill in using it. Finally, if a person comes to use a second language more than a first language, facility in the native language might be lost if it is not reinforced at home.

As you can surmise from this discussion of the social and cultural factors which influence language, no one variable operates independently of other variables. The language used during any speech event depends upon the simultaneous interaction of many social, cultural, and situational factors. Therefore, no one sample of a person's speech taken from a single situation, or from interaction with a single person, is likely to be representative of that individual's complete linguistic repertoire. While we may be able to identify a "typical" speech pattern, that pattern cannot be considered the only speech variety available to that person. The speech-language pathologist must recognize an individual's potential for language variation during both assessment and training.

DESCRIPTIONS OF SELECTED DIALECTS OF AMERICAN ENGLISH

As we mentioned a few pages earlier, several varieties of English are spoken in the United States. These variations are caused by several factors, central among which are (a) the languages brought to the country by various cultural groups, that is, speakers of English, Polish, Chinese, Wolof, and so on; (b) the indigenous Native American languages spoken in the country; (c) the mix of the various communities and regions where the cultural groups settled; (d) the political and economic power wielded by the various cultures settling in the regions; (e) the migration patterns of the cultural groups within the country; (f) geographical isolation caused by rivers, mountains, and other features, as in the dialects of the Ozark and Appalachian mountains; and (g) self-imposed social isolation or legal segregation. In particular, a cultural group which maintains a strong identity may develop a dialect of English as its children come into contact with standard English speakers in school. An example is the dialect spoken by Puerto Ricans in New York City.

In many parts of the southern United States, for instance, the original languages spoken were typically a type of English brought from the southern portion of Great Britain, indigenous Native American languages, and a number of languages brought from West Africa, including Wolof, Mende, and Fulani. Political and social power was usually held by the British settlers, and thus their language came to assume power in education and commerce. At the same time, English speakers were probably influenced by the languages spoken by the Africans and Native Americans. As a result, a particular type of English emerged in the region, which may be loosely called Southern English. Of course, within the South, there are further regional differences.

Within each speech community, we find other linguistic variations, each of which are influenced by the social variables discussed earlier—age, gender, socioeconomic class, and so on. Again, note that these variables are *not* biological, although certain speech communities coexist with biological (racial) groups, such as the Black community in the United States. Recall that the social variables are not mutually exclusive.

Many speakers are knowledgeable and sensitive to the linguistic expectations of varying audiences and, therefore, are capable of code-switching to different dialects—even dialects which are not indigenous to their speech communities—when the situation dictates. This interaction between structure and function might be an important pragmatic consideration of sociolinguistics generally and dialectologists in particular. For example, an articulate southern Black speaker might well use one dialect variety when communicating with working-class Blacks **(Black English Vernacular)**, another when communicating with educated Blacks **(Standard Black English)**, and still another when communicating with working-class Southern whites **(Southern White Nonstandard English)**. This process can work with languages as well as dialects; a teenager might use standard English with his employer, a vernacular English with his friends, and Chinese with his parents.

There are several excellent descriptions of dialects commonly spoken in the United States available (Allen & Underwood, 1971; Dillard, 1972; Smitherman, 1978; Wolfram & Fasold, 1974). Williams and Wolfram (1977) have prepared an excellent summary of most of the research in this area for six English dialects frequently encountered by speech-language pathologists in their professional practice—Standard English, Nonstandard English, Southern White Standard English, Southern White Nonstandard English, Black English, and Appalachian English. We will now look at some of these dialects.

Black English

Perhaps the most controversial and most frequently written about dialect of American English is **Black English,** variously referred to as "Black Dialect," "Black English Vernacular," and "Ebonics." Writings on this subject began to emerge in the sociolinguistic literature in the late 1960s and early 1970s.

Loosely defined as used in much of this research, *Black English* may be thought of as the linguistic code used by working-class Black people, especially for communication in informal situations within working-class Black speech communities. Its linguistic features, like those of any other dialect, are explained on the basis of social, cultural, and historical facts, not biological differences. Further, speakers of Black English are presumed to be knowledgeable in other dialects of English, notably standard English, as demonstrated by their comprehension of these other dialects.

Black English, like other dialects, is not exclusive of other dialects of English. In fact, linguistic analyses of transcripts of Black English speakers show that the overwhelming majority of their utterances conform with the rules of General American Speech (Loman, 1967).

A selected sample of the major characteristics of Black English, as described by the many writers on the subject, is presented in Table 3.1. Remember, these linguistic variations are not *errors* in the use of English. Instead, they are characteristics of linguistic systems with their own rules, which are as complex and valid as those of standard English. We can actually identify at least 29 linguistic rules of Black English that differ from standard English (Williams & Wolfram, 1977). Careful review of these 29 linguistic rules shows considerable overlap between Black English and several other dialects, notably Southern English and Southern White Nonstandard English. Because of this overlap, we need to be very careful not to assume that a particular linguistic feature used by a Black speaker is a feature of Black English. Because Blacks in the United States have a strong historical link with the Southern states, it is not surprising that there appears to be considerable overlap between Black English and the numerous dialects spoken in the South.

Several theories have been advanced to explain the development of Black English. One of the most popular of these theories is the *creolist* theory. Briefly stated, the creolist position holds that Black English is a complex hybrid involving several African languages and four main European languages—Portugese, Dutch, French, and English. These hybrids are believed to have

TABLE 3.1

Selected Phonological and Grammatical Characteristics of Black English (B), Southern English (S), Southern White Nonstandard English (SWNS), and Appalachian English (A). (Drawn from R. Williams and W. Wolfram, *Social Dialects: Differences vs. Disorders.* Washington, D.C.: American Speech and Hearing Association, 1977. Used by permission.)

Features	Descriptions	Examples	B	S	SWNS	A
Consonant cluster reduction (General)	Deletion of second of two conso-nants in word final position belong-ing to same base word	tes (test)	X		X	
	Addition of past tense (-ed) mor-pheme to a base word, resulting in a consonant cluster reduction	rub (rubbed)	X		X	
	Plural formations of reduced conso-nant cluster; assume phonetic repre-sentations of sibilants and affricatives	desses (desks)	X		X	
/θ/ phoneme	/f/ for /θ/ between vowels and in word final position	nofin (nothing) Ruf (Ruth)	X			
/ð/ phoneme	/d/ for /ð/ in word initial position	dis (this)	X			
	/v/ for /ð/ between vowels and in word final positions	bavin (bathing) bave (bathe)	X			
Future tense forms	Use of "gonna"	She gonna go (She is going to go)	X		X	
	"Gonna" reduced to 'ngna, 'mana, 'mon and 'ma	I'ngma go I'mana go I'mon go I'ma go (I am going to go)	X			
Double modals	Cooccurence of selected modals such as "might," "could," "should"	It liketa scared me to death (It almost scared me to death)	X		X	X
Intensifying adverbs	Use of intensifiers, i.e., "right," "plumb," to refer to completeness	right large (very large)	X		X	X
Negation	"Ain't" for "have/has," "am/are," "didn't"	He ain't go home (He didn't go home)	X			
Relative clauses	Deletion of relative pronouns	That's the dog bit me (That's the dog that bit me)	X		X	X
Questions	Same interrogative form for direct and indirect questions	I wonder was she walking? (I wonder if she was walking)	X		X	X

developed in Africa, as well as on American plantations, in the form of pidgins and creoles.

According to DeCamp (1971), pidgin languages develop when peoples speaking different languages come in contact with each other and have a need to find a common language, usually for commerce. Typically, a pidgin is developed by speakers of a nondominant cultural group who are in direct contact with a dominant group which speaks another language. Good examples include the pidgins still used by many Chinese and Hawaiians. At the outset of its development, a pidgin language may be very informal, consisting of single words, a simplified grammar, and many gestures.

Over time, pidgin languages may become more formal, in that vocabulary items selected primarily from the dominant language are embedded into a phonological and grammatical system derived from the nondominant language. When this happens and the pidgin is accepted as a native language, the language is referred to as **creole** language. Eventually, as the speakers of creole languages become more assimilated into the dominant culture, creole languages tend to move toward the standard language, through an intermediate stage referred to as *decreolization.*

There are some problems with the creole theory of Black English. For instance, it tends to view the language as being European-based rather than African-based. Despite its problems, however, the creolist explanation of Black English at least provides a historical orientation for the analysis and understanding of Black American speech.

Several researchers dispute the validity of the concept of Black English on other grounds. Some of their objections are based on the argument that it is impossible to assume that a single variety of speech accurately describes a population as culturally and geographically diverse as American Blacks. Still others reject the notion of Black English on the grounds that it only describes the speech of the working classes, while implicitly denying the existence of more educated forms of speech spoken by the Black middle class. Finally, writers such as Smitherman (1978), Labov (1972), and Kochmann (1971) argue that focus on the study of the structure of language, rather than on use of language as a communication tool, has prevented scholars from appreciating the richness of Black communication behavior. Oral traditions, for instance, such as proverbs, rhetorical style, and verbal contests are totally ignored by the formal structured analyses of contemporary linguistics.

Taylor (in press) is among a small group of scholars who have attempted to define Black English so as to account for the language and communicative behaviors of the full range of Black people in the United States. In this model, Black English is defined as the totality of speech spoken by Blacks in the United States, ranging from the standard (Standard Black English) to the nonstandard (Nonstandard Black English). Taylor's model is broad enough to take the situation or context into account, as well as the rules pertaining to language structure and to language use in the sense of interpersonal interaction.

English Influenced by Other Languages

Obviously, Black English is not the only social dialect of English used in the United States. Any cultural group's acquisition of a new language is influenced by the linguistic characteristics of that group's native language. Because there are people in the United States from so many different backgrounds, it is impossible to identify and describe all the varieties of English which have been influenced by other languages. On the other hand, these native languages typically *interfere* with the speaking of English when they do not contain elements which are part of English, or when the elements take a different form in the native language. For example, we are all familiar with the stereotype of the Oriental who cannot produce the English /r/ and so substitutes the /l/ instead.

Examples of language interference are commonly found in the United States among Hispanic, Native American, Pan Asian, French Cajan, Gullan, Hawaiian, and Virgin Islands populations. In all cases, the linguistic processes

TABLE 3.2
Examples of Spanish Interference on English Phonology.

Features	Environments	Examples
/c/ phoneme	/š/ for /č/ in all positions	share (chair); wash (watch)
/z/ phoneme	/s/ for /z/ in all positions	sip (zip); racer (razor)
/ŋ/ phoneme	/n/ for /ŋ/ in the word final position	sin (siŋ)
/v/ phoneme	/b/ for /v/ in all positions	bat (vat); rabbel (ravel)
/θ/ phoneme	/t/ or /s/ for /θ/ in all positions	tin or sin (thin)
/ð/ phoneme	/d/ for /ð/ in all positions	den (then); ladder (lather)
/ɪ/ phoneme	/iy/ for /ɪ/ in all positions	cheap (chip)

TABLE 3.3
Examples of Spanish Interference on English Syntax.

Features	Environments	Examples
Forms of "to be"	Absent in present progressive	He getting hungry (He is getting hungry)
Pronouns	Absent as subjects of sentences when subject obvious from preceding sentence.	"Carol left yesterday. I think is coming back tomorrow" (Carol left yesterday. I think she is coming back tomorrow.)
Third person (-s)	Absent in third person verb agreements	He talk fast (He talks fast)
Past (-ed)	Absent in past tense inflections	He walk fast yesterday (He walked fast yesterday)
"Go" with "to"	Future markings	He go to see the game tomorrow (He is going to see the game tomorrow)
"No" for "don't"	Imperatives	No do that (Don't do that)
"The" for possessive pronoun	With body parts	I hurt the finger (I hurt my finger)
Present tense markings	Progressive environments	I think he come soon (I think he is coming soon)
Locative adverbs	Placed near verb	I think he putting down the rifle (I think he is putting the rifle down)

underlying the variations are identical, the only differences being related to the actual languages involved, and the social, political, and economic histories of the speakers.

The largest group in the United States today with native language interference with English consists of people from Spanish-speaking backgrounds (including both Mexican Spanish and Puerto Rican Spanish). Tables 3.2 and 3.3 present some examples of how Spanish can interfere with English phonology and syntax respectively.

LANGUAGE DIFFERENCES AND COMMUNICATION DISORDERS

The question now is "how does a knowledge of language differences contribute to the practice of speech-language pathology?" Some possible answers to this question are discussed below.

Attitudes

Perhaps the most important recent contribution of sociolinguistics to the field of communication disorders has to do with attitudes toward language variation. The literature clearly suggests that speech-language pathologists must view language variety as a normal phenomenon, and not necessarily as an indication of a communication problem. This is a critical prerequisite for providing clinical services that fit the language codes and expectations of clients, their parents, and their communities.

Definitions

Another important recent contribution of sociolinguistics to the professional practice in communication disorders has to do with defining disordered communication. A sociocultural perspective toward communication disorders argues that all communication—normal or disordered—can only be defined, studied, or discussed in a cultural context. Since disordered communication is defined as a deviation from the norm, that norm has to be culturally based. In a large Black community, for example, the standards against which individual communication behaviors are evaluated must obviously include rules of Black communication in order to be valid. Of course, some biologically Black persons communicate according to the rules of some other community, usually the non-Black community that is economically, politically, or socially dominant.

There is also some evidence that societies have different values for defining minimally proficient (or normal) communication and, more importantly, what to do about conditions of abnormal communication. In some societies, for example, mild deviations in communication behavior may hardly be considered cause for alarm in the context of other priorities. Indeed, they might even be considered assets.

Our point here is that societies may have different criteria for determining when a difference makes a difference and what to do if one exists. Some feel that little or nothing should be done about a communication disorder except to keep it hidden from the public, because these disorders are perceived as acts of gods or demons. Unfortunately, there has been little research reported on what different societies consider disordered communication and what to do about it, especially in Third World countries. In the absence of data, the resourceful speech-language pathologist can, nonetheless, use imaginative interviewing techniques to determine definitions of communication disorder from clients, parents, family, or other members of the home community.

Testing and Diagnosis

Because there are varying communication rules among different cultural groups, your examination and diagnosis of a person with a communication disorder is much more likely to be effective if you use instruments, interpersonal interaction, testing, and interpretation of findings which are consistent with the communication rules of the group from which the person comes. For this reason, effective testing and diagnostic work is directly related to sensitivity to and use of culturally relevant materials and clinical orientations.

To begin with, speech-language pathologists rely heavily on standardized tests to determine the presence or absence of communication disorders. Most tests currently used in speech-language pathology are based on Northern Midland Standard English. For this reason, many of these tests, when administered and scored according to the prescribed norms, yield results which unfairly penalize speakers of nonmainstream dialects. They give the inaccurate impression of communication disorder when, in fact, no pathology exists.

Auditory perception is the process of identifying a sensory stimulus without necessarily attaching meaning to that stimulus.

An excellent example of the cultural bias in communication tests may be found in many tests of auditory perception. This process is believed to be a prerequisite for the normal decoding of auditory messages. For example, a task of discrimination might require a child to tell you whether the following two nonsense syllables sound alike or different: "id" /ɪd/ and "ed" /ed/. The expected answer for a standard English listener, of course, is "different." We know, however, that people tend to perceive incoming sounds according to the phonological rules of their native language. Thus, if the /ɪ/ speaker is not familiar with the /ɪ/ phoneme, although he does know the /e/ phoneme, he

This might be the case for a Chicana, since there is no /ɪ/ in Spanish.

may report the word pair as "same" instead of "different." This problem is particularly apparent when speakers of nonstandard English dialects are tested for their auditory discrimination abilities in standard English. In many cases, more errors than normal are recorded; therefore, the speech-language pathologist might inaccurately conclude that a child or adult is 1 to 2 years behind in auditory perceptual function when, in fact, there is actually no delay. Several recent researchers (e.g., Seymour & Seymour, 1977) have shown that, when cultural and sociolinguistic factors are taken into account in designing and administering language tasks, there are no statistically significant differences among cultural groups.

Taylor (in press) is among those authors who have discussed in some detail sociolinguistic dimensions in standardized tests. Drawing upon his work with researchers in several related disciplines, he lists seven distinct sources of possible bias in tests.

(1) Social situational bias—Violation of a situation/context rule for the test taker
(2) Value bias—Mismatch between values assumed in test items and the values of the test taker
(3) Phonological bias—Mismatch between phonological rules assumed in a test item and the phonological rules of the test taker
(4) Grammatical bias—Mismatch between grammatical rules assumed in a test item and the grammatical rules of the test taker
(5) Vocabulary bias—Mismatch between words and their use between test maker and test taker (may include underlying cognitive mismatches)

(6) Pragmatic bias—Mismatch between rules of communication interaction between test maker and test taker
(7) Directions/format bias—Confusions or misunderstandings created for test taker by the use of unfamiliar or ambiguous directions and/or test formats

In interpreting assessment data and diagnosing communication disorders, there is some evidence that, since different cultural communities define communication pathology differently, the speech-language pathologist must use this information. Let us take the case of stuttering to illustrate this point.

Leith and Mims (1975) note a sharp difference in stuttering patterns between Blacks and Whites. Whites, they report, show a strong tendency for what they call "Type I" stuttering, which is characterized by overt (audible) repetitions and prolongations with a moderate number of overt secondary characteristics, such as word phrase repetitions and accelerated speaking rates. Blacks, in contrast, show a strong tendency for "Type II" stuttering, which is characterized by more covert (nonaudible) prolongations and repetitions and a large number of relatively severe secondary characteristics, including total avoidance of speech. Black stutterers, like all Type II stutterers, often appear to have either a mild handicap or no handicap whatsoever, although they appear tense and anxious. That is, the Type II stutterer works very hard to appear not to stutter.

Leith and Mims (1975) argue that Blacks engage in Type II stuttering far more than Whites because, as pointed out by sociolinguists such as Mitchell (1969) and Kochman (1970), the Black culture in the United States places a high premium on oral proficiency and on being under control. Indeed, a substantial part of the Black male self-concept is built around proficiency in oral skills like ritual insults, rapping, and verbal routines with girls, and around being "cool," so as to always appear to be in control and never ruffled. Obviously, stuttering runs counter to these social values; therefore, the Black stutterer would naturally do everything possible to mask stuttering and the way it makes him feel.

A related problem deals with the child who appears to have delayed language development. The speech-language pathologist must determine whether the child has a true language disorder/learning disability or has mastered the rules for a nonstandard dialect and is simply missing some rules for Standard English. Being familiar with the child's native speech community is the first step in the assessment process.

Clinical Management

In the actual delivery of therapy and education, the speech-language pathologist can also apply sociocultural principles of language and communication. This area is only beginning to receive attention by researchers in communication disorders. However, significant changes in traditional approaches are beginning to appear.

First, the interpersonal dimension is a vital component of any type of effective clinical management of a communication disorder. For this reason, differences in the verbal and nonverbal rules used by the speech-language pathologist and the client can cause unintended episodes of insult, discomfort, or hypersensitivity, which could negatively affect the interpersonal dynamics needed for effective clinical work (Adler, 1973; Taylor, 1978).

Second, knowledge of developmental patterns of a particular language or dialect can help the professional determine differences between developmental variations and pathological deviations, the appropriate time to begin speech or language therapy for pathological features, and the course of therapy once it has started.

Seymour and Seymour (1977) have developed one of the few models for providing therapy for speech or language disorders which take language variation into account. Using Black English as their point of departure, the Seymours argue that, since many of the features of so-called Standard English and Black English Vernacular in the United States overlap, therapy goals for Black English-speaking children should fit with educational goals and social expectations. Therefore, their model is constructed so that particular linguistic features of both Black English Vernacular and Standard English are modified. The model recognizes the possibility of pathological deviations from both vernacular and the Standard English and that true linguistic competency in the culture probably requires people to be proficient in both systems.

Language Education

In some professional settings, the speech-language pathologist needs to instruct speakers of nonstandard dialects in Standard English. This is in addition to the usual professional responsibility of providing therapy for people with communication disorders. In these instances, the pathologist must keep in mind that teaching a second dialect is *not* the same as correcting a disorder. In teaching a second dialect, the goal is to establish a parallel linguistic form to stand alongside an already existing legitimate form for use in certain situations. In correcting a disorder, the goal is to eradicate unacceptable linguistic forms in favor of those which are considered "normal."

Feigenbaum (1970) is one of the major writers on the subject of second dialect instruction. Using principles from Teaching English to Speakers of Other Languages (TESOL), Feigenbaum has outlined a part "audiolingual" or "pattern practice" approach to teaching Standard English as a second dialect. The components of the program involve the following steps:

(1) Presentation of explicit examples of the two dialects, highlighting distinguishing characteristics.
(2) Discrimination drills between the two dialects, requiring the learner to determine sameness and difference between pairs of utterances.
(3) Identification drills which require the learner to properly categorize utterances as being from one dialect or the other.
(4) Translation drills requiring the learner to translate utterances presented in one dialect into the opposite dialect, that is, standard to nonstandard to standard.
(5) Response drills in which the learners respond, in quasispontaneous situations, to a stimulus presented in one dialect with a response consistent with that dialect or, eventually, with a response inconsistent with that language.

Unfortunately, the decision of whether to teach English as a second language, or Standard English as a second dialect, is not always clear-cut. It is one thing to determine, for instance, that a child from a Chinese family does not have the /r/ phoneme in his phonology or that a Chicano child does not have the /i/, but it is quite another thing to determine what, if anything, should be done about these dialects educationally, who should do it, and when it should be done. Some professionals and community leaders feel that community dialects should be perceived as culturally adequate and that children should be "left alone" to use the language of their home speech communities (the "No Intervention" view). Others, while respecting and preserving community dialects, feel that all children should also master the prevalent dialect, that is, Standard English, at least as a tool, so that they can use it in those situations where it is either expected or required (the "Bidialectal" view). A few even hold the counterproductive view that community dialects have little value and should, therefore be eradicated and replaced with Standard English (the "Eradication" view). This rather controversial issue is not likely to be resolved in the near future. The speech-language pathologist who deals with children from any minority group—be they Blacks, Hispanics, Orientals, Hawaiians, whatever—must be sensitive to these questions and, again, provide services to individuals in the context of the family or community expectations, the state of the art in educational linguistics, sociolinguistics, and the law.

The issue of teaching Standard English to speakers of nonstandard dialects of English, notably Black English Vernacular, has recently taken on legal ramifications. In 1977, a group of parents in Ann Arbor, Michigan, filed a suit in Federal Court, on behalf of 15 Black preschool and elementary children, charging that teachers in a local school had failed to adequately take into account the children's home dialects in the teaching of the language arts. Among their charges, the parents claimed that the teachers were not sufficiently knowledgeable about these dialects and, as a result, did not fully appreciate their intrinsic worth and usefulness in the educational environment. In several cases, children of the plaintiffs had been inappropriately enrolled in speech programs to "correct" their home dialects. The judge in the case concurred with the parents and ordered the Ann Arbor School Board to develop an educational plan which, among other things, would educate the teachers in the students' dialects and in how knowledge and value of the dialects can be used constructively in the language arts curriculum.

The Ann Arbor case places many of the issues pertaining to dialects and education into perspective. First, the fact that the parents sued to force the school to teach Standard English while preserving the home dialects corroborates data from several studies on parents' language attitudes and aspirations. Second, the arguments on behalf of the plaintiffs clearly support the bidialectal posture toward language education for nonstandard-English-speaking children. Throughout the trial, the plaintiffs' parents reiterated their belief that their right to equal protection of the laws, guaranteed by the 14th Amendment to the U.S. Constitution, requires schools to teach students Standard English, but not at the expense of eradicating or disrespecting home and community languages and dialects. Third, the plaintiffs' lawyers attacked the inappropriate placement in speech therapy of students who only demonstrate differences, not disorders, in language and communications. Fourth, the judge's ruling in this case suggests that professionals who offer language instruction to nonstandard speakers must be properly trained in the area of language variables and in applying that training to language arts education. Training of this type may be secured in disciplines such as sociolinguistics and bilingual education. Of course, the speech-language pathologist who assumes this role should remember that his or her function is that of a teacher and not of a therapist. First and foremost, the language professional must keep in mind that *different does not mean disordered.*

See, for instance, Taylor, 1973.

P.L. 94-142 also prohibits inappropriate placement into speech therapy and the use of discriminatory tests to make such placements. Because some children with language differences may, in addition, have communication disorders, the speech-language pathologist must be able to clearly distinguish between dialect and disorder.

SELECTED READINGS

Bell, R. T. *Sociolinguistics: Goals, approaches and problems.* London: B. T. Batsford, 1976.

Feigenbaum, I. The use of Nonstandard English in teaching standard: Contrast and comparison. In R. W. Fasold & R. W. Shuy (Eds.), *Teaching Standard English in the inner city.* Washington, D.C.: Center for Applied Linguistics, 1970.

Hymes, D. *Foundations of sociolinguistics: An ethnographic approach.* Philadelphia: University of Pennsylvania Press, 1974.

Seymour, H. N., & Seymour, C. M. A therapeutic model for communicative disorders among children who speak Black English Vernacular. *Journal of Speech and Hearing Disorders,* 1977, *42*(2), 247–256.

Taylor, O. L. Toward a definition of Black English. In C. Gibson (Ed.), *The black child,* in press.

Wolfram, W., & Fasold, R. W. *The study of social dialects in American English.* Englewood Cliffs, N.J.: Prentice-Hall, 1974.

REFERENCES

Adlam, D. S. *Code in context.* London: Routledge & Kegan Paul, 1977.

Adler, S. The reliability and validity of test data from culturally different children. *Journal of Learning Disabilities,* 1973, *6*(7), 429–434.

Allen, H. B., & Underwood, G. N. *Readings in America dialectology.* New York: Appleton-Century-Crofts, 1971.

Anastasiow, N. J., & Hanes, M. L. *Language patterns of poverty children.* Springfield, Ill.: Charles C Thomas, 1976.

Bee, H. L., Van Egeren, L. F., Strissguth, A. P., Nyman, B. A., & Leckie, M. S. Social class differences in maternal teaching strategies and speech patterns. *Developmental Psychology,* 1969, *1*, 726.

Bell, R. T. *Sociolinguistics: Goals, approaches and problems.* London: B. T. Batsford, 1976.

Bernstein, B. Socialization: With some reference to educability. In B. Bernstein (Ed.), *Class, codes and control: Theoretical studies towards a sociology of language.* London: Routledge & Kegan Paul, 1971.

Brandis, W., & Henderson, D. *Social class, language and communication.* Beverly Hills, Calif.: Sage Publications, 1970.

Bruner, J. Learning the mother tongue. *Human Nature,* 1978, September, 42–49.

DeCamp, D. The study of pidgin and creole languages. In D. Hymes (Ed.), *Pidginization and creolization of language.* London: Cambridge University Press, 1971.

Dillard, J. L. *Black English.* New York: Random House, 1972.

Edwards, A. D. *Language in culture and class.* London: Heinemann Educational Books, 1976.

Ervin-Tripp, S. Wait for me, roller skate! In S. Ervin-Tripp & C. Mitchell-Kernan (Eds.), *Child discourse.* New York: Academic Press, 1977.

Feigenbaum, I. The use of Nonstandard English in teaching standard: Contrast and comparison. In R. W. Fasold & R. W. Shuy (Eds.), *Teaching Standard English in the inner city.* Washington, D.C.: Center for Applied Linguistics, 1970.

Ferguson, C. Baby talk in six languages. *American Anthropologist,* 1964, *66*, 103–114.

Gleason, J. B. Code switching in children's language. In T. E. Moore (Ed.), *Cognitive development and the acquisition of language.* New York: Academic Press, 1973.

Greenberg, J. H. Language universals. In T. Sebeok (Ed.), *Current trends in linguistics: Theoretical foundations* (Vol. 3). Hawthorne, N.Y.: Mouton, 1966.

Gumperz, J. J., & Hymes, D. (Eds.). *Directions in sociolinguistics: The ethnography of communication.* New York: Holt, Rinehart & Winston, 1972.

Hollingshead, A. B. *Two factor index of social position.* Cambridge: Yale University Press, 1965.

Hymes, D. *Foundations of sociolinguistics: An ethnographic approach.* Philadelphia: University of Pennsylvania Press, 1974.

Kochman, T. Toward an ethnography of Black American speech behavior. In N. E. Witten & J. F. Szweo (Eds.), *Afro-American anthropology.* New York: Free Press, 1970.

Kochman, T. *Rappin and stylin out in the Black community.* Champaign: University of Illinois Press, 1971.

Labov, W. Rules for ritual insults. In D. Sudnow (Ed.), *Studies in social interaction.* New York: Free Press, 1972.

Lawton, D. *Social class, language, and education.* London: Routledge & Kegan Paul, 1968.

Leith, W. R., & Mims, H. A. Cultural influences in the development and treatment of stuttering. A preliminary report on the Black stutterer. *Journal of Speech and Hearing Research,* 1975, *40*(4), 459–466.

Loman, B. *Conversations in a Negro American dialect.* Washington, D.C.: Center for Applied Linguistics, 1967.

McCormack, W. C., & Wurm, S. A. (Eds.). *Language and man: Anthropological issues.* The Hague: Mouton, 1976.

Mitchell, C. *Language behavior and the Black urban community.* Unpublished doctoral dissertation, University of California, Berkeley, 1969.

Mitchell-Kernan, C., & Kernan, K. T. Pragmatics of directive choice among children. In S. Ervin-Tripp & C. Mitchell-Kernan (Eds.), *Child discourse.* New York: Academic Press, 1977.

Moerk, E. L. Changes in verbal child-mother interaction with increasing language skills of the child. *Journal of Psycholinguistic Research,* 1974, *3*, 101–116.

Newport, E. L. Motherese: The speech of mothers to young children. In N. J. Castellan, D. B. Pisoni, & G. R. Potts (Eds.), *Cognitive theory* (Vol. 2). Hillsdale, N.J.: Lawrence Erlbaum, 1976.

Nist, J. *A structural history of English.* New York: St. Martin's Press, 1966.

Rosch, E. Style variables in referential language: A study of social class difference and its effect on dyadic communication. In R. O. Freedle (Ed.), *Advances in discourse processes.* Norwood, N.J.: Ablex, 1979.

Seymour, H. N., & Seymour, C. M. A therapeutic model for communicative disorders among children who speak Black English Vernacular. *Journal of Speech and Hearing Disorders,* 1977, *42*(2), 247–256.

Shatz, M., & Gelman, R. The development of communication skills: Modification in the speech of young children as a function of the listener. *Monographs of the Society for Research in Child Development,* 1973, *38*(5, Serial No. 152).

Smitherman, G. *Talkin' and testifyin': The language of Black Americans.* Boston: Houghton Mifflin, 1978.

Snow, C. Mothers' speech to children learning language. *Child Development,* 1972, *43*, 549–565.

Snow, C., Arlman-Rupp, A., Hassing, Y., Jobse, J., Jootsen, J., & Vorster, J. Mother's speech in three social classes. *Journal of Psycholinguistic Research,* 1976, *5,* 1–20.

Taylor, O. L. Teachers' attitudes toward Black and Nonstandard English as measured by the Language Attitude Scale. In R. Shery & R. Fasold (Eds.), *Language attitudes: Current trends and prospects.* Washington, D.C.: Georgetown University Press, 1973.

Taylor, O. L. Language issues and testing. *Journal of Non-white Concerns,* 1978, *6*(3), 125–133.

Taylor, O. L. Toward a definition of Black English. In C. Gibson, *The black child,* in press.

Trudgill, P. *Sociolinguistics: An introduction.* New York: Penguin Books, 1974.

Wardhaugh, R. *The contexts of language.* Rowley: Newbury House, 1976.

Williams, F. (Ed.). *Language and poverty.* Chicago: Markham, 1970.

Williams, R., & Wolfram, W. *Social dialects: Differences vs. disorders.* Washington, D.C.: American Speech and Hearing Association, 1977.

Wolfram, W., & Fasold, R. W. *The study of social dialects in American English.* Englewood Cliffs, N.J.: Prentice-Hall, 1974.

ANATOMY AND PHYSIOLOGY OF SPEECH 4

Willard R. Zemlin

The phone rings, you pick it up, and say "Hello!" Between the thought and the spoken message lies a complex chain of events. To produce the sound /helo/, you use a whole series of nerves, muscles, and body organs.

Our task in this chapter is to explore how intact human beings speak. We will examine the processes by which dormant air in the lungs is transformed into the meaningful sequence of sounds we call *speech.* This information about the anatomy and physiology of normal speech will serve as a basis for the evaluation of people with disordered speech. In many cases, a speech-language pathologist is called upon to determine whether a speech problem has a physical basis or not. In other cases, the professional must predict to what extent a child or adult can overcome a physical problem or whether a different set of skills for coping with the resultant language problem is in order. In dealing with victims of strokes, with children with articulation problems, with infants born with cleft palates, with students with cerebral palsy (the list goes on), you will need to understand the process by which we speak.

But one note of caution is in order. In the human vocal organs, as in all human characteristics, there is a broad range of "normal." We will look at "typical" characteristics, but in practice you may see a wide span, just as adults from 5 feet to 7 feet can be called "normal" in height.

To begin, let's look at an overview of the organs we use in speech. Then we can move on to more depth in each system. The highly integrated and incredibly complex structures of speech production are confined primarily to the head, neck, and trunk. The *trunk* (or torso) is by definition the body, except for its free extremities (arms, legs, and head). It is divided into an upper **thorax** and a lower portion, the **abdomen,** which are separated by an important partition called the **diaphragm.** The diaphragm is the principle muscle of inhalation.

The structures illustrated in Figure 4.1 constitute the human vocal organs. They include the lungs-diaphragm-thorax complex, the **larynx,** and the vocal tract. The vocal tract can be broken down into a number of components which will be described later. For the present, we can think of the vocal tract as consisting of the throat or **pharynx,** the mouth or oral cavity, and the nasal cavities.

FIGURE 4.1
The Human Vocal Organs.

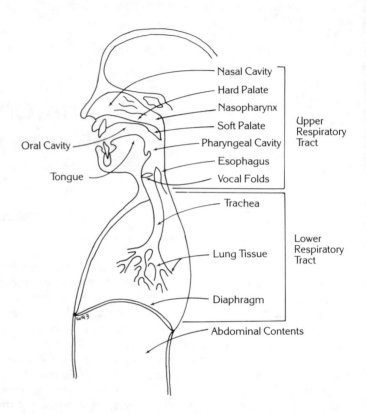

Nasal Cavity
Hard Palate
Nasopharynx
Soft Palate ⎤ Upper Respiratory Tract
Oral Cavity
Pharyngeal Cavity
Esophagus
Tongue
Vocal Folds

Trachea

Lung Tissue ⎤ Lower Respiratory Tract

Diaphragm

Abdominal Contents

Air, which is drawn into the lungs during inspiration, is placed under a modest amount of pressure in the expiratory phase of **respiration.** Appropriate adjustments of the internal larynx result in vibrations of the vocal folds, and that vibration transforms the dormant pressurized air in the lungs into a fairly regular series of air pulses during **phonation.** These quasiperiodic pulses, in turn, excite the air column within the vocal tract. This air column resonates for a very short time with each pulse of the larynx to produce a **glottal** or laryngeal **tone.** The process is somewhat like generating a short tone in a long-necked bottle by rapping the palm of your hand over its mouth. The difference is that the larynx generates such a rapidly occurring series of short-duration tones that each successive excitation begins before its predecessor has died away. As a result we hear what seems to be a sustained tone.

Changes in the shape and length of the vocal tract are mediated primarily by tongue, jaw, and lip movement in the process of **articulation.** These changes affect the resonance properties of the vocal tract, and we perceive the acoustical results as various meaningful sounds, in particular the vowels. Constrictions along the vocal tract may cause turbulent sounds to be generated, or the outward air flow may even be momentarily halted, with a mild explosive release of impounded air, to produce an entire category of sounds classified as consonants. The vocal folds may or may not be vibrating during consonant production, and so we recognize voiced and unvoiced consonants. Vowels, of course, must always be voiced (except in a whisper).

Disorders of articulation are discussed in the next chapter.

Since we are talking animals, the respiratory, phonatory, and articulatory structures shown in our model play dual roles for us—biological and nonbiological or biosocial. From a purely biological viewpoint, the body is little more than a complex array of pumps, valves, and levers that function quite automatically to sustain life. One of the remarkable features of speech production is that many of the biological roles of the respiratory, pharyngeal, and articulatory structures can be at least temporarily relinquished and "reassigned" a social or biosocial role. For example, highly specialized chemoreceptors which are located in the large arteries of the thorax and neck are sensitive to the relative concentrations of carbon dioxide and oxygen in the blood, and they automatically trigger the respiratory muscles to become active whenever an imbalance occurs. This accounts for our very regular and rhythmical breathing patterns when we are sleeping or quietly reading. Speech, however, is a conscious act. When the occasion arises, the roles of the respiratory, phonatory, and articulatory structures are suddenly transformed into elaborate and effective voluntary sequences of motor acts, and the biological functions, in a very real sense, assume a secondary role.

We must acknowledge, then, the contributions of the nervous system, especially as they relate to voluntary motor acts which result in speech. We can construct a model of the act of speech, incorporating the nervous system. Of paramount importance in this model is the role of various feedback avenues which permit an on-going monitoring of muscle contractions and the sounds produced as a consequence of muscle activity. One almost obvious feedback channel is provided by our sense of hearing. *It is very difficult to say something in the way you intend it to be said, without hearing what is being said, while it is being said.*

The communication problems of people with hearing disorders are covered in chapter 10.

Our tasks for the remainder of the chapter are clear-cut: to examine the anatomy of the vocal and related organs, to learn under what circumstances they become active, and to specify the acoustical consequences of their activity. Bear in mind that our descriptions are highly idealized ones and that the delicate chain in our model can be broken at any link, and sometimes more than one.

RESPIRATION

Aside from having something to say, the first requisite for speaking is a supply of pressurized air, which means we should begin by exploring the breathing mechanism and the respiratory process, in breathing to live and to produce speech.

See chapters 12 and 13 for discussions of problems resulting from faulty respiration.

The **respiratory tract** begins at the mouth and nose openings and terminates deep within the lungs. As illustrated in Figure 4.1, the larynx, pharynx, and oral and nasal cavities comprise the upper respiratory tract. These same structures are associated with phonation and articulation, so we will begin with the lower respiratory tract, the skeletal framework for which is shown in Figure 4.2. Its major components include the vertebral column, the ribs and sternum or breastbone, and the bony components of the *pelvis*. The seven cervical (neck) vertebrae provide attachments for postural muscles, in addition to supporting the head. The 12 thoracic vertebrae also provide attachments for postural muscles, in addition to important contributions to the rib cage. Twelve pairs of ribs attach to the thoracic vertebrae behind, while 10 pairs attach to the sternum in front. The lowest two pairs have no attachments in front and are called floating ribs. The five lumbar vertebrae support the upper part of the body and provide attachments for a complex array of postural muscles.

FIGURE 4.2
Skeletal Framework of the Lower Respiratory Tract and of the Torso.

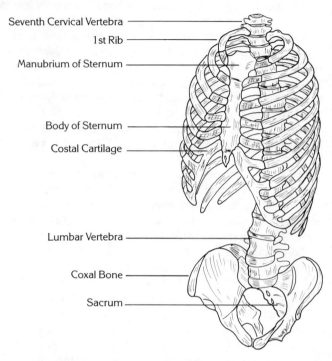

Seventh Cervical Vertebra

1st Rib

Manubrium of Sternum

Body of Sternum

Costal Cartilage

Lumbar Vertebra

Coxal Bone

Sacrum

The lowest part of the vertebral column consists of a single structure, the sacrum. It is actually composed of five vertebrae which become fused very early in life. The sacrum, together with the coxal bones, make up the pelvis. One of its functions is to act as a basin for the abdominal organs.

The Bronchial Tree and Lungs

Remember, the thorax is the part of the trunk above the diaphragm.

The thorax is largely occupied by the cone-shaped lungs. Between them, in a space called the *mediastinum,* lie the heart, esophagus, and great blood vessels. The heart has the vitally important role of pumping blood to the lungs, where it gives up its carbon dioxide and takes on a fresh supply of oxygen. The heart also receives oxygen-poor blood from the body through the veins, and delivers oxygen-rich blood by means of the arteries. The biological role of the lungs, then, is to extract carbon dioxide from the blood and to supply it with oxygen for bodily needs.

The larynx and part of the "bronchial tree" are shown in Figure 4.3a, and the bronchial tree in relation to the lungs is shown in Figure 4.3b. The trachea is composed of about 16 to 20 imperfect rings of **cartilage** which divide (*bifurcate*), giving rise to two main-stem **bronchi.** They in turn divide into smaller secondary or lobar bronchi which supply the lobes in the lungs (three in the right and two in the left lung). The 10 right-lung and 8 left-lung segments are supplied by the next division, which gives rise to the tertiary (third stage) bronchi. These divisions continue for about 20 more generations, until finally the passageway verges on the microscopic.

The smallest of the tubules leading to the depths of the lung are known as **bronchioles.** The terminal bronchioles open into alveolar ducts, which are characterized by numerous (about 300,000,000 in each lung) minute pits

FIGURE 4.3

(a) The Larynx and Bronchial Tree. (b) Bronchial Tree in Relation to the Lungs.

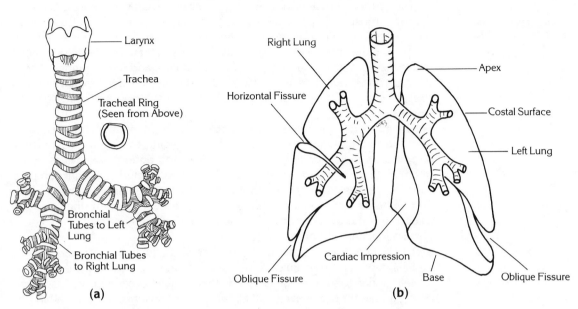

called **alveoli.** It is here that the actual gas exchange takes place between the blood and oxygen-rich air in the lungs. The combined surface area of the alveoli amounts to about 70 m^2, an area equal to that of a tennis court. Lung tissue is usually described as spongy and highly elastic. The elasticity is due to a framework of fibro-elastic tissue, which supports the respiratory structures, and to the properties of the alveoli, which are responsible for about ⅔ of lung elasticity. Each alveolus is lined by a layer of secretory tissue, only a single cell thick. Because of the universal attraction of molecules for one another at the surface between liquid and air, the alveoli tend to collapse, and it is the combined force of all the alveoli which makes the lungs so resistant to expansion. The lungs are prevented from collapsing, however, because of the **pleural membranes.**

Each lung is closely covered by a visceral pleural membrane, while the thorax is lined by a similar costal pleural membrane. It is tightly adherent to the inner walls of the thoracic cavity and to the surface of the diaphragm. These membranes are moist, which means the lungs can move freely in the thorax, and the rich network of pleural capillaries tends to absorb gases and fluids. This absorption results in a powerful negative pressure between the two pleural membranes, and this pressure links the costal and visceral membranes together with a force so great that the lungs cannot pull away from the thoracic walls, no matter how deeply we might inhale. Thus, when the diaphragm descends, and the dimensions of the rib cage increase, the lungs are literally forced into expanding.

When we are not talking, we breathe quietly about 12 times a minute, for the principal purpose of aerating the blood stream and cleansing it of carbon dioxide. The mechanics of air exchange during quiet breathing can be stated quite simply. Through contraction of the thoracic muscles, the depth, width, and height of the chest cavity are increased. Since the lungs are bound to the thoracic confines by virtue of the pleural membranes, they too must expand.

Atmospheric pressure
is the pressure of the
atmosphere, approxi-
mately 14.7 lbs/sq in
at sea level.

An increase in the size of the lungs creates a slight negative pressure within the bronchial tree and the pulmonary alveoli. With the airway open, about 500 to 750 cm^3 of air rushes into the lungs, until the alveolar pressure is the same as the atmospheric pressure. At the same time, the abdominal organs are compressed by the descending diaphragm, intra-abdominal pressure is elevated, and the anterior abdominal wall distends slightly. The muscles of inhalation then cease to contract somewhat gradually; and the expanded thorax-lung complex rebounds, usually without the assistance of any expiratory muscles, to create a slight positive pressure within the lungs. The result—the air rushes out.

Quiet breathing requires muscle activity during inspiration, but the expiratory forces are purely passive. As expiration begins, the *highly* elastic lungs contract as rapidly as the rebounding chest and abdominal cavities permit them to do so, and so the air within the lungs is subjected to a slight compression. Air rushes out of the lungs until once again alveolar pressure becomes the same as atmospheric. During each cycle of respiration, then, alveolar pressure is the same as atmospheric at the beginning of inspiration, end of inspiration, and end of expiration.

The biomechanics of breathing for speech production or for singing are a radical departure from quiet or vegetative breathing, and they are not completely understood. One difference is that in quiet breathing the inspiratory and expiratory phases each last about 2.5 seconds; but when breathing for speech, a short 2- or 3-second inspiration may be followed by as much as a 15-second expiration phase (while we are talking). Another difference is that when breathing for life purposes, the entire respiratory tract is open and air flow is relatively resistance-free; but when breathing for speech production, the expiratory air flow is met with resistance by the vocal folds located within

The articulators are
discussed and illus-
trated in chapter 2.

the larynx, by the articulators, or both. The pressurized air requirements for speech production place complex demands on the lower respiratory tract, and its associated muscles; but for most of us it all happens unconsciously.

Before we can proceed to the process of breathing for speech, we should briefly examine the muscles responsible for air exchange.

The Respiratory Muscles

The muscles responsible for increasing and decreasing thoracic dimensions are shown in Figure 4.4. Although there are about 100 muscles in the human torso (all paired except the diaphragm), only a small number contribute directly to the respiratory process. Muscles in general function as a power source in various types of lever systems, and they are described as having an origin, course, and insertion. The **origin** is usually the less mobile of the attachments, while the insertion is the structure acted upon. A joint (the fulcrum in the lever) typically lies between the origin and insertion.

The most important of the inspiratory muscles is the diaphragm. It alone can account for most of the thoracic expansion necessary for quiet breathing, and yet complete paralysis of the diaphragm does not handicap a person very much, so great is the compensatory potential of muscles which otherwise play virtually no role in breathing. The peripherally located muscular portion of the diaphragm arises from the lower margin of the rib cage and from the lumbar part of the vertebral column. These muscle fibers course upward and inward to insert into a tough broad sheet of central **tendon,** fibers of which are continuous with the fibrous pericardium that encases the heart. When the muscular portion contracts, the entire diaphragm moves downward and

FIGURE 4.4

Schematic of the Respiratory Muscles. (a) The Diaphragm in Relationship to the Rib Cage and the Vertebral Column. (b) The Costal Elevators, Posterior Serratus, Superior and Inferior Muscles. (c) The Intercostal Muscles of the Rib Cage and the Superficial-Most Abdominal Muscles.

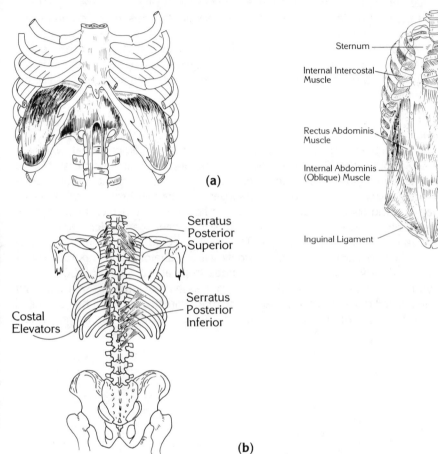

(a)

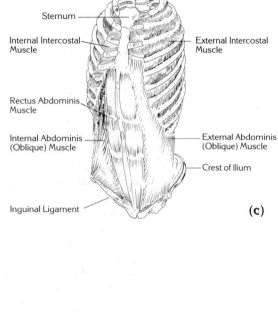

Rib No. 1

Sternum

Internal Intercostal Muscle

External Intercostal Muscle

Rectus Abdominis Muscle

Internal Abdominis (Oblique) Muscle

External Abdominis (Oblique) Muscle

Crest of Ilium

Inguinal Ligament

(c)

Serratus Posterior Superior

Serratus Posterior Inferior

Costal Elevators

(b)

somewhat forward, compressing the abdominal organs, and at the same time distending the lungs vertically. When we breathe deeply (yawning for example), the limits of compressibility of the abdomen may be approached, and the lower rib cage will actually be elevated and expanded by the contracting diaphragm.

Other muscles of the rib cage include the internal and external intercostals. As the name implies, they are located between the ribs. The internal intercostal muscles are well developed in front but poorly developed in back. The opposite is true for the external intercostal muscles, which are very well developed on either side of the vertebral column. The course of the internal intercostals is down and outward in front. Since the thorax is somewhat circular, the course is down and inward behind, *but* the muscles fail to continue to the vertebral column. The external intercostals also course down and outward, next to the vertebral column, and in front course down and toward the midline; but these muscles fail to continue as far as the union of the ribs. This means contraction of the intercostal musculature will exert an upward force on the ribs. Because of the complex geometry of the ribs, however, upward rotation not only increases the side-to-side diameter of the rib cage, but its front-to-back diameter as well.

Twelve stout slips of muscle, the levatores costarum (costal elevators), arise from the vertebral column, course down and outward, in much the same manner as the external intercostal muscles, with which they are continuous. As their name implies, these muscles elevate the ribs, complementing the intercostal muscles.

A powerful group of neck muscles, the scalenes, attach to the cervical vertebrae above and to the upper two ribs below. When they contract, on one side or the other, the head is tilted to the side, but when acting bilaterally they help elevate the rib cage.

Basic Respiratory Physiology

A person breathing quietly exchanges about 500 to 750 cm^3 of air with each respiratory cycle. This air is called *tidal air,* and the quantity is **tidal volume.** Other lung volumes and capacities are recognized, and most of them can be measured with a wet **spirometer.** As a person breathes through a mouthpiece, air is withdrawn from and returned to a floating drum, which rises and falls accordingly. The drum is coupled to a recording pen which registers the quantity of air exchanged in cm^3. The graphic recording is called a *spirogram,* and the example in Figure 4.5 is largely self-explanatory. One important measurement is **vital capacity,** which ranges from about 3500 to 5000 cm^3 in young adult males, and about 1000 cm^3 less in adult females. Another measure, called **residual volume,** cannot be made directly, but must be computed. It is the *air remaining in the lungs after a maximum expiration,* and it

Vital capacity is simply the maximum quantity of air exhaled after a maximum inhalation.

FIGURE 4.5
Schematic Spirogram.

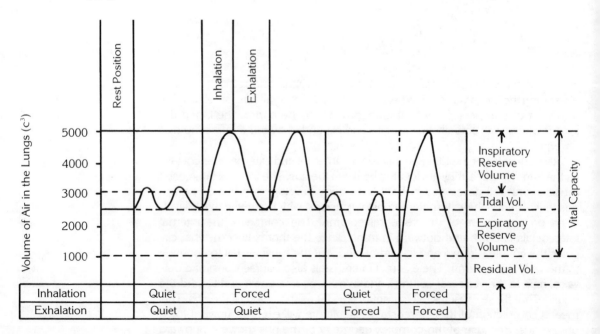

amounts to about 1000 to 1500 cm^3 in young, healthy lungs. In old age, residual volume can double. A short explanation as to why residual air remains in the lungs may provide some insight into the very fundamentals of respiratory physiology.

At birth, a baby's lungs are disproportionately large, but they are nevertheless bound to the thoracic walls by pleural linkage. At the end of a quiet exhalation, an infant's lungs are virtually empty of residual air. Growth of the thorax far exceeds that of the lungs, however; with increasing age, the lungs, linked to the thoracic walls, are placed under increased stretch, until finally, even after a maximum expiratory effort, they are still distended to the extent that almost ¼ of total lung capacity remains. With increased inspiratory efforts, the lungs are placed under even greater stretch and their inherent elasticity *tends* to pull the lungs away from the thoracic walls. Pleural linkage is so powerful, however, that the lungs simply cannot pull away. The lungs cannot assert their inherent elasticity until the rebounding thorax permits them to do so. And this extremely important point brings us to breathing for speech.

Speech Breathing

The amount of air remaining in the lungs after a passive exhalation amounts to about 38% of the vital capacity. At that lung volume, the inward pull of the lungs is opposed by the chest wall by an equal amount, so the lung-thorax unit is at equilibrium. By contracting abdominal muscles, our expiratory reserve can be completely exhaled, until only residual air remains. A simple experiment will illustrate the significance of thorax-lung recoil. A water **manometer** can be constructed from a bent glass tube with water in it, connected at the bottom to a short length of rubber tubing. If you inhale maximally (100% vital capacity) and then completely relax and breathe into the tube, the elastic recoil of the thorax-lung complex will generate enough air pressure to raise the column of water over 50 cm. At 80% vital capacity, the elastic recoil will raise the column about 30 cm; at 38% nothing happens; and at 0% vital capacity, the recoil of the thorax is outward, while the lungs pull inward. About 30 cm of negative pressure is generated, and the water backs up the tube toward you.

Usually we inhale about 70% of our vital capacity prior to speaking. The **"relaxation pressure"** amounts to about 20 cm of water pressure. The pressure requirements of the larynx, it turns out, are very modest, only 5 to 10 cm of water pressure. This means that, even without any muscle contraction, the relaxation pressure exceeds the requirements of the larynx by 10 to 15 cm of water pressure. In other words, there is easily enough outward pressure to produce speech. The excessive relaxation pressure is defeated by the partial sustained contraction of the inspiratory muscles during the speech act, which simply prevents the thorax from recoiling too rapidly. At about 55% vital capacity, the inspiratory muscles cease to contract. If we are to maintain adequate breath pressure, the expiratory muscles will be called into play, with a gradual increase in their activity as we encroach on the expiratory reserve volume. The result of all of this is that we can maintain an amazingly constant breath pressure throughout the entire lung volume range. During loud speech, or in singing, the breath pressure requirements may be as high as 20 cm of water pressure. In that event, the inspiratory muscles need not counteract excessive relaxation pressure.

THE LARYNX AND PHONATION

Anterior means toward the front, as contrasted with posterior, toward the back.

That is, if you start to inhale food, you cough.

The highly vulnerable lower respiratory tract is well protected by the larynx, a complex structure which is located in the **anterior** neck on a level with cervical vertebrea 3 through 6. The larynx is extremely sensitive to irritation. The vocal folds contained in it close, by a powerful **reflex,** to prevent the intrusion of foreign substances which might otherwise be accidently inhaled (while eating, for instance). This is usually accompanied by a reflexive contraction of the expiratory muscles to forcefully expel the invading material. If, after a moderately deep inhalation, the vocal folds are tightly closed, the air in the lungs is pressurized, as we have seen, which acts to stabilize the rib cage. Contraction of the abdominal muscles stabilizes it even more. Since abdominal pressure is also elevated, "thoracic-fixation" facilitates heavy lifting as well as those functions which demand high abdominal pressure (such as bowel and bladder evacuation and childbirth).

Dealing with people who have had their larynx removed is covered in chapter 6.

Besides its vitally important biological functions, the larynx also serves as the principal source of sound for speech. Approximated (tightened) vocal folds offer resistance to the outward flow of air; and because of the elastic recoil of the lung-thorax complex, pulmonary air is placed under pressure. When the pressure is sufficient, the resistance offered by the vocal folds is overcome, and they are literally blown apart to release a strong puff of air into the vocal tract. The vocal folds quickly snap together, only to be blown apart once more. This series of events occurs about 250 times each second for an adult female, and about 130 times per second for an adult male. The vibration rate determines the fundamental frequency or what we perceive as the **pitch** of the voice. The vocal folds must comply with basic laws of physics; and each of us, depending upon structural size, length, and muscular tension, has a particular range of natural frequency of vibration. There is an optimum frequency of vibration for each of us, and it is here our larynx operates most efficiently. This is why we ought to make the optimum frequency habitual.

Chapter 6 also discusses problems people have in controlling loudness, pitch, and other voice characteristics.

The loudness and pitch of the voice can be varied, of course, over a wide range, depending upon the force with which the vocal folds are approximated (which influences the air pressure requirements by the larynx) and the degree to which they are stretched.

No matter how we view the larynx—as a magnificently versatile musical instrument, or as an effective source of sound for speech production—from a mechanical standpoint it is not much more than a variable resistance to air flow. Perhaps we can liberate the larynx from this unglamorous description by becoming better acquainted with it.

Anatomy of the Larynx

See Figure 4.6.

The human larynx is an extremely variable structure from person to person, so much so that only a generalized picture can be presented here. Descriptions of the skeletal framework of the larynx often begin with the hyoid bone, even though it is not a laryngeal structure. It forms the point of attachment for a number of muscles of the tongue and neck, but it is nevertheless instrumental in maintaining the larynx in its proper position. The hyoid bone consists of a body and two major and two minor horns. The larynx is said to be "suspended" from it, which is partly true.

The laryngeal skeleton per se is composed of cartilage that does, however, become bone-like with age. The major cartilages are the ring-like cricoid, the shield-like thyroid, the flexible Delphian epiglottis, and the paired arytenoids.

FIGURE 4.6
*The Skeletal Framework of the Larynx—An "Exploded" View from the Front,
from Behind, and from the Side.*

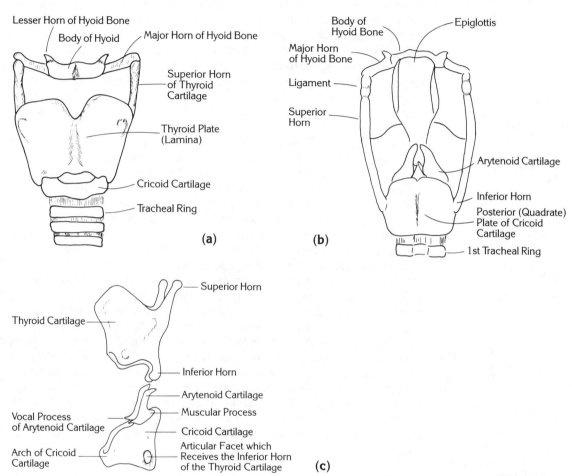

The cricoid cartilage surmounts the uppermost **tracheal** ring and is securely fastened to it by connective tissue. This almost circular cartilage has the shape of a truncated cylinder, with a narrow arch in front and a rectangular plate or lamina behind. Two pairs of important articular facets are found on this cartilage. Facets at the side accommodate the inferior horns of the thyroid cartilage, while the sharply convex and elliptical facets on the upper rim of the **posterior** plate receive the muscular processes of the arytenoid cartilage. These facets slope downward and laterally by about 40°.

*The **trachea** is the tube which extends from the larynx to the bronchi.*

The arytenoid cartilages, which are **tetrahedral** in shape, are each capped by a small cone-shaped corniculate cartilage. Each artenoid cartilage has a vocal process which projects into the larynx, and a muscular process laterally, the underside of which has a concave articular facet on it. It fits onto the convex elliptical facet on the cricoid, and the architecture of this cricoarytenoid joint has an important bearing on the movements of the arytenoid cartilages. When a downward force is exerted on the muscular process, the arytenoid cartilage rotates around the long axis of the cricoid articular facet. Thus the vocal process (to which the vocal **ligament** and muscular vocal fold are

A tetrahedron is a solid contained by four triangular planes, a triangular pyramid.

attached) swings outward and upward. When a forward force is exerted on the musuclar process, the vocal process rotates inward and downward. The cricoarytenoid joint also permits a certain amount of upward-inward, or outward-downward gliding action, but a very strong posterior cricoarytenoid ligament imposes constraints on the extent of movement. Rotation and gliding actions are the mechanisms by which the vocal processes (and vocal folds) are approximated at the midline (**adducted**) and separated (**abducted.**)

A single muscle, the posterior cricoarytenoid, abducts the vocal folds. It arises from the greater part of the posterior cricoid plate, and its fibers converge to insert on the muscular process of the arytenoid cartilage. A fairly substantial muscle, it acts to pull downward and back on the muscular process, causing the arytenoid cartilage to rotate on the long axis of the cricoarytenoid joint. This swings the vocal ligament and vocal folds upward and away from the midline. Usually, when breathing quietly, the space between the vocal folds, or *rima glottidis* (or simply, the **glottis**), remains fairly static; but when breathing deeply, the glottis suddenly dilates to reduce the effects of air friction, an action mediated by the posterior cricoarytenoid muscle.

See Figure 4.7.

Two muscles, the lateral cricoarytenoid and the interarytenoids, act in opposition to the abductor. The lateral cricoarytenoid is a small slip of muscle arising along the upper rim of the cricoid cartilage, just in front of the muscular process into which it inserts. When acting alone, it simply swings the vocal process downward and toward the midline. The vocal ligaments and vocal

See Figure 4.8.

folds attached to the thyroid cartilage, on either side of the midline in the front. When rotation occurs at the cricothyroid joint, they are subjected to varying degrees of tension, the principal mechanism by which voice pitch is regulated.

A single muscle, the cricothyroid, acts on the cricothyroid joint. Arising along the arch of the cricoid, the fibers fan out somewhat to insert along the lower border of the thyroid cartilage and on the inferior thyroid horn. Its action, illustrated in Figure 4.9, is to reduce the distance, in front, between the cricoid and thyroid cartilages. This action *increases* the distance between the vocal processes of the arytenoids behind and the thyroid angle in front. This in turn increases the tension of the vocal folds, and consequently the pitch of the voice is raised.

FIGURE 4.7

Abductor and Adductor Muscles of the Larynx.

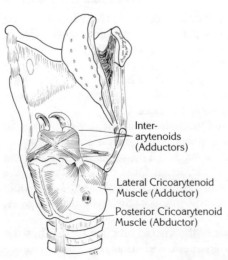

Inter-
arytenoids
(Adductors)

Lateral Cricoarytenoid
Muscle (Adductor)

Posterior Cricoarytenoid
Muscle (Abductor)

FIGURE 4.8
Rotational Movement at the Cricothyroid Joint.

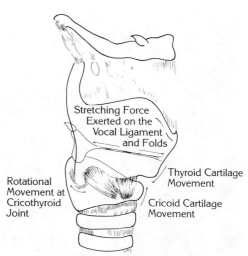

The action of the cricothyroid muscle is opposed by the thyroarytenoid muscle. It constitutes the muscular portion of the vocal fold. This muscle arises along most of the extent of the thyroid angle in front and courses back toward the arytenoid cartilage, to insert along the entire base. Many anatomists regard this muscle as being composed of two functionally separate parts. The **medial**-most portion (adjacent to the vocal ligament) is called the vocalis muscle. It is the vibrating part we can see when the larynx is examined by a mirror placed in the back of the throat. The lateral portion of the thyroarytenoid muscle is usually called the thyromuscularis. There is no anatomical basis for this division, but the thyroarytenoid does seem to be capable of segmental contraction, so a functional division seems justified.

Medial means toward the axis or midline.

See Figure 4.10.

FIGURE 4.9
Action of the Cricothyroid and Thyroarytenoid Muscles.

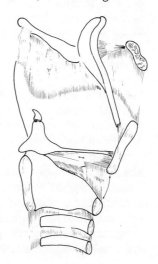

FIGURE 4.10

The Larynx as Seen in Indirect Laryngoscopy.

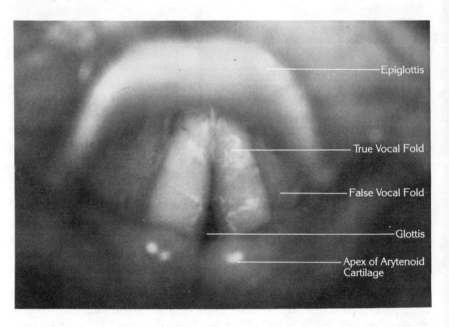

Epiglottis

True Vocal Fold

False Vocal Fold

Glottis

Apex of Arytenoid Cartilage

Basic laws of vibrating strings (vocal folds are sometimes called *cords*) tell us that an increase in tension will increase the frequency of vibration and thus pitch, as anyone who has tuned a stringed instrument well knows. The vibrating portion of the vocal folds can be relaxed to lower the pitch of the voice by relatively unopposed contraction of the thyromuscularis portion. Normally the vocal folds vibrate with quite precise regularity, but they are subject to inflammation, tumors and other neoplasms, abuse from tobacco and industrial smoke, and a host of insulting factors; and then the voice can become weak, rough, or just downright unpleasant.

See chapter 6 on voice disorders.

Increased tension of the vocal folds, then, results in a higher rate of vibration, but increased tension also demands an increase in subglottal pressure in order to maintain vibration. Here is where we begin to see the subtle and delicate interplay between the respiratory and phonatory mechanisms. (Just imagine the complexity of the interaction when the articulators enter the picture!)

Subglottal refers to below the glottis.

The loudness of the voice is controlled primarily by the force with which the vocal folds are approximated at the midline. Heightened activity of the lateral cricoarytenoid and interarytenoid muscles results in forceful adduction, and that *demands* an increase in subglottal pressure. But, in this instance, the pressurized air which forces the folds apart delivers a more powerful burst of air into the vocal tract. The larynx is also capable of sound production without vocal fold vibration. In the production of a *whisper,* the glottis assumes the shape of a more-or-less thin slit, and sometimes the vocal processes are toed inward so the glottis looks like the letter Y. Sustained production of a vowel at conversational pitch and loudness requires an air expenditure of about 125 cm^3/sec, while whispering requires over 300 cm^3/sec.

We have been describing the role of **intrinsic** laryngeal muscles, those which are confined to the larynx proper. Three **extrinsic** muscles also act on the larynx. These muscles, which have one attachment outside the larynx, include the sternothyroid, the thyrohyoid, and inferior pharyngeal constrictor muscles. The exact consequences of their action are only partly understood, but they influence the position of the larynx and help stabilize it.

Laryngeal Physiology

From our description of the larynx, we have learned that the vocal folds can be brought together at the midline with varying degress of force and can be placed under varying degress of stretch. Approximation of the vocal folds is often called *medial compression,* while the stretching force (which may or may not elongate the folds) is called *longitudinal tension.* Various combinations of the two, plus a *variable pressurized* air supply, account for the incredible versatility of the voice.

During quiet breathing, the vocal folds are relatively motionless and a triangular chink is formed by their leading edges. This opening between the free margins of the vocal folds is called the *rima glottidis,* or simply the *glottis.* The glottis is extremely variable in its configuration and dimensions, and as a consequence is capable of offering varying degrees of resistance to the outward flow of pressurized air from the lungs.

See Figure 4.11a.

During forced inhalation, something we do just prior to speaking, the vocal folds are widely separated, and so the larynx offers little resistance to the *inward* flow of air. As phonation begins, however, the vocal folds are brought very quickly *towards* the midline, so they offer a certain degree of resistance to the *outward* flow of pressurized air, when the forces of exhalation are released. The extent of resistance is highly variable, of course, depending upon the degree of medial compression and longitudinal tension. Medial compression is due to the relative activity of the adductors, while longitudinal tension is brought about by the **antagonistic** action of the cricothyroid and the muscles of the vocal folds.

See Figure 4.11b.

The adductors are the lateral cricoarytenoid and the interarytenoid muscles.

You may want to look back at Figure 4.9.

Now, as air pressure builds up beneath the vocal folds (subglottal pressure), it very quickly overcomes the laryngeal resistance. The folds are blown apart

The Bernoulli effect states that pressure

FIGURE 4.11
Glottal Configurations during Quiet Breathing and Forced Inhalation.

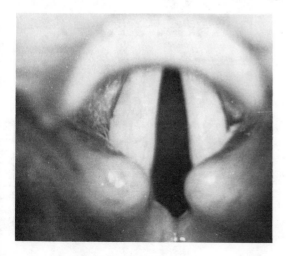
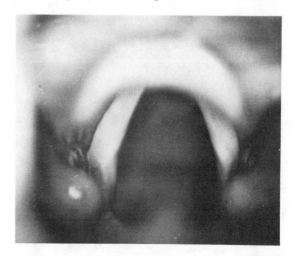

between the vocal folds (or any other constriction in the airway) results in a negative (sucking) pressure which becomes increasingly powerful as the velocity of air flow increases. A fairly complex phenomenon, it is covered in detail by introductory physics textbooks.

Adult female vocal folds are about 13 to 14 mm long; male vocal folds about 21 to 22 mm.

Figure 4.12 shows a subject in position for such a film.

to release a puff of compressed air into the *supraglottal* or *epiglottal* space. The quantity of compressed air which is released only amounts to 1 or 2 cm³, but nevertheless it results in a momentary drop in the pressure across the vocal folds (the transglottal pressure), and they snap back together. An aerodynamic phenomenon known as the *Bernoulli effect* contributes to the drawing of the vocal folds to the midline. The process of phonation, then, is primarily an aerodynamic phenomenon. This building up of subglottal air pressure and the blowing apart and snapping together of the vocal folds constitutes one complete cycle of vocal fold vibration. In adult females, this occurs about 200 to 260 times/sec; in adult males, who tend to have larger larynxes and longer vocal folds, the vibration rate is about 120 to 145 times/sec. During colloquial speech, however, when we might express surprise or delight or emphasize a point, the vibration rate (fundamental frequency of the voice) may exceed a range of two octaves for any given person. The fundamental frequency is the principal determinant of the pitch of the voice.

Ultrahigh speed motion pictures (4,000 frames/sec) have proven to be a valuable research technique in the study of the internal larynx during phonation. When the film is projected at the standard 16 frames/sec, we see a super slow-motion view of vocal fold vibration. A typical single cycle of vibration is described in terms of an opening phase, when the folds have been blown apart, a closing phase, when they are snapping back together again, and a closed phase, when the folds are fully approximated (or nearly so) and air pressure beneath them is once again building up. The relative durations of these three phases, and the magnitude of glottal area under various phonatory conditions, provide valuable insight into the mechanics of voice production. A single cycle of vocal folds vibration is shown in Figure 4.13, and a graph of glottal area as a function of time is shown in Figure 4.14.

FIGURE 4.12

A Laryngeal Physiology Laboratory. This photograph was taken through a sound-insulated booth which houses the (noisy) camera.

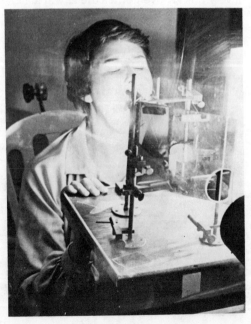

FIGURE 4.13

A Single Cycle of Vocal Fold Vibration, Photographed at 4,000 Frames/Sec. The vocal folds are together in the upper left frame, which represents the beginning of the cycle. They are maximally separated in the middle row of frames, and then begin to close, until in the frame in the lower right they are nearly completely approximated. The entire event, from closed through opening, and closing again, represents one complete cycle of vocal fold vibration and took about 1/140 sec.

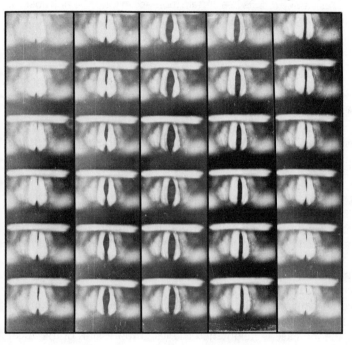

FIGURE 4.14

Fairly Representative Graph of Glottal Area as a Function of Time.

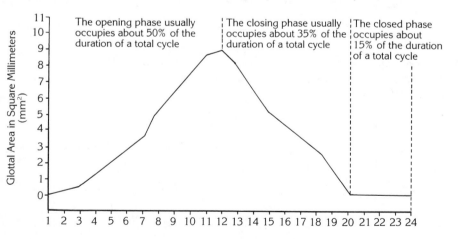

The Pitch-Changing Mechanism

We learned earlier that action of the cricothyroid muscle tends to elongate the vocal folds and to increase their longitudinal tension. Two factors account for the resistance to stretch that is offered by the vocal folds. One is the inherent elasticity of the vocal ligament and the vocal fold muscles, and we can identify it as inner passive resistance. The second is the inner active resistance, which is the result of contraction of the muscles of the vocal folds. An additional factor which influences the frequency of vocal fold vibration is their thickness, or mass, which decreases with increases in length.

When the vocal folds are placed under stretching force, they become thin, the inner passive resistance results in a certain increase in longitudinal tension, and the frequency of vibration (pitch) is raised. Inner passive resistance, however, cannot account for the full range of the human voice; the active resistance due to contraction of the vocal fold muscles further increases the longitudinal tension.

When the stretching force is removed from the vocal folds, their inherent elasticity tends to restore them to their original condition, and the pitch of the voice decreases. Furthermore, the muscles of the vocal folds contract without opposition (by the cricothyroid); they become shorter, somewhat flaccid, and the pitch drops further. The delicate interaction between the stretching force and the resistance (both active and passive) accounts in large part for the versatility of the human voice.

The Loudness Mechanism

See Figure 4.15.

The loudness of everyday speech is continuously changing, just as pitch is continously changing. If we examine ultrahigh speed films at high intensity (loud) phonation when compared to conversational intensity, the single difference is an increase in the duration of the closed phase. The glottis opens quickly, closes quickly, and then remains closed for a longer time than during phonation at conversational levels. In fact, the closed phase may occupy as much as 1/2 the total duration of an individual vibration cycle. The mechanism responsible for the increase is heightened medial compression of the vocal folds, and it is mediated by activity of the adductor muscles (lateral cricoarytenoid and interarytenoid). Increases in medial compression produce an increase in laryngeal resistance to air flow, and so once again the lung-thorax

FIGURE 4.15

Graph of Glottal Area as a Function of Time, Comparing Conversational to Loud Phonation. Note the substantial increase in the duration of the closed phase for loud phonation, an indication of the increase of the resistance to air flow at the laryngeal level.

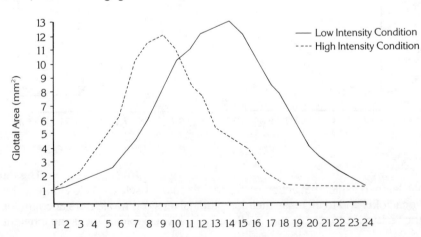

complex must compensate. During phonation at conversational levels, subglottal pressure requirements are modest, amounting to 2 to 4 cm of water pressure, while loud speech requires 10 to 15 cm of pressure. Each puff of air released by the vibrating vocal folds results in an increase in the "enthusiasm" of vibration of the air column of the supraglottal spaces (pharynx, oral, and at times, the nasal cavities).

To summarize, we have seen primarily that three factors influence the mode of vibration of the vocal folds. They are medial compression, longitudinal tension of the vocal folds, and subglottal air pressure. A number of additional factors can influence the behavior of the internal larynx. Many of them contribute to problems with the quality and pleasantness of the voice. The mass of one or both of the vocal folds may be modified by infections (laryngitis) or by growths on the folds (neoplasms); as a consequence the folds may vibrate irregularly (aperiodically), which imparts an unpleasant and rough quality to the voice. A loss of mobility at the joints of the laryngeal cartilages or loss of muscular strength may impose constraints on medial compression and longitudinal tension, so the pitch range is adversely affected. If the vocal folds fail to meet at the midline with sufficient force, they will offer inadequate resistance to air flow. A weak, breathy voice may result. A great many of these negative factors can be attributed to vocal abuse. Smoking, alcohol, polluted air, yelling in noisy environments are but a few of the abuses the larynx may be subjected to. And finally, the aging of the tissues of the speech mechanism will ultimately impose constraints on the ability of the elderly to communicate verbally as they once did. Proper care of our bodies, however, will often defer the aging effects for a long, long time.

ARTICULATION

As puffs of air are released into the vocal tract by the vibrating vocal fold, the dormant air column above the larynx is driven to produce a complex sound called the *glottal* or *laryngeal tone.* The lowest frequency component in this tone is numerically the same as the vibration rate of the vocal folds. All of the remaining components have frequencies which are integral multiples of this lowest or fundamental frequency. The intensities of the higher frequency components fall off rather sharply, so that not much acoustic energy exists at frequencies above 3,000 Hz. This harmonically rich glottal tone is the raw material from which all of our vowels and many of our consonants are formed.

With the articulators and the vocal tract in a neutral configuration, the cross-section of this "acoustic tube" is fairly constant throughout its length. Because of the comparatively high resistance at the glottal end, the vocal tract behaves acoustically like a tube closed at one end and open at the other. When excited, the air column in closed-open tubes oscillates or vibrates (resonates) at a frequency which has a wavelength that is four times the length of the tube, and at odd-numbered multiples of this first frequency. For example, an adult male vocal tract is about 17.5 cm in length, so the first resonant frequency is one which has a wavelength (λ) four times the length, or 70 cm (or .70 m). From basic physics we learn that

*Hz stands for **hertz,** which is a unit expressing "cycles per second"; i.e. 3,000 Hz = 3,000 cycles/sec.*

$$f = \frac{V}{\lambda} = \frac{340 \text{ m/sec}}{.70 \text{ m}} = 485.7 \text{ hz}$$

The first resonant frequency of our male vocal tract is 485.7 Hz. The resonances in the vocal tract are commonly called **formants,** and their frequencies are called *formant frequencies*. The second formant frequencies (an odd-numbered multiple of the first) is about 1,457 Hz, while the third formant frequency is about 2,428 Hz.

When the harmonically rich glottal tone is fed into the frequency-selective vocal tract, frequency components which correspond to, or nearly correspond to, the formant frequencies are reformed while the other frequencies tend to dissipate. Sounds which emerge from the lips will have frequency regions which are reinforced by the natural formant frequencies of the vocal tract.

See Figure 4.16.

Changes in the length, or in the cross-sectional area along the vocal tract, result in changes in the frequencies of the various formants. Lip rounding, lowering or raising of the larynx, changes in tongue and jaw position, or any combination of these gestures will influence the formant frequencies of the vocal tract; and we hear different vowel sounds.

Our task now is to examine the mechanisms by which the various dimensions act and how, therefore, the acoustical properties of the vocal tract can be modified.

The Skeletal Framework of the Vocal Tract

The skull, which forms the skeletal framework for much of the vocal tract, is composed of 22 individual bones, all rigidly joined together except for the

FIGURE 4.16

Schematic Tracing of an X-Ray of a Person Producing a Neutral Vowel, Vocal Tract Response Characteristics, and Spectrum of Glottal Sound. The radiated vowel spectrum is shown at the top of the figure.

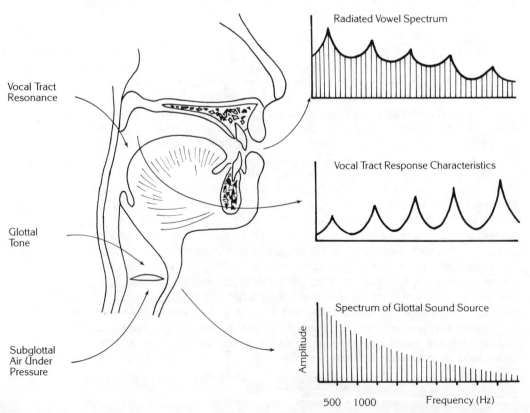

mandible. It articulates with the temporal bones by means of a complex "double-joint" that permits rotation, gliding, side-to-side movements, or various combinations of the three. The skull can be divided into two major parts: (*a*) the cranium (braincase), which houses and protects the brain, and (*b*) the facial skeleton, which forms the framework for the organs of mastication (teeth, jaws, and tongue), speech production (the articulators), and special senses (smell, vision, taste), and the muscles of facial expression. These two parts of the skull have entirely different growth patterns. The braincase, which triples in volume during the first 2 years, grows back and away from the geographic center of the skull and reaches 90% of its full size by the 10th year. The facial skeleton, which grows downward and forward, shows bursts of growth that are related to the times of eruption of the teeth, and it continues to grow until the middle or late teens.

*The **mandible** is the lower jaw.*

The results of these differential cranial and facial skeleton growth patterns can be seen in Figure 4.17.

Both the **maxillae** (upper jaws) and mandible (lower jaw) are characterized by an alveolar ridge or process, which is the bony housing for the teeth. The maxillary bones are very important contributors to the facial complex and to speech. Their horizontal processes meet at the midline to form the bony hard palate, which also forms the floor of the nasal cavities. The maxillae articulate with the temporal bone by way of the zygomatic bone and zygomatic arch, which together are sometimes called the *cheekbone.* In addition to forming points of articulation for the mandible, the temporal bone houses the hearing mechanism, and the mastoid and styloid processes are points of origin for some important muscles for speech production.

The skull rests on the first cervical vertebra (the Atlas), which together with the second (Axis) vertebra forms a complex joint that is responsible for the mobility of the head.

The Cavities and Associated Structures of the Vocal Tract

The cavities of the vocal tract form the resonant acoustic tube that is responsible for shaping the laryngeal tone into recognizable vowel sounds. In addi-

FIGURE 4.17
Skulls of an Adult and a Newborn. Note the difference in proportion of facial height and the braincase.

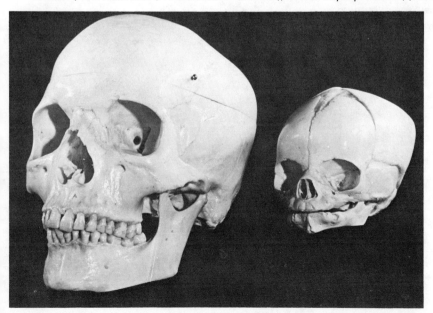

tion, when constrictions along its length cause air turbulence or momentarily halt air flow, consonants can be generated.

The small but variable space between the gums and teeth is called the *buccal cavity.* Its dimensions change when, for example, we round our lips for the production of the word *who.* A circular muscle, the orbicularis oris, surrounds the mouth opening and is largely responsible for the pursing of our lips. Additional muscles (of facial expression) which insert into the corners of the mouth influence the lips. The most superficial of the facial muscles, the platysma, is very active during speech production, but its actual contributions are poorly understood. It arises alongside the neck and inserts in part into the corner of the mouth. Beneath it can be found two important muscles of expression, the levator labii superior and depressor labii inferior, which elevate or depress the corners of the mouth. When acting together, they help compress the lips for production of the bilabial /p/ in *pop.* The deepest of the facial muscles is called the buccinator, which forms the muscular wall of the cheek. Because its fibers insert into the corner of the mouth, it is largely responsible for retracting the lips and assists in compressing them.

The oral cavity is bounded in front and on the sides by the teeth, gums, and alveolar bone and above by the hard and soft palates; the tongue forms

See Figure 4.18.

Thus the buccinator is referred to as the bugler's muscle.

FIGURE 4.18
Some Muscles of Facial Expression. The functions of muscles 1-12 are, briefly:
 1. *Frontalis wrinkles the forehead.*
 2. *Orbicularis oculi assists in closing the eye and in winking.*
 3. *Nasalis constricts the nostrils (twitches the nose).*
 4. *Levator labii superior elevates and everts the upper lip.*
 5. *Levator anguli oris elevates the corner of the mouth, as when sneering.*
 6. *Zygomatic major assists in elevating the corner of the mouth.*
 7. *Risorius retracts the angle of the mouth, and helps compress the lips.*
 8. *Orbicularis oris purses the lips in a sphincter-like action (puckers).*
 9. *Depressor anguli oris draws the corner of the mouth downward, as in pouting.*
10. *Depressor labii inferior draws the lower lip directly downward.*
11. *Mentalis wrinkles the chin, as in pouting.*
12. *Platysma helps retract the lips and compress them.*

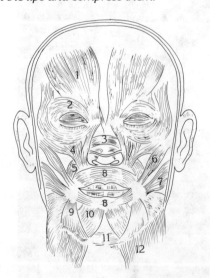

its muscular floor. The back of the oral cavity is set by the anterior fauces, behind which are the tonsils, especially in youngsters.

Figure 4.19 shows the parts of the oral cavity.

FIGURE 4.19
Schematic of an Oral Cavity.

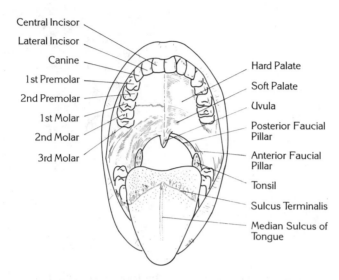

Central Incisor
Lateral Incisor
Canine
1st Premolar
2nd Premolar
1st Molar
2nd Molar
3rd Molar

Hard Palate
Soft Palate
Uvula
Posterior Faucial Pillar
Anterior Faucial Pillar
Tonsil
Sulcus Terminalis
Median Sulcus of Tongue

Dentition

The **deciduous** or temporary (baby) teeth develop very early in the embryo, and 20 of them (10 in each jaw) ultimately appear. The lower central incisors usually erupt first, followed shortly by the upper central incisors. The second molars, the last to appear, *usually* erupt by the end of the second year of life. Children begin to shed their deciduous teeth in their sixth year, and they are slowly replaced by permanent teeth. The shedding and eruption processes may continue into the early twenties, until the full equipped permanent dental arch has 16 teeth. The deciduous arch has no premolars (bicuspids) and no third molar, which explains the difference in numbers.

The set of teeth on one jaw is called the dental arch.

Aside from their obvious biological functions, the teeth play an important role in articulation, especially for the labiodental consonants /f/ and /v/ and the linguadental /θ/ and /ð/ sounds. The dentition also strongly influences facial growth throughout the developing years and facial balance all during life. The deciduous teeth are particularly important in contributing to the proper spacial relationships of the permanent teeth.

The configuration of the oral cavity is highly variable, more so than any other of the cavities of the vocal tract. Its ability to quickly and dramatically adjust for speech sound production can be largely attributed to the mobility of the tongue and jaw.

A tongue as seen from above is shown in Figure 4.20. Anatomically it is divided into a blade and root, with the **sulcus** limitans forming the boundary between the two. A shallow midline longitudinal groove runs the length of the blade, and the perimeter of the blade has numerous papillae which contain taste buds. They are specialized modifications of the epithelium. Beneath the epithelium is a tough layer of connective tissue called the lamina propria. It forms much of the skeleton for the tongue and its musculature. A vertically directed midline septum (partition) of connective tissue courses through the extent of the tongue; it also contributes substantially to its "skeleton." In

The epithelium is the tissue which lines the oral cavity and covers the tongue.

FIGURE 4.20
The Tongue as Seen from Above, Showing its Relationship to Some Adjacent Structures. (Drawing courtesy of Therese Zemlin.)

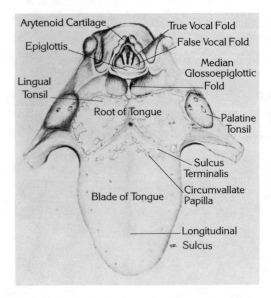

addition, toward the sides of the tongue on either side, the entering lingual artery-vein-hypoglossal nerve complex and its attending connective tissue form secondary septa, all of which increase the flexibility of the tongue.

Tongue Musculature

Changes in the shape of the tongue are often attributed to the intrinsic muscles, while the extrinsic muscles, which have an outside attachment, are said only to influence its position in the mouth. However, this construct is oversimplified and does not let you appreciate the intricate interrelationships of these muscles.

See Figure 4.21.

The superior longitudinal muscle is located just beneath the lamina propria of the dorsum. Its fibers extend from the hyoid bone to the tip of the tongue. Along the edges of the tongue, its fibers are interwoven with the longitudinally coursing fibers of extrinsic muscles (styloglossus and hyoglossus) and with fibers of the inferior longitudinal muscle. Its function is to shorten and assist in retraction. The inferior longitudinal muscle is located on the underside of the tongue at the sides. It is also interwoven with longitudinal fibers of extrinsic muscles, and its general function is to retract and depress the tip of the tongue. The transverse fibers originate from the lamina propria on one side of the tongue, traverse it, and insert into the lamina propria on the opposite side, fanning out somewhat as they approach the sides of the tongue. The verticalis fibers arise from the lamina propria of the dorsum and course vertically to insert into the connective tissue on the under surface. Its general function is to decrease the vertical dimensions of the tongue and at the same time to flatten it. When these four intrinsic muscles work with, or against, one another, an incredible number of shapes and tensions are possible. All in all, the intrinsic muscles are responsible (at least in part) for shortening, narrowing and elongating, elevating and depressing the tip, flattening and retracting, as well as pulling the tongue from side to side.

FIGURE 4.21
Schematic of Extrinsic Tongue Muscles.

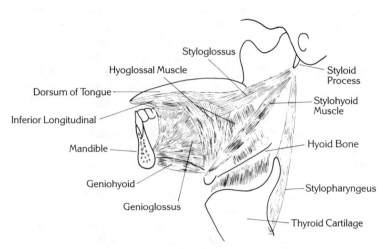

The extrinsic tongue muscles include the genioglossus, styloglossus, palatoglossus, and hyoglossus. The genioglossus arises from the inner surface of the mandible and radiates fan-like throughout the tongue, ultimately converging toward the tip. Some fibers attach to the hyoid bone and so can influence its position (and perhaps the larynx as well). The genioglossus comprises the bulk of the muscular core of the tongue. Probably its most important function is to protract the body of the tongue. The styloglossus arises from the base of the styloid process of the temporal bone as a slender slip which begins to radiate as it approaches the tongue, where its fibers interact with muscles at the side. Its principal function is to elevate the body of the tongue, an important gesture for such sounds as the /k/ and /g/. It also retracts the tongue. The fibers of the hyoglossus are found at the sides of the tongue. Although their course is initially vertical, from their origin at the body and greater horn of the hyoid bone, they turn to run longitudinally along with those of the styloglossus and the intrinsic longitudinal muscles. Its function is to depress the main body of the tongue. In doing so, it makes the back of the tongue convex. The palatoglossus muscle is a very slender slip which arises from the undersurface of the soft palate (to be described later). It inserts into the sides of the tongue, where the fibers interlock with transverse and longitudinal fibers. Although this is not really a tongue muscle, upon contraction it can either depress the soft palate (for production of nasal sounds such as the /m/, /n/, and /ŋ/), or it *may* influence the sides of the tongue to elevate them. Since the muscle forms a mechanical link between the soft palate and tongue, low tongue position seems to draw the velum downward along with it.

Mandibular Movement

The lips, teeth, tongue, and mandible are all structures associated with biting, tearing, grinding, and swallowing food, yet they serve us well for the subtle processes of speech production. Mandibular movement consists of opening-closing-gliding action. It is important because of the way the tongue is carried along with it, affecting the resonance properties of the vocal tract, and because this movement may be transmitted by way of the hyoid bone to the larynx.

*Figure 4.22 shows
these muscles.*

The muscles responsible for mandibular movement can be grouped functionally into elevators, depressors, and a single protractor. The elevators consist of the masseter, temporalis, and internal pterygoid muscles. The masseter is a powerful muscle, coursing from the zygomatic arch above to the angle of the mandible below. Its elevator action is complemented by the temporalis, a fan-shaped sheet of muscle which courses under the zygomatic arch to insert into the coronoid process of the mandible. It is not a very efficient muscle in humans, but it is responsible for the fast snapping action in meat-eating animals with long jaws. The third mandibular elevator, the internal pterygoid, arises from the base of the skull, just in front of and medial to the temporo-mandibular joint. Its fibers course downward and somewhat back to insert on the inner surface of the angle of the mandible.

Mandibular depression requires little in the way of power, but speed *is* important. Depression of the mandible requires that it be slipped a little forward in its articular capsule, a task that is accomplished by the external pterygoid. A stout muscle, it arises from the base of the skull in front of and medial to the condyle of the mandible, into which it inserts. Its action is to slide the condyle forward, on one side or the other, or both, which means it is responsible for protraction or the side-to-side grinding action that takes place when we chew our food.

FIGURE 4.22
Some Mandibular Muscles.

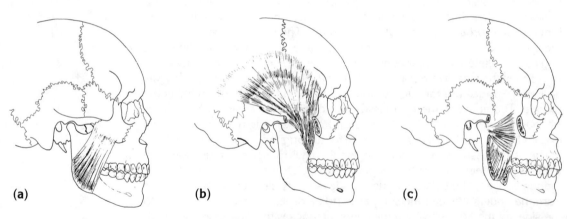

(a)   (b)   (c)

The roof of the oral cavity, formed primarily by the horizontal shelves of the maxillae, is covered by a tightly adherent connective tissue (mucoperiostium), which is thrown into a series of transverse ridges called rugae just behind the alveolar ridge. Rugae are thought to facilitate articulation for lingua-alveolar sounds such as /t/, /d/, the nasal /ŋ/ and the lateral /l/. Behind, the hard palate is continuous with the soft palate or **velum.**

The Soft Palate

*Speech problems
associated with cleft
palate are discussed
in chapter 11.*

The role of the soft palate is to couple or uncouple the nasal and pharyngeal cavities. When elevated, the soft palate acts as a valve and simply closes off the nasal cavity. This gesture is essential for the production of any consonant sound but especially for such plosives as /p/, /t/, and /k/. The soft palate can also be actively depressed for the /m/, /n/, and /ŋ/ sounds, and at times it is lowered for vowels adjacent to the nasal sounds. When that happens, the complex nasal cavities act as a secondary resonator and impart the quality we identify as nasality.

Four muscles act directly on the soft palate, two from above and two from below. The tensor palatini arises from the base of the skull and from the cartilaginous framework of the auditory tube. Its fibers wrap around a tiny hook-like extension of bone called the hamulus and from there insert into the palate as a thin tendinous sheet. Its function is to tense the soft palate. In doing so, it lowers the front part of it. The levator palatini is the muscle chiefly responsible for elevating the soft palate to establish velopharyngeal closure.

See Figure 4.23.

FIGURE 4.23

Schematic Representation of the Function of the Soft Palate (Velopharyngeal Muscles). The arrows indicate the approximate direction of their action and influence on the soft palate.

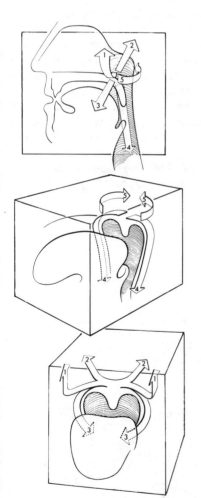

1. *Tensor palatini.*
2. *Levator palatini.*
3. *Palatoglossus.*
4. *Palatopharyngeus.*
5. *Superior pharyngeal constrictor.*

From Fritzell, "The Velopharyngeal Muscles in Speech," *Acta Oto-Laryngologica Supp.,* 1969, No. 250.
Used by permission.

It arises from the base of the skull and from the cartilaginous framework of the auditory tube. The palatoglossus was described with the extrinsic tongue musculature. The fibers of the palatoglossus arise from the substance of the soft palate and course vertically down toward the tongue, entering it at its sides where they blend with intrinsic muscle fibers. It is a very slender slip, comprising the muscular portion of the anterior faucial pillar. The significance of this muscle lies in the mechanical linkage it provides between the tongue and soft palate. This is one reason vowels formed with a low tongue position (such as /a/, /ɔ/) tend to be nasal when compared with the high tongue position vowels (/i/, /ɪ/). The palatopharyngeus also arises within the substance of the soft palate, but its vertically descending fibers blend with the muscles which form the upper part of the pharynx.

The Pharynx

See Figure 4.24.

The pharynx is essentially a muscular tube suspended from the base of the skull. Based on the relationship of its cavity to the cavities of the remainder of the vocal tract, the pharynx is divided into a nasopharynx, oropharynx, and laryngopharynx. It is largely connective tissue above, becoming increasingly muscular below, where its cavity is continuous with the larynx in front and the esophagus behind, and about the level of the sixth cervical vertebra. Its lowest fibers (the inferior pharyngeal constrictor) arise from the cricoid and thyroid cartilages and fan out somewhat as they course obliquely upward and toward the midline. The middle constrictor arises from the hyoid bone, while the superior constrictor fibers have a complex origin from the sides of the tongue, from the soft palate, and from the base of the skull. The superior constrictor is overlapped to some extent by the middle constrictor, and it in turn is over-

FIGURE 4-24

Schematic of the Pharynx as Seen from the Side. Note that the cervical vertebra and associated muscles are not shown.

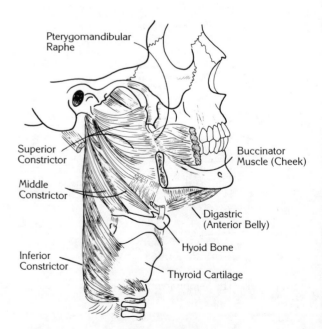

lapped by the inferior constrictor. This multilayered architecture gives the pharynx the strength required to initiate swallowing.

The principal contribution of the pharynx to speech production is as a resonator. It is not very dynamic as an articulator, and the changes which take place in the configuration of its cavity are mediated by tongue and jaw movement and by elevation and depression of the larynx. The upper portion (superior constrictor) is capable of dilating somewhat, however, due to some lesser muscles which enter from above and the side.

The least dynamic of the resonators are the nasal cavities, which are two narrow, somewhat symmetrical chambers, separated by a bony and cartilaginous (in front) nasal septum. The cavities communicate with the exterior by way of the nostrils (or nares) and with the nasopharynx by way of the choanae. The roof of the nasal cavities is formed by a very narrow plate of bone located between the orbits of the eyes, while the floor is formed by the same structures which comprise the roof of the oral cavity. The cavities are extremely complex in their overall configuration, which is attributable to the almost labyrinthine-like lateral walls. A superior, middle, and inferior nasal **concha** divides the air passageway into superior, middle, and interior **meatuses.** The conchae and septum are covered by a very vascular mucous membrane, which swells in response to very cold or dry air. Its function is to filter and bring inhaled air to body temperature during its brief passage into the nasopharynx, and it also functions as an extremely complex addition to the resonator system when the soft palate is lowered. Because of the elaborate mucous membrane lining and its complexity, the nasal cavities function as an energy-absorbing resonator which responds to sounds over a wide frequency range. These characteristics also contribute to nasality.

Look again at Figure 4.1 to see how the pharynx relates to the rest of the vocal tract.

*A **meatus** is an opening to a body passage.*

Articulatory Physiology

It is now time to put the anatomy lessons together and look at the overall picture. First, let us review a bit. We have seen that a steady state or unmodulated subglottal air supply can be placed under pressure by introducing air flow resistance when the forces of exhalation are released. We have also seen how resistance to outward air flow takes place at the laryngeal level to generate a glottal tone. We must realize that the vibrations of the vocal folds are not the source of those sounds we ultimately hear as speech. That is to say, whenever the vocal folds are blown apart by the elevated subglottal pressure, a short burst of pressurized air is released into the vocal tract. With the vocal folds vibrating at a rate of 150 times/sec, for example, a discrete burst of air is released into the vocal tract each 1/150 sec. The effect of these transient bursts of energy is to excite the dormant column of air above the larynx, and it vibrates for a short time. Although the amplitude of each vibration dies away quickly, the rapid succession of energy bursts serves to keep the air column vibrating. These short vibrations generated within the supraglottal air column constitute the glottal tone, and we have seen that it is rich in partials that are harmonically related to the fundamental frequency. We have also seen that the vocal tract, depending upon its configuration, is capable of resonating to or reinforcing some of the partials in the glottal tone. We might say that the glottal tone is shaped by the configuration, and therefore the acoustical properties of the vocal tract, to produce our voiced speech sounds. There are only three dimensions of the vocal tract which can be modified by the articulators: the overall length, the location of a constriction, and the degree of constriction.

Lip rounding, another variable, tends to increase the length of the vocal tract and at the same time impose a constriction on it.

Elevation and depression of the larynx has the effect of decreasing or increasing the length of the vocal tract, and the acoustic result is to lower or raise the frequencies of the resonances accordingly. Earlier we saw that the first three resonant frequencies of a male vocal tract 17.5 cm in length were about 485, 1,457, and 2,428 Hz. If the vocal tract were lengthened by just 2 cm, the resonant frequencies become 436, 1,308, and 2,179 Hz. As listeners, we could perceive that change easily.

The location and degree of constrictions in the vocal tract often determine whether the sound radiated at the mouth will be vowel-like or consonantal (turbulent or explosive). We should next examine the process by which vowels are formed from the glottal tone.

Vowel Production

For information on disorders of articulation, see the next chapter.

Each vowel in our language system is characterized by a unique energy distribution that is the consequence of the characteristic cross-sectional area and length of the vocal tract. Changes in the vocal tract are mediated by the articulators. For vowel production they are tongue, jaw, and lips, although the length can be modified by movements of the larynx and by lip protrusion and retraction. A tracing of an X-ray of a person producing a vowel with the vocal tract in a neutral configuration is shown in Figure 4.25. It also shows the intensity of an idealized glottal tone and the same tone after it has been shaped by the resonant characteristics of the vocal tract. The shape of the vocal tract during the production of an /i/ vowel is shown in Figure 4.26, along with the glottal tone, vocal tract response characteristics, and the radiated vowel after shaping. X-ray studies of speakers show that fairly predictable tongue positions can be associated with the individual vowel sounds. For example, a

See Figure 4.26.

See Figure 4.27.

vowel produced with the tongue high up and in front will be recognized as an /i/. If the tongue is moved to the opposite extreme of the oral cavity (low and back), it will probably be recognized as an /a/.

FIGURE 4-25

Vocal Tract in a Neutral Configuration and the Spectrum of the Sound Radiated at the Lips.

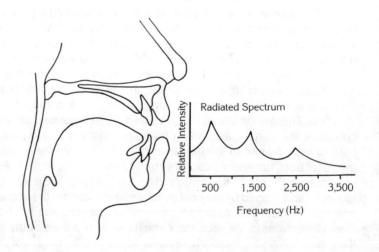

FIGURE 4-26

Vocal Tract in Configuration for Production of /i/ and the Spectrum of the Sound Radiated at the Lips.

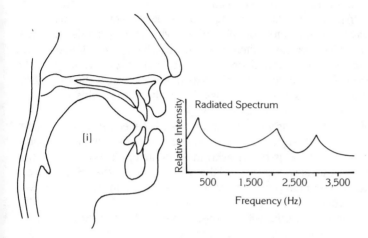

Eight vowel configurations which describe the extremes of tongue positions for their production have been recognized. All of the vowels we produce fall within the boundaries of these configurations. Vowels can also be classified according to tongue positions relative to the palate. For example, when the hump of the tongue is high and near the palate, the vowel produced is called a *close vowel;* when the hump of the tongue is low, pulled toward the bottom of the mouth, the vowel is called *open.* Vowels produced with the tongue near the center of the quadrilateral are called *central* or *neutral.*

Review Table 2.3 for the traditional vowel classification.

To round out our descriptive scheme, we also describe articulatory positions of the tongue as being either toward the front or toward the back of the oral cavity. The /i/ as in *need,* for example, is a *close-front* vowel, while /u/ as in *who* is a close-back vowel.

The degree of lip rounding and relative muscle tension in articulation are also used to classify certain vowels. Some vowels, for example, are produced

FIGURE 4-27

Vocal Tract in Configuration for Production of /a/ and the Spectrum of the Sound Radiated at the Lips.

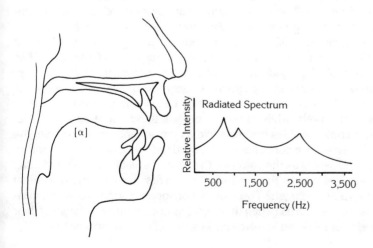

with the lips in a comparatively spread position. The vowels /i/ as in *team,* /ɪ/ as in *miss,* /ɛ/ as in *said,* and /ɝ/ as in *bad* are some examples. They are contrasted with rounded vowels such as /a/ as in *hard,* /ɔ/ as in *hawk,* /o/ as in *coat,* /ʊ/ as in *wood,* and /u/ as in *soup.* Some vowels seem to require more muscle activity for their production than others, which has given rise to tense-lax distinctions. They may help differentiate vowels which share almost exactly the same place of constriction, degree of constriction, and lip rounding. The /i/ (*team*) vowel, for example, is classified as a tense vowel, while its physiological neighbor /ɪ/ (*miss*) is a lax vowel. Much the same holds for the /e/ (tense) and /ɛ/ (lax), /ʌ/ and /ə/, /u/ and /ʊ/.

A group of speech sounds very similar to vowels is called *diphthongs.* They are often described as blends of two separate vowels, spoken within the same syllable. That is, a syllable is begun with the articulators in position for one vowel. They then shift smoothly toward the position for another. Say the word *boy* and listen to the changes in the vowel. The transition may bridge two, three, or more vowels in our everyday running speech. An example is the complex vowel in *boyandgirl,* with no break between the *boy-and.*

Consonant Production

See chapter 2, especially Table 2.4.

Consonants, which are characterized by constrictions or momentary occlusions of the vocal tract, are often described by place and manner of articulation and whether they are voiced or unvoiced. Consonants are said to be the constrictive gestures of speech, but many vowels are characterized by a certain degree of vocal tract constriction. Consonants often initiate and terminate syllables, and they comprise about 62% of all English speech sounds. They are not only more constrictive than vowels, they are more rapid and account in large part for the transitory nature of speech.

As we saw in chapter 2, places of articulation include the lips (bilabial), the teeth and lips (labiodental), the gums (alveolar), the hard palate (palatal), the soft palate (velar), and the glottis (glottal).

Manner of articulation describes the degree of constriction as the consonants initiate or terminate a syllable. For example, if closure is complete, the consonant is a *stop;* if incomplete, it is a *fricative.* Some voiceless consonants are produced as sustained sounds and are called *continuants.* When complete closure is followed by an audible release of the impounded pressurized air, the consonant is called a *stop-plosive* or simply a *plosive.* At other times complete closure is followed by a comparatively slow release of the impounded air, as the tongue sweeps along the palate backward. In this case, the consonant is called an *affricate.* Other sounds, called *glides,* are generated by rapid articulatory movement, and the noise or turbulent element is not as prominent as in plosives and fricatives. Some examples are /r/, /w/, and /j/. A small family of sounds, the *semivowels,* seem to qualify as vowel-like or consonant-like. They are sounds which may be syllabic in certain contexts and so serve as vowels, while in other contexts these same sounds either initiate or terminate syllables and so serve as consonants. For example, the semivowel /r/ serves as a consonant in the word *red,* while in the word *mother* this same sound serves as the vowel for the second syllable. In the word *little,* the semivowel /l/ serves as the consonant in the first syllable, and a vowel in the second syllable. Neat, eh? Three other consonant sounds /m, n, ŋ/, classified as *nasal consonants* (when they serve as consonants) because of their quality, are also considered semivowels in some classification systems.

Liquids are special semivowels because of the unique manner in which they are articulated. The liquid /l/ is produced with the tongue against the alveolar ridge so the breath stream flows somewhat freely around the sides of the tongue. Often a certain articulated gesture is associated with two consonants, which differ only in the voiced-voiceless category. The voiced /b/ and unvoiced /p/ constitute a cognate pair. Others are the /s/ (voiceless) and /z/ (voiced) and /f/ (voiceless) and /v/ (voiced) cognates.

Recall that these physiologically related consonants are called cognates.

Consonant production is very dependent upon the integrity of the speech mechanism, and very little leeway is allowed in their production. As listeners we seem to be far more tolerant of vowel coloration which occurs in regional and foreign dialects than we are of consonant variations in dialect. Now we should briefly examine the articulatory requirements for the various places and manners of consonant production.

Stop consonants are dependent upon *complete closure* at some point along the vocal tract. With the release of the forces of exhalation, pressure builds up behind the occlusion, until the air is released suddenly by the articulatory gesture. Closure for stop consonants occurs at the lips for the production of /b/ and its voiceless cognate /p/, with the tongue against the alveolar ridge for the /d/ and /t/ cognate pair, and with the tongue against the soft palate for the cognates /g/ and /k/. We must realize that elevated intraoral pressures are dependent upon an adequate velopharyngeal seal. If the soft palate is not brought into full contact against the back wall of the pharynx, an air leakage will occur and the ability to impound pressurized air behind the articulatory occlusion will suffer. Air pressure requirements for consonant production are actually quite modest, scarcely exceeding the pressure requirements for the larynx during vowel production. However, when we produce a voiced consonant, where intraoral pressure is elevated and the air pressure requirements of the larynx must be met, a compensatory increase in subglottal pressure is required to maintain voicing. The delicate balance and subtle interplay between the respiratory, phonatory, and articulatory mechanisms during the production of ordinary everyday speech is awesome, and yet it seems so simple—for most of us.

This happens with cleft palates and related disorders; see chapter 11.

Before leaving this topic, we should point out that the practice of contrasting stop consonants as voiced or voiceless is not without its hazards. Both voiced and voiceless stops are produced with a short interval of complete silence when they occur at the beginning of a syllable. When produced in the middle of a vowel-consonant-vowel sequence, a true distinction between voiced and voiceless stops may be perceived. A phenomenon called voice-onset-time (VOT) may be a useful perceptual cue. Voice-onset-time is the interval of time between the articulatory burst release of the stop consonant and the instant that vocal fold vibration begins. In English, the voice-onset-time is usually 30 milliseconds or less for a *voiced* stop consonant, and at times the voicing feature may actually begin slightly prior to the stop release. In that event, the voice-onset-time is said to be negative. Voiceless stops, on the other hand, usually have voice-onset-times of 30 milliseconds or more. In those instances when the release of air pressure is accompanied by a certain amount of aspiration, the voice-onset-times may range anywhere from 35 to 135 milliseconds.

A millisecond is 1/1000 second.

Fricative consonants are the result of a noise excitation due to a constriction somewhere along the vocal tract. Five common regions of constriction for the production of fricative consonants are used in the English language. Except for the /h/ consonant, which is generated at the glottis, all voiced fricatives have voiceless cognates.

The three nasal consonants /m, n/, and /ŋ/ are voiced, of course, but at the same time the vocal tract is completely constricted by the lips in /m/, by the tongue at the alveolar ridge in /n/, or by the dorsum of the tongue against the hard and/or soft palate in /ŋ/. The soft palate is lowered so that the acoustical transmission pathway is through the complex nasal cavities, and the sound is radiated at the nostrils. The lowered velum results in two resonant systems, with substantially different configurations and acoustical properties, placed side by side. The acoustical consequences are quite complex. The effective overall length of the vocal tract is increased, which lowers the frequencies of all the resonances. Because of the tortuous acoustic pathway through the nasal cavities, the amplitudes of the resonances are somewhat reduced. In addition, because of the complex acoustic interaction between the nasal cavities and the remainder of the vocal tract, the resonances are not as well defined as they are in vowel production. The importance of proper velopharyngeal closure cannot be overemphasized. During normal vowel and consonant production (except for the nasals), the nasal cavities are sealed off by the soft palate. In instances of tissue deficiency (a cleft palate, for example) or an immobile soft palate (paralysis), the nasal cavity coupling is inappropriate. Thus the person may impound pressurized air in the oral cavity for consonant production, and the vowels will be characteristically nasal.

See chapter 11.

THE NERVOUS SYSTEM AND SPEECH PRODUCTION

One communication disorder caused by failure of the brain and nervous system is aphasia, discussed in chapter 14; another is cerebral palsy, covered in chapter 13.

The ultimate mediator of almost all of our voluntary behavior—as well as our internal and external adjustments to changes in our immediate environment—is the nervous system. Composed of millions upon millions of individual cells called neurons and their supportive tissues, the nervous system instigates and transmits neural impulses which stimulate our muscles to contract. At the same time, muscle contraction and movements about the joints initiate neural impulses, and they in turn travel back to the coordinating centers of the brain to "tell it" what is going on and how well things are going.

Neurons are elongated cells (as are muscle cells) that are bioelectrically excitable (again, as are muscle cells). One important difference between neurons and muscle cells is contractability. Except for the extensions of its cellular substance, neurons are in many respects very similar to all of the other cells in the body. As shown in Figure 4.28, a neuron consists of a cell body and extensions of it. The neurons which supply muscles typically have a *single* relatively long extension called an axon, and numerous shorter extensions, clustered about the cell body, called dendrites. The terminal ending of an axon is characterized by numerous collaterals or branches (the end brush), which have little swellings or buttons at their tips. Depending upon their location, end brushes terminate either on the dendrites, on the cell bodies of other neurons, or on muscle fibers.

Whenever a neuron is stimulated, a chemoelectrical impulse is transmitted over the entire cell and its extensions or processes. As the impulse reaches the limits of the cell processes, a transmitter agent known as acetylcholine (which is manufactured by the neuron) is released by the end brush of the

FIGURE 4-28

Schematic of a Neuron.

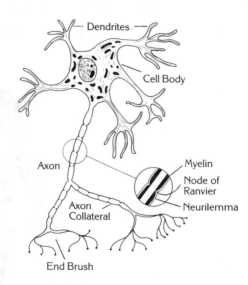

axon. It facilitates the transmission of the impulse to the cell body, its dendrite, or muscle tissue. Acetylcholine is released only at the axionic end of a neuron, in a region known as synapse in the case of a functional connection between two or more neurons or at the myoneural junction in the case of a functional connection between a motor-neuron and muscle. This helps explain why neural impulses pass from the axon of one neuron to the dendrite of another (and not the other way). The rule of thumb is that dendrites conduct toward the cell body and axons away from it.

The nervous system is divided into a central nervous system, which is that part enclosed and protected by the skull and vertebral column, and a peripheral nervous system, which is that part lying outside the bony confines of the skull and vertebral column. The central nervous system is in turn divided into the brain and spinal cord, while the peripheral nervous system is divided into a voluntary part (cranial and spinal nerves) and an involuntary part (the autonomic nervous system). A schematic nervous system is shown in Figure 4.29. Our immediate topic of interest here is in the central nervous system and the voluntary part of the peripheral nervous system. Neurons and chains of neurons which conduct impulses away from the central nervous system, usually to muscles, are called efferent or motor-neurons and those which conduct toward the central nervous system are called afferent or sensory.

A nerve can be thought of as a bundle of axons from individual neurons. Nerves may be composed exclusively of axons which are sensory, such as the optic (vision) and olfactory (smell) nerves; they may be essentially motor, such as the facial (facial muscles) and hypoglossal (motor nerve to tongue) nerves; or, as in the case of spinal nerves, they may be both motor and sensory (mixed nerves). Some nerves, then, may be composed of axons which have a variety of functions, such as reporting pain, temperature, muscle tension, limb movement, and limb position while delivering motor impulses to muscles at the same time. Within the central nervous system, bundles of axons called tracts have but one specific function.

FIGURE 4-29

Schematic of the Nervous System. Illustrations such as this one are based on a woodcut by Andreas Vesalius, an early 16th century anatomist (and artist) said to be the founder of modern anatomy.

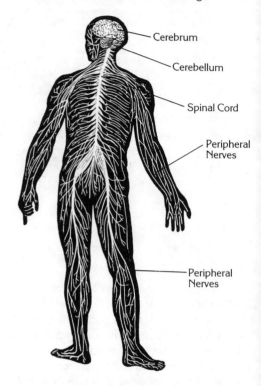

Cerebrum

Cerebellum

Spinal Cord

Peripheral Nerves

Peripheral Nerves

The Brain

The brain is probably best studied through its embryological development. In its very early stages, the brain consists of three hollow brain vesicles: the forebrain (prosencephalon), the midbrain (mesencephalon), and the hindbrain (rhombencephalon). With continued growth, the structures of the brain become increasingly elaborate and the three primary vesicles can be further divided.

The Forebrain and its Function

The forebrain (cerebrum) is by far the largest part of the human brain, consisting of two symmetrical cerebral hemispheres, the basal nuclei, and the center for olfaction (rhinencephalon). The outermost few millimeters of each hemisphere (the cortex) are characterized by a thin layer of cell bodies which appear dark in color and are called *gray matter.* Deep within the substance of each hemisphere are aggregates or clusters of nerve cell bodies (also gray matter) which collectively are called the *basal nuclei.* These structures are thought to play an important role in coordination of motor functions. The remainder of each hemisphere consists largely of nerve tracts which are extensions of the cortical gray matter. They appear light in color (due to a fatty deposit around them) and are called collectively *white matter.* Some of these fibers course (*a*) from the cortex downward (projection fibers), connecting the cerebrum with other parts of the brain and spinal cord, (*b*) from the front backward (association fibers), connecting the various parts of the cerebrum on the same side, and (c) from one side of the brain to the other (commissural fibers), connecting one cerebral hemisphere with the other. The surfaces of the cerebrum have numerous ridges and furrows which vary in depth. Deep furrows are called **fissures,** the shallow ones **sulci;** and the ridges between are called **gyri** or *convolutions.* Each hemisphere is divided into lobes which are named after the bones of the skull which cover them.

Vertebrate nervous systems are hollow and expand into ventricles in each cerebral hemisphere. In the spinal cord, a small central canal communicates with the ventricles of the brain. Cerebrospinal fluid, a clear liquid, circulates through the cavity system of the central nervous system, and obstructions to its circulation can lead to brain damage, mental retardation, and death.

The cerebral functions shown in Figure 4.30 are in part speculative, but some, such as sensory and motor, are well documented. It is largely by virtue of the development of the cerebral cortex, and association, projection, and commissural tracts that we are capable of that higher-order behavior that makes us human—reason, intelligence, memory, interpretation of sensation (correlation), and the very important speech and language. In addition to integrating and instigating voluntary motor behavior, the cerebrum places us in strong control of a lot of behavior that might otherwise be automatic or reflexive. Respiration during speech is an example. Talking with your mouth full of food is another. Consciousness and the ability to profit or learn from experiences (memory) are attributed largely to the cerebrum. However, the exact changes in the incomprehensibly complex chain of neural events which might occur for even the most simple speech act are largely unknown, and to even speculate staggers the imagination.

The remainder of the forebrain consists of the thalamus, a fairly large bulbous structure located just above the midbrain. It is a very important part of the forebrain. Although it is not completely understood, we do know that the thalamus receives sensory impulses from *all* parts of the body (except for smell). It also receives impulses from the cerebellum, cerebral cortex, and structures such as the basal nuclei, which are located adjacent to it. The

See also chapter 14.

The thalamus is supposed to tell us when we have had enough to eat, a reflexive func-

FIGURE 4-30

Diagrammatic Cerebral Functions. Some are well established; others are speculative or hypothetical.

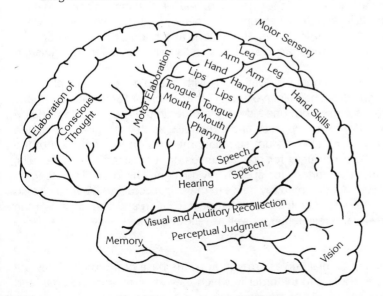

tion that we seem to have little difficulty overriding at the cortical level.

The Midbrain

The midbrain consists of paired, short thick stalks (cerebral peduncles) made up of descending and ascending fiber tracts. They connect the cerebrum with the hindbrain and with the spinal cord. The midbrain also contains (in the dorsal region) important visual and auditory correlation centers, as well as centers for motor coordination.

The Hindbrain

thalamus functions in an association role, as a synthesizer and relay center and as a sensory integrating center. It regulates water balance in the body, sleep and consciousness, body temperature, and food intake.

The hindbrain consists of the cerebellum, the pons (varolii), and the medulla oblongata. The cerebellum (little brain) is comprised of two richly furrowed hemispheres which are joined together by a central portion, the vermis. Three pairs of cerebellar peduncles connect the cerebellum with other parts of the nervous system; a cerebral connection by way of the superior peduncles, connections with the pons through the middle peduncle, and connections with the medulla oblongata by the inferior peduncle.

The vestibular apparatus are organs in the inner ear which produce the sense of equilibrium, movement, and body position. See chapter 10.

Inquiry to the cerebellum can be caused by strokes; for the effects on speech, see chapter 14.

The cortex of the cerebellum consists of gray matter, and a number of nuclei (gray matter) are contained within the deeper white matter. The cerebellum can be thought of as an elaborate integrating and coordinating center. Impulses from the motor center in the cerebrum, from the vestibular apparatus, and from our voluntary muscles enter the cerebellum through the peduncles, while out-going impulses are relayed to the motor centers of the cerebrum, down the spinal cord, and finally to our muscles. The cerebellum helps maintain muscle tone, posture, and equilibrium, as well as muscle coordination. Injury may result in difficulty in walking, producing coordinated voluntary movements, and speaking, due to a lack of coordination of the muscles of the articulators. In the event of cerebellar disease only parts of the body on the same side of the injury are affected. In spite of its importance, the activities of the cerebellum never enter into our consciousness.

The pons is located in front of the cerebellum, between the midbrain and the medulla oblongata. It consists of large numbers of transverse white fibers which join the two halves of the cerebellum and longitudinal white fibers which link the medulla with the cerebrum. Interspersed between the white fibers is gray matter. As its name implies, it functions as a bridge, but it also contains the nuclei of some important cranial nerves, as well as a center for regulation of breathing.

See chapter 10 for the crossover level of the auditory nerve.

The medulla oblongata is continuous with the spinal cord, and all of the ascending and descending nerve tracts of the spinal cord are found in it. Many of these tracts cross from one side to the other in the medulla. Descending motor tracts, for example, cross at the medulla, so that impulses generated on the left side of the cerebrum stimulate muscles on the right side of the body. A number of nuclei for cranial nerves are contained in the medulla, many of them important for speech production. The medulla oblongata serves as a conduction pathway between the spinal cord and the brain. It also contains centers for regulation of heart beat, dilation and contraction of the blood vessels, and respiration, as well as reflexive centers.

Cranial Nerves
See Figure 4.31.

Twelve pairs of cranial nerves emerge from the base of the brain. They are numbered according to the order in which they emerge from the brain and

FIGURE 4-31

Emergence of the Cranial Nerves from the Base of the Brain. The nerves are numbered from front to back, from I to XII, in accordance with the order in which they emerge.

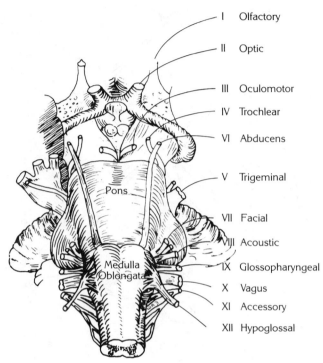

are named primarily according to function and distribution. Many of the cranial nerves important for control of the speech mechanism have their nuclei (of origin for motor nerves, of termination for sensory nerves) in the midbrain and hindbrain.

The Spinal Cord and Nerves
See Figure 4.32.

The spinal cord extends from the medulla oblongata above to the level of the second lumbar vertebra below. It diminishes in diameter somewhat as it descends, although it has two enlargements, one is the cervical and another in the lumbar region. The spinal cord is composed of both gray and white matter. The gray matter is located in the central region of the cord. When seen in cross-section, it resembles the letter H, or a butterfly. On each side of the midline, the gray matter is divided into ventral and dorsal columns or horns. The ventral column contains the cell bodies of the motor fibers of the spinal nerves, while the dorsal columns contain cell bodies from which sensory fibers ascend to higher levels of the cord and to the brain. Sensory fibers from the spinal ganglia enter the spinal cord and synapse with the dorsal horn neurons.

Thus any spinal nerve carries both sensory and motor fibers. Gray matter of the spinal cord also contains a large number of internuncial neurons which transmit neural impulses up and down the cord, from one side to the other, and from the dorsal to ventral roots of the spinal nerves. The spinal cord can be thought of as a great conducting pathway, to and from the brain, in addition to serving as an important reflex network for postural muscles and the limbs.

FIGURE 4-32

Cross Section of a Spinal Cord, Illustrating Dorsal and Ventral Horns (Gray Matter) and the Major Funiculi.

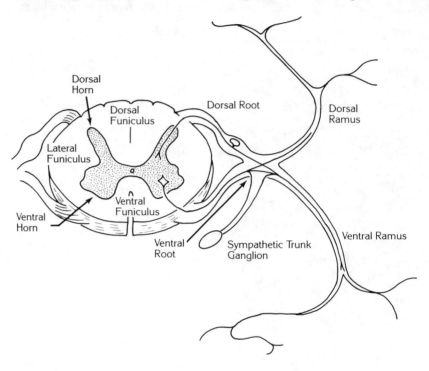

CONCLUSION

In the process of acquiring language and the rules for grammar and syntax, an awesome amount of information is somehow stored in the cerebral cortex. It is information we can retrieve at will, as often as we choose to, and it doesn't get used up or even wear out. Yet a tiny blood vessel can burst in the brain—and it's gone. We can automatically assemble meaningful thoughts, or we may search for words. Recall, judgment, coding, and decoding take place; almost instantly, these thoughts emerge as spoken words. And we know virtually nothing about the way in which cortical-level thought processes take place, and how they lead to sequential neural commands to the cranial and spinal nerves and then to muscles.

We do know that our respiratory muscles contract and relax voluntarily, to develop a reservoir of pressurized air. With almost perfect timing, the vocal folds are brought together at the midline to initiate phonation. Simultaneously, the articulators modify the configuration and therefore the acoustical properties of the vocal tract. Also at the same time, the train of speech sounds reaches our own ears as part of an integrated network of feedback channels. In the meantime, our muscles, tendons, and joints are transmitting a train of neural impulses back to the central nervous system to help complete the feedback information.

When stated this way, it all seems so simple—and it is, for most of us. For some people, however, something in this complex chain goes wrong. It falls to the speech-language pathologist to deal with the results.

We have briefly examined the anatomical and physiological bases for speech production. But no matter how exhaustive our pursuit of these particulars might be, ultimately each of us has to try to understand the whole picture as individuals. There *is* anatomical continuity between the tongue, hyoid bone, larynx, pharynx, soft palate, and even the lips. We can never discount what we know of the *functional* relationships between these structures, but we should also be aware that much has yet to be learned about the coordination of speech production.

The highly integrated and incredibly complex structures of speech production comprise a system we are just beginning to understand and fully appreciate. It is a delicately balanced, sensitive, and fragile system on one hand, resistant to disruption on the other, largely due to the human potential to compensate, a potential most of us will never put to use.

Finally, because of individual variability, our anatomical and physiological descriptions can at best be fairly representative and general in nature. This is good, because it is vitally important that our constructs about structure and function never become inflexible and stereotyped.

SELECTED READINGS

Hardcastle, W. J. *Physiology of speech production.* London: Academic Press, 1976.

Minifie, F., Hixon, T., & Williams, F. (Eds.). *Normal aspects of speech, hearing, and language.* Englewood Cliffs, N.J.: Prentice-Hall, 1973.

Tarkhan, A. Ein experimenteller Beitrag zur Kenntnis der Proprioceptiven Innervation der Zunge. *Zeitschrift für Anatomie and Entwicklungsgeschichte,* 1936, *105,* 349–358.

Zemlin, W. R. *Speech and hearing science: Anatomy and physiology.* Englewood Cliffs, N.J.: Prentice-Hall, 1981.

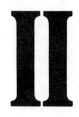

Disorders of Speech, Voice, and Language

EDITORS' COMMENTS

G. Paul Moore contributed to these editorial comments.

When you are introduced to a field of study, such as human communication disorders, by way of a college course and a comprehensive text book, you find yourself on a guided tour. The site might be pictured as an old mansion with several new wings. As you step into various rooms along the corridors, you become aware of certain features in each one, and you sense the mixture of old and new. The tour guide points out many of the important items that distinguish each area.

In Part I of this book, we have been trying to guide you through the landscape and history of the mansion—some background and perspectives for understanding problems of communication and how they can be dealt with. Your introduction to human communication disorders thus far has given you a view of our profession and the kinds of careers that are available, as well as basic concepts relating to the definitions of communication and language, the distinction between language difference and disorder, and the workings of the body in the process of communication.

It is almost time to take a look at the individual rooms in our mansion. Part II focuses on the major types of communication disorders—disorders of articulation, voice, fluency, and language. Each chapter starts with a case history to introduce you to a real person with the disorder. We also want to encourage you to listen to the portion of the audio disc that accompanies each chapter. As you read the cases, listen to the speech samples, and read the chapters, you will see that no single communication problem exists in isolation. A stutterer may have problems with phonation and voicing; a child with a language problem may have trouble with articulation as well. Furthermore, each child is unique. Although we can describe a normal pattern of language development, children acquire communication skills in functional units of varying dimensions and sizes. That is, they do not set out to systematically learn a certain distinctive feature or sound (like how to produce a voiced consonant) or a certain syntactical structure (like how to modify a word used for an object). Instead, they learn gradually to communicate—to make their ideas known to a listener, interweaving all the components of language. So when we reduce the communication process to specific fragments, we are doing it for our own convenience. We're dissecting a complex process in order to understand it.

But before we begin to look at individual types of communication disorders, we want to explain a little bit about certain theories of how they develop and some processes that apply to dealing with any person with such a problem. Each speech-language pathologist's beliefs about how communication and communication disorders develop can affect his or her choice of assessment techniques and intervention methods, so it is important that you be familiar with several different, commonly held perspectives.

PERSPECTIVES ON DEVELOPMENT OF COMMUNICATION DISORDERS

An on-going debate in the behavioral, biomedical, and clinical sciences is the relative contributions of heredity and environment to development of a specific trait in an individual. While we can say with certainty that the trait "blue eyes" is genetically determined, what about traits like mental retardation, neurosis, stuttering, perfect pitch? Here the answers are not so clear. We can identify at least four theories of the overall development of communication disorders: theories based on (a) medical or genetic causes, (b) psychological causes, (c) development or process defects, and (d) learning and conditioning.

Medical-Genetic Causes

Proponents of this theory feel that inheritance and biological structure play a major role in causing communication problems, although certain environmental stresses may trigger the appearance of the disorder. Thus a search for physical cause has two important functions. First, if we can identify the cause, we can try to treat it (rather than treating the symptoms). Second, we can try to prevent the disorder from developing in other people. A critical task of research would be to examine large numbers of people with a certain disorder and attempt to find any characteristics they share which could be causing the problem. These possible causes would include both physical factors, like brain damage or structure defects, and environmental stresses, which might determine why the condition develops in one person and not in another.

Psychological Causes

From this perspective, a person develops a communication disorder in order to satisfy some deep, unconscious need. In order to get rid of the problem, we would have to identify the underlying cause and help the person deal with that. In simplistic terms, once the underlying cause is dealt with, the surface problem should go away because the person no longer has a neurotic need for it. Intervention would focus on counseling, perhaps involving the family or other significant people in the child's or adult's life.

Developmental and Process Theories

Proponents of this approach feel that infants are born with the ability to develop language, and that disorders arise from a defect in the cognitive developmental processes a child uses. The environment is seen as facilitating or inhibiting the normal developmental pattern. Thus the first task of the speech-language pathologist would be to identify the defective process (for instance, auditory discrimination or visual reception) and then to help the person improve the process, modify the environment by developing the skill using a different process, or both. Again, concern focuses on causes rather than symptoms.

Learning and Conditioning

The final approach sees all behavior as learned. That is, infants are "blank slates" who learn because of what they experience. Advocates of this approach also feel that the critical factor in dealing with any type of disorder is the disordered behavior itself. An offshoot of stimulus-response psychology, the theory describes two processes by which behaviors are learned: classical conditioning and operant conditioning. In **classical conditioning,** a response is learned because it is consistently paired with a stimulus to which you already have an inborn or learned response. For example, one of my favorite foods is pizza. Because I've eaten and enjoyed it several times, I now begin to salivate as soon as I walk in the door of "Tony's" and smell tomato sauce and oregano. Salivation in response to food in the mouth is inborn; salivation in response to a smell is conditioned.

In **operant conditioning,** a response is learned because of the events which happen immediately after it (**consequences**). Any consequence which increases the probability that the target behavior will occur again is called a **reinforcer.** For example, when I work, I get paid; so I continue to work. The money is a reinforcer. I say "please pass the salt" because someone passes the salt.

The use of operant conditioning principles in education and clinical applications is often called **behavior modification.** In assessment and diagnosis, advocates of this approach describe the child or adult's current behavior as precisely as possible. This description includes the conditions under which the behavior occurs (called **antecedents**), the consequences which appear to reinforce the behavior, and the rate of the disordered behavior. This information is called **baseline** data and is used as a basis against which to evaluate progress. Intervention focuses on manipulating antecedents and consequences so as to decrease the undesirable behavior and increase selected target skills.

These four approaches overlap somewhat; in practice, the speech-language pathologist may choose the techniques from more than one in dealing with an individual problem. For example, while a certain voice disorder may have a distinct physical cause, the pathologist may use behavior modification to teach the person to compensate for it. As you read each chapter in Part II, you will see where these theories fit into the clinical management of each type of disorder.

For now, however, let us make one more brief stop, a look at a general process for assessing any communication problem.

THE ASSESSMENT PROCESS

No matter what the disorder, the process of assessment involves several steps, each of which depends upon the outcome of the previous step. The whole process may take several sessions, depending on the severity of the disorder. The accompanying model of the assessment process suggests that the depth of the assessment is inversely related to the number of individuals who go through each step. The process includes (*a*) screening, (*b*) diagnosis, (*c*) extension testing, (*d*) assessment for intervention, and (*e*) periodic assessment of progress. With school children who may be handicapped, current practice is to have a team conduct and review the assessment. The team makes all decisions about educational placement and special services.

FIGURE 1

Steps in the Clinical-Education Evaluation Process. (From E. M. Semel & E. H. Wiig, *Clinical Evaluation of Language Functions.* Columbus, Ohio: Charles E. Merrill, 1980. Used by permission.)

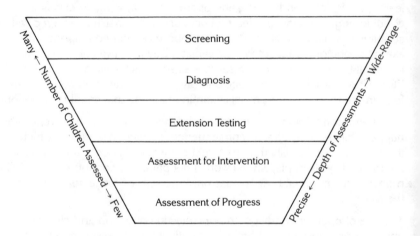

Screening

Screening involves testing a large number of people to identify those who show a significant enough problem to warrant in-depth testing. Most screening tests sample a wide range of skills, with only a few items per skill.

Diagnosis

Diagnosis attempts to identify those individuals with problems severe enough to call for intervention and, often, to specify the person's strengths and weaknesses in a given ability or range of skills. It also involves gathering detailed information about the individual, which includes a case history. The case history can include biographical, medical, psychological, social, behavioral, and environmental information. The history can usually be obtained by using questionnaires and interviews. The subject, his or her family, and other important people should all be interviewed.

In addition, diagnosis usually involves testing. Two main types of tests—norm-referenced and criterion-referenced tests—are used. A **norm-referenced** test is one which compares the individual's score to established norms, which are the scores of a large group of people. These norms are often presented by age level, and may include information on social, racial, ethnic, and economic background as well. The procedures for giving and scoring the test must be followed if the norms are to be valid, so the tests are also called *standardized*. In contrast, **criterion-referenced** tests compare an individual's score to a standard level, which is usually some sort of mastery of the skill. While there are some published criterion-referenced tests available, they are often constructed by individual speech-language pathologists and teachers. They can be especially useful in determining a person's strengths and weaknesses.

Extension Testing

Extension testing often follows diagnosis. It explores the primary variables which seem to be contributing to the communication problem. It can also involve determining which kinds of test tasks an individual has trouble with and which ones he finds easiest, so that the speech-language pathologist can be sure that the tasks used in intervention are helping rather than making learning more difficult. In essence, extension testing is used to establish the starting point for intervention. It allows the speech-language pathologist to judge the difference between the conditions at which the child or adult succeeds and the conditions under which he or she is expected to perform. It also allows the pathologist to specify the changes needed in input, in task formats, or in responses in order to help the individual succeed.

Assessment for Intervention

Once the strengths and weaknesses and the variables affecting success have been determined, objectives for intervention must be set. First, intervention areas and priorities are established. Second, long- and short-term objectives are set. Third, specific intervention strategies that correspond to the objectives are chosen. Finally, the levels of performance that will be considered acceptable must be identified. Without a clear picture of what the person can and cannot do, which skills should be targeted for intervention, and which conditions and strategies will facilitate progress, intervention may be directed at skills the child has already mastered.

Assessment of Progress

Since the goal of any intervention program is to improve the individual's abilities or to develop compensatory skills, the on-going assessment of progress (or failure to progress) is essential. Progress may be evaluated by methods similar to those used in diagnosis and extension testing, but it must be tied closely to the stated intervention objectives. The contents and procedures should be similar to those used in intervention, but not necessarily identical. Furthermore, the assessment should evaluate the transfer and generalization of the target skills. That is, it is not enough to be able to perform a new skill in the clinical setting with the speech-language pathologist; the child or adult should eventually be able to use the skill in everyday life, with all the people who are a part of that life.

Now that we've looked at some background issues, it is time to tour specific types of communication disorders. Keeping in mind the fact that the focus of our study is the whole individual person who has trouble making himself understood by the other people in his world, let us proceed.

FUNCTIONAL ARTICULATION DISORDERS

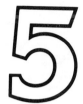

Leija V. McReynolds

Bobby, a 7-year-old, was referred to the Speech and Hearing Clinic by his classroom teacher and his parents. His problem was described as a severe articulation disorder.

Bob's birth and developmental history was unremarkable except for language. The mother reported that Bobby did not start talking until he was 3½ years old. Otherwise, his physical and motor development fell well within the normal range.

Bobby had suffered no unusual or prolonged illnesses or injuries. He had a number of colds and ear infections, but according to the pediatrician these were not any more numerous or severe than most children's bouts with the same illnesses. The pediatrician rated Bobby's health as average over the 7 years under his care.

No speech disorders have been observed in the immediate family members. Bobby has one sister who is 2 years older. According to the mother, the boy plays well with his peers and his relationship with the sister is quite good. Bobby participates in social and sporting activities in school and at home. Although he is not a leader, he participates as an equal in these activities. Bobby had not demonstrated any inhibitions in speaking to others until first grade. At that time he expressed annoyance when he was not understood by the teacher and some of his classmates. Until first grade he seemed unaware that his speech was different from others. His performance in school is slightly below the average, but IQ tests place him within the normal range.

Bobby was given a comprehensive assessment. Normal hearing acuity was noted for each ear with pure tone and speech stimulation. Word discrimination ability could not be tested due to the presence of numerous articulation errors in repeating discrimination test words. His receptive language was tested on the Peabody Picture Vocabulary Test and the Test for Auditory Comprehension of Language. In both measures, Bobby obtained scores well within the norms for his age group. His expressive language was assessed by administering the Carrow Elicited Language Inventory and the Expressive One-Word Picture Vocabulary Test. A conversational language sample was also obtained. On both formal tests Bobby scored at the 25th percentile, indicating that his performance fell within the boundaries of the lower 25 percent of the standardized populations. The numerous articulation errors made evaluation of his conversational *language sample difficult. However, Bob's expressive language consisted of complete sentences and phrases.*

The oral-peripheral physical examination revealed no structural abnormalities in the mouth. Tongue movements on nonspeech activities were appropriate. No malocclusion was evidenced in the alignment of teeth. Bobby's repetition of pa-ta-ka was slow, however. The oral-peripheral examination revealed no obvious physical or organic problems.

The Templin-Darley Articulation Test and the Goldman-Fristoe Articulation Test were administered. The following results were obtained:

	Substitutions	Omissions
Initial position	d/g, t/k/, t/s, d/z, p/f, b/v, t/ʃ, t/tʃ, d/dʒ, d/ʒ, w/r, w/l, t/θ, d/ð	-/r, -/l, -/dʒ
Medial position	n/d, d/g, d/k, t/s, n/tʃ, n/ʃ, d/z, t/dʒ	-/r, -/l, -/s, -/f, -/v, -/θ, -/ð, -/z, -/tʃ, -/ʃ
Final position	t/s, n/t, p/k, d/z, m/b, b/g	-/r, -/l, -/f, -/v, -/s, -/z, -/ʃ, -/dʒ, -/tʃ, -/g, -/k, -/θ, -/ð, -/t, -/d, -/p, -/b

According to Templin's normative data, Bobby's raw score is below the 3-year level of articulatory functioning on consonants. Stimulability was tested by requesting the child to imitate his error sounds. On this test Bobby correctly produced the /t/, /k/, /g/, /v/ and /f/ with instructional aid. A distinctive feature analysis revealed errors on (+) stridency and (+) continuancy at 90%. A high percentage of errors also occurred on the place features (+) back, (+) high, and (+) coronal.

A phonological process analysis of Bobby's conversational sample revealed that Cluster Reduction, Final Consonant Deletion, Stopping, and Assimilation were possible phonological processes present in his articulation errors. Further testing of processes was undertaken to determine whether the sounds affected by the processes were used by the child in any contexts contrastively. The analysis showed that most of the sounds were not in the child's spontaneous repertoire in any contexts; therefore operation of phonological processes was not supported.

Bobby's past history and present status indicate that physically he is performing adequately. Academically his performance is lower than average, but this may be due partially to his speech problem since his IQ has been established to be within the normal range. Socially the child is functioning normally and enjoys interacting with his family and peers. No medical reason for his speech problem has been identified.

On the formal hearing tests, Bobby evidenced no hearing problem. His language scores on the expressive language tests placed him in the lower 25th percentile but his articulatory deficit made it difficult to score the language tests. Articulation measures revealed numerous articulation errors of substitutions and omissions. These errors make his speech difficult to understand.

Bobby may be described as a child with a severe articulation disorder of unknown origin. Several recommendations were made. First, it was recommended that Bobby be enrolled in direct intensive articulation training. He should be seen by the speech-language pathologist individually 5 days a week. Next, it was recommended that a structured treatment program be developed to establish correct production of sound classes *through a selected sample of exemplars from two classes. Third, initially, contrast training between stops and fricatives should be administered. For example, the child can be trained to produce the /p/ and /f/ contrastively, first in nonsense syllable contexts and then in words. The /p/ and /f/ are likely targets because Bob can and does produce /p/ appropriately, and is stimulable on the /f/. Finally, generalization to other stops and fricatives should be tested frequently and always prior to initiating training on another sound pair. The generalization testing can be used to determine progress and to select future target sounds and contexts for training.*

You may now wish to listen to the speech sample accompanying this chapter, found on Audio Disc 1, Side 1 (sample #1).

As we have seen, in order for two people to communicate successfully, the sender must use a shared language to encode a meaning that the receiver can decode. If I'm talking to you, I must use words and structures that you understand. Furthermore, I must pronounce those words so that you can recognize them, at least with certain limits. **Articulation** is the process of producing the speech sounds of a language, and **intelligibility** is the quality that describes how readily my speech can be understood by listeners. The most precise words and the clearest structures are useless if you cannot understand them because the sounds are not intelligible. Unfortunately, problems with articulation are very common—in fact, they occur more often than any other type of disorder seen by most speech-language pathologists.

This chapter discusses the topic of functional articulation disorders, beginning with a short explanation of articulation and how it develops normally. A definition of disordered articulation follows, and later a definition of functional articulation disorders is offered. Next, we will summarize the most common explanations of the nature of functional articulation disorders and how remediation is approached within each explanation. The final sections are devoted to evaluation and treatment of articulation disorders. These sections describe the variables measured in assessing articulation disorders, with special emphasis on variables that seem to be useful in **prognosis** and in planning remediation programs. In this final section, general principles for planning remediation programs are also set forth.

*A **prognosis** is a prediction of how quickly and how well a person will recover from or overcome a condition with intervention.*

ARTICULATION AND ARTICULATION DEVELOPMENT

To be precise, the term *articulation* refers to the movements of the articulators in production of the speech sounds making up the words of our language. It is more than that, however, since production of each speech sound (phone) in each word needs to be related to the abstract representations (phonemes) of the language. That is to say, speech sounds are represented on two levels, the phonetic and the phonological level. As we saw in chapter 2, on the phonetic level there are many phones for one phoneme because individual speakers produce sounds differently. Further, the context (word or syllable) in which a sound is produced influences the phone as well. A child will produce a sound somewhat differently from the way an adult produces the same sound, because his vocal tract size is different from adults. Contextually, surrounding

To review, a phoneme is indicated with slash marks / /, and phones are enclosed in brackets [ ].

sounds influence production. For example, the phoneme /p/ will be produced differently in the words *pin* and *spin*. The [p] in *pin* is accompanied by aspiration (breath), while in the word *spin* the [p] is unaspirated. Thus, the phoneme for both productions is /p/, and the two ways of producing [p] in *pin* and *spin* constitute phones because the contexts in which they are produced influence their production.

On the phonological level, phonemes are linguistically important because they act as contrastive elements in the language; they serve to distinguish meaning, as the /p/ and /b/ do in the words *pin* and *bin*. Only the /p/ and /b/ are different in the two words; because they differ, we know that these are two words, each with a different meaning. The /p/ and /b/ thus contrast with each other. This contrast allows a differentiation of the two words in regard to meaning; therefore, the contrast is linguistic. Articulation, therefore, helps (*a*) to differentiate words from each other and (*b*) to make productions of sounds more precise.

You may wish to check Table 2.1 for a complete listing of consonants and vowels.

The English language consists of approximately 40 phonemes, categorized into vowels and consonants. Children learn these sounds gradually, and this gradual development has been studied in order to identify the sequence in which sounds are acquired (Poole, 1934; Prather, Hedrick, & Kern, 1975; Templin, 1957; Wellman, Case, Mengert, & Bradbury, 1931). The beginning of this gradual development has been studied by linguists, child development investigators, psychologists, and speech pathologists. At one time, linguists suggested that infant vocalizations, such as cooing and babbling, were unrelated to children's sound productions as they begin to produce meaningful words (Jakobson, 1968). This premise is the central idea in what is known as the *discontinuity theory* of phonological acquisition. However, recent research shows that infant vocal behavior is similar to child sound production in several ways. For instance, sound patterns of English are already present in infant babbling, and phonological processes used to describe young children's articulation error patterns can also be used to describe infant sound patterns (Oller, Wieman, Doyle, & Ross, 1974; Pierce, 1974; Stark, Rose, & McLagen, 1975). In addition, research has shown that infants tend to produce sounds which are within the language of their culture more frequently than sounds unlike the sounds of their language (Cruttenden, 1970; Rees, 1972). For these reasons, we now recognize that infant vocal behavior may have relevance to the sound acquisition patterns of children as they begin to acquire language. The similarities between infant vocal behavior and early language acquisition support a *continuity theory* of phonological acquisition (McReynolds, 1978). **Normative data** for infant sound patterns are not yet available, but investigations continue. These studies may offer important information for our understanding of how children gradually acquire the sounds of their language and how early acquisition begins. Thus far, data are available only for older children, that is, starting at about age 2.

***Normative data** result from the study of large groups of normally developing subjects to evaluate behavior at different age levels.*

Of primary interest to speech-language pathologists is the sequence of consonant acquisition, because consonants are more important to intelligibility than vowels. Normative data for ages at which particular consonants are usually present are reported in Table 5.1. These data are from two studies, one completed by Templin in 1957, and the other completed more recently by Prather, Hedrick, and Kern, in 1975. Younger children (ages 2 years to 4 years) were tested in the 1975 study, where in the Templin study the youngest age group was 3 years old and the oldest was 8. As you can see in the table, the sequence in which sounds appear in children's speech is similar in the two studies, but the Prather, et al., data indicate that sounds may be acquired at younger ages than we used to think. Prather and colleagues caution, however, that they tested each consonant in just two positions in words (initial and final), while Templin tested the consonants in three positions in words (initial, medial, and final). This difference may be responsible for the different results obtained in the two studies. Speech-language pathologists rely on developmental data like these to help determine if a child has an articulation problem (or has not yet reached the age where a missing sound should be present), and which sounds will ultimately be selected for treatment.

The initial position is the first sound in a word; the final is the last sound; the medial falls in the middle. A child may be able to produce a phoneme in only one or two of these positions.

TABLE 5.1

Ages (in Years and Months) at Which 75% of Children Correctly Produced Consonant Sounds.

Sound	Templin (1957) 3 Positions	Prather et al. (1975) 2 Positions	Sound	Templin (1957) 3 Positions	Prather et al. (1975) 2 Positions
m	3	2	g	4	3
n	3	2	s	4-6	3 +
h	3	2	r	4	3-4 +
p	3	2	l	6	3-4 +
ŋ	3	2	ʃ	4-6	3-8
f	3	2-4	tʃ	4-6	3-8
j	3-6	2-4	ð	7	4
k	4	2-4	ʒ	7	4
d	4	2-4	dʒ	7	4 +*
w	3	2-8	θ	6	4 +*
b	4	2-8	v	6	4 +*
t	6	2-8	z	7	4 +*
			hw	*	4 +*

*Sound tested but not produced correctly by 75% of subjects at oldest age tested.
+Reversal: Reported at earliest age level if only one reversal occurred and percentage at 11 older age levels exceeded 75%.

DEFINITION OF DISORDERED ARTICULATION

When an articulation error occurs, production of a phoneme is imprecise in one of several ways. Sometimes the intended phoneme is replaced by another phoneme. In that case, the error is one of **substitution;** the appropriate phoneme is replaced by an inappropriate phoneme. If a person says, "Don't *wet* me" when he means "Don't *let* me," he is substituting a /w/ for an /l/, and the substitution results in a shift from the word *let* to *wet*. This misproduction is likely to cause a misunderstanding of the intended word because the /l/ and /w/ function contrastively in the two words to differentiate them and their two meanings.

In other instances, a misproduction makes a phoneme sound different, but not different enough to shift the production into another phoneme. For example, a person might use aspiration in producing the [p] in *spin* when it should have been produced without aspiration. The aspirated [pʰ] in *spin* sounds funny, but the listener recognizes it as a /p/, not some other phoneme. The word is understood, although the [p] is distorted. This kind of production is referred to as a **distortion** because the sound has not been produced in the standard manner, but the production is perceived as the appropriate phoneme.

In disordered articulation, sounds within words are sometimes omitted entirely. If so, it is not always possible to determine what the phoneme should have been; and of course, since nothing is produced, it isn't possible to determine if the phone was produced in a standard manner. If a child says, "My ca___ is lost," you wouldn't know if the word was supposed to be *cat* or *cap*, because in this case the final sound in the word identifies what the word is and that sound is missing. These errors are called **omission** errors. The error types with examples are summarized in Table 5.2.

TABLE 5.2
Kinds of Articulation Errors.

Error Type	Definition	Example
Substitution	Replace one sound with another sound	Standard: The ball is <u>r</u>ed Substitution: The ball is <u>w</u>ed
Distortion	A sound is produced in an unfamiliar manner	Standard: Give the <u>p</u>encil to Sally Distortion: Give the <u>p</u>encil to Sally (the /p/ is nasalized)
Omission	A sound is omitted in a word	Standard: <u>Pl</u>ay the piano Omission: P_ay the piano
Addition	An extra sound is inserted within a word	Standard: I have a <u>bl</u>ack horse Addition: I have a bǝlack horse

Thus an articulation error may consist of a substitution, distortion, or omission of sounds (and infrequently, addition of extra sounds). At times a word is changed to another word because the error is a substitution which changes the intended phoneme. An articulation error may also result in distorting a sound without changing the intended phoneme, thus leaving the intended word unchanged although strange. Finally, sounds my be omitted entirely from words, and the omission is an articulation error.

But of course, it takes more than just one substitution, distortion, or omission to diagnose articulation errors as articulation disorders. We do not have standard criteria for determining how many or what kinds of errors comprise a disorder, but several variables are considered by speech-language pathologists in arriving at the conclusion that a child or adult has an articulation problem. Foremost in arriving at a decision is a judgment about how severely intelligibility is affected. This judgment of severity depends on a number of variables such as number of errors, type of error, and consistency of errors.

These variables will be discussed in more detail in the evaluation section of this chapter.

Frequently, however, the decision that a person has an articulation disorder is also influenced by the speech-language pathologist's own views concerning functional articulation disorders. That is, individual professionals have personal opinions about what constitutes a functional articulation disorder. These biases influence the variables to be measured in evaluation and the weight given to each measured factor.

Definition of Functional Articulation Disorders

See chapters 11 and 12.

Sometimes articulation errors are accompanied by physical abnormalities such as are seen in cleft palate or in neurological deficits as in apraxia. It is generally accepted in these instances that the structural or neurological deficit is at least partially responsible for the articulation defect. The exact relationship between the physical condition and the defective articulation may not be easy to establish; nevertheless, there appears to be some observable evidence that the two are related.

However, a large group of articulation problems have no known, or obvious, organic, neurological, or physical factors. Since the cause or causes for these problems are unknown, they have been relegated to a category labelled **functional** articulation disorders. *Functional* may mean any number of things; mostly, the term *functional* serves as a wastebasket label denoting only that the **etiology** for the disorder is unclear and no causal components can be identified (Shelton, 1978). It isn't that investigators have not attempted to identify causes; as a matter of fact, many variables have been explored in the hope that one or more would be found to be responsible for articulation problems, or at least closely related to them. Variables such as intelligence, motor skills, auditory discrimination, auditory memory, socioeconomic status, sex, personality, academic performance, dentition, and many others have all been explored in the hope that one or more would reveal a causal link (Winitz, 1969). Unfortunately, very few of the variables were found to be related to disordered articulation.

*The **etiology** of a condition is its cause or causes.*

The lack of a relationship between articulation disorders and these numerous variables studied has led most experts to assume that articulation disorders have multiple causes. They have also abandoned their attempts to find causes. Attention has shifted to regarding these variables as factors important to describing articulatory behavior itself, to seeking ways in which the variables could contribute to evaluation for determining the presence of the disorder, to making statements about prognosis, and to developing efficient treatment programs.

Although no causal relationships have been uncovered, individuals interested in the problem have begun to propose possible causes and possible models which explain the nature of articulation disorders. As a result, several approaches to functional articulation disorders have emerged. Needless to say, most approaches are somewhat mixed in that no one cause is purported to be wholly responsible. Rather, proponents may suggest one strong causal factor accompanied by other less strong, but still influential, factors contributing to the disorder. Emphasis in most approaches is frequently placed on the nature of the articulation problem (is it a motor problem? a perceptual problem?), more than on what caused the problem originally. A brief discussion of some major approaches follows. However, you should note that these approaches are placed into broadly defined categories, and each category includes input from a number of specific approaches differing from each other on one or more dimensions.

Discrimination Approaches

This is a process *approach.*

The most common approach for a number of years, and perhaps still, was developed by Van Riper and Irwin (1958), and subsequently expanded. According to this model, the underlying problem is poor sound discrimination. That is, the individual is not able to match the auditory feedback from his or her own production with the auditory patterns others produce. He is unable to discriminate the differences between his error production and the correct production of the same sound by others. This failure to discriminate may be caused by a number of factors (such as by slow physical maturation, or by listening to other family members who misarticulate), but the authors do not specifically identify the factors. In remediation, particular attention is paid to training the person with an articulatory defect to discriminate acoustic differences, to evaluate the adequacy of his or her productions in comparison to standard productions, and to modify error productions until they match the standard.

Another approach which emphasizes discrimination has been proposed by Winitz (1975), who nevertheless indicates that articulation errors represent learned behavior. He thinks the approximations which children produce while they are acquiring the phonology of their language become stabilized in some children's speech. These children develop functional articulation disorders. Winitz suggests that articulation errors may emerge because the child's productions vary from correct to incorrect over time, and the parents do not correct these errors. Training, according to this approach, should follow the training given by parents as they help their children learn to talk. That is, it should be part of a natural communicative exchange between the speech-language pathologist and the child, with minimal instruction on how sounds are produced and emphasis on listening tasks. Errors are eliminated when the child becomes a better discriminator of his own productions because others in the environment do not understand him.

Some support for the discrimination approach may be found in the research on variables related to disordered articulation. We have seen that, of the many variables studied, few were found to be related. Speech sound discrimination performance was one of the variables that appeared in several studies (although not in all) to be relevant. Because of the discrepancy among studies, it is currently suggested that, if discrimination is important, it is probably important only for some people, and primarily in the form of self-discrimination. Self-discrimination involves a person's judgment of the correctness of his or her own productions. Self-discrimination may be practiced in one of two ways: (a) the child or adult produces words which are tape-recorded and played back so that he or she can judge whether the sounds were produced correctly or incorrectly; (b) the child or adult says words and tells the speech-language pathologist immediately after saying each word whether the sounds in the words were produced correctly or incorrectly.

Approaches in which faulty discrimination is a central theme may include a phase in which a child is taught to discriminate the target sound from other sounds, identify correct and incorrect production of the target sound when produced by others, and discriminate his or her own correct and incorrect productions. Training in producing the sound is administered only after the child completes the discrimination tasks. The extent to which discrimination training is used differs from professional to professional.

There is another group of approaches in which discrimination is not considered to be an important variable contributing to the functional articulation problem. In these approaches, emphasis is placed on training correct production with no specific discrimination training administered. These approaches are discussed next.

Production Approaches

Undoubtedly, articulation involves, at least in part, the learning of a motor skill. An articulation disorder isn't necessarily a case of motor disability; nevertheless, articulation consists of fine motor movements which need to be coordinated precisely if speech is to be accurate. Several experts consider the motor component to be the important variable in treatment of functional articulation disorders.

Probably the best known approach in this category is the model conceptualized by McDonald (1964). In this model, children with articulation errors are thought to be arrested at some stage in sensory-motor development. The model does not suggest that learning and other variables do not influence the articulation pattern they present; rather, it suggests that the primary problem is the sensory-motor arrest to which other factors may be contributing. McDonald contends that the syllable, not the isolated sound, is the smallest unit of speech. McDonald envisages articulation as consisting of a series of overlapping movements in which the tongue, lips, and other articulatory muscles and structures are moving almost simultaneously as a person produces a word. Essentially, sounds are not produced sequentially, one at a time in a word, but rather they overlap with each other. For example, the lips are beginning to protrude in preparation for producing the /u/ during production of the /t/ in the word *true.*

Presently, basic research appears to support, at least in part, McDonald's viewpoint regarding overlapping movements of the articulators in the form of coarticulation. Studies of coarticulation show that articulators begin to move to form a particular sound long before it is produced audibly (Daniloff & Hammarberg, 1973). However, this coarticulation occurs in other than syllable-size contexts, as proposed by McDonald; it occurs across word and sentence boundaries too. Speech-language pathologists are frequently encouraged to take advantage of the phenomenon of coarticulation in training. It has been proposed that some sounds can be used to form facilitating contexts for acquisition of particular target sounds. For example, if /s/ is taught in the context of /t/, as in the word *stay,* the /t/ may make acquisition of /s/ easier than if the /s/ were followed by some other sound. Therefore, the /t/ is thought to be a facilitating context for learning to produce /s/. Unfortunately, research in coarticulary effects in training has not demonstrated that these effects do occur. Very few coarticulatory training studies have been conducted to date (Elbert & McReynolds, 1975, 1978). Possibly, future studies will be more definitive.

What we have demonstrated is that, if a child can produce a target sound correctly in some contexts, these contexts may be used in training by pairing the correctly produced context with the incorrectly produced context (Irwin & Weston, 1975). This pairing may help the child shift the correct production to the incorrectly produced contexts. Contextual influence is a major component in McDonald's sensory-motor approach. An error sound will probably be produced correctly in some phonetic contexts because children's error productions are usually inconsistent. If production of the error sound is tested in a sufficient number of syllables, the sound will probably be produced correctly in one or more of them. In order to find contexts in which a child might produce the target sound correctly, McDonald (1964) designed a test in which each sound is tested in a variety of word pairs (contexts) to help find the context(s) in which production is correct.

McDonald's approach to training is to give extensive practice in overlapping articulatory movements. The practice is accomplished by requiring the child to produce many one-, two-, and three-syllable nonsense items consisting of different permutations of consonants and vowels (for instance, bi, bi-bi, bi-bi-bi). The purpose is to give practice in every conceivable combination of articulatory movements. Initially, practice is given on syllables containing sounds

Review chapter 4 for details on the many muscles and organs involved in articulation.

The size of the speech unit has become an interesting issue in speech science, linguistics, and speech pathology and is yet to be resolved.

Chapter 2 has defined coarticulation.

the child can already produce; later the practice is shifted to syllables containing the target sound. Clearly McDonald highlights production training, leaving little room for discrimination tasks.

Shelton's (Shelton & McReynolds, 1979) conceptualization of functional articulation disorders fits within the sensory-motor model because it stresses the motor skill aspect of articulation. Much of Shelton's research has been based on principles involved in development of skilled motor performance. Recently, he has discussed a perceptual-motor learning model in which perceptual and cognitive factors receive added attention. He proposes that children and adults be asked to think about their articulation before producing the target sound, and would provide as much information as possible about how a sound is produced both before and after the individual produces the target sound.

Another approach fitting into the production emphasis is application of operant conditioning to articulation remediation (Garrett, 1973; Mowrer, 1973, 1978). In this approach, little attention is paid to causal factors; instead, the accent is on careful programming in remediation to obtain maximal changes as efficiently as possible. Reinforcement is used to carefully define **shaping** procedures. Many ready-made programs for articulation remediation are founded on the principles of operant conditioning (programmed instruction) and are available commercially (Costello, 1977; Gerber, 1977).

Needless to say, a number of motor skills learning principles have been incorporated into specific articulation remediation plans by individual speech-language pathologists. It is not unusual, for example, for speech-language pathologists to offer detailed phonetic instructions on tongue placement or lip postures during the course of training a new sound. Feedback on the child's response is also a common practice in training.

Linguistic Approaches

Linguistic models were developed later than were the discrimination and production models—not that linguistic information was ignored in the two earlier models. In fact, reference is made to linguistics in both. The impact of linguistic theory on language acquisition and treatment of language disorders is well recognized and familiar to most speech-language pathologists. This is less true for articulation. It was only when professionals realized that phonology, as one component of language, was being neglected in the onslaught of interest in morphology, syntax, semantics, and pragmatics that a revival of interest in phonology occurred (Ingram, 1976). Today attention is being devoted to the relevance of linguistic theory to the understanding of functional articulation disorders. Two linguistic notions have aroused the interest of speech-language pathologists: distinctive features and phonological processes. These notions will be discussed individually.

The theory of distinctive features was introduced in chapter 2; you may wish to review that discussion.

The theory of distinctive features has been applied to the description of articulation errors (McReynolds & Huston, 1971; Singh & Frank, 1972). The idea is that each sound (each consonant and vowel) is composed of a number of articulatory elements. To give a rather gross example of the concept of features, consider that the production of /b/ involves, among other things, bringing the lips together firmly, building up air pressure behind the lips, forcing the lips open with a burst of air, and vibrating the vocal folds (voicing). All of these articulatory gestures might be thought of as articulatory features which compose the /b/ sound. Each sound is composed of several features which, when grouped together, comprise a phoneme. The interesting thing about features is that any one feature is present in several sounds; this common feature defines the relationship among a number of sounds. To give an example, voicing is a feature present in several sounds—/b,d,g,z,v,ð/ and others. Because the sounds are all voiced, they form a class of voiced sounds. Other features function similarly in that they help demonstrate relationships between sounds.

Application of feature theory to functional articulation problems enables us to describe a problem in terms of feature errors, which in turn helps to reveal relationships among error sounds. By comparing the features of the target sound with the features produced in the error sound, it is possible to identify which features are in error. If, for instance, a child produced /p/ for /b/, /t/ for /d/, /k/ for /g/, and /f/ for /v/, it would be possible to say that in all of these errors she is substituting a voiceless sound for a voiced sound. Obviously, her error is on voicing, a feature that is necessary to production of the /b,d,g/ and /v/. What the child needs to learn is to produce both the voiced and voiceless sounds in a cognate pair, that is /p/ and /b/, /t/ and /d, /k/ and /g/, /f/ and /v/. That is, she needs to learn the voiced and voiceless contrast. Possibly because the error is a feature error rather than unrelated errors on a number of individual sounds, the contrast can be trained in just one or two pairs and the voicing feature may transfer to the remaining pairs without specific training on each pair.

This kind of generalization has occurred when feature contrasts are trained (Costello & Onstine, 1976; McReynolds & Bennett, 1972). When first introduced, the concept of determining that error sounds are related and share some common attributes was a somewhat unique one for speech-language pathologists interested in articulation disorders. It offered the new prospect that errors are systematic, rather than haphazard. This new perspective on the nature of articulation errors was carried further when it was proposed that functional articulation disorders be described in terms of phonological processes. They will be discussed next.

Articulation errors frequently fall into patterns; a child or adult may show a pattern of omitting most final consonants in words, or always substituting stops for fricatives, and so on. These patterns may reflect phonological processes, and processes may represent the way children simplify production of sounds which they are unable to produce correctly (Ingram, 1976; Shriberg, 1980). To state it another way, children use phonological processes to simplify difficult productions. To illustrate, we might say that a child omits final consonants in words because they are difficult for him to produce; that is, the child is using the process of "final consonant deletion." Application of phonological processes simplifies productions and results in articulation errors.

Similar to distinctive feature theory, phonological processes reveal relationships among error sounds. A process is not applied to just one sound, but to several sounds. Returning to the process of final consonant deletion, several sounds may be affected. A child may omit the /t/ in words that end with /t/ as in *cat, put, let;* he may also omit the /p/ in words ending in /p/ as in *cup, mop, flip;* further, all final /f/ and /s/ sounds may be omitted in the same way. Consequently, final consonant deletion afects the /t,p,f/ and /s/ sounds; therefore, it is a general process. Because it is general and the errors are systematic, relationships among the error sounds are revealed, as in distinctive feature theory. Different sounds are affected in a similar manner by one process, which demonstrates how the sounds are related. Supposedly, the transfer principle demonstrated in distinctive feature training should hold true for training directed at processes in that all affected sounds need not be trained individually. The speech-language pathologist should be able to focus training on eimination of a process, say final consonant deletion, in only one or two of the affected sounds. When the process is eliminated on those sounds, the process should also disappear from the remaining affected sounds without training.

To date, only one training study has been conducted to determine whether transfer occurs if training is directed at elimination of processes (McReynolds & Elbert, 1981b). Thus far, the data do not support the theory. However, the linguistic notion of generalization owing to presence of a system has strong appeal because it offers possibilities for planning more efficient treatment programs. It has even been proposed that the label *functional articulation disorders* should be replaced by the label *phonological disorders* because the latter term describes the nature of the problem more accurately. However, more data are required before this change in labels can be supported (McReynolds & Elbert, 1981a, b; Shelton & McReynolds, 1979).

Psychological Approaches

One other category of approaches deserves mention, although they have not had as strong an impact on treatment of functional articulation problems. The category includes a variety of psychological constructs used by a number of therapists.

For more on psy-choanalytic concepts, see Rousey's chapter or texts on counseling techniques; a detailed description is beyond the scope of this book.

A psychoanalytic model of functional articulation disorders has been proposed by Rousey (1971). Depending as it does on psychoanalytic concepts to explain errors, the model has not received wide acceptance. Treatment within this model requires someone such as a psychiatrist, with knowledge and training in psychoanalytic concepts.

Other approaches include psychological components as central units. In one, the child or adult is first made comfortable and encouraged to become motivated to change the incorrect articulation patterns (Hahn, 1961). Direct work on articulation is undertaken only after the person appears psychologically prepared to work on the error sounds. In another, people with diverse speech problems are grouped together for therapy (Backus & Beasley, 1951). The speech-language pathologist's role is to provide direction and support to the people in the group while they help each other within unstructured situations.

Psychological approaches have been helpful in reminding speech-language pathologists to view their clients as worthwhile individuals. The procedures outlined in the psychological approaches can be readily adapted to other training programs. These procedures include taking time to establish understanding and communication with the individual, appreciating his or her concerns and needs, and encouraging each person to become an active participant in the therapeutic process.

Summary

Regardless of the speech-language pathologist's theoretical positions concerning the cause or causes of functional articulation disorders or the nature of the disorder, there is overlap in the approaches used in remediation. Most speech-language pathologists do not adhere to any one theory or model of functional articulation disorders. Indeed, there are few "pure" models; the majority are eclectic, incorporating ideas and variables that appear sound or have been evaluated through controlled research. Etiological factors seldom play an important role in planning remediation programs, perhaps because they aren't readily identified. Customarily, too, speech-language pathologists use what has been suggested from experientially derived information. We must work with the tools in hand, the materials available—the professional's behavior and the child's or adult's articulation.

But the overlap among approaches is partly a function of research findings. Earlier we mentioned that many variables have been studied for causal relationships, but none were demonstrated to be etiologically important. However, a few of the variables were found to be important to understanding articulatory problems. These variables are often used in evaluation for several reasons. First, they help in determining if an articulation problem is present and how severe it is. They sometimes contribute prognostic information. Finally, they contribute information for planning effective remediation programs. Let us now look at articulation evaluation and some of the variables found to be valuable.

EVALUATION

Evaluation of a child or adult with a possible articulation disorder is a critical process, with more than one important purpose. As we have seen, the first step is an evaluation to determine whether the individual does indeed have an articulation problem warranting attention. Second, if the initial evaluation indicates the presence of a problem, the speech-language pathologist conducts a more complete assessment which includes an in-depth exploration of the person, his background, and his articulatory status. Results of a properly conducted comprehensive evaluation will help the professional understand and describe the problem, outline an effective remediation program, and make some educated guesses regarding the kind and degree of improvement to be expected.

Initial Procedure

The first decision is whether the child or adult presents an articulation problem severe enough to warrant a more complete evaluation. In many cases this question has already been answered by other referral sources. In the case of children, parents may be concerned about their child's speech and intelligibility, or teachers may refer children for evaluation. Another source for referral is dentists or children's physicians who are concerned that a child is slow in developing speech. Adults frequently refer themselves for evaluation because they are concerned about their own speech.

In the public schools, referrals may come after the speech-language pathologist has conducted a screening test of children in the lower grades or (if the school has had no speech services) of all the children in the school. Screening may take one of several forms. Many language professionals prefer to converse casually and briefly with each child on topics of interest to the children. They may ask the children their names, addresses, and when their birthdays are. Frequently each child is requested to count until stopped, or as far as he or she can. At other times the children are requested to name the days of the week, and older children may read short passages such as "My

Grandfather" (Darley, Aronson, & Brown, 1975). These passages are chosen to contain a representative sample of consonants and vowels of the English language, and the speech-language pathologist listens for the child's production of the sounds in the words.

Published articulation screening tests are also available for this purpose. A number of complete articulation tests have a screening version. For example, *The Templin-Darley Test of Articulation* (Templin & Darley, 1969) has 141 items for testing consonants, vowels, diphthongs, and blends. From those 141 items, 50 have been set aside for screening purposes. One simple and briefly administered instrument that can be used for screening is *The Predictive Screening Test of Articulation* (Van Riper & Erickson, 1969). This test is designed to predict whether first-grade children will need treatment to correct their articulation errors or whether they will correct their articulation errors without assistance. It can be administered within a matter of minutes, but the test applies only to first grade children.

When a screening test indicates that a child's or adult's problem is severe enough to warrant further evaluation, we move on to diagnostic procedures.

Background Information (Case History)

The extent of the case history information collected will depend on the severity of the problem. For example, if a child is identified in a school screening as having articulation errors on only one or two sounds, the speech-language pathologist may choose to obtain only a minimum amount of background information. On the other hand, if a child is referred by other sources because he or she is unintelligible, or if she is found to be unintelligible in screening, the professional will want to obtain as much information as possible. The amount of information sought on each person is based on an estimate of the need for detailed information.

In the initial interview with an adult, or with the parent if the client is a child, it is important to try to establish a good understanding of the person's or the parents' viewpoint of the problem. It behooves the speech-language pathologist to establish good communication with the adult or the child's parents and the child himself, for in remediation their cooperation is essential if changes are to take place. Thus, a case history is important not only to obtain information on the variables that contribute to the articulation problem, but to get an idea of the variables which are of concern to the people involved.

In some cases it is essential that the speech-language pathologist obtain information from other professionals such as teachers, psychologists, nurses, social workers, and physicians. Reports from these specialists will help the speech-language pathologist to a better understanding of the problem. When several professionals are involved and after each individual's report has been read, the specialists most concerned about the person may gather to discuss their insights into the problems. They may attempt to formulate a plan together for intervention which will serve the person's needs the best. One of the specialists, the one most closely concerned, may assume primary responsibility for the overall treatment program.

Remember that P.L. 94-142 currently mandates a team approach to assessing and remediating the deficits shown by school-aged handicapped children.

After a case history has been obtained, the speech-language pathologist will administer a number of tests to obtain a comprehensive profile of the communication problem (or problems) and to gather information for planning remediation. The measures may include tests of skills thought to be indirectly related to articulation as well as direct measurement of articulatory behavior. We will examine some of the indirect measures next.

Performance on Related Skills

Earlier in this chapter, we mentioned some of the variables which have been explored as possible causal factors or factors closely related to articulation deficits. As we noted, few of the variables were found to be related. However, one variable which appears to have more relevance than others is auditory discrimination ability. This, then, is a skill that may be tested during articulation evaluation. Depending on the professional's opinion of which discrimination abilities are most important to articulation remediation, an appropriate discrimination test is chosen. If the speech-language pathologist believes that individuals with articulation disorders have problems in discrimination of speech sounds, regardless of whether they produce the sounds incorrectly, a general speech sound discrimination test may be administered. Several are available (for instance, *Wepman Auditory Discrimination Test,* Wepman, 1958; *Templin Speech Sound Discrimination Test,* Templin, 1957). Usually these tests require that the examiner pronounce word or syllable pairs and have the subject indicate whether the words are the same or different. If the speech-language pathologist is interested only in the person's discrimination of his or her own error sounds, the professional may develop a word-pairing test incorporating correct and incorrect productions of the sound. In all likelihood, the speech-language pathologist would try to simulate the error production. For internal discrimination (self-discrimination), the child's or adult's productions may be recorded for later evaluation. The subject is requested to judge the correctness of the responses when they are played back to him or is requested to tell whether the sound was correct directly after it is produced in a word (Lapko & Bankson, 1975). We do not yet know how important this kind of testing is; findings of research studies do not agree (Aungst & Frick, 1964; Williams & McReynolds, 1975), and articulation problems can be corrected by production training. Furthermore, it seems logical to assume that as a child or adult practices correct production of a sound, he or she is simultaneously learning to discriminate correct and incorrect productions. Nevertheless, it is currently speculated that, if any type of discrimination is important, it would be a form of internal discrimination rather than general speech sound discrimination. Therefore, internal discrimination is sometimes tested and included in planning treatment programs.

Speech sound discrimination has been discussed briefly in the description of discrimination approaches to functional articulation disorders.

Language

Speech-language pathologists are encouraged to measure children's language skills for syntactic and morphological performance. This is particularly true with preschool children and children with severe articulation problems. Young children with severe articulation problems frequently have language problems as well. In fact, some speech-language pathologists believe articulation problems to be part of a more global language problem. It is possible, of course, for the speech-language pathologist to record the child's conversation in order to do a complete linguistic analysis of the syntactic and morphological performance, but this is very time consuming. Language sampling for an extended analysis is probably best reserved for children with apparent language deficiencies. A more efficient way to measure language when the problem appears to be mild or moderate is to present a number of commercially available language tests (such as the *Peabody Picture Vocabulary Test,* Dunn, 1965; *Carrow Elicited Language Inventory,* Carrow, 1974; *Test for Auditory Comprehension of Language,* Carrow, 1973), which are less time consuming.

For details on normal language development of young children, see chapter 8.

Motor Skills

Sometimes speech-language pathologists assess a child's ability to perform motor activities that are not associated with speech activities. However, it is probably not profitable to do this kind of testing, since research has shown that the muscles used in speech activities are not the same as those used in nonspeech activities (Shelton, 1963). However, professionals do request clients to perform rapid movements of the articulators in alternating syllables such as *pa-ta-ka* to determine how well the person can shift the articulators from one position to another.

Sensory and Structural Factors

Of special importance to articulation disorders is hearing. The speech-language pathologist will usually have prospective clients screened for hearing loss. The screening may be done by the speech-language pathologist; if a complete hearing test is mandatory, an audiologist may administer the test. It is essential to rule out hearing loss as a possible cause of articulation errors. Hearing impairment has been shown to affect a person's ability to articulate sounds, particularly the fricatives (Ling, 1976).

This is called oral stereognosis.

Some attention has been directed to the ability of people with articulation disorders to use sensory information from manipulation of forms in the mouth. Forms of different shapes and sizes are placed in the mouth while the person's eyes are closed. Afterward, the person selects a picture of the form from an array of pictures. It seems that people with articulation problems do not perform as well on these tasks as people without articulation problems (Ringel, 1970). Nevertheless, little research has explored the effect of training identification of forms in the mouth on speech. Generally, research exploring the effects on speech of training has found little or no relationship between the two behaviors (Shelton, 1971).

Careful procedures for conducting an adequate oral-peripheral examination are offered in Darley and Spriestersbach's book on diagnostic methods (1978).

Of greater importance is an oral-peripheral examination to assure that there is no obvious physical reason for the articulation disorder. The alignment of teeth is checked, the palate is observed, the movement of the tongue is tested, and so forth. The oral-peripheral examination helps rule out organic bases for the articulation errors.

Some speech-language pathologists also check for a condition called *tongue thrust.* They believe that some people exert undue pressure against the teeth, which results in malocclusion and possible articulation disorders. The posture is sometimes changed through training. Tongue thrust is a controversial issue (Mason & Proffit, 1974), however; apparently the training is thought by some to be beneficial, while others think it is not. The Joint Committee on Dentistry and Speech Pathology (1975) has published a statement recommending that tongue thrust treatment not be used routinely and that at the present it should be considered an experimental procedure. Perhaps well-controlled research will contribute better information on this issue in the future.

Skills Needed for Intervention

Finally, the speech-language pathologist needs some sense of the individual's readiness for intervention. Areas which may be assessed, especially in children, include (*a*) ability to pay attention and attention span, (*b*) long- and short-term memory, and (*c*) ability to imitate. Each of these may be a prerequisite to intervention.

Although all of the related skills and sensory and structural factors are considered in evaluation, the most concentrated effort is directed toward obtaining as complete an inventory as possible of the individual's articulatory status. A comprehensive examination of articulatory behavior is essential.

Articulation Assessment

The purpose of the articulation assessment, of course, is to obtain an adequate sample of the person's speech in as many forms as possible in order to allow evaluation of the production of consonants and vowels. Usually, because consonants are more important to intelligibility, emphasis is placed on the articulation of consonants.

Articulation Sample

Ideally, the speech-language pathologist would like to get samples of speech in spontaneous conversation, in naming pictures, and in imitation of words modeled by the examiner. This information helps show if the same sound (the test sound) is produced differently in the three kinds of samples. If an older child or an adult is the client, reading is added to the list.

Speech-language pathologists have always attempted to obtain conversational samples as well as responses to structured test items, but in recent years conversational samples have been given more emphasis. We are accumulating data which indicate that there are differences in production of consonants and vowels in conversation and in single words, as in naming pictures (Faircloth & Blasdell, 1979). The production of sounds in single words does not represent habitual articulation in everyday speech. Conversational samples give a truer picture of an individual's articulation because, as we have seen, production of any sound is affected by phonetic context. This movement needs to be captured in conversational speech because coarticulation takes place not only within single words, but also across word boundaries.

Several problems would be encountered, however, if the speech-language pathologist were to rely totally on conversational samples for information on production of all speech sounds. The primary problem is that some sounds are so infrequent in our language that we would need an enormous sample to evaluate all the sounds. In addition, scoring or transcribing productions from a conversational sample is very time consuming. Finally, speech-language pathologists usually like to obtain several productions of any one sound, particularly if the sound appears in more than one position in a word. Since production may differ as a function of position in a word or syllable, it is preferable to obtain more than one production of the same sound, as a releasing or arresting sound in syllable and word contexts (for instance, /m/ in the word *mop,* in *dummy,* and in *zoom*). To fulfill that requirement, obtaining a representative sample of positions, a large conversational sample would be necessary. The larger the sample, the more time consuming is the analysis of error productions. Therefore, professionals most often use articulation tests to assess articulation. It is safe to say that the articulation test is the major vehicle used to assess articulation disorders. Other measures are generally used to obtain information to supplement the articulation test results. We will now take a brief look at a few commonly used tests.

For example, the /ʒ/ in the word azure *is found in only a few words.*

Articulation Tests

Almost all commercially available tests sample articulation in picture-naming responses. The pictures are of items which can be named by a single word. Commonly, each consonant is tested in three positions: initial (e.g., *s*un), medial (e.g., bicycle), and final (e.g., bu*s*). During testing, the child or adult is shown a picture and asked to name it. The speech-language pathologist records the response on score sheets provided in the testing kit.

In many tests, several forms for recording productions are available to the professional, who selects the one most suitable for his or her purpose in providing the information desired. One simple way to record responses is to note whether the target sound was correctly or incorrectly produced, giving a "right" or "wrong" score. Another recording form is a notation indicating whether the response was a distortion, substitution, or omission (DSO). In some DSO scoring, the substitutions are specified; that is, the professional records the incorrect sound produced for the test sound. A final way of scoring responses is a transcription of the productions. Transcribing a production requires the speech-language pathologist to write exactly what the child or adult said on the score sheet. Usually the symbols of the International Phonetic Alphabet (IPA) are used for transcription. IPA transcription demands greater skill than other forms of response scoring, but on numerous occasions the detailed information can be put to good use in developing treatment plans. The trend in recent years is toward transcribing the responses as carefully as possible, so that the speech-language pathologist has a clear idea of how the person is using the articulators in producing errors. In addition, current linguistic approaches to articulation disorders require close phonetic transcription in order to specify errors explicitly.

This book uses IPA transcription symbols.

Commercially available articulation tests come in slightly different forms, but they are essentially designed to elicit similar responses. For example, in the *Templin-Darley Articulation Test* (Templin & Darley, 1969), a mixture of stimuli is used. At times a sentence completion form is presented. The speech-language pathologist shows a picture, begins describing it, and allows the child or adult to finish the sentence by supplying the word depicted by the picture ("Wash your hands with _____"). Questions are also asked ("What swims in water?"). The picture portion of the *Templin-Darley* is suitable for testing younger children, while for older persons a sentence form is available. The client reads a sentence containing words with the target sound. For instance, to test the /s/ sound, the sentence reads, "Sam helped a passenger get on the bus." Many tests simply require the person to look at the picture and answer the question, "What is it?"

Refer to the description of his approach to articulation disorders earlier in this chapter.

A somewhat different kind of test was developed by McDonald (1964). A sound is tested in only two positions instead of three, as an arresting sound in a syllable and as a releasing sound in a syllable. Moreoever, each consonant and vowel included in the test is sampled in approximately 48 contexts. Each sound is tested in two-syllable contexts in which the syllables are formed by two one-syllable words. The words are names for two pictures displayed side by side. For instance, in a sample of /s/ items, pairs of words such as *cup-sun, tub-sun, kite-sun,* and so forth are presented to test the /s/ in a releasing position in a syllable. The /s/ forms an arresting position in word pairs such as *house-pipe, house-bell,* and *house-tie.* McDonald developed these numerous contexts in order to give the person an opportunity to produce the target sound correctly if it is present in the repertoire in some phonetic context.

An articulation test which assesses the severity of an articulation problem in relation to the frequency of occurrence of individual phonemes in the language is the *Arizona Articulation Proficiency Scale* (Barker, 1972). Like most commercial articulation tests, it uses pictures to elicit single-word responses. In addition to providing a description of a child's articulation errors, it allows the errors to be analyzed in terms of a numerical index of intelligibility.

Weighted scores are assigned to sounds according to the frequency of occurrence of each sound in the English language. They form the index of intelligibility. The percentage correct score describes the intelligibility of a child's articulation.

The Fisher-Logemann Articulation Test (Fisher & Logemann, 1971) was developed with distinctive features in mind. As in most standard articulation tests, pictures are named; but the responses are analyzed according to place, voice, and manner errors. Narrow phonetic transcription of the responses is required in order to identify the features in error.

Many other articulation tests, such as the *Goldman-Fristoe Test of Articulation* (Goldman & Fristoe, 1969), are also available. In addition, some speech-language pathologists develop their own articulation tests using pictures from books or magazines.

Stimulability Testing

In addition to eliciting spontaneous picture naming, children and adults are tested for their ability to imitate correct production of their error sound or sounds. This procedure is known as **stimulability** testing (Carter & Buck, 1958) and was introduced into evaluation procedures by Milisen (1954). The speech-language pathologist provides a model (a correct production of the sound) and asks the person to imitate the model in words, syllables, phrases, and isolation. Frequently the model is accompanied by instructions or other help concerning placement of the articulators for production of the sound. Stimulability can be used to discover if the individual has the phonetic ability to produce the sound. Stimulability is also used for prognosis. It is one of the variables found relevant to articulation disorders, principally as a predictive tool. Children who can imitate their error sounds correctly are thought to present a favorable prognosis. Speech-language pathologists may decide to delay treatment of stimulable children, with the expectation that correct production may develop without direct training. Even when stimulability information is not used predictively, a child's performance on this task assists in planning and treatment, especially in regard to procedures for initial training steps. For example, training imitation is unnecessary because the child already imitates well. Furthermore, involved instructions on production are not needed because the child knows how to produce the sound. Stimulable children are expected to move through treatment more rapidly than unstimulable children.

Conversational Sample

In addition to the articulation and stimulability tests, a conversational sample my be recorded for later analysis. For hesitant children, pictures are presented to elicit spontaneous speech. Speech-language pathologists learn to provide cues and prompts which work effectively for obtaining speech from children.

Use of Evaluation Information

A number of results from the evaluation can be used in decision making. Traditionally, the determination that an individual has an articulation disorder is based on a combination of factors. A few of the most important for this decision include (a) the person's age, (b) the number of sounds in error, (c) the consistency of error productions, (d) the form of the errors, (e) stimulability, and (f) dialectal distinctions. We will discuss the use of each of these factors.

With almost all children, speech-language pathologists use a developmental norm analysis to determine whether the sounds in error are produced correctly by most children of comparable age. If they are not, the professional may decide that the problem does not warrant treatment. Frequently in this case the child is placed on a list to be rechecked within a few months or a year, in order to determine whether the correct production has developed. However, if the sounds in error are sounds which most children younger than the client are producing correctly, the speech-language pathologist will probably decide that treatment is warranted. Developmental norms are less useful for older children and adults in deciding if training is needed. When developmental norms are used in the analysis and if they are the primary determiners, the speech-language pathologist will sequence training on the basis of sound acquisition. Sounds which are acquired early will be trained before later-appearing sounds.

Although age comparison is important, other factors are used in conjunction with the developmental time table. Among these may be the number of error sounds in the person's repertoire. Customarily, a child or adult with many sounds in error would be considered to be more urgently in need of treatment than a person with only one or two sounds in error. But that decision also depends on the form of the error and whether the incorrect productions are consistent. If the child shows an inconsistent pattern, producing both correct and incorrect forms of a target sound, the correct sound may be in a transition stage. It is possible that the correct production, which is now unstable, will stablize without training. And if the error sound appears more in the form of a distortion than a substitution or an omission, the correct production may emerge in time without direct training. One other variable is considered in sifting through the information obtained during evaluation—stimulability. If the child produced the sound correctly in imitation, training may be delayed in order to give the correct production an opportunity to emerge without training.

All of these variables are weighted singly and in combination in determining if an articulation problem is severe enough to require treatment. Information on other factors will influence the decision as well. Among these are the cultural and/or dialectal variations which are acceptable in the speech community in which the child or adult lives. People living in the South produce the vowels differently from people living in Northern states, and Northeasterners drop the /r/ after vowels. Black English Vernacular accounts for some articulatory differences from Standard English. These differences may not constitute an articulation disorder, particularly if they are not contrary to the speech practices of a given community; and speech-language pathologists must keep these variations in mind when diagnosing articulation disorders.

Recall the discussion on dialectal variations in speech in chapter 3.

Consideration also needs to be given to the person's own concern about his or her articulation; or, if the client is a child, concern expressed by parents or teachers. If these individuals feel that the articulation errors render the person unintelligible, or if other people find the person unintelligible, the speech-language pathologist must consider these concerns in evaluating the articulation errors. In addition, reports from other sources that articulation errors interfere with intelligibility will influence decisions by the speech-language pathologist. A factor of some importance in many cases is the person's own motivation for changing his or her articulation pattern.

Linguistically Derived Analyses

More in-depth analyses of evaluation results are used by those who believe that articulation problems arise from linguistic deficits more than other sources. Because these professionals suspect that a system is operating to account for the errors and that the errors are related to each other, their analyses are directed to revealing these relationships. As we saw earlier, two kinds of analyses may be performed: (a) a distinctive feature analysis (McReynolds & Engmann, 1975) and (b) a phonological process analysis (Hodson, 1980; Wiener, 1979).

In a distinctive feature analysis, features composing the target sounds are compared to the features composing the error sounds which replace the target sound. The purpose is to identify the one feature or the few features which are in error and account for a number of error sounds. If any such features are found, the speech-language pathologist would use the analysis results to select the features to be trained contrastively. For example, if a child were found to substitute discontinuant sounds such as /tʃ/, /dʒ/, /t/, and /p/ for continuant sounds such as /ʃ/, /ð/, /s/, and /f/, then the child would be trained to establish the discontinuant and continuant feature contrast in a pair of sounds which differ only on that feature. In our example, the pair might be the /tʃ/ and /ʃ/ sounds. Except for the features of continuancy and non-continuancy, these two sounds are composed of the same articulatory features. Because a distinctive feature analysis is time consuming, many speech-language pathologists do not use it unless a child has several error sounds which are difficult to explain without seeking a common factor among them.

In a phonological process analysis, all errors are categorized under the processes which appear to fit the description of the process (for example, all words in which the final consonant is omitted are placed in the category of "final consonant deletion" process; all words in which fricatives are replaced by stops are classified as being operated upon by the "process of stopping"). The analysis is usually performed on a conversational speech sample because all processes are supposed to be context-sensitive. For example, a final consonant deletion process can be demonstrated only in contexts requiring final consonants, as in words. After each word in the sample is carefully analyzed for processes (there are 8 to 40 or more processes possible, depending on the author), the speech-language pathologist selects the processes, one by one, which will be targets in remediation. The goal in treatment is to eliminate the processes, because these simplification processes are responsible for the articulation errors.

Summary

We have described a number of analysis procedures and variables to be taken into account in planning remediation, including:

(1) Analysis based on developmental sequence of sound
(2) Analysis of distortions, substitutions, and omissions
(3) Analysis based on distinctive features and
(4) A phonological process analysis.

Variables which will influence the decision, in addition to the results of the analysis, include:

(1) Chronological age
(2) Stimulability
(3) Consistency
(4) Number of errors
(5) The form of the error sound
(6) Dialectal influences and
(7) Client concern and motivation.

Customarily the speech-language pathologist attempts to place information derived from all of these measures into perspective. Decisions as to which sounds to train, where training should begin, and how training should proceed are usually founded on information from a combination of the factors.

Evaluation Report

When all the data from the initial interview and the audiological, peripheral, and other tests are in, and the articulation analysis has been completed, a summary speech evaluation report is written. The purposes of the report are to (a) indicate whether the person has an articulation disorder, (b) describe the articulation carefully, (c) make some statements, if applicable, about etiology and prognosis, and (d) make recommendations regarding the kind of training most suitable for the individual. If other professionals have been involved in the evaluation, copies of the report are distributed to them. When the evaluation report has been completed and treatment is indicated, a remediation program based on the recommendations is developed. Remediation is considered next.

REMEDIATION

We have already seen that speech-language pathologists emphasize testing of those variables which are most relevant to their particular approach to the nature of articulation problems. Remediation programs are also subject to the same biases. In addition, other variables enter into decisions about the direction training should take. For example, speech-language pathologists may choose specific procedures from a variety of approaches to develop a treatment package. Some tailor treatment programs to meet the needs of individual clients, while others administer similar treatment to everyone, regardless of the history, the nature of the problem, or the pattern of each person's articulation errors. Further, professionals differ in their opinions as to whether the articulation errors should be treated directly or indirectly. If indirectly, treatment may be aimed at causes or other problems which are thought to be responsible for, or to contribute heavily to, the articulation problem. Thus approaches to remediation are numerous and depend somewhat on the training received by the speech-language pathologist in his or her academic program. Since research has not been devoted to careful evaluation of the approaches or models which have been proposed, we cannot suggest that any one or several programs are more effective than others.

General Principles

Although, on the surface, diversity in remediation programs seems the status quo, there is some agreement on broad principles underlying treatment programs. Ordinarily, intervention is viewed in terms of learning principles (Bankson & Bernthal, in press; Winitz, 1969). Remediation may be thought of as training in learning a motor skill, a discrimination skill, an articulatory response, or a phonological rule, but regardless of what is thought to be trained—that is, the content of what is learned—it is generally recognized that learning takes place during treatment. Therefore, learning principles are used.

Treatment is usually divided into at least two phases: acquisition and generalization. Alternatively, some authors refer to three phases: acquisition, habituation, and automatization. In both cases, however, articulation remediation is considered to consist of a phase in which the person is made aware of how a sound is produced correctly and is provided with deliberate practice in producing the sound at a conscious level, and a phase or phases in which the person gradually learns to produce the sound effortlessly in a variety of contexts and situations.

Acquisition Training

Acquisition training consists of graduated training steps during which the child or adult is taught to produce the target sound consciously. During training, the person is guided carefully through a series of graduated steps from an incorrect production to approximation of the target response and finally to the correct response (Bankson & Bernthal, in press; Van Riper, 1978). Not only is the specific response developed gradually, so are the contexts in which the response is produced. For example, the progression may be from learning to produce the target sound in isolation, to learning to produce it in more complex units in a sequence from syllables to words to phrases and sentences. A sequence may also be followed in the kind of stimuli presented and the kind of response required. For example, in initial phases, if needed, the person is given a model of the sound and asked to imitate the model. When the imitation is accurate, the speech-language pathologist may shift control to spontaneous production of the target sound. This may be done in a number of ways; most commonly, pictures with the target sound in the names are presented, and the child responds to them. Control can be shifted from picture naming to supplying a word with the target sound in a sentence completion form or to reading (if the child can read). Adults may go directly from imitating to reading.

Within this general framework, speech-language pathologists apply their own specific procedures. For example, some who view articulation as learning a motor skill may give a person extensive instructions on placement of the articulators during production of a sound and detailed feedback concerning the adequacy of the production after he has responded. Others use a minimum of verbal explanation, relying instead on precise, immediate, and briefly presented feedback which indicates if the response was correct or incorrect. For those who believe in a structured approach to remediation (and they are probably in the majority), operant conditioning offers precise procedures for treatment. Emphasis is on presenting clear definitions of stimuli and using carefully controlled procedures which gradually shape the correct response through approximations in training. Special emphasis is placed on the role of consequent events. Correct responses are reinforced (with tokens, praise, or other desirables), and incorrect responses are either ignored or punished (the clinician may tell the client the response is wrong or take back tokens earned during the session). Many articulation programs applying principles of operant conditioning are available (Costello, 1977; Gerber, 1977). The programs are often written so specifically that they can be administered by an aide.

A general outline of training phrases is found in Table 5.3.

Generalization

Articulation remediation, of course, has the goal of changing error sounds to correct sounds which are used in everyday speech in all situations. After the sound has been trained so that the person can produce it readily, attention shifts to generalization of the sound to a variety of contexts, situations, and persons. We do not know much about how best to effect generalization (McReynolds & Elbert, in press). Therefore, speech-language pathologists attempt to conduct carry-over work by shifting from highly structured to less

TABLE 5.3
General Outline of Remediation Phases and Materials Used.

I. Acquisition
   A. Imitative production
      1. Responses
         a. Isolated sound
         b. Syllables—Sound in initial, medial, final positions
         c. Words—Sounds in initial, medial, final position
      2. Materials
         a. Clinician produces model
         b. Pictures
   B. Spontaneous production
      1. Responses
         a. Words
         b. Phrases
         c. Sentences
      2. Materials
         a. Pictures
         b. Completion sentences
         c. Short stories
II. Automatization or generalization phase
   A. Conversations with speech-language pathologist on topics of interest
   B. Conversation with speech-language pathologist in setting other than clinic or school
   C. Conversations with other individuals in clinic or school
   D. Conversations with other individuals in other settings

structured lessons involving reading or conversational speech. Occasionally professionals will bring in other people to participate in the sessions, in order to encourage carry-over of the correct articulation with other individuals. They also ask classroom teachers to remind a child or, if the client is an adult, ask family members to be alert to the person's articulation. However, we must be careful to caution others not to overdo their help, so that the person does not become overly self-conscious about the problem. Self-consciousness could result in the person talking less, which defeats the purpose of the treatment program.

The newer linguistic approaches to articulation disorders offer an opportunity to structure training so that untrained sounds and contexts may generalize. Recall that both the distinctive feature and the phonological disorders approaches assume that a system with rules is used. Thus, as in language, to change a rule, each item affected by the rule need not be trained individually. Instead, training on a few examples might lead to a change in the remaining items affected by the rule. The linguistic models are appealing in terms of the possibility of obtaining generalization with minimum training; however, data for this generalization are not abundant. Generalization has been shown to occur when features are trained (Costello & Onstine, 1976; McReynolds & Bennett, 1972), but no reports of generalization from phonological process training have yet been published (McReynolds & Elbert, 1981b).

In summary, remediation is an individual process for most speech-language pathologists. Mostly, it depends on each person's biases in regard to the nature of functional articulation disorders. Nevertheless, most speech-language pathologists, when they are exposed to procedures which have been shown to be effective, will incorporate them into the framework of their remediation principles. At this point, procedures used in acquisition training are specified better than are procedures which will facilitate generalization of the newly acquired target sound.

As we have seen already, of primary importance to any therapeutic endeavor is trust and understanding between the person with a problem and the helping professional. This is true in treatment of articulation disorders, too. The speech-language pathologist should put forth every effort to gain the child's or adult's cooperation. This is best done by recognizing that the client is a person to be respected, entitled to courteous treatment and understanding at all times. This will be aided if the speech-language pathologist tries to understand each person's unique needs, adjusting training so that it suits those needs. It is profitable to spend time encouraging the person to become an active participant in the remediation process, well-motivated to change the articulation pattern which is in error.

CONCLUSION

Articulation problems are successfully identified, assessed, and treated. At present many methods are used for these purposes, all with some degree of effectiveness. Recently the complexity of articulation and articulation problems has gained greater recognition. This awareness in turn has generated issues needing to be addressed in carefully controlled research studies. Happily, it has also resulted in new and exciting approaches to understanding and treating functional articulation disorders.

SELECTED READINGS

Backus, O., & Beasley, J. *Speech therapy with children.* Boston: Houghton Mifflin, 1951.

Bernthal, J. E., & Bankson, N. W. *Articulation disorders.* Englewood Cliffs, N.J.: Prentice-Hall, 1981.

Darley, S. L., Aronson, A. R., & Brown, J. R. *Motor speech disorders.* Philadelphia: W. B. Saunders, 1975.

Ingram, D. *Phonological disability in children,* New York: Elsevier, 1976.

McReynolds, L. V., & Elbert M. *Articulation disorders of unknown etiology and their remediation.* In N. Lass, L. McReynolds, J. Northern, & D. Yoder (Eds.), *Speech, language and hearing.* Philadelphia: W. B. Saunders, in press.

Winitz, H. *Articulatory acquisition and behavior.* New York: Appleton-Century-Crofts, 1969.

Winitz, H. *From syllable to conversation.* Baltimore: University Park Press, 1975.

REFERENCES

Aungst, L. F., & Frick, J. V. Auditory discrimination ability and consistency of articulation of /r/. *Journal of Speech and Hearing Disorders,* 1964, *29,* 76–85.

Backus, O., & Beasley, J. *Speech therapy with children.* Boston: Houghton Mifflin, 1951.

Bankson, N., & Bernthal, J. Assessment of articulation. In N. Lass, L. McReynolds, J. Northern, & D. Yoder (Eds.), *Speech, language and hearing.* Philadelphia: W. B. Saunders, in press.

Barker, J. *Arizona Articulation Proficiency Scale.* Los Angeles: Western Psychological Service, 1972.

Carrow, E. *Test for Auditory Comprehension of Language.* Austin, Tex.: Urban Research Group, 1973.

Carrow, E. *Carrow Elicited Language Inventory, Learning Concepts.* Austin, Tex.: Author, 1974.

Carter, E. T., & Buck, M. B. Prognostic testing for functional articulation disorders among children in the first grade. *Journal of Speech and Hearing Disorders,* 1958, *23,* 124–133.

Costello, J. Programmed instruction. *Journal of Speech and Hearing Disorders,* 1977, *42,* 3–28.

Costello, J., & Onstine, J. The modification of multiple articulation errors based on distinctive feature theory. *Journal of Speech and Hearing Disorders,* 1976, *41,* 199–215.

Cruttenden, A. A phonetic study of babbling. *British Journal of Disorders of Communication,* 1970, *5,* 110–117.

Daniloff, R. G., & Hammarberg, R. E. On defining coarticulation. *Journal of Phonetics,* 1973, *1,* 239–248.

Darley, F. L., Aronson, A. R., & Brown, J. R. *Motor speech disorders.* Philadelphia: W. B. Saunders, 1975.

Darley, F., & Spriestersbach, D. *Diagnostic methods in speech pathology* (2nd ed.). New York: Harper & Row, 1978.

Dunn, L. B. *Peabody Picture Vocabulary Test.* Circle Pines, Minn.: American Guidance Service, 1965.

Elbert, M., & McReynolds, L. V. Transfer of /r/ across contexts. *Journal of Speech and Hearing Disorders,* 1975, *40,* 380–387.

Elbert, M., & McReynolds, L. V. An experimental analysis of misarticulating children's generalization. *Journal of Speech and Hearing Research,* 1978, *21,* 136–150.

Faircloth, M. A., & Blasdell, R. C. Conversational speech behaviors. In N. Lass (Ed.), *Speech and language: Advances in basic research and practice* (Vol. 2). New York: Academic Press, 1979.

Fisher, H. B., & Logemann, J. A. *The Fisher-Logemann Test of Articulation Competence.* Boston: Houghton Mifflin, 1971.

Garrett, E. R. Programmed articulation therapy. In W. D. Wolfe & D. J. Goulding (Eds.), *Articulation and learning.* Springfield, Ill.: Charles C Thomas, 1973.

Gerber, A. Programming for articulation modification. *Journal of Speech and Hearing Disorders,* 1977, *42,* 29–43.

Goldman, R., & Fristoe, M. *Goldman-Fristoe Test of Articulation.* Circle Pines, Minn.: American Guidance Service, 1969.

Hahn, E. Indications for direct, nondirect, and indirect methods in speech correction. *Journal of Speech and Hearing Disorders,* 1961, *26,* 230–236.

Hodson, B. W. *The assessment of phonological processes.* Danville, Ill.: Interstate Printers and Publishers, 1980.

Ingram, D. *Phonological disability in children.* New York: Elsevier, 1976.

Irwin, J. V., & Weston, A. J. The paired stimuli monograph. *Acta Symbolica,* 1975, *4,* 1–76.

Jakobson, R. Kindersprache, Aphasie and Allgemeine Loutgesetze. *Child language aphasia and phonological universals* (1941). (A. R. Keiler trans.). The Hague: Mouton, 1968.

Joint Committee on Dentistry and Speech Pathology-Audiology. Position statement on tongue thrust. *Asha,* 1975, *17,* 331–340.

Lapko, L. L., & Bankson, N. W. Relationship between auditory discrimination, stimulability and consistency of misarticulation. *Perceptual and Motor Skills,* 1975, *40,* 171–177.

Ling, D. *Speech and the hearing impaired child: Theory and practice.* Washington, D.C.: Alexander Graham Bell Association for the Deaf, 1976.

Mason, R. M., & Proffit, W. R. The tongue thrust controversy: Background and recommendations. *Journal of Speech and Hearing Disorders,* 1974, *39,* 115–132.

McDonald, E. T. *Articulation testing and treatment: A sensory-motor approach.* Pittsburgh: Stanwix House, 1964.

McReynolds, L. V. Behavioral and linguistic considerations in children's speech production. In J. F. Kavanagh & W. Strange (Eds.), *Speech and language in the laboratory, school and clinic.* Cambridge, Mass.: MIT Press, 1978.

McReynolds, L. V., & Bennett, S. Distinctive feature generalization in articulation training. *Journal of Speech and Hearing Disorders,* 1972, *37,* 462–470.

McReynolds, L. V., & Elbert, M. Articulation disorders of unknown etiology and their remediation. In N. Lass, L. McReynolds, J. Northern, & D. Yoder (Eds.), *Speech, language, and hearing.* Philadelphia: W. B. Saunders, in press.

McReynolds, L. V., & Elbert, M. Criteria for phonological process analysis. *Journal of Speech and Hearing Disorders,* 1981, *46,* 197–204. (a)

McReynolds, L. V., & Elbert, M. Generalization of correct articulation in clusters. *Applied Psycholinguistics,* 1981, *2,* 119–132. (b)

McReynolds, L. V., & Engmann, D. L. *Distinctive feature analysis of misarticulations.* Baltimore: University Park Press, 1975.

McReynolds, L. V., & Huston, K. A. A distinctive feature analysis of children's misarticulations. *Journal of Speech and Hearing Disorders,* 1971, *36,* 155–166.

Milisen, R. A rationale for articulation disorders. *Journal of Speech and Hearing Disorders.* Monograph Supplement No. 4, 1954, 6–17.

Mowrer, D. E. Behavioral appilcation to modification of articulation. In D. Wolfe & D. Goulding (Eds.), *Articulation and learning.* Springfield, Ill.: Charles C Thomas, 1973.

Mowrer, D. E. *Methods of modifying speech behaviors.* Columbus, Ohio: Charles E. Merrill, 1978.

Oller, D. K., Wieman, L. A., Doyle, W. J., & Ross, C. *Child speech, babbling and phonological universals.* Paper presented at the Sixth Child Language Research Forum, Stanford University, Palo Alto, California, April, 1974.

Pierce, J. E. *A study of 750 Portland, Oregon children during the first year.* Paper presented at the Sixth Child Language Research Forum, Stanford University, Palo Alto, California, April, 1974.

Poole, I. Genetic development of articulation of consonant sounds in speech. *Elementary English Review,* 1934, *11,* 159–161.

Prather, E. M., Hedrick, D. L., & Kern, C. A. Articulation development in children aged two to four years. *Journal of Speech and Hearing Disorders,* 1975, *40,* 179–191.

Rees, N. The role of babbling in the child's acquisition of language. *British Journal of Disorders of Communication,* 1972, *1,* 17–23.

Ringel, R. L. Oral sensation and perception: A selective review. *ASHA Report #5.* Washington, D.C.: American Speech and Hearing Association, 1970.

Rousey, C. L. The psychopathology of articulation and voice deviations. In L. E. Travis (Ed.), *Handbook of speech pathology and audiology.* New York: Appleton-Century-Crofts, 1971.

Shelton, R. L. Therapeutic exercise and speech pathology. *Asha,* 1963, *5,* 855–859.

Shelton, R. L. Oral sensory function in speech production. In W. C. Grabb, S. Rosenstein, & K. Bzoch (Eds.), *Cleft lip and palate.* Boston: Little, Brown, 1971.

Shelton, R. L. Disorders of articulation. In P. H. Skinner & R. L. Shelton (Eds.), *Speech, language and hearing.* Reading, Mass.: Addison-Wesley, 1978.

Shelton, R. L., & McReynolds, L. V. Functional articulation disorders: Preliminaries to treatment. In N. Lass (Ed.), *Speech and language: Advances in basic research and practice* (Vol. 2). New York: Academic Press, 1979.

Shriberg, L. D. Developmental phonological disorders. In T. J. Hixon, J. H. Saxman, & L. D. Shriberg (Eds.), *Introduction to communication disorders.* Englewood Cliffs, N.J.: Prentice-Hall, 1980.

Singh, S., & Frank, D. A distinctive feature analysis of the consonantal substitution pattern. *Language and Speech,* 1972, *15,* 209–218.

Stark, R. E., Rose, S. N., & McLagen, M. Features of infant sounds: The first eight weeks of life. *Journal of Child Language,* 1975, *2,* 205–221.

Templin, M. C. Templin Speech Sound Discrimination Test. In M. C. Templin, *Certain language skills in children.* Minneapolis: University of Minnesota Press, 1957.

Templin, M. C., & Darley, F. L. *The Templin-Darley Test of Articulation* (2nd ed.). Iowa City: University of Iowa, Bureau of Educational Research and Service, Division of Extension and University Services, 1969.

Van Riper, C. *Speech correction principles and methods* (6th ed.). Englewood Cliffs, N.J.: Prentice-Hall, 1978.

Van Riper, C., & Erickson, R. L. *The Predictive Screening Test of Articulation.* Kalamazoo: Western Michigan University, 1969.

Van Riper, C., & Irwin, J. F. *Voice and articulation.* Englewood Cliffs, N.J.: Prentice-Hall, 1958.

Wellman, B. L., Case, I. M., Mengert, I. G., & Bradbury, D. E. Speech sounds of young children. *University of Iowa Studies in Child Welfare,* 1931, *5*(2).

Wepman, J. M. *Wepman Auditory Discrimination Test: Manual of Directions.* Chicago: Language Research Association, 1958.

Wiener, F. F. *Phonological process analysis.* Baltimore: University Park Press, 1979.

Williams, G. C., & McReynolds, L. V. The relationship between discrimination and articulation training in children with misarticulations. *Journal of Speech and Hearing Research,* 1975, *18,* 401–412.

Winitz, H. *Articulatory acquisition and behavior.* New York: Appleton-Century-Crofts, 1969.

Winitz, H. *From syllable to conversation.* Baltimore: University Park Press, 1975.

VOICE DISORDERS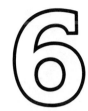

G. Paul Moore

Keith, a 27-year-old-high school football coach and teacher with an excellent physique and physical condition, referred himself to the speech and hearing clinic with a moderately severe breathy and hoarse voice and intermittent moments of total voice loss. His pitch range was limited to the low notes in his potential range. He had lost the higher notes with progression of the voice disorder. The coach reported that he was very verbal, which was confirmed by the fact that he talked almost continuously during the evaluation.

A medical report showed typical bilateral vocal nodules of moderate size. Both vocal cords were slightly inflamed. Keith reported a long history of hoarseness. He has always been active physically and vocally and noted that the hoarseness had recently become worse. An older friend and coach also had a hoarse voice and a laryngeal tumor of some sort that required surgery. This experience frightened Keith into attending to his problem.

His typical daily routine begins at 5:00 AM with 7 miles of jogging. At 6:30, he conducts football practice, which continues until the start of the regular school schedule. He teaches five classes each day in which he lectures most of the time. After school there is more football practice and sometimes he holds private classes in gymnastics. He arrives home around 8:00 PM; after dinner, he often reads bedtime stories to his 3-year-old son. During those evenings when his team has a football game, he shouts and yells almost continuously throughout the game. His voice is always extremely hoarse following a game.

A diagnosis of moderately severe breathy-hoarseness with intermittent loss of voice resulting from medium size, bilateral vocal nodules was made. These lesions were caused by excessive vocal use and abuse in his occupation as coach and teacher.

Keith lived in a region where he could not obtain direct aid from a speech-language pathologist. Consequently, we planned a program with him which contained the following parts. (a) Detailed description of the nature and causes of vocal nodules. This information was presented at the time of the voice evaluation with the aid of photographs of vocal nodules and the playing of his voice recording. The need to eliminate vocal abuse and reduce speaking to a minimum was stressed. (b) Review of the work situation to identify places where vocal abuse could be reduced. This discussion resulted subsequently in the following actions: elimination of all *except essential speaking (he put himself on almost complete silence for 10 days); introduction of a whistle and bull horn for signalling and giving instructions on the football field; alteration of his classroom methods to use students in instruction, more written work, and the like; and restraint of vocal output during games.*

After 1 month, Keith returned to the clinic for re-evaluation. His voice had improved substantially; and although the nodules were still present, the general inflammation had subsided and the nodules were somewhat smaller. A continuation of the same therapy regimen was recommended. Subsequent evaluations at intervals over the next several months revealed continued improvement except for temporary set-backs following games during which he had yelled.

One of the most important changes affecting the ultimate management of this voice problem was Keith's perception of his role as a coach. He came to realize that his excessive yelling was an extension of his own participation in the sport. During the games and practice sessions, he partially reverted to his playing days through his shouting and excessive verbal output. When his thinking became more mature, Keith was able to exert appropriate control of his voice.

You may now wish to listen to the speech sample accompanying this chapter, found on Audio Disc 1, Side 1 (sample #2).

The vocal sample on your audio disc could have been a rough, gravelly sound or some other dramatic illustration of a voice disorder. However, a deviation of moderate severity associated with vocal nodules was selected because it demonstrates a type of problem speech-language pathologists meet frequently. If possible, listen to the voice several times. Note particularly the persistent breathiness, the intermittent **aphonia,** and the subtle reduction in these features following therapy (as revealed in the second sample.) The next time you have a chance, listen to the voices of your family and friends, of sales people and waiters and other people you meet. Listen to your own voice. Do you hear any hoarseness, nasality, breathiness?

Aphonia *is complete loss of voice.*

What would you, as a speech-language pathologist, do with and for the man whose voice and case summary were presented? What about those other voices you listened to? Discovering answers to those questions and similar questions about other voice problems is the goal for this chapter.

VOICE PROBLEMS AMONG COMMUNICATION DISORDERS

Many people are difficult to understand or have speech that is unpleasant or unattractive to hear. Their manner of speaking may limit the type of work they can do and may affect their social acceptance by other people. Some omit or distort certain sounds of the language; others substitute one sound for another, as when someone says, "Mith thmith thent me to thee you." This type of speech, of course, is an articulation disorder. Other individuals speak with many interruptions in the flow of speech, with pauses where they do not belong and with meaningless repetitions of sounds or words. This kind of speech is called stuttering. The pitch of the voice of still others is inappropriate. For a man it might be too high; for a woman, too low. Some have voices that

See chapter 5.

See chapter 7.

are too weak; others, too loud. Still others have voice quality deviations such as hoarseness or too much nasal resonance. The last three kinds of deviations—pitch, loudness, and quality—are customarily classified as voice disorders. These problems sometimes exist by themselves, but frequently they are combined with other voice or speech problems to form a complex communication disorder. No one of the types of deviation can be considered more important than another, and the speech-language pathologist must be prepared to manage each or all, regardless of their combinations. The complexity of voice disorders and the negative emotional reactions they can produce in both the speaker and the listener make them a definite challenge for the language professional.

Normal and Abnormal Voice

How can voice disorders be recognized? How are they determined? Perhaps the easiest way to get at the question is to try to define the "normal" voice. Experience tells us that there are many normal voices. We distinguish the voices of babies, children, adolescents, adult men and women, and aged men and women. Each of these groups has distinctive characteristics, and they are different from each other; yet they are "normal" so long as they meet our expectations for the group. On the other hand, when the pitch, loudness, or quaity of a voice differs from that which is customary in the voices of others of the same age, sex, or cultural background, we classify it as deviant or defective. Obviously, the listener's personal criteria, which are derived from training and experience, are the bases for these judgments. Almost everyone will consider an extremely hoarse voice to be defective, but there are many degrees of hoarseness. Where on the continuum from severely defective to excellent will a particular voice be placed? For example, what about Rod Stewart—is his voice "too" hoarse? There are no electronic or other instruments that will place a voice on the scale for us. The listener must make the judgment. Though everyone has a set of criteria for vocal excellence, your evaluation skills will improve with training. Consequently, it is essential that people dealing with speech-language pathology learn to listen definitively. As one of the great early speech pathologists, Wendell Johnson, said, "Speech pathologists must grow long ears."

Prevalence of Voice Disorders

How many voice problems are there in the population? Do these deviations justify the attention of the speech-language pathologist? Many surveys have been made of school populations, but there are no firm figures for the general adult population. The studies in the schools report wide variations that range from a few percent to 20% or more (Milisen, 1971, p. 628; Senturia & Wilson, 1968; Silverman & Zimmer, 1975). These differences probably result from variables such as the grade levels surveyed, the procedures used to gather and evaluate data, the criteria used, and possibly the cultural environment. Children in the lower grades usually have more deviations than older children (Baynes, 1966; Sauchelli, 1979). When we consider all the variables, we can see that selecting even an approximate estimate of the number of voice problems in the schools is arbitrary. However, we need some reasonable estimate to use as a basis for planning remedial programs. Consequently, a compromise, based on the largest survey thus far reported, justifies our accepting 6% as a reasonable estimate (Senturia & Wilson, 1968).

Voice disorders are heard frequently in the adult population, but no reliable estimate of the numbers involved is available. Actually, since voice disorders rarely interfere with understanding what is said, lay people pay relatively little attention to most of them. One reason is probably that acute temporary conditions such as colds, laryngitis, and other upper respiratory disturbances that cause hoarseness, breathiness, hyponasality, and other vocal variations are so common that they are not a source of concern. Unfortunately the chronic and sometimes very serious conditions that affect the same areas and cause the same types of vocal deviations also tend to be ignored.

Another attitude often associated with voice disorders frequently impairs remedial work. A voice—whether it is good, poor, or in between—tends to be identified with the person who uses it. Many people have a strong resistance to change, even when the voice is clearly seriously defective.

Dysphonia describes any condition of poor or unpleasant voice quality.

A contrasting attitude is found universally among persons who depend upon their voices in their work. **Dysphonias,** whether resulting from disease or from no apparent organic cause, can be a source of great concern. When your income or social acceptance is threatened, you are highly motivated to correct the problem. Many singers, teachers, lawyers, and preachers seek help for voice problems.

There are also many other people in a variety of professions who as part of their work are vitally concerned with voice and its production. In music journals, you can find articles about voice written by singers and teachers of singers; there are many studies reported in the professional speech literature by speech pathologists, linguists, phoneticians, actors, and teachers of speakers; a number of medical journals publish reports by such specialists as laryngologists, neurologists, psychiatrists, and endocrinologists about disease and rehabilitation of the vocal mechanism; engineers, particularly acoustical and electrical engineers, write about vocal sound, its composition, analysis, synthesis, and transmission. Voice is an enormously complex phenomenon. Those who are primarily concerned with the remediation and prevention of voice disorders are fortunate that there is so much help. This broad involvement of other scientific and artistic disciplines challenges every speech-language pathologist to extend his or her own knowledge well beyond the confines of speech pathology.

PHONATION AND THE LARYNX

When a baby is born, it cries almost immediately. That squalling is music to the parents and others in attendance, but the voice cannot properly be called *musical.* The infant fills his lungs with air and expels it vigorously. As the air rushes out, the vocal cords in the larynx come together and are forced to flutter. This vibration may be regular or irregular, but it rapidly interrupts what would otherwise be a relatively continuous, rushing air stream. The rapid interruptions of the air flow create pressure changes or sound waves in the air, which radiate in all directions from the infant's mouth and stimulate the ears of the listeners. As the infant matures, he learns to vary the vocal sound to express hunger, pain, discomfort, or pleasure—by cooing, squealing, and laughing. Additional refinement in voice production occurs with the acquisition of language, which is linked to the parallel maturation of the awesomely complex hearing, vision, neural, and muscle systems.

As we saw in chapter 4, the larynx is a remarkably sturdy, yet sensitive, organ. It has four major biological protective functions: (*a*) closing the airway to protect the lungs from food and liquids; (*b*) impounding the breath, thereby stablizing the rib cage for more efficient muscle support in lifting; (*c*) impounding the air for increasing internal abdominal pressure, as in bearing down; and (*d*) opening the airway to allow easy inhalation and exhalation. The larynx also serves a social function—the production of voice for both verbal and nonverbal communication.

The process of phonation is quite complex; yet its major features can be described rather simply, as in the description of the infant's cry. The power for sound production comes from the breath stream, which is moved by the muscles that expand and contract the thorax. It follows that the initial phase of phonation is the inhalation of some air. Second, the air is expelled from the lungs rapidly or slowly as needed. When the air pressure against the mucosa of the trachea reaches the equivalent of only a few millimeters of water pressure, many reflexes are activated (Wyke, 1974). These reflexes, in combination with volitional nerve impulses from the brain, cause the vocal cords to close the glottis and to be adjusted for the intended pitch and loudness of the sound. The outflowing air stream meets the impeding vocal cords, is stopped momentarily by them, and then pushes them apart. Air spurts through the glottal opening, but is cut off by the elastic recoil of the muscles in the vocal cords which, in combination with the Bernoulli effect, close the glottis. After the glottis has been closed, the air pressure again increases on the underside of the vocal cords until the glottis opens again to release the air. This process of opening and closing may occur as slowly as about 70 times a second in low bass voices or more than 1,000 times a second in high sopranos. The motion of the vocal cords, combined with the air flow, creates trains of pressure waves in the air which move ear drums, microphone responders, and other flexible objects on which they impinge. When the pressure waves pass from the larynx through the upper respiratory tract, they are modified by the adjustments of the pharynx, tongue, velopharyngeal valve, and other structures into vowels and other sounds of language.

The muscles and cartilages that accomplish these functions have been described in chapter 4. You may want to review them carefully as a basis for understanding phonation.

Some of the vocal sounds produced by infants and adults are musical; others give the impression of roughness or noise which is often called *hoarseness.* Sometimes there is also a sound of the breath flow that is identified as breathiness. Occasionally, also, speech sounds that should come out through the nose do not do so, or the opposite may occur and sounds that should exit from the mouth seem to come from the nose. Almost everyone appreciates a musical voice, and most recognize nasality, hoarseness, or other deviant voices. Recognition and identification are important, but speech-language pathologists must also know what happens in the speech mechanism when normal and abnormal voices are produced. They must be able to answer such questions as: What happens in the larynx when a "musical" tone is produced? How do the vocal cords create hoarseness? What is the basis for breathiness? Why is some speech denasal? Why do some sounds escape abnormally through the nose?

The musical, or pleasant, or smooth vocal tone which is considered to be the "normal" voice occurs when the vocal cords vibrate regularly. That is, the glottis is opened and closed with a regular period to alternately stop and start the air flow. This action creates a series of evenly spaced pressure waves that stimulate the ear mechanisms in comparable sequences. When this normal or musical voice is produced, the vocal cords move through a vibratory cycle in which they separate, then come back together and remain together for a brief instant. This normal vibratory cycle can be represented graphically by

See Figure 6.1.

FIGURE 6.1

Normal Movements of the Glottal Borders of the Right and Left Vocal Folds at their Anterior-Posterior Midpoints. The zero line approximates the median sagittal plane; the curves above and below that line trace the motions of the right and left vocal folds respectively. The diverging lines represent separation of the vocal folds as the glottis opens, convergence indicates closure, and the single line shows contact and a closed glottis. The diverging lines that continue beyond the start of the converging phase represent waves that often continue laterally on the upper surface of the vocal folds after the maximum glottal opening has occurred. At that moment in the vibratory cycle the lower border of the vocal fold becomes visible in its closing motion. Consequently the interrupted line represents an instant in which the upper and lower borders of the vocal folds are visible simultaneously.

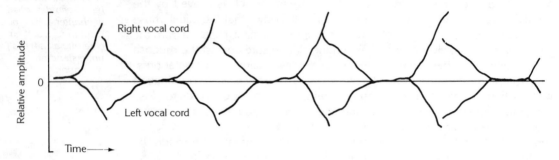

FIGURE 6.2

Normal Adult, Female Larynx with Vocal Folds Abducted for respiration (left) and Adducted for Phonation (right). The small white areas on the edges of the vocal folds are accumulations of mucus that often form at regions of excessive pressure or trauma. The major orienting positions and structures are:

(A) Anterior
(P) Posterior
(R) Subject's right side
(L) Subject's left side
(1) Epiglottis
(2) False vocal folds (or ventricular folds)
(3) True vocal folds (or vocal lips or vocal cords)
(4) Glottis
(5) Arytenoid area
(6) Trachea

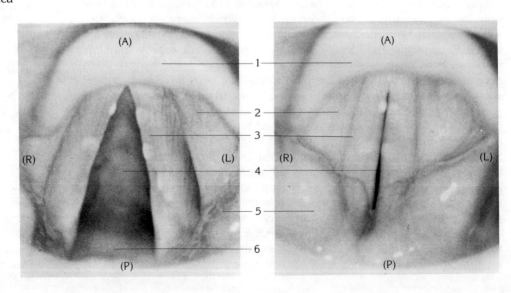

tracing the movements of points on the margins of the vocal cords as they go through several vibrations.

Diagrams are more meaningful when you can visualize the underlying or functioning mechanism. Figure 6.2 shows a normal larynx when seen with the aid of a small mirror placed in the pharynx. This is the image the laryngologist sees in an ordinary indirect or mirror examination. Figure 6.3 is an X-ray image that illustrates the placement of the mirror and its relationship to other structures.

FIGURE 6.3

Lateral X-ray Image of the Nose, Mouth, Pharynx and Larynx Showing a Laryngeal Mirror in Place for Viewing the Vocal Folds. The structures are:

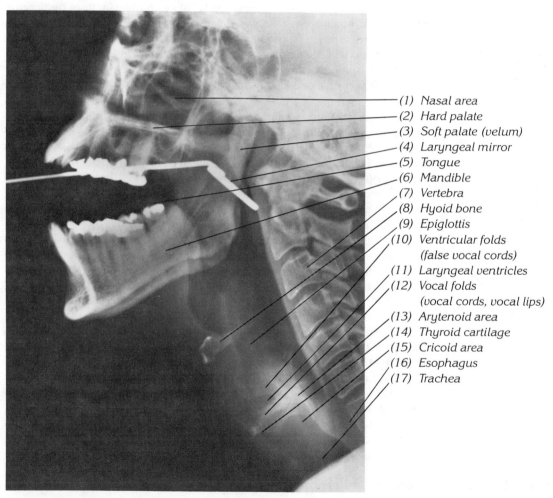

(1) Nasal area
(2) Hard palate
(3) Soft palate (velum)
(4) Laryngeal mirror
(5) Tongue
(6) Mandible
(7) Vertebra
(8) Hyoid bone
(9) Epiglottis
(10) Ventricular folds
(false vocal cords)
(11) Laryngeal ventricles
(12) Vocal folds
(vocal cords, vocal lips)
(13) Arytenoid area
(14) Thyroid cartilage
(15) Cricoid area
(16) Esophagus
(17) Trachea

The vocal cords extend from front to back and are approximately parallel with the ground when a person is upright; they are somewhat like lips and are separated posteriorly during respiration. The upper part of the mirror image shown in Figure 6.2 is toward the front of the larynx, where the epiglottis and anterior ends of the vocal cords (or vocal folds or vocal lips) can be seen. Since the patient faces the examiner during a mirror examination, his right vocal fold is at the viewer's left. The ventricular, or false, vocal cords can be seen as folds of tissue that form part of the lateral walls of the interior of the larynx. The lower part of the image shows the regions of the arytenoid cartilages to which the posterior ends of the vocal cords are attached. When the space between the vocal cords (the glottis) is open, it offers a view down into the trachea. The larynx and vocal cords ordinarily move almost constantly, slightly during quiet breathing and vigorously during coughing or speaking. Some concept of their gross movements toward and away from each other can be seen in Figure 6.4. This sequence of images was taken from a section of normal speed motion picture film which was made by substituting a camera for the eye of an examiner. The vocal cords can be seen moving away from each other during inhalation and approaching each other for phonation. However, normal speed motion pictures cannot show the separate vibratory movements that are represented in Figure 6.1. "Slowing" the vibratory motion for observation requires special procedures such as stroboscopy or ultra high speed photography. The filming rate of the ultra high speed photographs used in this chapter is approximately 5,000 pictures/sec. This means that 1 second of laryngeal photography is "slowed" on projection for viewing to about 200 seconds, or a little more than 3 minutes.

See Figure 4.13 for a sequence of ultra high speed photographs taken at 4,000 frames/ sec.

We have seen that a musical, smooth, or normal voice is associated with sound waves that are regular; each successive vibration occupies the same, or almost the same time. However, if the normal voice slides up or down the musical scale, each succeeding vibratory period is progressively shorter for the upward glide and longer for the downward glide. This type of pitch change is called *glissando* by singers. The important features of these normal phonatory vibrations are regularity in successive cycles and continuous progressive change. That is, there is no random irregularity in the length of amplitude of the vibration from one cycle to the next.

When randomness of period or amplitude does occur in successive vibrations, the voice is heard as hoarse. Figure 6.5 displays a series of pictures from an ultra slow motion film of a larynx producing a hoarse voice. Figure 6.6 represents the movements of those vocal cords. Note the random variation in length of consecutive vibratory cycles. This randomness creates an equally irregular acoustic wave that is heard as hoarseness or roughness.

The vocal cords may also produce a breathy voice, a voice that sounds as though it combines a whisper with vocal tone. This type of sound occurs when the vocal cords vibrate without complete glottal closure. The vibratory cycles are composed of opening and closing phases in which the vocal folds move laterally and medially, but do not meet along their entire lengths. Normal speaking contains frequent moments of breathy sound, as when a vowel follows a /h/ or other unvoiced consonant. However, some voices are predominantly or continuously breathy, which categorizes them as abnormal.

PARALLEL PERCEPTUAL AND PHYSICAL FACTORS

So far we have seen that the vocal cords can vibrate slowly or rapidly to create pitch changes; they can release a pulsing train of pressure waves with greater or lesser velocity to produce differences in loudness; they can vibrate regularly or irregularly and with various other differences to create several phonatory qualities. These changes in vibration are not haphazard; they have causes. They are underlying physical principles that determine pitch, loudness, and quality.

FIGURE 6.4

Normal Larynx. This sequence of photographs took approximately 0.9 sec and extended from the cessation of phonation in the upper left corner progressively through abduction for inhalation, adduction, and the resumption of vocal fold vibration in the lower right corner. The sequence of images progresses from top to bottom through the three columns.

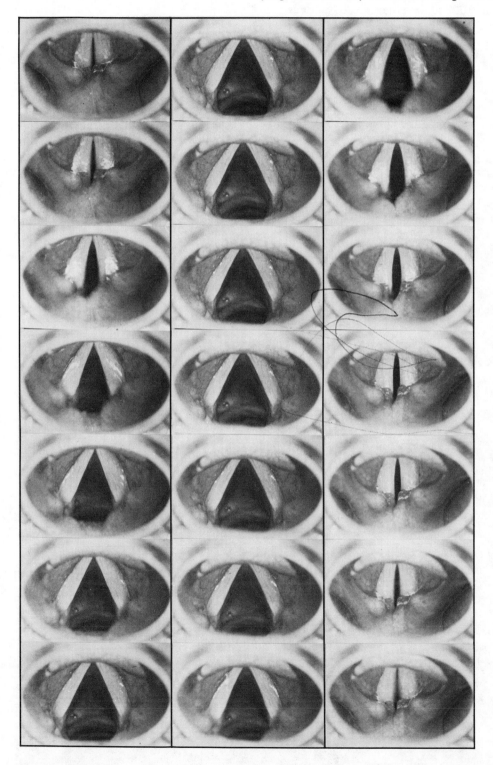

FIGURE 6.5

Ultra Slow Motion Film Sequence Demonstrating Random, Almost Chaotic Vocal Fold Vibration in a Larynx with Severe Laryngitis. The single, larger image in the upper left corner shows a swollen white area anteriorly on the right cord and edematous swelling posteriorly. The left fold is quite flaccid. The sequence of images progresses from above downward in each column and represents an elapsed time of approximately 0.007 sec at a rate of 5,000 pictures/sec.

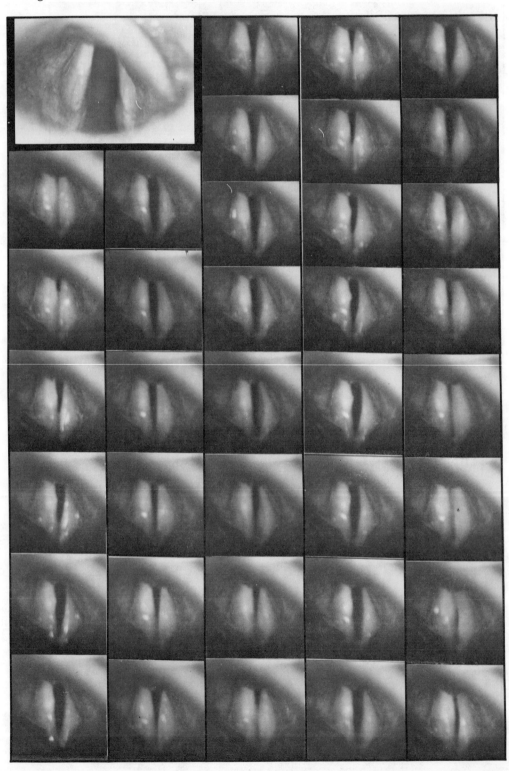

FIGURE 6.6

Vibratory Movements of the Glottal Borders at the Anterior-Posterior Midpoints of the Right and Left Vocal Cords in the larynx pictured in Figure 6.5. Irregularity of motion is revealed in aperiodicity, phase differences, and variable amplitude. (This graph was not generated from the series of photographs used in Figure 6.5.)

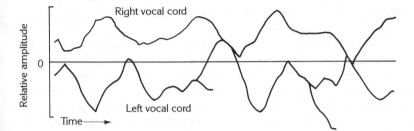

Pitch—Frequency

Pitch is a perceptual concept that refers to a musical scale. When a tone goes from a lower to a higher pitch, the vibrator, whether violin string, clarinet reed, or vocal cords, increases its frequency. That is, *frequency,* when referring to sound, is a physical concept that indicates the number of vibrations within a period of time. Raising the pitch, that is, increasing the frequency in a musical instrument such as a violin, occurs when elasticity (or tension) is increased, when the mass of the vibrator is made smaller, or when the length of a vibrator is shortened without changing its elasticity or mass. The pitch of the voice is raised when the vocal cords are elongated. This adjustment accomplishes two changes. First, it increases the tension or elasticity (which is defined as the relative speed of return of an object to its position of rest after it has been displaced). Second, elongation reduces the mass of the vocal cords at all points along their length. Lengthening the vibrator to raise pitch may seem at first to contradict the idea that a shorter vibrator produces a higher frequency. However, when the vocal cords are elongated, the increased tension and reduced mass counter the length factor and cause a higher frequency. You can observe the same phenomenon by stretching and plucking a rubber band.

Remember, the word that means vibration cycles per second is Hertz (Hz).

Loudness—Amplitude

Loudness is a perceptual concept that has a physical parallel in the amplitude of motion of the air molecules against the ear drum. That is, when the sound wave, which is represented by the forward and backward movement of the air molecules, displaces the ear drum a greater distance, the sound is said to be louder. Variation in amplitude is generated at the glottis by a combination of breath pressure and manner of vibration of the vocal cords. When the subglottal air pressure is relatively large and the resistance to glottal opening is substantial, the air is released in brief spurts that have both high velocity and high volume. When a high energy pulse hits the air above the glottis, it moves the molecules a greater distance than when the pulse has a lower volume–velocity combination. This greater distance is in effect a greater amplitude, which is propagated in the sound wave and heard as a louder sound. Since loudness is proportional to the pulse-volume of air and its velocity through the glottis, it is easy to understand how the same loudness could be heard if the volume and velocity were changed proportionately in opposite directions; that is, if the velocity of the air were decreased and the volume increased or vice versa. There is almost an infinite variation of laryngeal adjustments possible.

Quality—Complexity

The quality of voice cannot be completely separated from pitch and loudness, but the word *quality* designates the audible features of a voice that distinguishes it from another voice when both are at the same pitch and loudness. The perceptual concept of quality has a parallel physical representation in the complexity of the sound wave. Another way to express complexity is by referring to the number and relative intensities of the partial tones that constitute the sound.

Almost all the sounds we hear are complex sounds. An uncomplex, single, or pure tone is the kind that comes from a tuning fork or pure tone audiometer. When two or more tuning forks are sounded at the same time, the combined sound is complex. There are many other complex sounds, some of which contain **noise**. Some of these are the normal fricative sounds such as /f,v,θ,ð,s,z/. Noise is also a frequent component of hoarse and breathy voices. If several tuning forks are sounding and another is added, the quality of the sound will change. The quality of the sound will also change if one or more of the forks is made to produce a louder sound. In other words, as stated above, the quality of a sound is determined by the number and relative intensities of the partials that compose it.

*In technical use, **noise** is complex sound composed of irregular vibrations, to which a pure pitch cannot be assigned.*

The complex sound that is "voice" is determined by the way the glottal pulse is released and the modifications of that pulse sound in the pharynx, mouth, and nose. Not all of the vibratory factors are known, but we have reason to believe that the speed of opening and closing of the glottis during vibration, the length of the closed phase in the vibration cycle, and the undulatory configurations of the vocal cord margins influence the number and intensities of the partial tones.

RESONANCE

The sound generated in the larynx is modified by a process called *resonance*. As the complex sound passes through the upper respiratory tract, some of the partials are enhanced and others are suppressed. Perhaps the most obvious resonance effect is in the formation of vowels. The partials that are emphasized become apparent as formants that can be displayed by **sonograms** and other means of analysis. Each vowel requires a unique arrangement in the oral cavity; that is, the /i/ sound in *see* cannot be made when the mouth and tongue are adjusted for /a/ as in *father*. Sometimes the structures are impaired by paralysis or physical deformity, which alters the resonance patterns and creates speech or voice defects. For example, if the velopharyngeal closure cannot be made, sound comes out of both mouth and nose when only the oral route is normal. This open velopharyngeal port produces a hypernasal sound in the speech.

*A **sonogram** is a graph of a sound or sounds, produced by a special electromechanical device.*

There are many other resonance distortions possible; they are discussed later in this chapter.

Resonance is a physical phenomenon that occurs in cavities and elastic structures. The air in the respiratory tract is elastic; when the pulses from the glottis enter the airway, they strike adjacent air molecules, which causes them in turn to bump the next molecules and then the next and so on. This process creates longitudinal waves that are propagated through the air. After the molecules are displaced, they tend to return to their positions of rest; that is, they tend to oscillate forward and backward. However, if another pulse comes along, the molecules are disturbed again, sometimes before they reach their rest or neutral positions. When a series of impulses occurs, the fluctuations create what we call a *sound wave*. The fronts or advancing parts of the wave cycles travel in all possible directions. They run into the walls and other structures in the upper respiratory cavities and bounce back in widening circles, much like water waves in a tub or pool. Sound waves are even reflected by openings such as the channels between the tongue and palate and the lips. The reflected waves encounter the on-coming waves with varying effects. When waves traveling in opposite directions are moving the molecules in the same back and forth directions, the movement is enhanced and the waves become bigger. However, when the on-coming and reflected waves impinge upon the molecules in opposite directions, the motion is cancelled and no energy is transmitted. This simplified example explains what happens when a pure tone or a partial in a complex sound is resonated or suppressed. When augmentation occurs, the amplitude of the wave is increased and the sound is louder. In contrast, cancellation represses both the wave motion and the sound. In the case of the vowel sounds, augmentation and suppresion create the formants which determine the phonemes.

By extending this image into the act of speaking, you can be overwhelmed by the potential variations in wave configurations that accompany the changing resonator adjustments. The complexity of the sound is increased by another dimension when an organic defect or paralysis is present. The resonance phenomenon persists as a physical occurrence, but the sounds produced are atypical. Consequently, they constitute an articulation or voice disorder.

Another factor that relates to resonance and has an influence upon vocal sounds is absorption. When a resonator has hard walls, as in a brass tube, its response characteristics are different from those found in a soft-walled cavity. The hard-walled space resonates only sounds that are at or very close to its resonance frequency. In contrast, a soft-walled resonator responds to a broadened range of frequencies around the central frequency of the resonator. When you consider the changes in the linings of the nose, mouth, and pharynx related to moisture and dryness, excess mucus secretion, and abnormal contraction of the muscles, you can easily see the significance of this concept for the speech-language pathologist.

These comments about phonation and resonance imply that they are interrelated in voice production, even though they are distinct functions. This interrelation of the two processes is demonstrated in the production of vowel sounds. The distinction between phonation and resonance is illustrated by the fact that a person may have his larynx removed and still learn to speak. The requirement for speech without a larynx is a sound source that can substitute for the larynx. Any complex sound in the voice range that can be put into the mouth or pharynx will form intelligible speech when you perform the customary articulatory movements and adjustments.

The possibility of substituting another sound source for the larynx is discussed in some detail later in the chapter.

FACTORS THAT INFLUENCE VOCAL CORD VIBRATION AND VOICE

We have seen that vocal sound is specifically and closely associated with the way the vocal cords and the resonators function. There is always a reason, a cause (usually biological) for a malfunction and the associated faulty voice. Since the ultimate objective of courses on communication disorders is to develop preventive and remedial therapy, it follows that the speech-language pathologist must know how to find the causes which are the focus of therapy in order to provide appropriate remedial measures. However, before you can recognize causes, you must know what they are. You must have answers to the question "What can cause the vocal cords to vibrate abnormally or not to vibrate at all?"

There are many causes of abnormal vocal cord function and the consequent phonatory disorders. Some of them influence the manner of vocal cord adjustment and degree of glottal closure, others affect the vibrations of the vocal cords themselves, and many simultaneously impair both adduction or abduction and vibration. Various degrees of impairment in vocal cord adduction and abduction can be present, extending from maximum lateral positioning with a wide-open glottis to tight contact between the vocal cords with a completely closed glottis. Most of the voice problems associated with incomplete adduction have a prominent breath noise component that ranges between complete aphonia, as in whispering, and very slight breathiness heard as a lack of clearness in the vocal tone. At the other extreme of glottal adjustment, when the vocal cords are pressed together with excessive pressure, the breath stream as well as the voice is totally interrupted. The normal use of this adjustment is at the start of a cough or holding the breath during lifting, but some people attempt to use a slightly modified form of this tight closure for phonation.

The adjustments and vibration of the vocal cords can be impaired by one or more of the following five factors: (a) psychogenic or functional problems, (b) paralyses and joint diseases, (c) trauma and surgical modification, (d) debilitating diseases, and (e) masses that interfere with vibration or glottal closure. Let us now look at sketches of each of these types of disorders and relate them to aphonia and dysphonia.

Psychogenic or Functional Problems

The aphonic voice may occur when a person does not want to converse or sing. However, nonorganic aphonia and dysphonia are more apt to be related unconsciously to stress and anxiety. Emotional problems associated with overwhelming situations at home or at work or school may incapacitate the laryngeal function enough to prevent phonation. There are other instances where a true temporary laryngeal disease creates an aphonia that persists after full biological function has been restored. Possibly the aphonia provides a protection or relief somewhere in the individual's life and is, therefore, extended. However, prolonged aphonia following recovery from an organic laryngeal disorder sometimes results in an inability to adduct the vocal cords sufficiently for phonation. Some voices are aphonic all the time, but that degree of voicelessness is rare. Usually aphonia is intermittent; the voice often alternates irregularly between aphonia and dysphonia, which may be breathy-sounding or hoarse. The implication is that the laryngeal conditions that contribute to one type of voice may also cause others.

Functional dysphonia of the breathy type, which signals vocal cord vibration without a closed phase, may also be associated with home or work environments where an extremely quiet voice is required. This type of speaking can easily become habitual. A similar condition and voice may be developed also by young women in high school and college who try to emulate actresses and entertainers. In our culture, the breathy, low-pitched, female voice is often interpreted as "sexy."

As in articulation and other disorders, a functional voice disor- Another type of functional dysphonia occurs when the vocal cords are squeezed together so tightly that they cannot vibrate normally. A mirror view reveals the superior structures of the larynx to be pressed into the airway, often obscuring the view of part or all of the true vocal cords. The adjustment resembles the laryngeal closure in the first stage of a cough. When overadduction occurs, the vocal sound may be quite hoarse and low-pitched, as heard in some of the sterotyped gang-bosses in motion pictures. Occasionally the ventricular folds are adducted more or less completely and forced to vibrate. The voice usually is quite hoarse, is often called *dysphonia plicae ventricularis,* and creates the impression of effort. The several forms of hoarseness associated with excessive closure of the glottis are called in the literature *hyperfunctional dysphonia* (Boone, 1977; Froeschels, 1952).

der has no known physical cause.

Problems Related to Organic Factors

Many voice disorders are caused by **organic** impairments. Treatment of the underlying problem is usually the responsibility of such medical specialties as otolaryngology, endrocrinology, or neurology. However, when a person with an organic voice disorder comes to the speech-language pathologist for voice therapy, the professional must know whether to refer to the proper specialist or to conduct a remedial program. The preparation includes basic knowledge of the diseases and disabilities that may be involved.

*An **organic** impairment is one which has a physical cause.*

Paralysis and Ankylosis

A common organic cause for the failure of the vocal cords to close the glottis completely is paralysis. Paralysis is a disorder in which a muscle loses the ability to contract; consequently, the structures to which paralyzed muscles are attached cannot be moved voluntarily. Usually the cause is impairment of the nerves supplying the involved muscles. The nerves may be severed, crushed, squeezed, or inactivated by trauma, infection, or other disease.

When a vocal cord is paralyzed, it remains in approximately the same position; that is, it does not adduct or abduct. However, the stable position may vary in different larynges, according to the nerves involved. When one recurrent laryngeal nerve is severed, the vocal cord on the same side will usually rest in a paramedian position. The healthy vocal cord can approach and sometimes contact the paralyzed cord to achieve nearly complete glottal closure. If both recurrent nerves are involved, both vocal cords will be in paramedian positions, causing a narrow glottal aperture. When both the superior and recurrent laryngeal nerves on the same side are damaged, the involved vocal cord will remain in a lateral position, causing a large glottal space even when the unaffected cord is adducted to the maximum.

Para means beside or alongside of.

Since paralysis interferes with glottal closure, a certain amount of air is usually wasted during phonation, which causes a weak, breathy voice. The absence of firm glottal closure also affects the cough. Instead of the normal sharp or sudden change from no air flow to a burst of air, the cough with paralysis sounds like a forceful "huh." However, even though a breathy sound usually accompanies laryngeal paralysis, a nearly normal voice occurs when the healthy vocal cord approximates its paralyzed mate. A paralyzed cord vibrates almost as well as a healthy cord. When the vibrators are close together, the air stream activates both of them. During vibration they are pushed laterally; when they swing medially, their glottal margins go past their rest positions to contact each other more or less firmly. When this vibratory sequence takes place, the conditions for normal phonation are met.

If both vocal cords are paralyzed and they lie in paramedian positions, the vocal sound is usually relatively normal. The vocal cords are able to accomplish nearly normal glottal closure during vibration, which provides the necessary and typical train of pressure pulses. With bilateral recurrent nerve paralysis, the major problem is inadequate airway and difficulty breathing rather than sound.

Ankylosis, or impairment of arytenoid movement resulting from stiffness or fixation at the cricoarytenoid joint, is another cause for incomplete glottal closure and a breathy voice. If cancer, arthritis, or some other inflammatory joint disease prevents adduction and abduction, the function of the impaired larynx is essentially the same as that which accompanies paralysis. The amount of glottal opening varies among people, and the severity of the vocal deviations corresponds to the degree of opening.

Trauma and Surgical Modification

Occasionally movements of one or both arytenoid cartilages are limited or prevented by trauma. If the cartilages of the larynx are fractured in an automobile or motorcycle accident, they may heal in such a way that normal motion is not possible. The accompanying voice, of course, varies with the type and extent of the physical alteration.

The trauma problem is illustrated by the case of an 18-year-old student who was in a motorcycle accident. He was traveling about 40 miles an hour through a forest at dusk when he struck a chain that had been stretched across the trail at neck height. His larynx was crushed, but surgeons realigned the broken cartilages and placed a special splint called a *stent* into the larynx to support the parts while they healed. After the stent was removed, both vocal cords remained in lateral positions, causing a wide open glottis and total aphonia. Some months later, the right vocal cord regained the ability to adduct and abduct normally, but the left arytenoid cartilage and vocal cord remained somewhat lateralized. With the restoration of a partial glottal closure some vibration could be achieved, producing a weak and breathy but serviceable voice.

A laryngectomy is surgery to remove the larynx.

A similar case occurred in which the larynx was crushed so severely it could not be preserved. Consequently, a total **laryngectomy** was performed. This young man developed excellent esophageal speech. Additional information about speech without a larynx can be found later.

Occasionally the laryngeal surgeon finds it necessary to modify the larynx to improve respiration. One arytenoid cartilage may be removed, and the vocal cord on that side fastened laterally to provide an open airway. The accompanying voice is usually quite breathy.

Another surgical procedure that produces a chronically open glottis is a cordectomy. Sometimes the treatment of choice for a tumor on one vocal cord is to remove the diseased part with the underlying tissue. Frequently, scar tissue will replace the absent tissue, but a defect in the closure with a breathy, weak voice almost always persists.

Debilitating Diseases and Conditions

Incomplete or inadequate glottal closure can be caused by weak muscle contraction. A common cause of muscle weakness and relatively quick fatigue is anemia. This disorder results from an inadequate blood supply to muscles, organs, and other body parts. People who are chronically fatigued or who tire quickly with exertion often reflect this condition in the voice. It tends to be weak and breathy, which signals either the absence of glottal closure or very brief contact between the vocal cords during vibration.

Anemia may also contribute to vocal weakness through its effect on the muscles of respiration. Since the loudness of voice is directly related to breath pressure, and since breath pressure is determined by expiratory force exerted by the thoracic and abdominal muscles, it follows that fatigue of these muscles will diminish the vocal energy.

Myasthenia can interfere with gross adduction and also the finer adjustments of the intrinsic laryngeal muscles. The word *myasthenia* appears in two phrases, *myasthenia gravis* and *myasthenia laryngis,* which have markedly different meanings. Myasthenia gravis is also known as *myoneural junction disease.* This disorder is related to "reduced availability of acetylcholine at the myoneural junction" which "causes progressive flaccid weakness or paralysis with strenuous muscular effort. Sometimes muscles supplied by the vagus nerve are the first to be affected by this disease" (Aronson, 1980, pp. 87–88). The voice becomes progressively breathy and weaker, nasality increases, and articulation loses its precision with continuous talking. The symptoms can be relieved with medication.

Myasthenia means a muscle without strength.

Myasthenia laryngis was introduced by Jackson and Jackson (1937) to refer to muscles that are more or less chronically fatigued and which tire readily. The authors identify five classes of cases of myasthenia laryngis.

> Those due to (*a*) damage of the muscles by violent shouting, shrieking, screaming at football games, and other brutal abuses of the larynx; (*b*) muscular fatigue from prolonged excessive though not violent use; (*c*) excessive load imposed by a tumor, or an arthritic cricoarytenoid joint; (*d*) invasion by neighboring inflammatory conditions; and (*e*) association with chronic laryngitis caused by the abuse. (p. 313)

Although other authors may not classify these conditions as myasthenia laryngis, they recognize the damaging effects on the voice of all these conditions.

Protruding Masses

Closure of the glottis can be prevented by tumors or granulomas between the arytenoid cartilages or along the glottal borders. These abnormal structures interfere mechanically and result in an incompletely closed glottis or atypical vibration. The type of tumor or other obstruction need not be considered at this point, as they are discussed in the next section. The important consideration here is that the glottis remains open to some degree, and the voice will be breathy and sometimes hoarse.

LOCALIZED LESIONS AND OTHER DISORDERS

Frequently the conditions that impair glottal adjustment have a local influence upon one or both vocal cords to cause voice abnormalities. Earlier in this chapter, we mentioned that hoarseness can be caused by random variations in the consecutive vibrations of the vocal cords. As we stated, one cause for this vibration is abnormal increase or decrease in the size or mass of one or both vocal folds. Aronson (1980) has summarized the effects of mass in the following statement.

> Mass lesions of the vocal folds . . . produce one or more of the following pathologic changes.
> (1) Increase the mass or bulk of the vocal folds or immediately surrounding tissues.

(2) Alter their shape.

(3) Restrict their mobility.

(4) Change their tension.

(5) Modify the size or shape, or both, of the glottic, supraglottic, or infraglottic airway.

(6) Prevent the vocal folds from approximating completely along their anterior margins.

(7) Result in excessive tightness of approximation. (p. 57)

What are these masses that can influence the vocal folds, their vibration, and the voice? A few of the common ones need to be well understood by the speech-language pathologist. However, you must always remember that an abnormal voice and the aberrant vibrations associated with it can have a variety of etiologies. Putting it another way, you cannot diagnose a specific disease by the sound of the voice. A mass on a vocal fold exerts its influence variably according to its location, size, and firmness.

Tumors

Tumors usually come to mind first when you think about mass lesions of the vocal cords, but what is a tumor? The word *tumor,* like the word *automobile,* has a broad meaning encompassing many types. *Tumor* has been defined as a "neoplasm (new growth); an abnormal mass of tissue that grows more rapidly than normal and continues to grow after the stimuli which initiated the new growth cease" (*Stedman's,* 1976). They can be either benign or malignant. A benign ("kind") tumor is "one that does not form metastases and does not invade and destroy adjacent normal tissue" (*Stedman's,* 1976). *Malignant* means evil: "cancer; a tumor invading surrounding tissues and usually capable of producing metastases, likely to recur after attempted removal and to cause death of the host unless adequately treated" (*Stedman's,* 1976).

Metastasis means the transfer or migration of a disease from one location to another and the establishment of the disease in the new location.

Polyp

A polyp is a benign tumor commonly found in the larynx. This term is also very broad in its meaning. Polyp "is a general descriptive term used with reference to any mass of tissue that bulges or projects outward, or upward, from the normal surface level" (*Stedman's,* 1976). It may be broad-based (*sessile*) or be attached by a stalk (*pedunculated*).

> The (laryngeal) lesions included under this term include two distinct entities. One is the polypoid mass localized to the middle of the membranous vocal cord. The other type of lesion is the diffuse polypoid degeneration of both entire membranous vocal cords which has also been termed *localized hypertrophic laryngitis.* (Ballenger, 1969, p. 405)

Polyps may be found in the nose and other locations along the repiratory tract as well as in the intestinal tract.

> The localized vocal polyp is the most common benign lesion of the larynx. This lesion, like the vocal nodule, is due mainly to trauma secondary to vocal abuse.... Frequently the onset of the lesion can be related to a single episode of vocal strain. Polyps may also develop acutely following an upper respiratory infection. (Ballenger, 1969, p. 405–406)

If a polyp protrudes from the glottal border of a vocal fold, it tends to interfere with contact between the folds during vibration. The result may be a breathiness in the voice. If the polyp is large, it may rest partially on the opposite vocal fold, where it interferes with vibration. It may become an auxiliary vibrator contributing to the hoarseness.

Vocal Nodules

Vocal nodules, often referred to as *singer's nodes* or *screamer's nodes,* or with similar terms, are a type of polyp. However, most experts recognize the distinctiveness of the shape, location, and composition of vocal nodules and refer to them with one of those identifying names. Vocal nodules are usually small, sessile, slightly pink or grayish-white protrusions located bilaterally, opposite each other at the junction of the anterior and middle thirds of the entire length of the vocal folds. This position is the same as the midpoint of the membranous section of the vocal folds. The location of the nodules probably identifies the place of greatest trauma during vocal cord vibration.

These lesions tend to develop in people who yell themselves hoarse at football games and the like or who abuse their voices with other types of excessive use. The vocal abuse causes swelling that reduces the flexibility of the vocal folds, tends to increase vocal cord contact at the swollen areas, and may also prevent total glottal closure. Some small hemorrhages in the subsurface area (Reinke's space) may also contribute to the congestion. Swelling usually disappears in 24 to 36 hours with rest and moderate use. However, when vocal misuse continues, as with people who talk excessively, yell often, sing abusively (as in some popular entertainment groups), or abuse the vocal cords while making other sounds (for example, children imitating motorcycles), the swelling persists, tissue changes occur, and the traumatized area becomes organized, circumscribed, and protruberant. The larynx pictured in Figure 6.7 shows moderately large vocal nodules in a 21-year-old woman.

The special names such as *screamer's nodes* and *singer's nodes* emphasize their traumatic origins. The abuse is related to high vocal intensity, prolonged use, high pitch, and combinations of these factors. Vocal nodules are found in persons of all ages, but more prepubertal boys develop them than girls in the comparable developmental period. The ratio is reversed in the postpubertal period, when young women in their late teens and early twenties have a relatively high incidence of nodules. There is some evidence that vocal nodules in boys tend to disappear during the adolescent voice change (Ballenger, 1969; Kimelman, 1980).

The abusive vocal behavior associated with vocal nodules can be caused by both psychological and social factors. The typical child with nodules is a

FIGURE 6.7

Well-Defined, Moderately Large Vocal Nodules in a 21-year-old Female. These lesions were caused by a combination of yelling, singing, and excessive talking. The voice was breathy-hoarse.

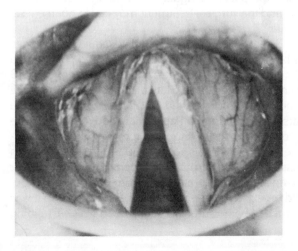
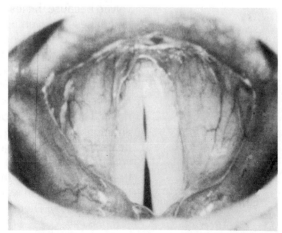

younger sibling who fights verbally with his brothers and sisters. He is usually competitive, aggressive, interested in sports, vocally loud, and has some personality adjustment problems. Aronson (1980) observes that the factors related to vocal nodules in children are basically similar to those in adults.

The severity of a voice deviation produced in the presence of nodules may vary with vocal tasks in the same larynx; it may also differ from one larynx to another without a close correlation with the size of the nodules. The vocal sound tends to have a prominent breathy component and frequently gives the listener the impression that the speaker is exerting excessive effort in speaking. The quality is essentially the same as that caused by polyps or any other mass that protrudes from the glottal border on one or both membranous vocal folds.

Hematoma

Hema- *means blood and* -oma *means tumor.*

A **hematoma** is a swelling filled with blood. These lesions usually result from trauma, as in the case of "blood blister" on a pinched finger. The laryngeal trauma is usually vocal abuse or violent coughing that causes a little hemorrhage just under the covering membrane. The blood is usually resorbed, and the structure returns to normal. However, the hematoma may be followed by fibrous changes that cause a polyp or nodule and the associated voice disorders.

Papillomata

Papilla *means nipple-like.*

A *biopsy is the surgical removal of a small sample of tissue that is then examined microscopically.*

There are two general kinds of papillomata; one kind is hard, the other soft. An example of a hard papilloma is the common wart. The soft papillomata do not look like warts, but instead tend to be glistening, pinkish-white, and irregular. However, sometimes they can be differentiated from polyps or carcinoma only by **biopsy.** These lesions arise from the mucous membranes and may be found in the pharynx, trachea and at other sites, including the larynx. "Papillomata are the most common laryngeal tumors of childhood; and although their presence is not unusual at birth, they are most often discovered between the ages of 2 and 4" (Aronson, 1980, p. 60). When these lesions are located on the vocal cords, they usually cause dysphonia; the type and severity of the voice deviation is related to the size and location of the lesion. The cause of papillomata is not known.

The usual treatment of papillomata is to remove them surgically. The procedure may need to be repeated, sometimes frequently, since papillomata tend to recur. Occasionally, the speech-language pathologist becomes involved because the lesions and the surgical treatment may cause hoarseness, breathiness, or even aphonia.

The case of a man now 43 years old illustrates a familiar sequence of stages with papillomata. He was born in Mexico and at the age of 3 had papillomata removed from his vocal cords. At 9, surgery was necessary again; after 19 more years, following his move to the United States, additional tumors were removed. The voice had been adversely affected, but during his 43rd year he noticed an increased hoarseness in his voice. Papillomata had regrown on the anterior portions of the vocal folds. Following their removal, the larynx appeared as shown in Figure 6.8. The glottis is somewhat "s"-shaped, and both vocal cords show scar tissue. The abnormal glottal configuration and scar tissue combined to create an inefficient vibrator. The voice was masculine but higher in pitch than would be expected in a man his age and size, and it was slightly breathy. There seemed to be no surgical modification or vocal training that could bring the voice closer to normal. Fortunately, his speech was serviceable and adequate for his work.

FIGURE 6.8

Adult, Male Larynx in which Papillomata Had Been Surgically Removed Several Times. A little vocal cord tissue had been excised and some scar tissue developed. The "S"-shaped glottis was an inefficient vibrator. Excessive mucus collected in this larynx, as revealed by the mucus string between the arytenoid cartilages and the bubbles on the superior surfaces of the vocal cords.

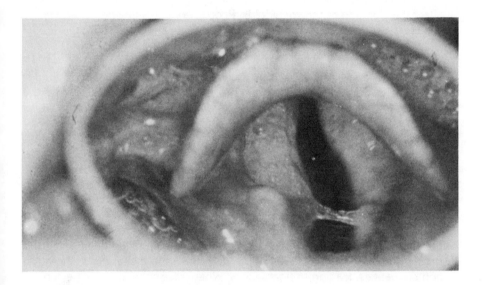

Carcinoma

A carcinoma (a type of cancer) is a malignant tumor and is indeed an evil thing. It can grow on one or both vocal cords and affect their vibration much as do polyps or papillomata. It is not possible to distinguish among carcinoma, polyps, papillomata, and the like, by the sounds produced. They all simply alter the manner in which the vocal cords are positioned and vibrate. Each can disrupt the behavior in the same way. The etiology of carcinoma is not known, but there is a well-established positive statistical relationship between laryngeal cancer and smoking. Furthermore, the chance of developing laryngeal cancer is increased substantially when alcohol is combined with smoking (Snidecor, 1970, 1971; Webb & Irving, 1964).

Carcinoma, which is a cancer that develops from surface tissue, may grow subtly in the larynx and not become apparent until it produces a change in the voice. However, this vocal change often appears early in the course of the disease and provides an opportunity for early, and frequently successful, treatment. Therapy is the responsibility of physicians, but what they do often creates a condition that requires the services of a speech-language pathologist.

The three major forms of medical treatment for carcinoma are irradiation, surgery, and chemotherapy. These procedures may be employed separately or in various combinations. When a malignant tumor in the larynx is discovered early, it can often be treated successfully with irradiation, which may leave no or only minimal, vocal disorder. If surgery is the treatment of choice, part or all of the larynx will be excised. When a total laryngectomy is performed, the open end of the trachea is brought to the surface of the neck, where it is attached to an opening in the skin called a *stoma*. The patient then breathes through this opening from the outside directly into the lungs, without having the air pass through the nose or mouth.

Chemotherapy is a procedure in which a chemical substance is introduced into the body either by tablets taken orally or by injection. There are many medications used in this kind of treatment. They are selected on the basis of the needs of the specific patient. Chemotherapy is not used often in the treatment of laryngeal carcinoma, primarily because the other procedures are more direct and effective.

There are many disorders other than tumors in the larynx that adversely affect the vibration of the vocal folds. People working with speech and voice disorders need to be familiar with these problems and their implications.

Edema

-itis means inflammation

Edematous *means filled with fluid or swollen.*

An edema is a swelling caused by excessive fluid in the tissues. This fluid is a pale, clear, amber-colored, watery component of the blood that carries the red cells and remains after the red cells coagulate. Its presence in the larynx signals a number of possible problems, which include vocal abuse, laryngitis, localized diseases, and systemic disorders such as endocrine disturbances.

The vocal cords contain a unique region that readily becomes **edematous** (Ballenger, 1969). The amount of swelling can vary from minimal to extensive, involving one or both entire vocal cords. The effect of the swelling also varies. When it is minimal, it may lower the pitch slightly as the result of increased mass and change in compliance. When swelling increases moderately, the enlarged surface areas may remain loose enough to slide back and forth over the underlying muscles which drag the mucosal surfaces back and forth during the vibrations. These deviations can cause some changes in the vibration sequences, leading to hoarseness. When edema becomes so extensive that the vocal cords are greatly enlarged, the arytenoid cartilages may be prevented from adducting, which could leave an opening between them and cause a breathy hoarseness. With this degree of swelling, the vocal cords may also be pressed together so tightly that they cannot vibrate. These comments indicate that edema is not a disease, but a symptom that can be caused by various etiologic factors. While the swelling and not the specific disease or disorder alters the vocal cord vibration, the therapy must focus on the underlying etiology wherever possible.

Contact Ulcer

Erythema is abnormal redness.

Another laryngeal disorder that is causally related to the way a person speaks and which may produce vocal deviations is contact ulcer. Vigorous glottal closure sometimes traumatizes the mucosal covering of the arytenoids of the vocal processes or other contacting areas, and an ulcer (a sore) forms on one or both cartilages. Frequently, as inflammatory processes continue, granulation tissue develops on the ulcer. The granulation may become large enough to prevent complete glottal closure. The condition sometimes causes **erythema** and edema on the membranous vocal cords. The person may feel sharp pain at the side of the neck over the posterior part of the thyroid cartilage, or the pain may radiate to an ear during swallowing or coughing.

Contact ulcer occurs usually in men in their forties who talk much, forcefully, at low pitches, but not necessarily loudly. There is some evidence that gastric reflux is a predisposing factor (Cherry & Margulies, 1968; Chodosh, 1977; Delahunty & Cherry, 1968). The voice will not be noticeably altered so long as the granulation tissue does not prevent glottal closure and the edema is limited to the posterior larynx. However, when a glottal opening persists or the vocal folds become swollen, the voice will be breathy or slightly hoarse.

Laryngeal Web

The term *laryngeal web* refers to a membranous partition, extending usually from one vocal cord to the other. However, it may occur at the level of the ventricular folds or below the glottis and be either **congenital** or scar tissue resulting from injury or surgical procedures. Webs are usually located in the anterior part of the larynx. They can vary in size from a small bit of tissue to a membrane that completely occupies the glottis. When the web (also called a **strider**) is extensive, it will impair respiration and require surgical intervention. Where it is smaller, it may cause striderous breathing or hoarseness or even aphonia. However, the presence of the smallest congenital webs may not become apparent until a child attempts to talk. When the child tries to talk, the voice may be hoarse and have a higher than normal pitch. This condition is another in which the laryngeal surgeon and speech-language pathologist must work together.

Congenital means present at birth.

The effects of a laryngeal web and other problems are illustrated in the case of an 11-year-old boy in the fourth grade who had hypernasality and a high-pitched voice. The other children called him "squeaky" as a result of his unusual voice and ridiculed him. The hypernasality reduced his intelligibility somewhat and contributed to his communication problem. All these conditions led to his withdrawal from his schoolmates and his reclusiveness.

The child was examined by several physicians over a period of years. They reported a bifid uvula (divided in two parts) and a normal larynx. The probable cause for the nasality was recognized as the uvular defect, but the speech-language pathologist who worked with the boy became convinced that there was also some laryngeal abnormality causing the high pitch. She arranged for another laryngeal examination. On this attempt, a small web was exposed between the true vocal cords at the anterior commissure. Appropriate laryn-

FIGURE 6.9

A Laryngeal Web in an 18-year old Boy. The web extends from the glottal opening to the anterior commissure.

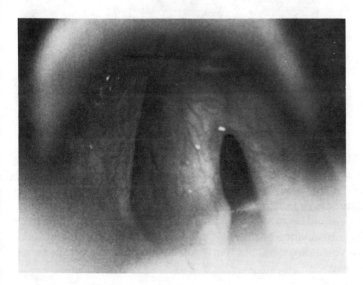

gological procedures eliminated the web and provided the basis for a normal voice, which the speech-language pathologist was able to help the boy develop and stabilize. The hypernasality was reduced through speech therapy, and the boy's personality improved markedly.

Figure 6.9 is found on page 163.

The 18-year-old boy whose larynx is shown in Figure 6.9 had had vocal cord polyps removed when he was quite small. Following that operation, the vocal folds became attached to each other, as shown in the figure. Special surgery corrected the condition and permitted the development of a relatively normal masculine voice.

Cysts

A cyst is "a closed bladder-like sac formed in animal tissues, containing fluid or semifluid morbid matter" (*American*, 1951). These lesions may occur in many parts of the body. In the larynx they "are most commonly formed in the false cord and aryepiglottic fold" (Ballenger, 1969, p. 310). However, they sometimes develop on a true vocal cord, as illustrated in Figure 6.10. Cysts usually result from the obstruction or occlusion of a duct or other outlet from a gland. Material and fluids tend to collect, causing the enlargement.

When a cyst is on the glottal border, the voice is usually breathy and not very loud, similar to that heard with a polyp or other protrusion. Other cyst locations can affect the voice differently.

FIGURE 6.10
A Cyst on the Left Vocal Cord of an Adult Woman.

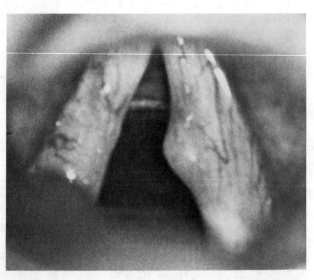

VOICE DISORDERS RELATED TO RESONANCE DEVIATIONS

The discussions in the preceding section emphasize phonatory problems; that is, voice disorders originating at the sound source. However, in the case report of the 11-year-old boy with a congenital web and bifid uvula, we referred to hypernasality, a resonance problem. Phonatory and resonance deviations may each cause voice disorders, but many vocal problems result from combinations of the two.

When the sounds /m,n,ŋ/ come out through the nose, they are considered normal. When part or almost all of the other sounds of English escape through the nose, the result is atypical and is classified as abnormal. There are two types of **hypernasality** that are accompanied by nasal emission. A third uses the nasal spaces for resonance, but little or no sound is emitted from the nose.

One of these hypernasalities is sometimes called *rhinolalia aperta,* which means nasalization caused by an opening between the oral and nasal cavities. This speech often accompanies a cleft palate, a short palate, or paralyzed soft palate, and may be difficult to understand. People with these disorders may also have a noisy escape of air from the nose, particularly on the plosives and fricatives, sounds which normally require an increase in oral breath pressure. With severe rhinolalia aperta, all sounds (including the vowels) are nasalized.

Rhino- *means nose;* -lalia, *speech;* aperta, *open.*

Chapter 11 discusses cleft palate in detail.

A mild form of hypernasality of the open type is found in many speakers who habitually use an imprecise form of articulation. The problem is most obvious during rapid speaking; it is usually absent when vowels and other nonnasal sounds are produced in isolation. These persons sometimes present a mixture of hyper- and hyponasality. This tendency to mix the forms is increased when the adenoids are enlarged.

A second type of hypernasality of the open type is frequently referred to as *nasal twang.* The voice is related auditorially to the nasal area, but there is no audible air flow through the nose. Some regional dialects involve nasal twang, and there, of course, the voice is not considered to be abnormal. Country and blue grass singing are often characterized by this sound. The "twang" hypernasality is caused by reduction of the size of the velopharyngeal opening in association with constriction of the pharyngeal and laryngeal muscles. It is almost without exception a functional or learned vocal quality.

The third type of hypernasality sounds a little like the twang, but it is caused by an obstruction in the anterior part of the nasal spaces. It can be produced intentionally by pinching the nostrils closed and attempting to "talk through your nose." When the nasal passages are occluded anteriorly and sound is allowed to enter the nasal cavities through an open velopharyngeal port, the posterior part of the nasal spaces and the nasopharynx resonate the sound jointly with the oral-pharyngeal space. The sound is emitted from the mouth. This arrangement of resonators is logically called *rhinolalia clausa* (closed) *anterior.*

Hyponasality

Another type of resonance problem related to the nose is called **hyponasality,** *denasality,* or *rhinolalia clausa posterior.* As the name implies, there is less than the expected amount of nasal resonance, which results from an occlusion of the nasal spaces either in the nasopharynx or at the posterior part of the nose. Almost everyone has had this type of voice with a severe head cold. However, when denasality is chronic, it is usually caused by enlargement of the adenoid. This structure, also called the *pharyngeal tonsil,* grows on the posterior wall of the nasopharynx just above the level of the soft palate. If it is enlarged, it can occlude the nasopharynx, thereby restricting the flow of air and sound through the nose. Theoretically, /m, n/ and /ŋ/ would be the only sounds altered by posterior nasal obstruction; those sounds would become /b, d/ and /g/ respectively, as in *bad* for *mad, dad* for *Dan,* and *sprig* for *spring.* However, many dialects of American English speech regularly have a slightly nasalized component which permeates most sounds. As a result, almost all of the voiced speech sounds—not just the /m, n, ŋ/—may be influenced by posterior blockage.

Muffled Voice

For want of a more precise term, a certain muffled quality is sometimes called a "hot potato" voice. This sound usually results from a mass in the valecula between the base of the tongue and the epiglottis or from a swollen epiglottis. A form of the quality is heard also when the tongue is habitually retracted toward the pharynx during speech. This type of speech tends to be dialectal and is characteristic of certain rural areas.

Closed Mouth Speech

One other type of resonance deviation deserves mention because it is quite common in all dialects and because it is combined with articulation problems that reduce intelligibility. This problem has no specific name, but it is often described as "closed mouth" or "clenched jaw" speech. Many people try to speak with their teeth almost in occlusion and their lips separated by only a narrow slit. These oral adjustments contribute to mild hypernasality, inaccurate formation of the vowel sounds, and imprecise consonant formation. This type of speaking also frequently signals laryngeal hypertension with its attendant hoarseness. Speaking with a relatively closed mouth requires extra effort to achieve easy intelligibility, an effort that is rarely exerted in the rapid, habitual speaking of everyday conversation.

ASSESSMENT AND DIAGNOSIS

Speech-language pathology is a direct, active clinical profession. The clinician's major objective is to provide effective therapy that will enable an individual with a speech or voice problem to speak more normally or adequately. To develop rational therapy, the voice clinician must understand the structure and function of the vocal mechanism and the disorders that may impair that mechanism. We have now sketched those factors. However, to know *about* it is not enough; you must also have a knowledge of *how to*. How to develop therapy begins with an assessment of the voice and a diagnosis, or determination of its cause, whenever possible. Starting therapy without a diagnosis is a lot like starting on an automobile trip in a strange place without a map.

The procedures of assessment and diagnosis of voice disorders are not codified into one best system; but a plan that works reasonably well can be described as having five steps: (*a*) listening, (*b*) looking, (*c*) asking questions, that is, obtaining a history, (*d*) seeking the help of specialists in other fields as necessary, and (*e*) assembling the data and establishing a diagnosis.

Listening

Earlier in this chapter you were urged to listen to the voices of your associates and strangers and your own voice. Now that we have described many of the causes of voice problems, you should be able to listen with greater precision and to have some insight into related causes.

How should you go about listening to a voice that may be defective or atypical? You should listen to a variety of samples to assess its conversational characteristics, its customary pitch and pitch range, its usual loudness, and its phonatory and resonance qualities. A simple way to "screen" the speech is to record it. This not only gives you an opportunity to hear the voice in its customary state, it also establishes a permanent record for reference. The child or adult should be asked to record the name, address, and date; a slow, measured count from 1 to 10 and from 80 to 100 (if you note a sibilant deviation, add a count of the 60s or 70s; if either a /θ/ or /f, v/ problem is heard, ask for a count of the 30s or 40s). A count is used because almost everyone can do it, it does not depend upon reading skill, it offers a wide variety of language sounds, and the familiarity of the material reduces the reticence people often feel in recording sessions. The 80s provide words beginning with a vowel, which readily display the habitual tightness of glottal closures. Initial vowels tend to be released sharply and explosively after a tight glottal closure in what is called a *glottal attack*. Counting the 90 sequence emphasizes tendencies toward either hyper- or hyponasality.

Next the child or adult should be asked to hum a tone at a comfortable pitch and to slide it up and down the scale. A vowel /o/ or /a/ should also be intoned in the same pitch changes. The speech-language pathologist may need to demonstrate what is intended. Maximum prolongation on at least three trials with a vowel should be obtained to assess phonatory efficiency. This is not a precise tool, but by timing the trials, air use can be estimated. If the prolongation is less than 7 to 8 seconds in children and 15 seconds in adults, either the air supply is deficient or there is air wastage in the larynx.

Throughout this recording process, the customary loudness of the voice is usually demonstrated. However, an indication of the ability to produce a loud voice can often be obtained by requesting a count of 1 to 5, with each number being louder. Sometimes people find it difficult to speak loudly in a small room (where recordings are usually made). When the client shows this reluctance, the speech-language pathologist may need to estimate loudness capacity by asking questions about shouting at football games and similar occasions.

To complete a screening of the voice for the recording, the clinician should encourage the child or adult to talk in his customary manner. Questions about the voice problem and its development usually elicit both a satisfactory sample of the voice and a useful history. However, with children or others who do not have much information about themselves, talking about after-school activities, sports, and hobbies customarily generates an adequate sample. If possible, a short standard paragraph should also be read aloud and recorded. This is particularly useful in later evaluations of the voice to assess improvement.

By the time the speech-language pathologist has heard the speech samples from preliminary conversations and during the recording, he should be able to describe the major features of the problem and its probable source, that is, the larynx or resonance areas or both. Any other deviations in speaking, such as articulatory abnormalities, should have been noted also.

Large-scale screening for voice disorders is rarely needed.

Looking

Usually what you hear is not an adequate basis for assessment; observation of the organs and structures that produce the speech is also necessary. The speech that comes from a person's mouth is only as good as the motions and adjustments of the structures that produce the speech.

Looking means observing the size, shape, color, and mobility (where applicable) of the face, lips, teeth (and mandible), tongue, hard and soft palate, pharynx, and larynx. Casual observation of the face while the child or adult talks and smiles will usually identify asymmetries or sluggish movements. The purpose here is to identify weakness or paralysis which may have a relationship to the speech or voice disorder. Looking at the regularity and occlusal relationships of the teeth can also be valuable. This type of observation, as well as noting other internal structures, can be aided by a flashlight.

The mobility of the tongue can be observed when the person is asked to protrude the tongue, move it from side to side, and to repeat such sounds and words as "la, la, la," "kitty, kitty, kitty," and "puh, tuh, kuh." If the tongue swings to one side when the person is instructed to protrude it in the midline or if it moves sluggishly during the production of speech sounds, some neural problem can be suspected. This type of problem needs the attention of a physician. When some hyper- or hyponasality is present, particular attention should be paid to the soft palate. When the person says "ah" or yawns, the soft palate should lift toward the posterior pharyngeal wall, and both sides should move symmetrically. If palatal movement appears to be inadequate and hypernasality is present, whatever impairs the motion is probably the cause of the problem. Conversely, if palatal movement is inadequate but hyponasality instead of hypernasality is present, there probably is an enlarged adenoid or some other mass obstructing the movement of the soft palate. Occasionally, you will see two uvulas instead of one hanging down from the posterior border of the soft palate. This condition is called a *bifid uvula* and is important to voice because the space between the two uvulas may extend up into the velum (or soft palate) far enough to prevent adequate velopharyngeal closure. Furthermore, the bifid uvula sometimes signals a submucal cleft of the soft palate. When hypernasality of the rhinolalia aperta type is present, the speech professional must make a referral to an otolaryngologist with questions about the bifid uvula. However, bifid uvulas often have no adverse effect on the speech.

Figure 6.2 shows a mirror view of a larynx.

The vocal cords cannot be seen when looking directly into the mouth. However, they can be viewed with the aid of a small mirror, similar to those used by a dentist, when it is placed in the pharynx. The procedure is not difficult, and some advanced speech-language pathologists become skillful observers of the vocal cords. Even with this skill, the speech-langue pathologist does not attempt to diagnose disease. His interest is in seeing the size, shape, mobility, and color of the laryngeal structures and how they may affect speech, just as he observes structural features and movements of the lips or tongue. Observation should always be considered in addition to, and not a replacement for, the otolaryngologist's examination. The appropriate information relating to the health of the larynx, pharynx, and ears must be obtained from an otolaryngologist.

We stress the use of a specialist rather than a general medical practitioner because they are usually not skilled in laryngcal examination.

The History

In cases where you are assessing a child, you may have to obtain the history from the parents.

The history of a voice disorder often contributes importantly to the planning and conduct of the remedial program. In those instances where the cause of the problem is obvious, such as an accident, surgery, or a specific disease, the collection of background data will concentrate primarily on current attitudes about the problem, expressed need for remedial help, motivation, and capacity to undertake a remedial program. However, when the cause of the vocal difficulty is not evident, careful questioning is essential. The speech-language pathologist attempts to obtain the following five types of information: (a) the individual's opinion of the nature and seriousness of the problem, (b) the start and course of development of the problem, including previous speech treatment, (c) medical and health history, (d) family structure and interrelationships, and (e) history of voice and speech deviations in the family. Answers to these questions will tell how precisely the child or adult perceives the problem as compared with what the examiner has heard and seen. It will also reveal the length of time the disorder has been present, plus the suddenness or gradualness of onset. Learning about previous remedial experience will give insight into the concern for the problem felt by the person and the family. The medical and health history, particularly prior to and around the time the voice problem seemed to begin, may reveal not just the diseases that could have influenced voice production, but also the feelings of the family toward the person and the problem. The family structure, including the number of siblings or children, the position of a child in the sequence of children, and the stability of the family, will reveal the presence or absence of verbal competition and compatability. These factors are often associated with vocal abuse and voice disorders. When voice disorders are apparently present from birth, as evident in the cry sound or possibly striderous breathing, the etiology may be developmental lag, structural abnormality, or disease. The developmental and structural deviations may be inherited, and questioning sometimes reveals voice problems elsewhere in the family.

Obtaining a good case history requires broad knowledge about speech and voice disorders and skill in formulating questions. It is a process designed to aid the person with the problem, but he or she may not always perceive it as such. Questioning is an art that improves with self-evaluated experience.

It can be facilitated by careful reading of the pertinent books listed at the end of the chapter.

Referral

As we have seen, voice disorders have different and often quite complicated etiologies. This chapter has suggested that the causes may be found in heredity, disease, injury, learning ability, family structure, and environmental models, or a combination. While speech-language pathologists are required to know the potential significance of etiologic factors, they are not qualified to explore all of them. Fortunately, there are skillful professional colleagues in special areas of medicine, psychology, and education who are ready to help. Frequently, a complete diagnosis of a voice disorder cannot be made until one or more of the specialists has contributed a second evaluation.

Ideally, every person with a voice disorder should be examined by an otolaryngologist before receiving a voice evaluation. This medical specialist is the custodian of the health of the organs of communication. Unfortunately, for various reasons, the voice evaluation sometimes must precede the medical examination. However, no harm is done if an otolaryngologist assesses the laryngeal, pharyngeal, oral, nasal, and otological conditions and conducts whatever medical treatment is indicated before vocal therapy begins. In addition to the guidance these examinations can provide for therapy, they also keep the speech-language pathologist from being responsible or legally liable if a vocal rehabilitation program is conducted in the presence of an unrecognized serious disease.

Usually otolaryngologists are alert to problems related to allergies, metabolic disturbances, anemia, neurologic problems, and other disorders that may adversely affect the respiratory tract. Consequently, referral by the speech-language pathologist to other medical specialists is rarely necessary. However, since evaluation and diagnosis are continuous processes, the speech-language pathologist may wish to make referrals after a period of voice therapy if a need for additional assistance becomes evident.

Summary and Diagnosis

The cause of voice disorders can usually be determined when the description of the vocal sound is evaluated along with observations made by the speech-language pathologist and physician and with information from the history. Of course, during the voice evaluation, the examiner constantly relates what is heard with what is seen and reported, so that establishing a diagnosis may not require a separate, formal assembly process. However, when referral data are not available at the time of vocal assessment and where several persons are involved in the evaluation, a systematic amalgamation of information is desirable. The first focus is on a description of the voice and an indication of its relative severity; second, a statement should be made of pertinent medical, social, and psychological information; finally, an opinion should be stated that indicates the probable causal chain. The case study and recording presented at the beginning of this chapter illustrate a typical summary and diagnosis.

THERAPY FOR VOICE DISORDERS

The real reason for learning about voice disorders and their causes is to help either prevent or remedy these disorders. We have seen that voice problems almost always occur when the vocal cords vibrate abnormally or when the resonators are shaped or linked atypically. The altered vibration and resonance can be caused either by organic changes affecting the size, shape, texture, tonicity, and position of the critical structures or by learned changes, which can also determine position as well as dimensions and contractile tensions in the antagonistic muscle groups. The organic changes originate in disease, heredity, injury, and aging; the learned changes are based on speech models, personal beliefs, and methods of adjustment to environmental requirements and stresses. Obviously, the organic and nonorganic causes are frequently intertwined. Whenever possible, therapy is directed toward the underlying causal factors. However, sometimes the direct causes are no longer active or are not amenable to change. Consequently, therapy must often be directed partly or entirely to symptoms. Unfortunately, the term *voice therapy* is synonymous with *voice exercises* in the thinking of many people. Voice exercises *are* important, but they constitute only a small part of voice therapy. One of the major objectives of this chapter is to stress that vocal rehabilitation is an overall process affecting the individual's health and life-style as well as the voice itself.

For an example, see the case study at the beginning of the chapter.

Therapy for voice disorders encompasses three distinct but interdependent procedures. One is medical, which includes surgery, radiation, medication, and psychiatry; the second is environmental, which encompasses both modification of the environment for the benefit of the child or adult and the related program of helping the individual to adjust to the environment; the third is direct vocal rehabilitation, which includes the training activities for reducing the disorder and improving the voice.

The Medical Approach

Surgical treatment may completely eliminate a voice problem, or it may unavoidably leave an impaired structure and a voice defect. In this situation, speech rehabilitation may be able to help the person achieve maximum effectiveness with the structures that remain. Speech-language pathologists should be vitally concerned about the surgical procedures, even though they play no direct role in them. The more you know of the past surgical treatments and their implications in voice production, the better you will be able to develop a rational voice therapy.

Medications and other nonsurgical techniques may help cure a disease or bring a condition such as anemia or allergic response under control, thereby restoring physical vigor or reducing swelling. This kind of aid provides a more normal vocal mechanism and the possibility of a normal voice.

The Environmental Approach

Earlier in this chapter we suggested that school or employment and living environments sometimes cause people to use their voices excessively or traumatically and thereby create behavioral or organic changes in the larynx that produce voice disorders. Environments may also contain physical irritants or allergens that are detrimental to the larynx or resonators and consequently cause problems.

Voice therapy must consider, and when possible alter, these detrimental factors. One procedure that can be used where appropriate is consultations with the family, teachers, or employer to explain the effects of vocal abuse and to gain cooperation in reducing the amount and loudness of the individual's speaking, yelling, singing, and other excess use. When a person's occupation requires him to speak in a noisy setting, as at a desk in a factory, a small microphone and amplifying system can reduce vocal strain. Help in comparable circumstances can also come from ear stopples, which reduce the sound to the ear and thereby lessen the tendency to shout excessively. Air pollution from particulates, dust, pollen, and the like can often be reduced by the use of air conditioners or masks. The speech-language patholgist usually initiates these types of environmental therapy, but great help can be provided by the physician, social worker, or teacher.

Helping the individual adjust to his environmental situations is an aspect of the "direct approach" which is discussed in the next section.

The Direct Approach

Many and varied activities can be employed by the speech-language pathologist working directly with a person with a voice disorder. These procedures constitute the therapy of the clinical sessions and the carry-over of the person into practice and daily use. For convenience, the activities are grouped under seven headings which are listed alphabetically. Each has its function, and none is inherently more important than the others. Since several are often used together, there is no set sequence of introduction into the therapeutic process.

Whole books have been written on each of these seven items; the discussion here is limited to concepts involved.

Listening Skills or Ear Training

Most people do not hear their own voices as others hear them when they speak or sing. People are almost always surprised (and frequently shocked) when they hear a recording of their voices for the first time. Fortunately, clinical experience shows that a person can learn to modify his or her voice toward a more normal or target voice after becoming aware of its sound (Van Riper, 1978).

Teaching a person to listen is an important and early step in voice therapy. The process should be systematic and usually begins with pitch recognition and discrimination. Some people with voice problems identify and match pitches easily, but there are many who find these tasks to be very difficult.

Training in identifying various features of pitch can begin by trying to distinguish between higher and lower tones sounded on a piano or pitch pipe. The speech-language pathologist can construct tapes of recorded sound-pairs, some of which are separated widely on the musical scale and others progressively closer together, to give tasks of graduated difficulty. Identifying the sounds can be followed by attempts by the child or adult to match them.

Mental Hygiene

This old-fashioned term, which has been replaced in current literature by *mental health*, is used here on purpose to parallel the concept of physical hygiene. It implies healthy thinking and the means of both achieving and maintaining it. Everyone must confront problems and decisions, and some form of resolution is always made, whether appropriate or inappropriate. When people have a way to resolve difficulties, they do it easily and appropriately. When they do not have a "normal" or acceptable solution, they may acquire some substitute such as withdrawal, aggressive behavior, worrying, or even a voice disorder.

Many people with voice disorders do not understand what is happening in the larynx or resonators when they produce deviant sounds. Furthermore, they do not readily associate their vocal disorders with their anxieties and frustrations. Careful explanations using diagrams, photographs, and models or other illustrations where appropriate, often help people understand their problem. Detailed descriptions also provide insight that can lead to modified behavior or relief of anxiety about possible disease. The person who is worried or anxious about his or her voice or state of health will tend to be hypertense and will have poor control over the voice.

Another procedure in mental hygiene is careful, sympathetic, unhurried listening by the speech-language pathologist. When the person learns that what he says is held in strict confidence, he may reveal worries, frustrations, and anxieties that adversely affect his life and his voice. Many of these problems are not deep-seated or of long duration, but they can interfere with the restoration of a normal voice. With proper management by the speech-language pathologist, the basic problems can often be talked through with relief and voice restoration.

In this aspect, treatment of voice disorders is no different from treatment of any other speech or language problem. See the other chapters in Parts II and III of this book.

You may wonder about the appropriateness of using interviewing, counseling, and guidance techniques in therapy for voice disorders. This concern is appropriate, because it should encourage you to seek instruction in these techniques of clinical psychology. They are essential. Aronson (1980) expressed the need in the following statement:

> Any in-depth study of voice disorders forces us to conclude that so long as clinicians obtain privileged information from patients; so long as people have voice problems because of life stress and interpersonal conflict; so long as voice disorders produce anxiety, depression, embarrassment, and self-consciousness; so long as patients need a sympathetic person with whom they can discuss their distress, will speech pathologists need to consider their training incomplete until they have learned the basics of psychological interviewing and counseling. (p. 239)

Physical Hygiene

Good physical hygiene encompasses those activities and practices that promote good health. The presumptions underlying our emphasis on physical well-being are that a healthy person learns more easily, his muscles respond more readily, and he has greater stamina. Conversely, muscles that lose tonus and strength as the result of sedentary living, poor diet, or illness are less capable of performing properly than when they are strong and in good condition. Voices of weakened or ill persons reflect their disabilities. The speech-language pathologist can contribute to the health of the child or adult by encouraging a proper diet, adequate rest, and sufficient exercise. Many persons with voice disorders, particularly functional disorders, are not aware of the potential relationship of the voice to physical health.

Posture and Movement

Good posture could be considered an aspect of physical hygiene, but it is so vital in voice therapy that it deserves special emphasis. The term *good posture* as used here means maximum efficiency in body movement and positioning. It does not mean a rigid military position. This concept is emphasized by two experts in physical education, who wrote,

> Postural fitness may be defined as that fitness which each individual should seek to achieve, whereby he may assume and maintain proper segmental relationships in all movements of the body. Such a state of fitness provides functional efficiency in handling the body in all postural positons undertaken in work, play, or everyday living. . . . No definite standard of postural fitness for all is proposed, other than the suggestion of urgency for individual effort in striving toward the ultimate in body build and in efficiency of movement. (Lowman & Young, 1963, p. 9)

People who have sedentary occupations without compensatory physical activity typically lose strength in the muscles of their abdomen, back, and legs. This weakening allows the anterior abdominal walls to protrude and the shoulders to droop forward. When they stand or walk, the abdominal protrusion and shoulder droop are often accompanied by a rounded upper back, forward head carriage, and a forward curving of the lumbar spine. This postural change tends to interfere with respiratory efficiency.

The speech-language pathologist can help a person improve his or her posture by encouraging him to institute a physical education program at a local gymnasium or at least do routine daily calisthenics at home. Poor posture and reduced tonus of the skeletal muscles cannot be identified as a direct cause of voice disorders, but general physical fitness certainly will augment the remedial process.

Regulation of Breath Pressure

The lung capacity can be increased somewhat by regular practice in deep breathing. A second type of breathing exercise is associated with phonation. It focuses on efficiency and is concerned with the particular muscles used in inhalation and exhalation. Expansion of the thoracic space seems to be accomplished most efficiently by the combined action of the diaphragm and lower ribs in association with good posture. When the muscular sections of the diaphragm contract, they pull the entire structure downward, which displaces the contents of the abdomen slightly downward and forward to protrude the upper, anterior abdominal wall (the epigastrium). When the ribs move outward and upward to help draw the air inward, the central area of the body expands. In contrast, the most inefficient movements for inspiration are lifting the upper chest, along with the clavicles and shoulders, in combination with an inward motion of the epigastrium. Efficient expiration for phonation is accomplished by depressing the ribs concurrently with the inward movement of the abdominal wall, primarily at the epigastrium. The association of efficient breath movement with good posture and muscle strength should be obvious. Achieving breath control for speech can be accomplished effectively by inhaling as described and then prolonging sounds for as long as possible. These sounds should be timed occasionally and charted to obtain an objective record of progress. Changes in loudness during prolongation should also be practiced (Moncur & Brackett, 1974).

Relaxation

Many voice problems are associated with too much tension in the muscles used in speaking, a hypertention that is found often also in other musles throughout the body. Earlier in the chapter we referred to stressful situations causing hypertension. The resolution of conditions causing anxiety, worry, and the like is certainly important in reducing hypertension, but the satisfactory management of psychogenic factors often is not possible. Furthermore, the reduction of psychological and social pressures may leave a void; many people would not know how to relax even when they had nothing specific to cause hypertension. Consequently, direct and specific training in relaxation is usually helpful and often necessary in the management of a variety of voice problems.

There are many procedures in use today through which people try to achieve a state of relaxation. For general purposes, *relaxation* is defined as the absence of muscle contraction. This state can be induced throughout the entire body, where it is used as therapy for both muscular and circulatory hypertension, for digestive disorders, for "nervousness," and for a host of other illnesses. The techniques commonly used to achieve relaxation can be grouped into four categories: (*a*) meditation and/or deep breathing, (*b*) biofeedback, (*c*) suggestion, and (*d*) muscle sense with voluntary reduction of contraction.

Meditation techniques emphasize quiet surroundings and a mental state of peacefulness and calm. Frequently deep breathing and various postures are employed to help achieve the desired state. Biofeedback uses the phenomenon of electrical activity in muscles, which is directly proportional to the degree of muscle contraction. When sensors are placed on the skin (usually the forehead) and the sensed excitation is amplified and connected to a meter or other responder, an individual can be informed visually or audibly of the extent of muscle contraction. This feedback monitoring allows the person to learn how to reduce muscle contraction. Subsequently, the individual should be able to control this tension without the electronic aid. Relaxation by suggestion is a very old procedure that depends importantly on imagination. The person pictures himself in a quiet, peaceful place, or imagines his arms, legs, and so forth as being either very heavy or very light. He may listen to a rhythmic sound generator that creates the effect of waves on a beach, or another peaceful setting. Often an instructor who is guiding the relaxation procedure heightens the effect of suggestions by directing attention to, for example, heaviness in the arms and legs, while speaking in a quiet, monotonous voice. The fourth listed technique, which teaches the person to become aware of muscle contraction and to release the tension, is called *progressive relaxation* and is associated most closely with Jacobson (1976). Jacobson developed a systematic procedure in which each of the major muscle groups is contracted, one at a time in a progressive sequence, usually beginning with the arms, so that the sensation of the particular contraction can be identified and subsequently released. As a person practices relaxation, the amount of tension progressively diminishes; practice facilitates relaxation. A refinement of total body relaxation is called *differential relaxation*. In this process, the individual learns to recognize and release muscle contractions in a limited area such as the face or an arm. The objective step-by-step, sensory approach of the Jacobson procedure associated with the differential relaxation feature has caused *progressive relaxation* to be used widely in speech-language pathology.

We urge you to read one of the Jacobson books or chapter 7 in Moncur and Brackett (1974), listed at the end of the chapter.

Voice Training: Vocal Exercises

The six procedures of the "direct approach" we have discussed so far have not included much discussion of the voice proper and what can be done to rehabilitate or improve it. The first six procedures focus on the reduction or elimination of both mental and physical impediments to efficient voice production. In contrast, vocal training is designed to improve the voice to the maximum extent possible with the mechanisms available. The literatures of speech, music, and theater are rich with suggestions for training the voice. Many of the exercises and drills used in vocal therapy have come from these backgrounds. When these suggestions are combed from the literature, modified for rehabilitative purposes, and augmented by additional speech therapeutic techniques, the array is impressive. We will illustrate the use of a few of them.

Eliminating Vocal Abuse   So long as vocal abuse or excessive vocal use is present, exercises for vocal improvement that do not address the abuse problem directly will have little beneficial effect. There are many ways to reduce vocal abuse, such as some of the following procedures for improving voice production, but in some situations a direct attack on abuse as such is indicated.

A proven technique for reducing vocal abuse and thereby providing the vocal mechanism an opportunity to restore itself and the voice is behavior modification. This aid to learning is successful when an individual has the desire to eliminate a habit or to modify some activity and when he or she can both observe and count the particular behavior. For example, when a person has vocal nodules resulting from screaming, yelling, excessive talking, and the like, he can eliminate the lesions by counting the episodes of vocal abuse in selected situations, charting them, and systematically reducing the number and length of the periods of vocal abuse. Several effective programs for modification of vocal abuse have been reported. One of these, which has been particulary successful in elementary schools, was developed by Johnson (1976) and his associates. After abuse has been eliminated or when vocal problems remain following disease, external trauma, and the like, positive voice training procedures are usually necessary.

Finding the Best Sounds   Everyone (except someone who is mute) has a repertory of vocal sounds. Some sounds will be produced more easily and with better quality than others. The best sounds can be located by asking the child or adult to produce a variety of vowel sounds at low, medium, and high pitches and with different loudness levels. The most pleasant or least effortful phonation is selected as a guide or target vioce (Boone, 1977). This "best" should not be thought of necessarily as the target for the regular speech pattern for the person with hoarseness or other dysphonia, since a voice may sound least hoarse at a pitch that would be too high for general use. The person is taught to feel and hear optimum production, and an effort is made to produce other sounds equally well. The person also attempts constantly to improve the target voice. Finding the best voice is closely related to the listening training we have described.

Finding the best voice is also related to a concept called *optimum pitch*. This term refers to a note or small cluster of notes on the musical scale at which vocal tone can be produced with relatively little effort and considerable loudness. Everyone has a pitch range that extends from a lowest to a highest note, extremes at which little or no change in loudness can be produced. As the pitch is moved upward from the lowest tone, the dynamic range (loudness) can be increased progressively with each scale step to a maximum. After the maximum, the dynamic range decreases with rising pitch. Vocal training increases the ranges of both pitch and loudness, but the average voice reaches its maximum dynamic range at four to five full tones above the lowest pitch (Coleman, Mabis, & Hinson, 1977; Damsté & Lerman, 1975; Schutte, 1980). This region is where the voice seems to be produced maximally; it is the optimum pitch for speaking.

Exercises for Reducing Hypertense Phonation   Hypertense phonation signals overly tight glottal closure during phonation, or excessive effort to close the glottis when an organic problem interferes. This pattern can usually be relieved by the combination of general relaxation and the following types of phonation drills.

"Yawn–Sigh" Phonation.   The person is instructed to yawn as naturally as possible and, after a full inhalation, to expel the air while producing a breathy, sighing sound. This and other exercixes should be repeated successively several times and also at intervals throughout a clinical session, as well as at home between sessions.

Aspirate Initiation of Vowel Sounds.   When the [h] sound precedes a vowel as in "ha," the vocal cords begin to vibrate while they are adducting and consequently do not begin to vibrate from a tightly closed glottis. The maneuver leads to laryngeal relaxation and a desirable, slightly breathy voice when carried over into words and sentences. Drill sentences such as "Hold hope high," "How high is that house?" and "He hid Harry's hat in a hurry" are useful transition devices.

Breathy Phonation.   People who can relieve laryngeal hyperfunction with aspirate initiation can usually speak with an excessively breathy voice when used as a drill. If imitation of the speech-language pathologist's intentionally breathy voice is not satisfactory, ask the person to substitute short sentences during the sigh-type exhalation. Sometimes "acting a part" or role-playing where a breathy voice is typical of the character will help the hypertense person to substitute more relaxed phonation.

The Chewing Method.   This "method" is a widely used exercise in which the person exaggerates real chewing. While performing this act, he phonates sounds which are "chewed." The activity usually reduces tension in the laryngeal area (Froeschels, 1952; Wyatt, 1977).

Increase in Phonatory Efficiency   Phonatory efficiency implies maximum balance between air supply and adjustment of the laryngeal mechanism. Stated negatively, if there is air wastage or the vocal cords are adjusted with too much or too little glottal opening, phonatory efficiency is reduced. When excessive air is used during phonation or, in contrast, when the inefficiency of phonation reflects a glottal closure that is too tight, efficiency may be increased by several means. One of the most useful procedures for both forms of phonatory inefficiency is tone prolongation. In this type of drill, the child or adult practices vocalizing as long as possible on each breath, at various pitch and loudness levels, and while as relaxed as possible. Usually this type of exercising helps the person increase the air supply and improve laryngeal control of the phonatory airstream. Sounding tones quietly up and down a musical scale on a single breath also helps to increase phonatory efficiency. The tonal drills can be extended into phrases and sentences, where the number of words on one breath can be gradually increased. The point should be made that there is no virtue in speaking long sentences on one breath during conversation; exercises that increase that ability simply supply the speaker with both an extra capacity when needed and a more efficient mechanism. Some speech-language pathologists might quite properly associate the prolongations of phonation time with breath control. As steady-tone phonation is extended and phrase length increases, there is usually an accompanying reduction in both laryngeal hyper- and hypofunctional phonation.

Vocal Pitch Training   The pitch deviations that speech-language pathologists see most frequently are levels that are higher than normal for the age and sex of the speaker, lower than normal under the same expectancy factors, or monotonous (that is, there is relatively little pitch variation). When the pitch is high in the male adolescent or adult, and the larynx has been medically diagnosed to be normal, the following procedures are appropriate.

(1) Listen to the pitch and quality of the cough and to "clearing the throat." If these vocalizations sound essentially normal, there is a strong implication that the vocal potential is good.
(2) Ask the man to "clear his throat" and prolong the sound into a continuous humming tone. This sound frequently stays within the normal range.
(3) Sometimes the man with habitually high pitch can voluntarily produce a tone in the normal range in certain circumstances, such as singing or imitating another voice. When this is the case and the man genuinely wants to have a normal voice, he should practice the lower pitch frequently. Concurrently, the speech-language pathologist should reinforce the tone by matching it and uttering it loudly near the man's ear. Recording of the voice with playback also often helps him identify and maintain the target voice.
(4) If the preceding techniques do not produce satisfactory results, laryngeal manipulation should be introduced. Men with functionally based high pitch usually carry the larynx high in the neck; the thyroid notch frequently touches the hyoid bone, which is also elevated. Palpation of the thyroid cartilage when the man is relaxed and not phonating will permit the speech-language pathologist to identify the notch and borders of the thyroid lamina. The clinician should then place an index finger on the notch, with the thumb and fingers at either side, and gently press downward toward the chest while the man "clears his throat" or coughs gently. Of course, the clinician explains that the high pitch is associated with the high carriage of the larynx and that the repositioning is important. Occasionally, pressing downward and backward simultaneously will cause

the voice to break into a lower pitch and register. The man should be attempting to lower his own pitch at the same time. If he achieves a lower pitch, a period of intensive practice should follow immediately. However, several therapy sessions may be necessary to achieve and stabilize the major change. When a lower pitch occurs with the speech-language pathologist's finger on the thyroid, the pressure should be reduced gradually over successive trials. If the desired pitch is maintained, the man should be taught to use his own finger. Usually the finger contact can be reduced and removed completely within a brief time. The man should practice the new voice several times each day, and attempt to use it all the time as soon as the control is relatively stable.

When the vocal pitch is too low in the individual's probable range and the larynx is normal, the boy or man is usually trying to imitate another voice or is attempting to "sound more masculine." This type of phonation often incorporates **glottal fry,** which is a grating or popping sound that occurs most often toward the end of sentences of phrases where the pitch and breath pressure customarily drop. Men who speak at the low end of their pitch ranges will not readily accept the concept of a higher pitch. However, they will welcome an opportunity to increase their speaking effectiveness. This objective can be met in part by focusing on prosodic elements such as stress and phrasing.

Another technique that may help people who have habitually low pitch is role-playing. Ask them to read the part of an appropriate character in a play script. Additional assistance can come from intoning musical scales, matching pitches, and practicing reading or speaking with a moderately loud voice.

When the pitch of a woman's voice becomes low enough to cause her to be falsely identified as a male in a telephone conversation, the basic problem almost always is a hormonal imbalance. Medical treatment may arrest the change, but does not reverse it. Voice therapy can assist mostly in an emphasis on female prosodic patterns, particularly an increase in upward pitch changes in word stress.

When an individual speaks with little pitch variation, the voice may reflect an identity problem such as that of men who wish to sound "more masculine" by speaking monotonously at the bottom end of the pitch range. Another type of relatively inflexible, monotonous pitch pattern signals a listless, weak, or depressed person. If these individuals want to change their vioces, they usually can do so through ear training, self-monitoring, and pitch flexibility drills of the type mentioned previously. Obviously, combinations of mental hygiene and pitch drills are needed.

Procedures for Increasing Vocal Loudness   People who do not speak loudly enough for their needs do so for one or a combination of four reasons: (*a*) there is an organic problem that impairs normal function, (*b*) the person is shy and reticent about speaking, (*c*) there is a hearing loss, or (*d*) the person does not know how to use a big voice without damaging the mechanism. When an individual has an organic problem such as paralysis, a postsurgical condition, or some other disability that prevents glottal closure during vocal fold vibration, the voice may never be loud enough. However, we do have a few procedures that often prove helpful. One is greater air flow, which improves the approximation of the vocal cords by increasing the amplitude of their vibration. With greater amplitude the medial as well as the lateral excursions are extended. Furthermore, the Bernoulli effect probably contributes some additional medial deflection when the vocal cords approach each other.

Improvement in the movement and control of the breath stream for increased loudness can also be achieved through exercises with unvoiced and voiced fricatives. For example, the /ʃ/ sound should be produced quietly and then as loudly as possible. Subsequently the /ʒ/ should be practiced with similar variations. The /f, v, θ, ð, s, z/ and /tʃ, dʒ/ are equally applicable.

Another suggestion made frequently for the improvement of vocal cord approximation is to tense the muscles of the arms or legs, which heightens the muscle tonus elsewhere in the body—including the larynx. The effect is to increase feeble muscle contractions and thereby improve glottal closure. The person is instructed to squeeze the arm of the chair or to pull upward on the seat of the chair or to try some similar isotonic exercise. A variant is the pushing exercise in which the person lifts clenched fists to the upper chest, elbows extended laterally, and then thrusts the fists downward vigorously while uttering a vowel sound as loudly as possible (Froeschels, Kastein, & Weiss, 1955).

Further assistance for the person with a continuously weak voice is improvement in articulatory precision. When words are spoken with precise movements of the tongue, lips, and soft palate (this does not mean overly precise, pedantic speaking), the speech is easier to understand and there is less demand on the phonatory mechanism.

You might wish to review the suggestions for improving articulation in chapter 5.

The person who is capable of producing adequately loud sound, but who is reluctant to speak with sufficient voice, usually needs help with personality adjustment and the development of more self-confidence. In addition to mental hygiene procedures, we have some speech exercises that directly reduce the voice problem and contribute to self-confidence. The fricative drills for loudness described above provide a good, nonthreatening start in a clinical setting. Another approach is to supply masking noise through headphones while the person reads aloud. When the person reads appropriately loud, it should be recorded and subsequently played back along with recordings of the habitual voice. This kind of demonstration that a louder than usual voice can be produced is a great encourager.

A third useful procedure is role-playing with a play script. Sometimes hand puppets facilitate the shift to other characters and their voices, particularly with high-school age and younger children.

The person who must be able to use a loud voice, such as a minister, lawyer, athletic coach, or actor, but who is unable to do so for more than a few minutes without feeling discomfort or becoming hoarse needs help in building a voice. Those who have this problem usually come to the speech-language pathologist with hypertense muscle adjustments in the larynx and also in the tongue, soft palate, and jaw. These adjustments are often accompanied by general muscular hypertension, poor posture, and respiratory habits that are inadequate for sustained loud speaking. These people also often have vocal nodules or a chronic laryngitis.

Remediation is a long-term process. This fact often surprises or even irritates people with a problem; they want something done to them or for them immediately. They frequently find it difficult to accept the concept that whatever is done is done *with* them, not to them; remediation is a collaboration between client, speech-language pathologist, and other professionals. These people accept the fact that change and improvement in their tennis will take time and practice. But they fail to realize that the coordination needed for good voice production is probably more subtle and less easily modified than movements of arms, legs, and torso. Voice therapy, particularly when designed to build a big voice, goes on 24 hours a day, 7 days a week.

The specific procedures to be instituted, in addition to explanation, relaxation, respiration, and posture, include drills for easy phonation, unvoiced-voiced fricative production at minimum and maximum intensities, and the drills for prolongation to increase the efficiency of breath usage. In addition to these exercises, practice should be gradually carried over into a large room such as an auditorium. When the person begins to practice the exercises in the large hall, he or she should phonate gently as though attempting to reach only the first few rows of seats. Gradually, over a period of weeks, as each loudness level becomes established, the loudness should be increased to reach successive rows. The period of time at each new loudness level should also be extended progressively, as the voice and larynx will permit. Efficient, relatively relaxed, loud voice for long periods of time is the ultimate objective. The capacity to produce a big voice provides a luxury of vocal energy that improves vocal quality and flexibility, even when the louder voice is not needed.

Modification of Resonance   The resonance characteristics of the vocal tract have a marked influence on the quality of the voice. Where organic variations do not interfere, resonance is modified primarily by movements of the tongue, positioning of the lips, opening or closing of the velopharyngeal valve, and changing the size of the parynx. When the tongue is carried forward in the mouth, the voice has a "thin quality." Frequently, this faulty voice quality also features articulation on the back lip rounded vowels with broad smile or slit-shaped lip positions. The "thin voice" gives the impression of immaturity (Fisher, 1969). This voice is also characteristic of the effeminate male voice. In contrast, when the tongue is retracted, the voice tends to sound throaty. These resonance problems can be relieved with exercises in which the person is taught to sense the tongue positions and hear the deviant sounds by exaggerating the malpositions and distorted sounds. Of course, the "cute young thing" who uses a "thin voice" to wheedle her father or boy friend or who is reluctant to accept a more mature role will need to change her perceptions of herself. The effeminate male will also need counseling to help him recognize the abnormal impression he conveys. The direct voice quality drills for the "thin quality" will stress the back vowels with appropriate lip rounding. The voice and diction literature contains many useful drills (Fisher, 1969; Moncur & Brackett, 1974).

The throaty quality is heard most frequently in men, particularly those who attempt to speak near the bottom of their pitch ranges. Direct drills that stress front vowels are beneficial, particularly when used with the bilabial and lingua-alveolar consonants. The throaty quality resembles the "muffled" voice mentioned earlier and the remedial measures, except for the treatment of organic problems, are similar.

The most obvious resonance disorders are hyper- and hyponasality. Hypernasality of the open type (rhinolalia aperta) almost always results either from a cleft palate, in which the roof of the mouth is incomplete, from a short palate, or from paralysis. Surgical procedures have been developed to the point that most children with a cleft palate or short palate can be successfully treated. A wide range of prosthetic speech appliances can also be constructed to supplement or substitute for surgical treatment.

See chapter 11.

When hypernasality is present without an apparent organic cause, the speech usually responds to voice treatment. The basic objective, of course, is to achieve closure of the velopharyngeal port at the proper time. We have many procedures that can help meet this objective. They can be illustrated in the following five types of exercises.

(1) One of the most basic is ear training, which implies learning to recognize nasalized and nonnasalized sounds in both isolated vowels and continuous speaking. Recordings are played for identification of gross and subtle contrasts. This procedure is extended to listening to the person's own recordings and then to monitoring of on-going speech.

(2) Contrast of nasal and nonnasal production. When the person learns to hear differences, drills that alternate nasal and nonnasal sounds such as /ba-na/ /mba/ /kudnt/, and so on can be introduced. After some control has been achieved, negative practice can be used. In negative practice, the child or adult intentionally produces an extreme hypernasalization. This sound should be alternated with both the normal (good) production and a completely denasal version.

(3) Open mouth drill. When the mouth is open widely for sound production, there is less tendency for the sound to be forced through the nose, even when a complete velopharyngeal closure cannot be made. Furthermore, the velum seems to increase its activity when contraction in other muscle groups is exaggerated.

(4) Vigorous sound production. When the plosives are spoken vigorously, the velopharyngeal closure is made firmly and increased air pressure in the pharynx adds to the tightness of the closure. Energetic whispering of /pa, ta, ka/ as well as vigorous utterance of the voiced syllables /ba, da, ga/ is very useful, even with slight velopharyngeal leakage.

(5) Lower pitch. Occasionally, when the pitch of the voice is lowered, the perceived hypernasality is reduced. Drills of the type recommended for pitch change are applicable.

So far we have emphasized reducing excessive nasal resonance. Occasionally a person needs to increase nasal resonance. Usually denasality is associated with an obstruction in the nasal passages or nasopharynx. However, in some cases medical treatment cannot remedy the situation, or the person maintains a denasality which was learned by imitation. Increase in appropriate nasal resonance requires ear training and drills for emphasizing the /m, n, ŋ/ sounds. Humming each of these sounds, combining them with vowels, and intentional, vigorous exhalation through the nose usually produce good results. Additional practice should be conducted with phrases and sentences that are rich in the nasal sounds.

SPEECH WITHOUT A LARYNX

Earlier in this chapter, in the review of the relationship between phonation and resonance, we described the larynx as the generator of linguistically undifferentiated sound that is modified into meaningful speech by the movements and positions of the organs of resonance and articulation. We also said that any complex sound could substitute for the laryngeal sound if it were put into the upper airway. Loss of the larynx occurs rather frequently, usually as the result of surgical treatment for cancer. And on occasion, external trauma also requires laryngectomy as a life-preserving measure. After the larynx has been removed, the laryngectomized person has three possible substitute sound sources: a natural vibrator created surgically, an artificial larynx instrument, or an existing or natural vibrator at the sphincter at the junction between the pharynx and esophagus. This third mechanism is the source of burp sounds.

Surgical Procedures

*A **pseudoglottis** is simply an artificial glottis.*

Many surgical procedures to aid voice production have been developed, with varying degrees of success. These operations can be classified into one of three categories: (a) those that construct a vibrator which is activated by the pulmonary air as it passes through the **pseudoglottis** and on into the pharynx at about the location of the original larynx; (b) those that provide a shunt that carries the pulmonary air from a special opening in the upper part of the trachea to the esophagus, where vibration occurs; and (c) those that incorporate an external device in combination with a surgical passage through which the air is redirected into the pharynx.

*The **stoma** is the new opening in the neck through which laryngectomee breathes.*

When a pseudoglottis is constructed, pulmonary respiration occurs through a customary **stoma** in the neck which joins as opening in the side rather than the end of the trachea. The upper end of the trachea, or sometimes part of the cricoid cartilage, is covered by a portion of the esophageal wall or other membrane in which a small slit opening is made. This opening joins the pharyngeal cavity to the trachea to allow exhaled air to pass from the trachea to the pharynx when the stoma is closed. Vibration of the slit mechanism or the tissues in the hypopharynx creates a sound which is articulated into speech. Unfortunately, the several varieties of pseudoglottis are rarely successful because liquids and food tend to leak through them and go into the lungs to cause congestion or pneumonia.

The shunts vary somewhat in type and surgical methods, but essentially they are small, surgically created channels that extend from the upper part of the trachea into the esophagus. When the stoma is closed by a finger during exhalation, the air is forced through the channel into the esophagus. There it sets the sphincter at the top of the esophagus into vibration to create sound. Leakage has been a problem with the shunt procedures, but ingenious valve prostheses which promise a successful solution to the problems are constantly being developed and refined.

The third type of surgical procedure, the use of an external devise and surgical passage through the side of the neck, has had only imited use. In this system, the pulmonary air is carried from the stoma through a tube to a valve mechanism that is housed in a small enclosure that lies on the chest. The air then passes into a small tube that enters the pharynx through a surgically created channel located high on the side of the neck. The sound is created either by a reed in the housing, or by the vibration of the tissue when the air enters the pharynx. When ordinary, quiet respiration occurs, the air flows into and out of the trachea through a valve in the enclosure. However, when the person wishes to speak, he or she exhales air suddenly to close that outlet valve. This directs the air to the channel. The valve eliminates the need for the laryngectomee to close the stoma with a finger and thus frees both hands for other purposes.

Artificial Larynges

Artificial larynges are of two general types, classified according to their source of power: pneumatic and electronic. The pneumatic instruments are hand-held, have an air supply tube, a sound source, and a sound conducting tube. When a laryngectomee speaks with one of these instruments, he or she connects the air supply tube to the stoma to conduct the exhaled air to the sound source. The sound source is a container that houses a vibrator, either a reed or a piece of broad rubber band. These vibrator elements are activated by the air flow and generate a sound which is conducted into the mouth through a small tube that passes between the lips. Intelligible speech is made by articulating in the usual manner.

The electronic artificial larynges are more common than the pneumatic instruments, primarily because they are easier to use and maintain. These units take several forms according to the manufacturer's designs, but their function in speaking is similar. The instruments generate a buzzing sound that comes from one end of the unit, which is held in one hand and can be turned on and off with a thumb switch. Its pitch can be varied somewhat. When a laryngectomized person speaks with this type of instrument, he or she places the sounder end firmly against the upper part of the neck at a location which has been experimentally determined to produce the loudest speech. The sound passes through the skin and other tissues of the neck into the pharynx and mouth where it is available for speech. The articulatory movements in speaking are essentially the same as they are for normal speech.

Several other electronic devices combine certain features of the pneumatic and electronic instruments. One of these is an electronic unit on which a funnel-like attachment covers the sounder and leads the sound into the mouth by way of a small tube. This device is useful for those people who cannot tolerate vibrator contact on the skin of the neck or who are unable to transmit sufficient sound through the tissues. Another device conducts the sound from an earphone-type sounder through a tube into the mouth. The sounder unit is held in the speaker's hand and can be turned on and off with a little push-button switch. The power for the unit comes from a battery pack carried in a pocket or other convenient container.

A variant of this concept has the sounder located in the bowl of a tobacco pipe and uses the step to transmit the sound into the mouth. This unit has not been used widely; we have mentioned it here to show the extent of the aids that have been developed to assist the laryngectomee.

Esophageal Speech

The third option for a sound source available to a laryngectomized person is a natural vibrator within the individual. This sound source is usually the sphincter at the junction of the pharynx and esophagus. The sound produced has been made by everyone at sometime in their lives; it is called *burp, belch,* or *eructation.* The sound occurs when air in the esophagus is forced through the constriction at the top of the esophagus and causes it to vibrate. Obviously, this sound, like any of the artificial sounds mentioned previously, could be used in speaking if it were prolonged and available whenever desired. The problem then, is to learn to take air into the esophagus and to return it with sound as needed.

There are two means by which air is introduced into the esophagus; it may be pushed in or it may be drawn in. When the larynx has been removed, the channel between the pharynx and lungs is closed, which leaves the lips, velopharyngeal port, and the pharyngeoesophageal sphincter as the remaining exits and entrances to the mouth and pharynx. If the air pressure is increased sufficiently in the mouth and pharynx, the air will escape through the least resistant exit. Fortunately, the constriction at the top of the esophagus can be relaxed somewhat with training, which allows the pressurized air to flow into the esophagus. The air pressure can be increased by tongue and jaw movements. When the tongue is placed against the alevolar ridge, as for the production of /t/ or /d/, air is impounded behind it. If the back of the tongue is lifted to the roof of the mouth, the air is pushed into the pharynx and on into the esophagus when the sphincter permits it. Immediately after that injection, the air is expelled to vibrate the sphincter and produce a sound. With practice, larger amounts of air can be injected and the expulsion prolonged.

A second form of the injection technique was developed in the Netherlands (Moolenaar-Bijl, 1953). This procedure emphasizes the plosive sounds, unvoiced fricatives such as /s/ and /ʃ/, and combinations such as /ts/ and /tʃ/ that require relatively high intraoral pressure. When a larngectomized person produces syllables or words containing these pressure sounds, a little of the momentarily impounded air injects into the esophagus to add to the air supply. Experiments have demonstrated that more syllables can be uttered on a single expulsion when there are many pressure sounds in the sentences than when there are none.

The second method for obtaining air in the esophagus is a form of inhalation. Air is drawn into the esophagus about the way it is taken into the lungs. If the upper opening into the esophagus normally remained open in everybody, air would be drawn into the esophagus concurrently with the lungs by the expansion of the chest. If a laryngectomized person could learn to open the esophagus voluntarily, or relax it to minimal resistance, he or she could draw into the esophagus when the breath is inhaled for pulmonary respiration. This procedure is learned by a large number of laryngectomees, many of whom have excellent esophageal speech. Frequently, fluent esophageal speakers use both injection and inhalation techniques interchangeably and automatically without being aware of the specific technique of the moment. Some of these speakers develop voices that are nearly normal, but most laryngectomees maintain some hoarseness. Furthermore, their speech is marked by short phrases, caused by the limited air supply from the esophagus.

No alaryngeal form of speaking is as desirable as normal speech, but any of the forms, when used well, can be extremely useful. In addition to the undesirable presence of the short phrases of esophageal speech and the atypical vocal quality and pitch accompanying all substitute voice production, a further limitation with surgical reconstructions and artificial larynges is the need to use one hand to assist the voice production. However, one offsetting advantage of the reconstructions and artificial larynges is the capacity to use normal phrasing. Almost all alaryngeal speech lacks pitch variation; the exception is the few esophageal speakers who achieve some pitch change.

The most frustrating problem for all alaryngeal speakers is low vocal intensity. Trying to compete against the ordinary social and environmental noises is difficult and fatiguing. A parallel problem exists when these people attempt to communicate with hearing impaired spouses and others. Working with the laryngectomized person requires patience, understanding, and sensitivity to these social results of a physical problem.

CONCLUSION

Voice disorders, which encompass abnormalities of pitch, loudness, and quality, are found among people of all ages. The atypical voice can arise either at the sound source, usually the larynx, or in the resonators, the spaces of the upper respiratory tract. For various reasons, the sound generator or the resonators may not function normally. These malfunctions are not capricious—they have causes, but the causes are not always apparent. There is much evidence that the factors underlying faulty operation of the vocal mechanism are extremely varied. They range from psychosocial disorders that show themselves in atypical adjustments and movements of the organs of communication to actual structural modification of these organs by disease or trauma.

Remedial programs for voice disorders must recognize the etiologies in each individual case and attempt to modify those causes where possible. Therapy programs must also incorporate the means for increasing function to maximum efficiency. The full restoration or development of normal voice is not always possible, but usually we have remedial techniques available that can at least help a person to more intelligible speech, to more normal vocal sound, and to more efficient, trauma-free voice production. In a society such as ours, which depends heavily on spoken communication, every step toward better communication is a valuable improvement.

SELECTED READINGS

Boone, D. R. *The voice and voice therapy* (2nd ed.). Englewood Cliffs, N.J.: Prentice-Hall, 1977.

Diedrich, W. M., & Youngstrom, K. A. *Alaryngeal speech*. Springfield, Ill.: Charles C Thomas, 1966.

Hejna, R. F. *Speech disorders and nondirective therapy*. New York: Ronald Press, 1960.

Moore, G. P. Voice disorders organically based. In L. E. Travis (Ed.), *Handbook of speech pathology and audiology*. New York: Appleton-Century-Crofts, 1971.

Wilson, D. K. *Voice problems of children* (2nd ed.). Baltimore: Williams and Wilkins, 1979.

REFERENCES

American college dictionary. New York: Random House, 1951.

Aronson, A. E. *Clinical voice disorders*. New York: Brian C. Decker, 1980.

Ballenger, J. J. *Diseases of the nose, throat, and ear* (12 th ed.). Philadelphia: Lea and Febiger, 1977.

Baynes, R. A. An incidence study of chronic hoarseness among children. *Journal of Speech and Hearing Disorders,* 1966, *31,* 172–174.

Boone, D. R. *The voice and voice therapy* (2nd ed.). Englewood Cliffs, N.J.: Prentice-Hall, 1977.

Cherry, J., & Margulies, S. Contact ulcer of the larynx. *Laryngoscope,* 1968, *78,* 1937–1940.

Chodosh, P. L. Gastro-esophago-pharyngeal reflux. *Laryngoscope,* 1977, *87,* 418–427.

Coleman, R. F., Mabis, J. H., & Hinson, J. K. Fundamental frequency—Sound pressure level profiles of adult male and female voices. *Journal of Speech and Hearing Research,* 1977, *20,* 197–204.

Damsté, P. H., & Lerman, J. W. *An introduction to voice pathology*. Springfield, Ill.: Charles C Thomas, 1975.

Delahunty, J. E., & Cherry, J. Experimentally produced vocal cord granulomas. *Laryngoscope,* 1968, *78,* 1941–1947.

Fisher, H. B. *Improving voice and articulation.* Boston: Houghton Mifflin, 1966.

Froeschels, E. Chewing method as therapy. *Archives of Otolaryngology,* 1952, *56,* 427–434.

Froeschels, E., Kastein, S., & Weiss, D. A. A method of therapy for paralytic conditions of the mechanisms of phonation, respiration and glutination. *Journal of Speech and Hearing Disorders,* 1955, *20,* 365–370.

Jackson, C., & Jackson, C. L. *The larynx and its diseases.* Philadelphia: W. B. Saunders, 1937.

Jacobson, E. *You must relax* (5th ed.). New York: McGraw-Hill, 1976.

Johnson, T. S. *Vocal abuse reduction program.* Logan: Utah State University, 1976.

Kimelman, M. D. Z. *The effect of puberty on vocal cord nodules in males.* Unpublished Masters thesis, University of Florida, 1980.

Lowman, C. L., & Young, C. H. *Postural fitness: Significance and variances.* Philadelphia: Lea and Febiger, 1963.

Milisen, R. The incidence of speech disorders, In L. E. Travis (Ed.), *Handbook of speech pathology and audiology.* New York: Appleton-Century-Crofts, 1971.

Moncur, J. P., & Brackett, I. P. *Modifying vocal behavior.* New York: Harper & Row, 1974.

Moolenaar-Bijl, A. The importance of certain consonants in esophageal voice after laryngectomy. *Annals of Otology, Rhinology, and Laryngology,* 1953, *62,* 979–989.

Sauchelli, K. R. *The incidence of hoarseness among school-aged children in a pollution-free community.* Unpublished Masters thesis, University of Florida, 1979.

Schutte, H. K. *The efficiency of voice production.* Druk: Kemper, Groningen, 1980.

Senturia, B. H., & Wilson, F. B. Otorhinolaryngic findings in children with voice deviations. *Annals of Otology, Rhinology, and Laryngology,* 1968, *77,* 1027–1042.

Silverman, E. M., & Zimmer, C. H. Incidence of chronic hoarseness among school-age children. *Journal of Speech and Hearing Disorders,* 1975, *40,* 211–215.

Snidecor, J. C. Speech without a larynx. In L. E. Travis (Ed.), *Handbook of speech pathology and audiology.* New York Appleton-Century-Crofts, 1971.

Stedman's Medical Dictionary (23rd ed.) Baltimore: Williams and Wilkins, 1976.

Van Riper, C. *Speech correction: Principles and methods* (6th ed.). Englewood Cliffs, N.J.: Prentice-Hall, 1972.

Webb, M. W., & Irving, R. W. Psychologic and anamnestic patterns characteristic of laryngectomees: Relation to speech rehabilitation. *Journal of American Geriatric Society,* 1964, *12,* 303–322.

Wyatt, G. L. The chewing method and the treatment of the speaking voice. In M. Cooper & M. H. Cooper (Eds.), *Approaches to vocal rehabilitation.* Springfield, Ill.: Charles C Thomas, 1977.

Wyke, B. D. Laryngeal neuromuscular control systems in singing: A review of current concepts. *Folia Phoniatrica,* 1974, *26,* 295–306.

DISORDERS OF FLUENCY

7

George Shames
Cheri Florance

When she first came to the clinic, Laura was 30 years old. She is a college graduate and trained as an occupational therapist. She had then been married for 10 years, with three children—8, 5, and 2. Her husband was a young, successful attorney with offices in a large Eastern city some 30 miles from the small urban community in which the family resided. Laura had worked, but never as an occupational therapist. Before her marriage, she worked for a short time on an assembly line in a factory and as a waitress while in college. She applied for a job as an occupational therapist only once, but was turned down, she felt, because of her speech. She never again applied for such a position. Laura is graceful, poised, mature, and articulate. She would be considered overall as an attractive and sensitive person. She has an open and ready smile for her children and her husband, and a very easy and comfortable manner with them. However, during her first interview, we could see the traces of sadness in her face and eyes. She projected a sense of helplessness which generated a great deal of nurturance from those who are around her. Two years before, soon after the birth of her third child, she became extremely depressed and attempted to commit suicide; but it was thought to be more of a gesture than a bona fide attempt. Her psychiatric therapy was brief and apparently successful. Laura attributed her depression in part to having a very severe problem of stuttering.

As she related the history of her stuttering, she openly cried as she recalled the occasions as a young child that her parents forbade her to talk when guests were in the home. Her embarrassment and sadness and anger over these thoughts overwhelmed her. Wherever she went, she carried little index cards on which she had written out brief messages as substitutes for oral communication, in case she needed information, was lost, or was in an emergency situation that required communication. She reported on one occasion, in an airport, when she had wandered around for 30 minutes trying to physically locate a gate and flight without talking or asking for help. She had finally found her destination in silence. She tearfully stated that, because she stutters, she can never say "thank you" to people, who in turn mistakenly think she is rude, aloof, or ungrateful. She never uses the phone, depends on her husband for talking, shopping, and so on, and constantly stays at his side during social outings. She feels she is a failure as the wife of a professional man and as a mother. She recognizes her overdependence on others and how she has benefited from her own posture of helplessness.

She reported several previous encounters with therapy for her problem. These ranged from parent counseling, psychiatric therapy, and hypnosis to more traditional speech therapy in schools, in hospitals, and in universities. She had been in and out of therapy for some 25 years. Although her hopes for help had been dashed many times, and she carried the scars of many years of disappointment and futility, she was still more hopeful than skeptical. She came in for her initial interview literally pleading for help to be free from her agonies, both public and private, about her stuttering.

One could not help but be impressed with her motivation, her need for support, and her fragility as she was about to initiate still another duel with her problem. It was with these awarenesses of her and a sense of my own responsibility that I joined her in this clinical relationship.

You may now wish to listen to the speech sample accompanying this chapter, found on Audio Disc 1, Side 1 (sample #3).

In our examinations of articulation and voice, we have seen that a broad range of characteristics can be considered "normal," and that the line between "normal" and "disordered" is often fuzzy—depending upon the subjective opinion of the person doing the evaluation and the reactions of the person being evaluated and the other important people in his or her life. This is also the case with disorders of fluency. Fluent speech contains all the appropriate nuances of meaning associated with variations of rhythm, phrasing, stress, inflection, and speed, without inappropriate pauses, interjections, or fragmenting of the communication act. We use the term for people who speak a foreign language—"Oh, yes, Jonathon speaks four languages fluently." We readily accept many forms of **disfluency,** such as pauses to edit and compose utterances. We accept interjections like "um" and "uh" while a speaker gathers his thoughts. We accept the fragmenting associated with being interrupted and the repetitions of sounds and words of an excited speaker. Clearly, not all disfluencies are part of a disorder or a problem. But we also recognize some limit to acceptable disfluency, and once a speaker goes outside of these broad, imprecise boundaries, we say he has a fluency disorder. As do other communication disorders, fluency disorders come in an assorted array of types, forms, and circumstances, and they cause a broad array of reactions in both listeners and speakers.

Disfluencies include pauses, hesitations, interjections, prolongations, and repetitions which interrupt the smooth flow of speech. Some professionals use disfluency *and* dysfluency *interchangeably.*

Finding the line between normal disfluency and fluency disorders can be quite difficult. Most normal disfluencies are either repetitions of whole words, or pauses and interjections. But if a speaker repeats words quite frequently or repeats the same word again and again in the same phrase, her speech may be considered abnormal. If her pauses are too frequent or too long, they may also be considered abnormal. As listeners, we are accustomed to hearing speech in a certain way, which lets us respond to the content of the message. But sometimes we find ourselves paying attention to how the speaker is talking instead. If we are paying attention to the disfluencies in the speaker's speech, then the speaker may have crossed the line over to "disorder." Furthermore, listener reactions are a significant dimension of a disorder of fluency.

Cluttering is characterized by a very rapid speech, often so rapid as to be unintelligible. The speaker may clip off his speech sounds,

Fluency disorders are seen in both children and adults. They can be associated with such neurological and physical problems as cerebrovascular accidents (strokes), cerebral palsy, epilepsy, and other forms of brain damage, as well as mental retardation. Very often, people with neurophysiological problems have the fluency disorder of **cluttering.**

Disorders of fluency are also observed in the absence of any identifiable neurophysiological problem. These disorders of fluency are commonly known as stuttering. Some theories about the cause of stuttering suggest that it has an organic basis, even though none has been conclusively identified. Stuttering and its associated problems can be quite complex. Because the fluency disorders associated with identifiable neurophysiological problems are considered elsewhere in the book, we will focus primarily on the problem of stuttering in this chapter.

Stuttering is the major subcategory of fluency disorders. It is a problem for approximately 1% of the population, over 2,000,000 children and adults in the United States alone. About 85% of all cases of stuttering start during the preschool years. Boys outnumber girls who stutter by a ratio of four to one. Interestingly, about 80% of those who have stuttered at one time or another spontaneously recover from it (Sheehan & Martyn, 1966).

The longer stuttering persists in any given person, the more likely it is that associated emotional problems will develop. As listeners react to a developing stutterer's speech, the young stutterer also reacts to his speech and to the reactions of others. He may feel embarrassed, guilty, frustrated, angry. Many stutterers come to feel helpless, which often damages their sense of personal value and worth. Stuttering frequently leads to confusion and any number of social and emotional conflicts for the child or adult speaker, for his family, friends, teachers, and anyone else who interacts with him. The normal disfluency that is a relatively simple and effortless developmental milestone can be compounded into a serious social, emotional, and communication handicap. It can profoundly affect an individual's basic self-concept, his sense of his own worth and value as a human being, his goals, aspirations, and expectations for himself, and his basic style of coping with life.

Many stutterers respond to their problem by being overaggressive, by denying its existence, by projecting reactions in listeners, or by feeling anxious and timid. They often avoid talking or avoid any social circumstance where talking is expected, to the point of socially isolating themselves. A child's potential for an education, for an occupation, and for a fulfilling social and emotional life can be seriously reduced by long-term, persistent stuttering. Stuttering can easily become the focal point around which a person and his family organize their life. The speech-language pathologist, therefore, must address this problem within all the developmental, familial, and social contexts that the individual functions.

omit sounds and words, and fire rapid bursts of speech— almost with the speed of a machine gun. The exact causes of cluttering have not been identified, but it may have physical as well as emotional components.

See chapters 12, 13, and 14.

For this reason, we will often use "he" in reference to a single stutterer.

DEFINITION

A precise quantitative definition of stuttering is difficult to present. It is a multidimensional problem. Some aspects lend themselves to reliable and quantitative measurement, with other aspects being more elusive. Perhaps stuttering is best characterized as a problem that involves a cluster of a particular kind of speech behaviors, feelings, beliefs, self-concepts, and social interactions. Each of these components of the problem vary from person to person. In each person, they influence one another to generate a terribly complicated problem involving disruptions of speech and the associated reactions. The speech-language pathologist *must* deal with the emotional and social problems as well as the disordered speech itself.

Here is the way one stutterer saw his problem. For him, the following statement was a personal definition of stuttering.

> Well, I recall many times that I had been in restaurants and wanted to order something of my choice and anticipated a block or anticipated stuttering and would select something else from the menu because it was easier to say that word at the moment. Another time I might be OK with ordering that. It was such an uncertain thing, and I never knew when I would be all right an hour from now or five minutes from now.

Stuttering affects the fluent, smooth, and effortless flow of words emitted by a speaker. In reports of early civilizations, we find that Moses reportedly stuttered, as did Demosthenes of the early Greeks. This complex and unusual disorder has perplexed the victims and their families as well as professionals from those days to the present. We still do not know what causes stuttering, and effective therapy for it has been quite elusive—in spite of the pervasive and powerful impact it can have on all aspects of a person's life.

Because of the complex nature of the problem, no two stutterers have exactly the same difficulties. As early as 1889, Saikorski stated that "the varieties of stuttering are so many and complex that the person interested in this neurosis must ask himself whether it is a single disorder or a nmber of disorders. . . . The overt behaviors differ so much that it is impossible to compare and classify symptoms" (p. 44).

Review chapter 3 for a discussion of some cultural differences in stuttering symptoms.

Stutterers present a wide variety of symptoms, both visible and hidden. Overtly, they may repeat sounds or words; they may prevent their vocal cords from vibrating, resulting in a block or absence of sound; or they may prolong sounds abnormally. In addition, they may show secondary behaviors such as eye blinking, head jerking, or facial grimaces. Many stutterers show a great deal of muscular tension and forcing when they try to speak. Covertly, they may substitute words, talk indirectly around a topic, or reply with incorrect information to avoid certain words. We must be careful not to categorize a stuttering problem as mild, moderate, or severe based on overt behavior alone. A stutterer with only covert behaviors may have as many difficulties as one who has an overtly severe problem. Although other people may not recognize the person as a stutterer, he may be avoiding speaking situations or giving incorrect information to avoid stuttering. For example, stutterers have told me about giving an incorrect name when asked, ordering hamburger when they wanted steak, answering "I don't know" to questions as simple as "What is your address?" The problem of stuttering can have an extreme effect on a person's life, whether or not the problem appears severe on the surface.

Basic Issues and Questions

As an area of study, the topic of stuttering has had a varied history. If we were to attempt to write its history, we would need to write about several simultaneous developments that at times interacted and at times were quite independent of one another. The simultaneous developments in the theory, research, and clinical management of stuttering parallel many developments in the behavioral, biomedical, and clinical sciences. We are still trying to answer one basic question—whether one learns to stutter or inherits the condition (or tendency) from ancestors. This question relates to a number of other significant questions. If stuttering is a neurosis, what are its basic personality characteristics? What about the psychodynamics? If it is learned, how is it learned? Are there basic physiological and organic factors operating which contribute to its development? What are the roles of anxiety, family, and culture in the development and maintenance of stuttering?

These types of theoretical questions have led researchers to ask whether stutterers as a group differ from fluent speakers by any identifiable characteristics. Are there certain characteristics that distinctly and uniquely differentiate stutterers from nonstutterers that could give us clues to the cause of stuttering? Relating to these questions are questions about clinical management. Do you attempt to identify and treat the cause of stuttering, or do you treat its symptoms, independent of its cause? Do you treat the emotional aspects or the motor aspects of the problem? If both, then in what sequence? Can you apply the principles we have learned in experimental laboratories to the actual clinical management of the problem? These are some of the many issues and questions which continue to face the theorist, the researcher, the clinician, and the stutterer.

THEORIES OF CAUSATION

As with other communication disorders, we can classify the numerous theories of stuttering as being based on inheritance, child development, neurosis, and learning and conditioning. These categories of theories overlap somewhat, and a specific theory may fit into more than one category. Let us now turn to the content of some major representative theories.

Cerebral Dominance

Dysphemic theories view stuttering as a symptom of some inner, underlying complicating neurophysiological or biological disorder.

The Orton-Travis Theory of cerebral dominance (Orton & Travis, 1929) is one of the better known **dysphemic** theories of the cause of stuttering. It states that a child is predisposed to stutter because neither side of his brain is dominant in controlling the motor activities involved in talking. This theory generated a great deal of reserach on laterality, handedness, the shifting of handedness, electroencephalographic (EEG) studies of the brain, and electromyographic (EMG) studies of the speech muscles. It also led to specific clinical management techniques involving the use of rigidly programmed unilateral motor activities (Bryngelson, 1935, 1939). Although the theory was popular and generated great interest, the evidence does not support it. The research evidence is equivocal, and the clinical results have been found wanting.

Biochemical and Physiological Theories

West (1958) also viewed stuttering as involving an inherited predisposition. He felt that it is primarily a convulsive disorder, related to epilepsy, with instances of stuttering being seizures that could be triggered by emotional stress. West related his theory to a blood-sugar imbalance observed in stutterers while they were stuttering. This theory in particular is associated with a great deal of research on basal metabolism, blood chemistry, brain waves, twinning, and neurophysiological correlates to stuttering.

Related theories have been developed by Wingate (1969), Perkins, Ruder, Johnson, and Michael (1976), Schwartz (1974), and Adams (1978). They discuss the physiological and aerodynamic events occurring in the vocal tract during speech, and view stuttering as problems with phonation, respiration, and articulation. Adams, Wingate, and Perkins and colleagues separately discuss the problem in terms of phonetic transitions which make it difficult for the stutterer to start, time, and sustain air flow and voicing in coordination with articulation.

*In reference to stuttering, a **block** is a complete or partial interruption of the smooth flow of speech.*

Schwartz discusses the possibility of an uninhibited airway dilation reflex, which is the stuttering **block.** Where Schwartz feels that there may be a genetic predisposition to this problem, Adams leans toward an explanation of classical conditioning.

All of these studies have been reviewed by Bloodstein (1975). His general conclusions are that "the results of this type of research do not appear to demonstrate conclusively that the average stutterer exhibits any clinical pathology within the range of the factors that have been investigated." The few differences that have been reported in cardiovascular functioning and metabolic rate as well as autonomic reflexes and brain potentials have not been confirmed.

Much earlier, Hill (1944a, b) concluded that suspected physiological and biochemical differences between stutterers and nonstutterers could just as easily be caused by excitement, emotion, muscular effort, or fatigue. However, the theories of Wingate and Adams, dealing with abnormal laryngeal activity, are still very new and tentative. They may help us develop a broader understanding of the dynamics and cause of stuttering.

Genetic Theory

It is difficult to attribute the development of any trait or behavior to effects of genetics or the environment, because all traits develop in some context. The question is rather to determine the relative contributions of each—in this instance, to the problem of stuttering (Kidd, 1977). Up to this time, we have not been able to identify any biochemical defect as a cause for stuttering, and it seems unlikely that we will do so in the foreseeable future. Even if one were to be discovered, any determination of its contribution to the development of stuttering might be confounded by environmental factors. However, we do have research models that have been applied to the data we have on the concentration of stuttering in families. That data sometimes enable us to predict stuttering and suggest that there may be an important genetic basis for this problem. We still need research to sort out these genetic factors and derive clinical applications for dealing with the stuttering problem.

Diagnosogenic-Semantogenic Theory

Perhaps the most widely embraced theory of the cause of stuttering is Wendel Johnson's diagnosogenic-semantogenic theory (Johnson, 1938, 1942, 1944, 1961). This theory has been called a developmental theory (Ainsworth, 1945) and an "anticipatory struggle" theory (Bloodstein, 1975). Following his research and interviews with parents of young stuttering and nonstuttering children, Johnson stated that:

> Practically every case of stuttering was originally diagnosed . . . by usually one or both of the child's parents. What these laymen had diagnosed as stuttering was by and large indistinguishable from the hesitations and repetitions known to be characteristic of the normal speech of young children . . . Stuttering as a definite disorder was found to occur, not before being diagnosed, but after being diagnosed. (1944, pp. 330ff.)

In Johnson's view, this diagnosis by the parents creates an environment of "difference" and "handicap." The child soon begins to speak abnormally in response to the parents' anxieties, pressures, help, criticisms, and corrections. Both child and parents respond to the idea of handicap more than to the child's actual speaking behavior. As Johnson stated so aptly, stuttering begins "not in the child's mouth but in the parent's ear."

This theory inspired à great deal of research. We have a great deal of evidence showing that most normal young children exhibit disfluent speech (Davis, 1939, 1940; Winitz, 1961). We also know that parents of stutterers are sometimes anxious and perfectionistic and have high standards. However, there is some question about the dynamics of the "original diagnosis" (Bloodstein, 1975). And there are serious questions about whether calling attention to disfluency necessarily results in an increase in its frequency (Wingate, 1959).

Outgrowths of Johnson's diagnosogenic-semantogenic theory include ideas dealing with stutterer's feelings that they are helpless and victimized (Williams, 1957), as well as the concept of stuttering as anticipatory struggle (Bloodstein, 1958). It also directly influenced cognitive therapy, which focuses on faulty beliefs about self-control and the reinforcing pay-offs of stuttering (Rubin & Culatta, 1971).

Neurotic Theories

The neurotic theories of causation of stuttering focus on a number of different personality and psychological attributes of stutterers. Through observation, interviews, projective tests, and paper-and-pencil tests, attempts have been made to understand the stutterer's personality, psychodynamics, social adjustment, and inner, unconscious needs. Stuttering has been viewed as a need for oral gratification, as a need for anal gratification, as a covert expression of hostility, as an inhibition of threatening feelings and messages, as a fear of castration, as repressed aggression and hostility, as a device for gaining attention and sympathy, as well as an excuse for failure. According to these theories, stuttering can become a well-integrated, purposeful defense against some threatening idea. From a psychoanalytic point of view, stuttering acts as a mechanism to repress unwanted or threatening feelings (Abbott, 1947; Barbara, 1954; Glauber, 1958; Travis, 1957).

Research on these ideas has had a very spotty history. Formal tests given to stutterers to identify their unique personality characteristics suffer from problems of validity and reliability, while observations of behavior suffer from the theoretical biases and subjectivity of the observers. These theories might best be evaluated in terms of their utility in clinical management, rather than in research activity. However, psychoanalysis and traditional psychotherapy for the problem of stuttering, especially in adults, have not been effective on a large scale.

Conditioning Theories

You may wish to review the types of conditioning, described on page 109.

As applied to stuttering, classical conditioning theories suggest that an originally unconditioned breakdown in speech fluency becomes associated with a speaker's anxiety about talking. If this happens often enough, the person will stutter in any anxiety-provoking circumstances; the stuttering becomes classically conditioned. Wolpe's (1958) view of stuttering as a symptom of classically conditioned speech fears led him to use systematic desensitization in therapy. Techniques of systematic desensitization include counterconditioning and reciprocal inhibition. That is, the stutterer, who has learned to stutter, learns not to. This, in turn, influenced Brutten and Shoemaker (1967), who formulated a two-factor theory of stuttering. They state that speech disruptions, triggered by automatic fear reactions, are classically conditioned responses to speech, to talking situations, to listeners, and so on. However, they see the nonspeech behaviors of stutterers (the muscle tension, blinking eyes, grimaces, etc.) as being operantly conditioned. These behaviors are designed to avoid stuttering or to cope with fluency failures.

We have seen that stuttering is often (if not always) associated with anxiety. Some theorists feel that anxiety reduction is an important component of the conditioning process that results in stuttering. One such theory sees Johnson's view of stutterers as doing those things that would avoid stuttering or would avoid negative listener reactions as the core of the problem (Wischner, 1950, 1952a, 1952b). That is, stutterers build up fears before they begin to speak. Once they have spoken (stuttered), those fears are reduced simply because the problem is no longer in front of them. This reduction in anxiety reinforces the stuttering.

Sheehan (1953, 1958a, 1958b) applied approach-avoidance conflict theory to the problem of stuttering. In this theory, the stutterer is seen as vacillating between the desire to speak and the desire not to speak. The stutterer also vacillates between wanting to be silent and wanting not to be silent. When the drive to avoid talking is stronger, he is silent. When the drive to approach talking is stronger, he is fluent. When the drives are equal, he is in conflict and he stutters. According to Sheehan, whether they choose to be silent or choose to talk, stutterers are reinforced for their choices by an immediate reduction in their anxieties.

Still another group of theories are derived from operant conditioning. Flanagan, Goldiamond, and Azrin (1958) demonstrated that stuttering could be increased and decreased in the laboratory as a function of its consequences. At least some overt stuttering behaviors could be controlled through operant conditioning. Based partly on these experiments, Shames and Sherrick (1963) analyzed and discussed various hypotheses relating Johnson's diagnosogenic theory to operant conditioning. They found continuity between the conditioning processes operating in normal disfluency and those operating in stuttering.

Another spin-off from the Flanagan et al. research was several therapies known as *rate control* therapies. These techniques use delayed auditory feedback as a vehicle for initially changing a stutterer's speech (Curlee & Perkins, 1969; Goldiamond, 1965; Ingham & Andrews, 1973; Perkins, 1973a, 1973b; Ryan & Van Kirk, 1974; Shames & Florance, 1980).

The Shames and Sherrick theoretical analysis also led to several therapies which apply operant conditioning techniques within actual clinical interviews. Shames, Egolf, and Rhodes (1969) demonstrated that the specific content of stutterers' speech in therapy could be increased by reinforcing the content with verbal approval or reduced by mildly verbally punishing with disapproval. Other research has dealt with parent-child verbal interactions (how parents and children talk to each other) (Kasprisin-Burrelli, Egolf, & Shames, 1972; Shames & Egolf, 1971, 1976). This research showed that it is possible to change the way the parents and children verbally interact and to reduce stuttering with these tactics. These results can be interpreted as indicating that stuttering is reinforced on an individualized basis in parent-child verbal interactions.

To backtrack a bit, a persistent question in the study of stuttering has been the role of punishment in its development. For years, under the influence of Johnson's diagnosogenic theory, it was generally felt parents' punishment of or attention to the normal disfluencies of their children aggravated the problem and led to the development of stuttering. However, some operant conditioning research (Siegel, 1970) has shown that stuttering and disfluency can be reduced by **punishment.** Thus there has been a professional as well as humanitarian conflict about the role and functioning of punishment in stuttering and its management.

In the terminology of operant conditioning, **punishment** *is the opposite of reinforcement; that is, it denotes a consequence that weakens the preceding behavior.*

Two separate studies have demonstrated that the usual laboratory reduction of stuttering as a function of punishment could be reversed (Brookshire & Eveslage, 1969; Halvorson, 1971). Both of these studies are excellent laboratory simulations of the sequences of events that may well go on in the homes of young early stuttering children. Most parents who use punishment as a way of managing their children use it at their own convenience—often some time after the behavior they want to decrease. The research suggests that, to be effective, punishment must be prompt, administered as soon as possible after the undesirable behavior. Also, most parents use the type of punishment with which they are most comfortable at the time. Sometimes they take away privileges, sometimes they arrange for social isolation of their children, sometimes verbally abuse and scream at their children, and sometimes they spank them. The research indicates that, to be effective, punishment must be consistent from incident to incident. Finally, after punishing their children, many parents either reward the child for performing an alternative desirable behavior or (in a fit of guilt) lavish the child with affection. Punishment which is paired with positive reinforcement tends to strengthen rather than weaken the original behavior.

That is, the "punishment" is technically a reinforcement.

We can summarize by saying that it is not the punishment per se which may generate stuttering, but rather its poor control when used, in terms of timing, consistency, and pairing with positive reinforcement. Young children show both fluent and disfluent speech. Poorly controlled punishment of disfluency may well help explain why disfluency is strengthened and fluency is weakened in these children. Note that we are not suggesting that punishment is a viable therapeutic or preventive tactic for early stuttering. Rather, we are suggesting that punishment is difficult to control in the home as a way of managing children. Therefore, it should be avoided. In this sense, Johnson's diagnosogenic theory may well be valid, even though it did not provide a complete analysis of the role of punishment. Where Johnson was commenting on the *use* of punishment, Brookshire and Eveslage and Halvorson could be interpreted as commenting on the *misuse* of punishment as a cause of stuttering.

Summary

The cause or causes of stuttering have not been established, although there have been many studies of its symptoms, its correlates, and tactics for modifying it. Fortunately, the methods of therapy have grown and we have improved our success rates in spite of our basic lack of understanding of the cause of this problem. We cannot help but wonder how much further along we might be in its prevention and management if such knowledge were available.

NORMAL DISFLUENCY

The act of speech is, as we have seen, enormously complicated. Lenneberg (1967) has conservatively estimated that there are 140,000 neural events required for each *second* of motor speech production.

> Since the passage from any one speech sound to another depends ultimately on differences in muscular adjustments, 14 times per second an "order must be issued to every muscle," whether to contract, relax, or maintain its tonus. . . . It is clear, however, that the readjustment does not occur simultaneously for all muscles but that various groups of muscles have characteristic timing; some are active shortly before the onset of the phoneme, some during, and some shortly after. Thus we gather that the rate at which individual muscular events occur (throughout the speech apparatus) is of an order of magnitude of several hundred events every second.

Thus, if the speaker produces 14 phonemes per second, using about 100 muscles involved in speech requiring 100 motor units apiece ($100 \times 100 \times 14$), very complex motor behavior results (Darley, Aronson, & Brown, 1975).

It is within this context that stuttering develops. Because of the difficulty and complexity of learning to talk and learning language, young children often make errors. Normal disfluency may begin in the infant's early babbling, as he begins to imitate the rates, rhythms, sequences, and melody of his language. Usually during his second year, a child may use jargon as he plays. That is, he may utter a stream of nonsense syllables, but use the inflections and stress of developed language. This may well be a "fluency rehearsal" state for the child, as we hear and recognize smooth transitions from nonsense syllable to nonsense syllable, many of which resemble adult patterns of fluency. But as they move from babbling to early jargon to early speech, some children develop a pattern of disfluency that makes their speech difficult to understand. Thus, rather than the normal disfluency of occasional pauses and repeated words, they may use more distracting repetitions of syllables.

We can sum up with several hypotheses regarding the function of speech disfluency.

(1) Disfluency appears to be a type of speech behavior toward which the human being is physiologically predisposed. Such speech disfluencies would more likely account for pauses and hesitations in speech as accommodations to the basic rhythms and limitations of our physiological systems.

(2) One general class of speech disfluency behavior, speech repetitions (sound, syllable, word, and phrase), appears to be learned.

(3) As learned behavior, normal speech repetitions are not randomly emitted but are controlled in an orderly system through various environmental circumstances.

(4) Some of the circumstances, processes, and functions suggested as being involved in normal disfluency are:
   (a) Obtaining a listener's attention;
   (b) Composing and editing speech responses;
   (c) Filling silences created by pauses to prevent the listener from speaking;
   (d) Various states of deprivation and aversive stimulation;
   (e) Competition for talking time;

    (f) Interruption;
    (g) High levels of emotional arousal and excitement.
(5) Fluency and disfluency may be two distinctly separate classes of speech responses. Each of these classes of responses may have its own history of original emission (fluency in early jargon and disfluency in early repetitious babbling) and later reinforcement and stimulus control. They coexist, but compete in time and physiology for their actual behavior occurrence. You cannot be fluent and disfluent at the same exact instance in time. Both are a part of normal speech development and are elements in the speaking repertoires of normal nonstuttering as well as stuttering children and adults. (Shames, 1968, p. 700)

THE DEVELOPMENT OF STUTTERING

Bloodstein (1960a, 1960b) describes four general phases of development of stuttering. These phases may overlap, and there is a great deal of individual variation. In its earliest phase, Phase I, the stuttering is episodic, occurring most often when the child is upset, has a great deal to say, or is under pressure to communicate. The stuttering is characterized mostly by repetitions of words or syllables at the beginning of an utterance, on function as well as content words. Usually in this phase the child shows little concern or reaction to the speech disfluencies.

In Phase II, the stuttering has become more chronic, and the child thinks of himself as a stutterer. The stuttering occurs on the major parts of speech, increasing under conditions of excitement or rapid speech. However, the child still shows very little concern about his difficulties in talking. This phase is usually characteristic of elementary school children.

In Phase III, the stuttering may vary with specific situations. The stutterer may regard certain sounds and words as more difficult than others. He may avoid saying certain words and substitute easier words in their place. There is very little avoidance of talking situations, and no outward evidence of embarrassment. However, the child may show the beginnings of anticipatory stuttering and react with irritation to his difficulty.

In Phase IV, the stutterer has very fearful anticipation of stuttering, fears words, sounds, and situations, has frequent word substitutions, avoids speech situations, and feels afraid, embarrassed, and helpless. This phase is usually seen in late adolescence and adulthood.

Van Riper (1954) has suggested a three-stage developmental process: primary stuttering, transition, and secondary stuttering. Primary stuttering (the effortless repetition and prolongations of speech which Johnson called *normal disfluency*) is followed by the transitional stage. This is characterized by repetitions and prolongations which are faster, longer, and less regular in occurrence. Some children also begin to struggle and feel frustrated. This stage is sometimes followed by the third stage, secondary stuttering, which is characterized by struggle reactions, fear, and avoidance. Van Riper (1971) has modified this original view of development by discussing how stuttering changes over time. He has identified four tracks of development, change, and probable ultimate outcome. A given child will show only one of these patterns, progressing through the track sequentially.

Table 7.1 summarizes and illustrates the four tracks described by Van Riper.

TABLE 7.1
Four Tracks of Development of Stuttering. (Drawn from C. Van Riper, The Nature of Stuttering.
Englewood Cliffs, N.J.: Prentice-Hall, 1971, pp. 116–117. Used with permission.)

		At Onset	**Developmental Progression**
	Track I	Begins 2½ to 4 years	Repetition of syllables increases in frequency and speed and becomes irregular
		Previously fluent	
		Gradual onset	
		Cyclic	Repeated syllables begin to end in prolongations
		Long remissions	
		Good articulations	Prolongations show increased tension, tremors, struggle; evidence of frustration
		Normal rate	
		Syllabic repetitions	
		No tension; unforced	Overflow of tension, facial contortions, retrials, speech output decreases, signs of concern
		No tremors	
Loci refers to placements of a disfluency with the speech stream.		Loci: First words, function words	Situation fears and avoidance behavior develop. Word fears and fears of certain words arise; use of tricks to disguise and cover up; speech attempts often hesitant; poor eye contact; output of speech decreases; both repetitions and prolongations as core behavior
		Variable pattern	
		Normal speech is well integrated	
		No awareness	
		No frustration	
		No fears; willing to talk	
	Track II	Often late; at the time of first sentences	Behaviors remain the same but the speed increases; number also increases
		Never fluent	
		Gradual onset	Little change in form
		Steady	Little change, little awareness, little frustrations
		No remissions	
		Poor articulation	Duration of nonfluencies increases, more syllabic repetitions, little awareness
		Fast; spurts	
		Gaps, revisions, syllabic and word repetitions	Occasional fears of situations, not of words or sounds; long strings of syllabic repetitions at fast speed added to other behaviors; some fears of situations; good eye contact; no disguise; output of speech; increases; little avoidance; primarily repetitive; unorganized
		No tension	
		No tremors	
		Loci: first words, long words, scattered throughout sentence, content words	
		Variable pattern	
		Broken speech with hesitation and gaps even when no disfluency	
		No awareness	
		No frustration	
		No fears; willing to talk	
	Track III	Any age child has consecutive speech	An increase in frequency but behavior changes little at first; signs of frustration
		Previously fluent	
		Sudden onset, often after trauma	More retrials, lip protrusions and tongue fixation appear; prolongations of initial sounds
		Steady	

TABLE 7.1 (cont.)

	At Onset	Developmental Progression	
	Few short remissions	Tremors, struggling, facial contortions, jaw jerks, gasping, marked frustration	
	Normal articulation		
	Slow, careful rate		
	Unvoiced prolongations	Interruptor devices become prominent, rate slows, more hesitancy, more refusals to talk	
	Laryngeal blockings		
	Much tension	Intense fears of words and sounds; many avoidances; patterns change in form and grow more bizarre; much overflow; output of speech decreases; will cease trying to talk; poor eye contact; normal speech becomes hesitant; frequent nonvocalized blockings; primary tonic blocks with multiple closures	
	Tremors		
	Beginning of utterance after pauses primary		
	Consistent pattern		
	Normal speech is very fluent		
	Highly aware		*A **tonic block** is a speech stoppage with prolongations and hesitations.*
	Much frustration		
	Fears speaking situation and certain words		
Track IV	Late, usually after 4 years	The number of instances increases; shown in more situations	
	Previously fluent		
	Sudden onset	Little change in form, monosymptomatic and symbolic	
	Erratic		
	No remissions	Little change	
	Normal articulation	Little change in type but duration and visibility increase, no interruptions of new forcings, increased output of speech	
	Normal rate		
	Unusual behaviors		
	Variable tension	Very few avoidance or release behaviors; not much evidence of word fears; few consistent loci; very aware of stuttering; stutters very openly; good eye contact; little variability in the stuttering behavior; normal speech very fluent; talks a lot; consistent pattern; few silent blockings; either tonic or clonic	
	Few tremors		
	First words, rarely on function words, content words especially		
	Consistent pattern		
	Normal speech is very fluent		
	Highly aware		*A **clonic block** is characterized by repetitions.*
	No frustration		
	No evidence of fear, willing to talk		

THE ASSESSMENT PROCESS

There is no one right way to assess a stuttering problem. The choice of tactics will vary with the unique problems presented by the stutterer. They may vary from person to person, with the theoretical and professional training of the speech-language pathologist, and with the interpersonal styles of both participants. Let's take a look at some examples to see how individual diversity may affect assessment.

William Fancis has had a stuttering problem for 35 years. During elementary school, he was seen in a group with children with articulation problems in the public schools. His speech did not improve. Over the years, he has been told by a variety of professionals that "there is no cure for stuttering; you must learn to accept your disability and make the best of it." Nevertheless, he has not been able to accept his problem gracefully and fulfill his vocational and personal goals in spite of it. Rather, he has isolated himself from others, living as a social recluse with no friends, avoiding nearly all communication, even with his parents and relatives. Although he achieved scholastically as an engineer, nearly completing his PhD, he was painfully afraid of entering the competitive job market, blaming his speech for his difficulty. Thus, he took a low-paying job as a library aide at a university, living a meager, lonely existence. William heard a news program about a stuttering clinic which offers hope for treatment of the problem. Very skeptically, he called the clinic for an appointment.

Dorothy Jean is 3½ years old, the first child in her immediate family as well as the first grandchild for both sets of grandparents. Dorothy is a bright, vivacious, energetic child with unusual charm and attractiveness. About 3 months ago, however, Dorothy began to show difficulty when attempting to express herself. It was as though the words suddenly "got stuck in her throat," and she was momentarily unable to speak. The family physician told her mother not to be concerned, as most children will go through a developmental phase of normal disfluency. The doctor said that as long as the family does not react to her abnormal behavior, she will simply outgrow the problem. Although Dorothy's parents have done their best "not to react," her problem has worsened. Recently she has begun to struggle overtly; she blinks her eyes and jerks her head when trying to produce certain words. At this point, her mother called the clinic for a speech evaluation.

Jack Rolfe is a 13-year-old stutterer, a member of the junior high football team and a good student. His mother and father are extremely concerned about his severe stuttering, which has been a problem since early childhood and seems to have worsened over the last few years. Jack does not feel that he has a problem at all. Although his stuttering is very frequent and very severe in terms of duration and form, he denies its existence, stating that with his friends or in the classroom he *never* stutters. He says that occasionally he may have a slight problem at home, but it doesn't bother him and he can see no reason to do anything about it. Jack's denial of his problem is very frustrating to his mother. She wants to impress upon him the value of good speech, trying to convince him that if he doesn't change his speech the consequences could be disastrous. He may never have dates, may be cut off from school parties and functions, may not be able to enter fully in class discussions, lessening his chances for future social, academic, or vocational success. Jack, however, rejects his mother's concern, insisting that the problem does not interfere with any aspect of his personal or scholastic activities. At this point, against his wishes, Jack is brought by his parents to the speech clinic for an evaluation.

Clearly, different techniques of assessment would be called for in these three cases. Assessment of a stuttering problem in a young child like Dorothy would be vastly different in purpose and style than assessment of an adult like William Francis. With a child, the speech-language pathologist must first decide whether or not a problem exists, and then evaluate the child's awareness and reactions to his speech and the child's here-and-now environment. With most adults, stuttering has been a problem for quite some time, so diagnosis is not an issue. The assessment tasks are to choose therapy strategies and develop a prognosis.

The most valid and reliable assessment procedures are based on direct observation. With direct observation we need not worry about the memory lapses of Dorothy Jean's parents, about Jack's distortions of the extent of his problem, or about intervening theoretical interpretations by William's previous speech-language pathologists. However, if we limit our assessment to observing current behaviors, we may lose a picture of the historical development of the problem or any long-term pattern of behaving, feeling, and interacting. At best, any assessment procedure is a short-term compromise. Recognizing that we cannot directly observe everything that is currently happening, that we cannot go back and watch the problem develop, and that we cannot always see the person fantasize or get angry or frustrated, we try to sample the client's and family's behaviors, feelings, interactions, and personality. We do this with direct observation, interviews, and tests, trying to tap representative and pertinent dimensions of the problem. Most of the time this process of substituting small samples during an evaluation for long-term observation is recognized as a compromise. Most speech-language pathologists talk about assessment as being a long-term, on-going process, continuing even as therapy is going on. They temper their formal test interpretations with information learned during the therapy process.

The speech-language pathologist's personal view of the causes of stuttering will affect the assessment process (and the therapy process as well). The professional approach should provide guidance as to *what* should be evaluated. This should result in a *description* of the problem. If the original causes of the problem and reasons for its maintenance are significant elements in the theory and if they are to be dealt with in therapy, they ought to be part of the basic description of the problem. On the other hand, if these factors *are not* significant targets during therapy, then the search for causes may have little purpose. From the general description, we should be able to develop a general strategy of therapy, including short-term and long-term goals as well as special tactical procedures.

No matter what the speech-language pathologist thinks about the causes of stuttering, certain types of questions need to be asked during the assessment.

Description of the Problem and Baseline Measurement

The evaluation of the stutterer includes a description of the disordered behavior. Many speech-language pathologists tally the frequency and type of stuttered words during spontaneous speech or oral reading. The severity of the problem may also be assessed using a rating scale or descriptive category such as mild, moderate, or severe. Other behavioral baselines used include measurement of talking time, speech content selection, and secondary symptoms.

An interview with the person or family often provides information regarding the current impact of the problem on the person's social and school or vocational life, as well as his self-concept. Further exploration of certain personality variables may be important for planning therapy. During therapy, adults, especially, may be encouraged to take risks in revealing their feelings about themselves and about people they know and love. They may be confronted with their own rigidity about what they feel about their problems. For these reasons, the speech-language pathologist needs a feeling for the client's tolerance of ambiguity, his rigidity or flexibility, how comfortable he is taking risks. These variables can be assessed and may help indicate how the client will handle the stress associated with personal change during therapy. How does the person see himself? If he sees himself as a helpless victim of fate, controlled by his environment, and is a person who needs a lot of support and nurturance, he may require very different treatment than a person who feels in control of himself and his life. These types of personality differences may be important to understand before therapy begins, so that appropriate treatment can be offered and the potential for success improved. Further, the coping and defense mechanisms the person has developed to help him adjust to living with stuttering may influence the rate of change. The person who has used his stuttering as the primary (if not sole) excuse for his failures or fears may need more time in therapy, progressing more slowly than someone with a more realistic self-concept.

The assessment of the environment may play an important part in understanding the current problem. Especially when evaluating the young child, the speech-language pathologist may wish to examine the specific events that occur before and just after incidents of stuttering. Analyzing video- or audio-tape samples of parent-child interaction in the home and therapy setting may be time well spent. The environment of the adult stutterer may also contribute to prognosis. Factors such as resistance to progress from the spouse and time or job constraints may affect therapy. Unfortunately, these factors may be difficult to assess at first.

The client's reinforcement history may have a strong impact on the current problem as well as on the prognosis. Generally, the longer the person has had the problem, the worse the prognosis. However, many adolescents experience more difficulty in therapy than many adults, perhaps because it is harder for them to admit that they are different from their peers (as in the case of Jack Rolfe). Further, from previous therapy experiences, the older client may have developed negative attitudes toward the problem as well as toward his own ability to succeed and change. These attitudes may influence the prognosis and treatment. As with evaluating personality, assessment of a case history is dynamic. It does not end after the first session, but continues actively on the parts of both therapist and client throughout therapy.

The speech-language pathologist's approach to causation may lead him to certain questions to be answered during the assessment. At the same time, a preoccupation with causation can create clinical near-sightedness. For example, if you believe that the stuttering is the result of irrational beliefs, then you may evaluate how the person talks about and characterizes the problem. If you believe that the environment may affect the development and maintenance of the problem, you may choose to do a home analysis. If you see stuttering as a learned behavior, you may elect to obtain baseline behavioral tallies. In general, as we have seen, any speech problem is very complex, affecting all aspects of the person's life. The wise speech-language pathologist keeps an open mind during the assessment, being vigilant and attentive toward any behavior, attitude, or belief held which may contribute to the current difficulties.

Determination of Goals

When a stutterer decides to have his stuttering evaluated, he has certain expectations and objectives that he hopes will be fulfilled. At the same time, the speech-language pathologist also generates goals for the evaluation. For the most part, the stutterer comes to a clinic hoping to have his problem treated effectively—to the point that he no longer stutters, no longer has to be careful or vigilant about talking, no longer sees himself as a stutterer. However, he may have some unconscious need to remain a stutterer. He may have enjoyed certain rewards because of his problem, such as not being called on in class, receiving individual attention from listeners, and gaining nurturance and sympathy for his helplessness. Further, he may have learned to use stuttering as an excuse for an unsuccessful social life, poor grades, lack of athletic ability, and so on. Thus, giving up stuttering may be more difficult and complicated than would first appear, especially for people who avoid risk-taking and who are afraid of change. Thus, the stutterer may have one set of goals at a conscious and reasoned level and a very different set of goals at the hidden, subconscious level.

The speech-language pathologist's goals generally are the result of the therapeutic philosophy. He may believe that the best a stutterer can achieve is to accept himself as a stutterer. He may believe the person can become a fluent stutterer by monitoring and being careful at all times. On the other hand, the speech-language pathologist may believe that the person can completely rid himself of his problem. Generally, during the initial period, the client and speech-language pathologist communicate their goals to each other. If they are able to agree about their objectives, they can form a tacit contract implying that the stutterer will submit to the therapist's care for help.

More about how these goals affect therapy is presented later in this chapter.

Treatment Plan and Prognosis

During the assessment, the speech-language pathologist determines a general treatment plan. For the young, such as Dorothy Jean, he may plan to spend a great deal of time with the parents in the home and clinic. The goal may be to manipulate the child's environment so that the stuttering reduces and ultimately disappears, rather than directly treating the child. For clients like Jack Rolfe or William Francis, the professional may decide to describe the proposed treatment as completely as possible in advance, giving the client the opportunity to make a knowledgeable and informed choice to enroll in therapy.

Questions regarding prognosis may also be raised during the assessment. The prospective client (or the child's parent) is often concerned with issues such as "What are the chances of success?" "How long will therapy last?" "How often must I attend?" "How much will it cost?" Although these questions can be of vital importance to the person, they are usually difficult to answer directly or precisely. Generally, everyone progresses through the therapeutic process differently. Nevertheless, predicting outcome and duration of treatment is important. The baseline measures made before therapy may be helpful here. Such variabes as how the person views his ability to control his destiny, his tendency to reinforce himself, his ability to cope with stress, as well as speech characteristics, may predict how rapidly he will make progress. Some clinical programs do not place a lot of emphasis on measuring speech behavior before therapy, because they do not intend to move away from these behaviors as part of therapy. Rather their therapy may plan to teach new behaviors which in essence are absent at the time of the assessment (Shames & Florance, 1980). In these instances, progress is measured as movement toward a goal rather than away from the pretherapy status. In other therapies, where the focus is on modifying stuttering, a pretherapy baseline assessment of types, form, frequency, and duration of instances of stuttering may be important, as progress will be determined by the person's ability to improve from the baseline state. For example, if a person stuttered on 50% of the words on a reading passage, improvement could be documented by giving the same sample after treatment and noting that he now stutters on only 25% of the words.

Summary

Assessment is a complicated, long-term process. Not all assessment is done prior to therapy. The speech-language pathologist must reassess the person's stuttering during each session as well as during pre- and postprobes. At the same time, the client and significant people in his environment will also be evaluating the progress. All of these variables interact as the person moves toward his goal.

THERAPY FOR STUTTERING

There are probably as many perspectives toward therapy for stuttering as toward its causation. Some of our ideas have recently changed, while others have remained fairly constant over time. As you might expect, the ideas that have remained constant are generally those that have proven to be successful and effective. Those strategies that have changed and are still changing are those that have been less effective or unsuccessful. In general, the approach to treatment will depend first and foremost on the age of the stutterer; different techniques are used for young children, who are just developing the problem, and for adolescents and adults, who have had fluency problems (and often unsuccessful therapy) for years.

Therapy for the Young Developing Stutterer

Therapeutic strategies for the young, preschool aged, developing stutterer have been fairly constant and have had high success rates. There are several approaches to therapeutic intervention for early stuttering—environmental manipulation, direct work with the child, psychological therapy, desensitization therapy, parent-child interaction therapy, fluency-shaping behavioral therapy, and parent and family counseling. The choice of which one to use in individual cases depends upon the results and information gained from an assessment and evaluation of the problem. Some of the different strategies can be used in combination with each other, and some may also be useful for more advanced stages of the problem in older stutterers. A critical variable in dealing with young children is always the family, as the family can either reinforce or counteract the efforts of the speech-language pathologist.

Environmental Manipulation

Environmental manipulation is a therapeutic procedure which focuses on those variables operating in the child's environment which are thought to be contributing to the maintenance of the stuttering. Through both direct observation and parent and family conferences, the speech-language pathologist tries to identify these factors and to change the child's environment so that their function in maintaining stuttering is reduced or eliminated. Variables that can affect stuttering include:

(1) General excitement level in the home
(2) Fast-paced activity
(3) Communicative stress

  (4) Competition for talking time
  (5) Social and emotional deprivation
  (6) Sibling rivalry
  (7) Excessive speech interruptions, and talking attempts aborted by family members
  (8) Standards and expectations that are unrealistically high or low
  (9) Inconsistent discipline
  (10) Too much or too little structure for acceptable child behavior
  (11) Availability of parents
  (12) Excessive pressure to talk and to perform
  (13) Arguing and hostility among members of the family
  (14) Negative verbal interactions between the child and the family
  (15) Use of the child as a scapegoat or displacement of family problems onto the child.

Clearly, the list could go on and on. Each of these variables could be potent in maintaining stuttering. And each, if a factor and if reversed, could help eliminate stuttering as a problem. By helping a family become aware of these elements and their effects on the child's fluency, by helping each family member to determine his or her own individual influence, and by establishing a high priority for changing the child's environment, the speech-language pathologist may be able to reduce or eliminate the stuttering. But to accomplish this, the family has to agree upon a goal—to eliminate the child's stuttering. The needs of each family member and their direct influences on the child's fluency have to be reconciled with the process of changing the family environment. Often this process opens up totally new and unexpected problem areas that relate to the child's speech. It may also lead into different interpersonal or psychological problems of the family. The speech-language pathologist should be prepared to deal with these problem areas or to refer the family for appropriate intervention, such as family therapy, marital counseling, or psychological therapy.

Direct Therapy

Direct therapy involves actively and regularly seeing the young developing stutterer for therapy. Sometimes this means directly working on the speech symptoms of the child, but more often it means seeing the child, while working around the child and not directly on disfluency behavior. The theoretical assumption is that the child's stuttering is symptomatic of a more basic underlying problem, usually of a psychological and interpersonal nature.

Psychological Therapy   Children who are thought to have psychological or emotional problems which affect stuttering may be referred to play therapy or psychiatric therapy. These therapies assume that the disfluent speech is a symptom of a deeper, underlying psychodynamic problem. In this therapy, very little attention is given to the speech symptom per se. Rather, the focus is on the child's psychological coping and defense mechanisms, personality development, anxieties, other feelings, and interpersonal relationships. Advocates of this approach feel that, through the theoretical perspectives and clinical tactics of these therapies, psychological problems will be eliminated, thereby getting rid of the symptoms of stuttering. These therapies, of course, are carried out by trained specialists.

Some children have been helped by these psychologically oriented therapies, but for the most part, they have not generally been effective in reducing or eliminating stuttering behavior. However, there might be some value to psychotherapy as an adjunct to other forms of speech therapy (Bloodstein, 1975).

Desensitization Therapy   Another form of direct work with the child but not directly on the child's speech disfluency is desensitization therapy (developed by Egland, 1954). The theory behind this therapy is similar to the theory which underlies environmental manipulation. The child's stuttering is a response to environmental stresses. However, a distinction is made between unusual or unreasonable stress (the criterion for electing environmental manipulation) and the expected or reasonable stress which is found in the typical family situation. Stuttering which is judged to be a response to "normal stress" may be reduced by increasing the child's tolerance for stress. Desensitization therapy attempts to gradually increase the child's tolerance for stress. This is usually done in individual activities—often play—that reduce disfluency to its lowest level, known as the *basal level* of disfluency. Often stuttering can be completely eliminated during these activities. The speech-language pathologist keeps as many stress factors as possible from operating. The desensitization sessions might involve eliminating talking altogether for a while and interacting nonverbally, not asking direct questions, silent parallel play, avoiding stressful content themes while talking, maintaining a low excitement level, maintaining a slow pace of interaction, and so on. Very gradually, the speech-language pathologist reintroduces these stress factors (usually identified by watching the child interacting with family members and by conferring with parents) into the therapy session. The professional closely monitors the child's behavior for signs of emotional reactions and tries to stop just short of precipitating speech disfluency. This may happen three or four times in a session (introduction of stress followed by reduction). The speech-language pathologist introduces more stress into each session without precipitating stuttering, with the goal of extending the child's tolerance for the process. In this way, the child is "desensitized" to these normal stresses. Eventually, family members may be brought into the session to help the child generalize the fluency to the home environment, where these stresses probably occur naturally. The child is gradually nurtured into the normal stress of the family. The family can learn this nurturing process and become amenable to it and even to reducing some of the stress, when the end goal is helping to change the child rather than changing something about themselves.

Parent-Child Verbal Interaction Therapy   Related to the tactics of desensitization therapy is a therapy based on parent-child verbal interactions (Shames & Egolf, 1976). The assumption underlying this therapy is that childhood disfluencies develop in the social context of verbal interactions with parents, with the parents inadvertently reinforcing and maintaining the child's disfluency. After observing specific and individualized parent-child verbal interactions, the speech-language pathologist can mirror-image the process and do just the opposite of what the parent was observed to do following instances of disfluency. When the child's stuttering is reduced to 1% or less with the speech-language pathologist, the parents are introduced into the therapy to learn the more productive forms of verbal interaction with their child and to carry it on in the home.

Fluency-Shaping Behavioral Therapy   For many years, under the influ-ence of the diagnosogenic-semantogenic theory of stuttering, direct work on the speech of young stutterers was avoided. Experts thought that direct work on a young child's early stuttering could result in awareness of disfluency by the child, in anxieties and guilt, and in a feeling of being different. There is logic to this line of thought, especially if the focus of direct therapy is on stuttering and its acceptance and control. However, more recently, some ther-apies have been developed that focus on fluency, that is, on helping children learn to do those things while talking that nonstuttering children do.

Williams (1979) has developed a therapy which emphasizes "easy, normal" talking and actually encourages children to attend to the smooth and easy behavior they are capable of performing. Ryan and Van Kirk (1974) have developed a therapy which gradually increases the length and complexity (GILCU) of the child's utterances. Shames and Florance (1980) have also developed a "slowed-down" speech pattern which is keyed to continuous phonation between words and which is shaped to normal processes of speaking behavior. The Ryan-Van Kirk and the Shames and Florance therapies also organize a system of reinforcement to facilitate generalization to the child's everyday environments (Ryan & Van Kirk, 1974; Shames & Florance, 1980).

Parent and Family Counseling

We have just seen that many aspects of the child's environment cut to the core of the family and its individual members. Identifying and ultimately changing some family behavior patterns might well require a close and caring counseling relationship for the group as a whole as well as for its individual members. To meet the final goal, the needs of the family as well as the child must be considered. Parent and family counseling is designed to help family members understand how their behaviors and feelings interact with the stut-terer's behavior and feelings and recognize, accept, and act on these feelings.

In some instances the speech-language pathologist may feel that the speech of the child is within the boundaries of normal disfluency, while the anxieties and concerns of the parents persist. In these instances, parent con-cern is a legitimate target for therapeutic intervention. This intervention is not simply a matter of providing parents with information about normal devel-opmental disfluency. The speech-language pathologist also acknowledges and deals with the parents' feelings. In these circumstances the parents, not the child, are the clients. The focus may start out on the child, but the coun-seling situation often redefines the problems and issues in terms of the par-ents, their histories, their interactions, feelings, and behaviors, with a much broader perspective than speech and/or parenting. The issues start to focus on the parents as individuals.

Skills in interviewing and counseling, as well as a knowledge of stuttering, child management, and family dynamics, are prerequisites for this type of therapeutic intervention. Without these skills, the speech-language pathologist might better serve the family by a referral to someone who has the proper training and skills. The combination of parent and family counseling with environmental manipulation probably represents the highest rate of thera-peutic success for the problem of stuttering. This success may be due to the short history of the child's stuttering problem and its early form and development.

Therapy for Advanced Stuttering

Advanced stuttering can be much more complicated in its dynamics, in its overt symptoms, in its hidden aspects, as well as in its interpersonal and psychological correlates, than early stuttering. The problem has existed longer, and thus the stutterer, his family, and his listeners have had more opportunity to develop negative reactions to the stuttering. Most advanced stutterers evolve a number of coping strategies in their attempts to survive the problem. The stutterer's speech is typically characterized by muscular tension and forcing, fragmenting of utterances, and superfluous motor activity, sometimes remote from the speech mechanism. He is painfully aware of his speech and of reactions to it. He may be embarrassed or may feel inferior, guilty, hostile, anxious, aggressive, or timid as he vacillates between approaching and avoiding talking. Given the possibilities for such complex compounding of a problem which feeds on itself motorically and emotionally, it is not surprising that the therapies for this problem have also vacillated between the mysterious, the complex, and the simplistic.

Therapy for advanced stuttering ranges from tactics such as putting stones in the mouth, oral surgery, waving the hand rhythmically in the air, chewing one's breathstream, superstitious incantations, deliberate stuttering, and electric shock, to psychotherapy, biofeedback, controlled fluent stuttering, and sophisticated conditioning techniques. Even within each of these broad therapeutic techniques, there have been numerous variations and combinations involving counseling, desensitization, stuttering controls, and fluency-inducing procedures.

If you are interested in pursuing this topic in depth, several available volumes describe specific therapeutic tactics and principles. See the Selected Readings at the end of this chapter.

Space in a single chapter does not permit a detailed discussion of these various therapies in any descriptive detail. Many are no longer in use. We will discuss a few of these therapies as they may illustrate some specific issues and principles about therapy.

As we have seen, variations in therapeutic practice are in part a function of how the problem has been defined and perceived theoretically. If stuttering is seen as a symptom of anxiety, then therapy will deal with anxiety. If stuttering is seen as an anticipatory struggle, then therapy legitimately deals with the stutterer's expectancies. If stuttering is seen as being conditioned, then therapy deals with components of the conditioning model.

When we talk about therapeutic practice, we are including several components that are critical to overall clinical management. These include:

(1) Goals of therapy
(2) Tactics of therapy, including:
    (a) Target behaviors
    (b) Style of therapy
    (c) Self-management
    (d) Transfer and maintenance
(3) Follow-up studies.

General Goals of Therapy

The goals of each therapy program are a function of how the problem is perceived, which in turn should be reflected in the specific therapeutic tactics used. Generally the goals of therapy focus on:

(1) Changing the way the stutterer talks
(2) Changing the way the stutterer feels
(3) Changing the way the stutterer interacts with the environment.

Within these broad categories, we find much polarization of thinking.

For example, in the past, some therapies assumed that stuttering was a chronic and permanent condition that would be aggravated by any therapeutic attempts to reduce or eliminate it—"once a stutterer–always a stutterer." Stutterers were counseled to accept their problem, in "a reasoning of resignation" (Shames, 1979). These therapies employed tactics of negative practice (Dunlap, 1932), voluntary stuttering (Bryngelson, 1955), and controlled and fluent stuttering (Van Riper, 1954).

Other therapies have as their primary goals the reduction of anxiety about speech. These would include systematic desensitization (Brutten & Shoemaker, 1967; Lanyon, 1969), psychotherapy (Barbara, 1954; Glauber, 1958; Travis, 1957), semantic-based therapy (Bloodstein, 1975; Johnson, 1933; Shames, et al., 1969, Williams, 1957), and role enactment (Sheehan, 1975).

Therapy work on stutterer's anxieties was also a part of these programs, as well as other systems which focus primarily on changing speech. Advocates felt that, by learning to control stuttering and do it voluntarily, stutterers would develop a sense of control over their behavior that would result in their not feeling helpless and anxious.

This same indirect focus on anxiety characterizes some of the therapies that more prominently concerned with developing stutter-free speech. With the accumulation of stutter-free talking time, the person's expectations should eventually change from anticipating stuttering to anticipating fluency, which would result in a reduction in speech anxieties.

Goals for Changing Speech   There are at least four approaches to changing the way stutterers talk.

(1) Help the stutterer to become a fluent stutterer. With this goal in mind, the stutterer learns to deliberately emit disfluencies in a predesigned and controlled way (Van Riper, 1954).

(2) Help the stutterer to learn monitored fluency, with a small residue (1% to 3%) of stuttering still allowed. In this therapy the stutterer deliberately performs behaviors that compete with stuttering. It requires continuous and long-term vigilance and control of fluency-inducing behaviors (Schwartz, 1976; Webster, 1980).

(3) Help the stutterer to learn monitored fluency with no residue of stuttering. This is like goal (2) except for the residue of stuttering. It results in what Perkins calls "Speech Actors," because the stutterer maintains fluency by virtue of his being deliberate and vigilant about his speaking behaviors, quite unlike nonstutterers (Perkins, 1979; Ryan & Van Kirk, 1974).

(4) Help the stutterer to develop automatic, nondeliberate, stutter-free speech. In this therapy, deliberate monitoring of fluency-inducing behaviors may be an intermediate step, which is eventually replaced by automatic stutter-free speech (Shames & Florance, 1980). Systematic desensitization, which focuses on manipulating the stutterer's anxiety through visual imagery and fantasy, has the same goal of stutter-free speech.

Goals for Changing Feelings   The polarization and variation of thinking we have just seen is also present in the goals which deal with changing the way the stutterer feels. These goals for changing feelings are generally paired with the goals for changing his speech.

(1) In those therapies that include voluntary stuttering and have as a goal becoming a fluent stutterer, there is usually a goal of helping the stutterer to become more comfortable in accepting his permanent destiny as a stutterer, and learning to live with his problem without guilt, embarrassment, social avoidance, or feelings of inferiority. The stutterer learns to feel a sense of control over the stuttering, even without striving for fluency.

(2) With those stutterers whose goal is monitored fluency, feelings may not necessarily be directly worked on. Under these circumstances, the goal regarding feelings may be somewhat ambiguous and left to the individual. Because of the slight residue of stuttering associated with monitored fluency, the stutterer would probably be left with the feeling of being a "mild and infrequent stutterer" who needs to monitor his speech continuously to keep from stuttering. The uncertainties of having stuttering lurking just beyond the next utterance are still present, whether the person stutters frequently or infrequently. Again, however, feelings of confidence about his ability to monitor his fluency are encouraged and may develop.

(3) Those stutterers who are stutter-free but continue to monitor their talking have feelings of being in-between or in transition. These people may or may not call themselves stutterers, but they cling to a "special" status for themselves, for any number of personal reasons as well as the reality of their special efforts to maintain fluency.

(4) Those stutterers who become stutter-free and do not monitor their fluency with any special effort find a reality base in their talking and can change how they feel about themselves as speakers. They often no longer think or feel about themselves as stutterers. They begin to interact from a posture of strength rather than a posture of apology and weakness. They develop new and sometimes frightening expectations for themselves and generally see many more choices for themselves socially, educationally, and vocationally. Speech no longer is a constraining factor in fulfilling their goals for living. However, such a radical change can carry much stress, and the person may need to readjust some interpersonal relationships as well as his personal identity. Even positive changes need to be nurtured, assimilated, and integrated into a person's self-concept and life system. As these changes occur, the person may feel that the past was safe and the future is frightening. Counseling may well help the person deal with feelings about the past as a stutterer, feelings about the present, and fears about the future (Shames & Florance, 1980).

(5) Psychologically oriented therapies such as psychoanalysis, counseling, and psychotherapy (as well as systematic desensitization) focus directly and almost exclusively on the feelings of the stutterer. However, where counseling and psychotherapy *do not* focus on feelings or factors associated with stuttering or talking, systematic desensitization focuses on those anxieties that are associated with speech. The goals in psychotherapy are to redefine the stutterer's problem; stuttering is viewed as a symptom of a basic emotional or interpersonal conflict. The goals are to recognize, understand, and confront these basic issues. In systematic desensitization, the goal is to reduce anxieties about talking.

Goals for Interpersonal Relationships

Goals of therapy which pertain to interpersonal interactions are generally quite similar from therapy to therapy. Most of the therapies seek to provide the stutterer with more choices regarding social activities and relationships with people. At the very least, it is hoped that the stutterer's posttherapy speech status is not a factor in his interpersonal relationships. On paper, this sounds reasonable. With new talking skills, the stutterer should be in a better position to relate, to socialize, and to interpret the nature and quality of his relationships without stuttering being a factor. Our society tends to put high value on being gregarious, out-going, and talkative, with much less value on being relatively quiet and deliberative. Naturally, the hope is that the person would be comfortable in both circumstances and could make choices according to his comfort rather than superimposed expectations.

Tactics of Therapy

Tactics in therapy, like goals of therapy, should relate to the general dynamics of the problem. Tactics refer to how the therapy is carried out, as well as to the specific content variables.

Teaching and Learning   In some therapies, the speech-language pathologist functions as a teacher or instructor and the client as a student. The tactical questions come down to what is to be learned by the stutterer and how is it to be learned. We must recognize that everything that is to be learned does not necessarily have to be taught. In these circumstances, the speech-language pathologist tries to organize and arrange an optimum environment for learning during therapy. The professional may impart information to the stutterer, show him how to do something by demonstrating it, or provide instructions and feedback to behave in certain ways. These functions are much more clinician-centered than client-centered and assume that the speech-language pathologist has the major responsibility for leading the stutterer through the therapeutic experiences.

The speech-language pathologist may also function merely as a "reinforcer" of various attempts by the client to improve or change with little advance information about alternatives or choices of "right" or "wrong" ways to do things during therapy. This therapy is decidedly client-centered; the client is free to define his problems and to choose and to learn from both experience and from the professional the most productive and effective activities for improvement. The speech-language pathologist's reinforcing activities offer directive guidelines. However, because they are provided *after* rather than *before* the client's activities, the client rather than the clinician takes on the responsibility for moving and directing the therapy.

These teaching, instructing, demonstrating, and reinforcing tactics in therapy are usually used in combination. The directive teaching functions are usually employed in early phases of therapy, when the stutterer is first learning how to change the motor aspects of his speaking behavior. However, in later stages of therapy, when the stutterer is faced with the tasks of using and integrating his new skills into his real, nonclinical world, the direction and responsibility may be shifted to or be more mutually shared with the stutterer.

The need to help the stutterer become responsible for managing the problem and for managing certain aspects of the therapy has been considered in most therapy regimes for some time, but the question of the best way to accomplish this is still open. Some people may need a great deal of structure and organization from the speech-language pathologist and may have to be gradually nurtured into becoming responsible for managing their problems and therapy. Others may quite easily develop their own therapeutic strategies and problem-solving styles. Some stutterers can be classified as **high self-**

reinforcers who need to evolve their own strategies, while others tend to function as **low self-reinforcers** who need a great deal of support and structure from the therapist (Shames & Florance, 1980). As a result, Shames and Florance added a therapy phase which provides training in self-regulation and self-monitoring techniques, based on the principles of self-reinforcement developed in programs for weight reduction and smoking reduction. Eventually the stutterer must become free of any special therapeutic support systems. Otherwise his destiny is to be forever dependent on the monitoring, feedback, and thinking provided by the speech-language pathologist. The professional must take care that his comments and interpretations do not deprive the stutterer of opportunities to think and interpret for himself. Therapeutic tactics at all stages should maximize opportunities for the stutterer to grow and to express his potential for independent problem solving.

Our discussion of *how* stutterers may learn about themselves, about their problem, or from the various experiences organized by the therapy still leaves open the question of *what* is to be learned. What stutterers learn relates directly to how the problem is perceived and to the goals of therapy that relate to those perceptions. Some stutterers may learn to stutter fluently, and some may learn to speak without stuttering by emitting behaviors which compete with stuttering. These behaviors include controlling the rate of talking, controlling phonation and breathstream, and developing a gentle onset of speaking. Some stutterers may learn to accept their stuttering and to understand the detailed dynamics of their stuttering motorically, emotionally, and interactionally. They learn to be comfortable and unembarrassed as a stutterer. Other stutterers may learn about being a nonstutterer and all of the emotional elements of changing their basic self-concepts.

Different stutterers under differing therapeutic regimes obviously learn different things in different ways. These variations reflect the variations in individuals as well as the variations in professional thinking about the problem. They are also a reflection of how much is yet to be learned about the nature of therapy for this problem.

Transfer and Maintenance   Most of the early therapies for advanced stuttering which focus on learning to accept and control stuttering paid a great deal of attention to transferring these skills, behaviors, and attitudes to the stutterer's nonclinical environments. Often the bravery and resolve that operate in the clinic room must be carefully moved into the stutterer's outside world, or the new skills would not be functional in any real-life situation. The transfer of these new skills may meet with resistance from the stutterer, especially when the stuttering has been emotionally useful. Therefore, in these programs, stutterers were given talking assignments, homework, and situational desensitization experiences to facilitate their carry-over.

Unlike the older therapies, many of the newer therapies which emphasize fluency-inducing behaviors focus primarily on tactics for initially changing the stutterer's speech in the clinic, with much less attention to transfer and maintenance. These therapeutic regimes can be seriously and severely criticized as being nothing more than laboratory exercises in fluency with little or no impact on the real problem. Any therapy program must involve transfer.

One technique mobilizes the stutterer's family, friends, and teachers as agents of reinforcement in their therapy for children (Ryan & Van Kirk, 1974). The child is scheduled for a series of experiences in his nonclinical environment under reinforcement contingencies that are carried out by people in the home, at school, and so on.

In another scheme, the stutterer systematically rates himself on how well he monitored his new speaking skills during the day (Perkins, 1973b). The stutterer would rate his breathstream management, prosody, rate of speech, and self-confidence. If the ratings were low on any of these components, the stutterer would give extra attention to that component in practice and conversational settings.

Another approach invokes the principles and use of behavioral contracting (Shames & Florance, 1980). In this regime, the stutterer commits himself in advance to monitoring his stutter-free speaking behaviors in a progressively expanding array of comfortable social and emotional circumstances, using explicit self-reinforcement procedures. The contract is generated daily by the client. It spells out in detail where, when, to whom, and for how long he will monitor his speech. The stutterer also rates the difficulty level of the contract and evaluates his performance. Gradually, the detailed contract is expanded in time, duration, frequency, and difficulty. Eventually most of the stutterer's talking time is deliberately monitored under his own self-regulated contingencies.

Depending upon the stutterer and his disposition toward self-management, a balance among these types of transfer activities and processes, involving one or all of them, may be the most effective way to approach this critical phase of therapy.

Maintenance and Relapse   When a stutterer first enters therapy, he is capable of emitting many different kinds of behaviors, of having many different kinds of feelings, and of generating many different kinds of interactions and reactions in his environment. Some of these are quite desirable and productive and contribute to the stutterer's happiness and well-being. Others may be quite undesirable and nonproductive, and contribute to feelings of despair and desolation.

As a result of therapy, the desirable and productive behaviors and feelings should become more prominent, while the undesirable and nonproductive behaviors and feelings should become less functional. However, at any point, each of us is capable of bringing out any prominent or obscure part of ourselves, depending on the circumstances of the moment. This directly relates to issues of maintenance and relapse in therapy for stuttering. There is no quantitative criterion for deciding whether or not a relapse has occurred. If a stutterer stutters once, 6 months after therapy, has he relapsed? How many times, with what frequency, duration, form, and time intervals after therapy does it take to constitute a relapse? In spite of the problem of precisely defining the nature of a relapse, we can say that relapses occur with an alarming and discouraging frequency following therapy for advanced stuttering. Those behaviors called *relapse* come under the same behavioral controls that any other behavior does (Shames, 1979). At any time, before, during, and after therapy, the stutterer can stutter, can use monitored stutter-free speech, and can speak without stuttering or monitoring speech. The probability of each of these behaviors may be a function of the events occurring at the time. Our evaluation of their desirability (related to the goals of therapy) dictates whether or not each instance is called *maintenance* or *relapse*.

There are a number of different possible explanations for relapse (Boberg, Howie, & Woods, 1979). One rather pessimistic view holds that relapse is a part of the human condition and occurs almost invariably after treatment for most (if not all) human behavior problems. Another view is that relapse might be prevented if clinic support were maintained longer and withdrawn more

Maintenance *refers to the continued emission of the target behaviors acquired during formal therapy. It may also refer to the continuing experience*

*of certain desirable
feelings and social
patterns that were
acquired during ther-
apy.* Relapse *refers to a
return to the prether-
apy state. It may also
refer to substitution of
new undesirable
behaviors for the old
ones.*

slowly. Still another view is that change in personality must take place before a lasting change in fluency will result. Another view is that, in intensive therapy programs, the stutterer cannot cope with the speed of changes in his speech and he therefore relapses. Boberg and colleagues further suggest three significant theoretical possibilities for relapse. One is that stutterers use very small disfluencies that are barely recognizable in therapy, but grow in magnitude and form the seeds for later relapse after therapy ends. A second possibility is that posttherapy speech monitoring is a nonrewarding experience and is eventually not continued by the stutterer. Third is the inevitability of relapse if there is a heavy genetic and therefore physiological basis for stuttering in a given person.

Many experts have proposed techniques to promote maintenance. Ryan and Van Kirk (1974) encourage daily monitoring of stuttering, fading out home practice but continuing clinical contact for evaluation and reinstruction. Ingham and Andres (1973; Ingham, 1975) encourage the stutterer to continue practicing prolonged speech and to maintain clinical contact. Perkins (1971) suggests a continuation of periodic clinical contacts for speech practice and counseling. Webster (1980) encourages the initial overlearning of the behaviors necessary for fluent speech, toward the goal of making these behaviors automatic. Shames and Florance (1980) tend to agree with Webster that the best way to combat relapse is to make those behaviors which compete with stuttering automatic. However, they approach that goal not through initial overlearning, but through processes of generaliztion and systematic scheduling of unmonitored speech as a formal part of therapy.

Different therapies have reported different maintenance and relapse rates, ranging from 50% to over 90% maintenance, depending upon the ages of the clients, the tactics employed for initially changing the stutterers' speech, and whether transfer and maintenance procedures were employed. All therapies seem to have a significant drop-out rate. In spite of these data and the drop-out rates, we are making significant increases in successful therapeutic outcomes. The prognosis for the problem of stuttering has been undergoing a gradual change from pessimism to tempered optimism.

Counseling

Another tactic that is generally found in most therapies is counseling. Counseling does not mean "lecturing" a stutterer about himself. Rather, it refers to providing an opportunity for the person to explore, verbalize, think, and express his feelings about himself and his problems, about his therapy, about the process of changing, about his expectations and fears about the future, and about anything else that is of significance for him. The process is usually a client-centered one that respects the individual's potential for finding solutions. It encourages the person to take the responsibility for setting the topical agenda and for setting the pace for talking about himself and his problem. As we have seen, therapeutic change can bring with it stress and therefore the need for a caring companion through the change process. Therapeutic change in psychotherapy may also be directly related to how susceptible the client is to the influences of the therapist (Strupp, 1962, 1972). As the client learns to trust the therapist and learns that the therapist will not abuse him, some very powerful bonds of affection may develop between them. It is out of this climate of trust and love that the client makes changes in himself. Although the client may bring his own "will to recover" to the therapeutic experience, it is this powerful and close interpersonal relationship which nurtures and sustains that "will" through the sometimes painful aspects of therapy.

Very often, counseling tactics are combined with some of the teaching tactics we have mentioned to deal with the multiple aspects of the stuttering problem. The content of the counseling sessions will vary with each individual, how he sees his problem, its impact on his life, his general expectations about his future, and his understanding of himself. The content may also vary with the specific emphases relative to his speech goals. As such, in those therapies which focus on learning to become a fluent stutterer, some of the counseling time may focus on feelings of acceptance of being a stutterer and on the specific dynamics of stuttering episodes, reactions to listeners, and reactions to stuttering. There is a heavy focus on "stuttering." In therapies which focus on the development of stutter-free speech, the counseling may not necessarily dwell on stuttering, but rather on the experiences of stutter-free talking and on all of the possible positive and negative aspects of becoming a fluent speaker.

In the total clinical management of advanced stuttering, whether the therapy is based on conditioning or not, there is little doubt that counseling is a necessary component. The changes in speech which are accomplished through direct teaching process, the clinical relationship, and the support of a caring speech-language pathologist, as well as the self-understanding that emerges from the counseling process, can be combined into a powerful and effective facilitating force in providing for the total needs of the stutterer in therapy.

PREVENTION

For many good reasons, there has been no work directly attacking the issue of prevention of stuttering. Without any conclusive evidence about the etiology of stuttering, it is difficult to eliminate the causes to prevent its development. Unlike the medical sciences, we cannot immunize children against developing stuttering. From a humanitarian and ethical standpoint, we cannot attempt to cause a child to stutter (even if we knew how), because we are not certain that we could reverse the process. Furthermore, direct research on the prevention of a problem that may have an environmental base is extremely difficult to conduct. However, except for the genetic theory of stuttering, most theories imply a message of prevention.

Johnson's semantogenic theory (1944) tells us that if we can arrange the appropriate semantic environment relating to a child's normal, developmental disfluencies, stuttering could be prevented from developing. Shames and Egolf's work on parent-child verbal interactions (1976) suggests that, as a general preventive measure, positive verbal interactions between parents and children could prevent a stuttering problem. But these ideas are only infer-entially related to prevention. Both commonsense and research tell us that part of the answer to prevention is in good child-rearing and parenting prac-tices, along with providing parents with information about child development in general and about speech and language development in particular. Perhaps the most successful preventive measures are those which pay attention to parents' concerns (well-founded or not) in conferences and counseling, so that any untoward factors operating in the home can be promptly and compassionately handled before they start to affect how fluently a child communicates.

CONCLUSION

The problem of stuttering continues to present a number of challenges to theorists, to researchers, to speech-language pathologists, and to stutterers themselves. The cause of the problem is still not clear. As a result, prevention has received almost no attention. The problem has had a history of controversy and inconsistency. Experts have argued and disagreed over its theory, causation, definition, dynamics, measurement, and clinical management. However, emerging from all of this controversy has been a history of growth and improvement. Some parts of the problem are obvious and available for all to see; other parts are hidden and private. There are many facets to its study, understanding, and management. We can look at its behavioral components, its physiological components, its emotional components, and its interactional components.

As these various components of the problem are conceptualized, integrated, and related to broader perspectives in the cognitive, developmental, behavioral, and biomedical sciences, the potential for its ultimate resolution is accordingly enhanced. There is yet much to do. Fortunately, we have time to do it.

SELECTED READINGS

Bloodstein, O. *A handbook on stuttering.* Chicago: National Easter Seal Society for Crippled Children and Adults, 1975.

Brutten, E. J., & Shoemaker, D. J. *The modification of stuttering.* Englewood Cliffs, N.J.: Prentice-Hall, 1967.

Emerick, L., & Hamre, C. *An analysis of stuttering: Selected readings.* Danville, Ill.: Interstate Printers and Publishers, 1972.

Florance, C. L., & Shames, G. H. Stuttering treatment: Issues in transfer and maintenance. In J. Northern (Ed.) & W. Perkins (Guest Ed.), *Seminars, speech language hearing, strategies in stuttering therapy.* New York: Grune & Stratton, 1981.

McFall, R. M. Parameters of self monitoring. In R. Stewart (Ed.), *Behavioral self management, strategies, techniques and outcomes.* New York: Brunner/ Mazel, 1977.

Shames, G. H., & Egolf, D. B. *Operant conditioning & the management of stuttering.* Englewood Cliffs, N.J.: Prentice-Hall, 1976.

Shames, G. H., & Florance, C. L. *Stutter-free speech: A goal for therapy.* Columbus, Ohio: Charles E. Merrill, 1980.

Shames, G. H., & Sherrick, C. E., Jr. A discussion of nonfluency and stuttering as operant behavior. *Journal of Speech and Hearing Disorders,* 1963, *28,* 3–18.

Sheehan, J. G. *Stuttering: Research and therapy.* New York: Harper & Row, 1970.

Siegel, G. M. Punishment, stuttering and disfluency. *Journal of Speech and Hearing Research,* 1970, *13,* 677–714.

Stewart, R. Self help group approach to self management. In R. Stewart (Ed.), *Behavioral self management, strategies, techniques and outcomes.* New York: Brunner/Mazel, 1977.

Strupp, H. Patient-doctor relationship: Psychotherapist in the therapeutic process. In H. J. Bachrach (Ed.), *Experimental foundations of clinical psychology.* New York: Basic Books, 1962.

Strupp, H. On the technology of psychotherapy. *Archives of General Psychiatry,* 1976, *26,* 270–278.

Van Riper, C. *The nature of stuttering.* Englewood Cliffs, N.J.: Prentice-Hall, 1971.

Van Riper, C. *The treatment of stuttering.* Englewood Cliffs, N.J.: Prentice-Hall, 1973.

Williams, D. E. A point of view about stuttering. *Journal of Speech and Hearing Disorders,* 1957, *22,* 390–397.

REFERENCES

Abbot, J. A. Repressed hostility as a factor in adult stuttering. *Journal of Speech Disorders,* 1947, *12,* 428–430.

Adams, M. R. Further analysis of stuttering as a phonetic transition defect. *Journal of Fluency Disorders,* 1978, *3*(4), 265–271.

Ainsworth, S. Integrating theories of stuttering. *Journal of Speech Disorders,* 1945, *10,* 205–210.

Barbara, D. *Stuttering: A psychodynamic approach to its understanding and treatment.* New York: Julian Press, 1954.

Bloodstein, O. Stuttering as an anticipatory struggle reaction. In J. Eisenson (Ed.), *Stuttering: A symposium.* New York: Harper & Row, 1958.

Bloodstein, O. The development of stuttering: I. Changes in nine basic features. *Journal of Speech and Hearing Disorders,* 1960, *25,* 219–237. (a)

Bloodstein, O. The development of stuttering: II. Developmental phases. *Journal of Speech and Hearing Disorders,* 1960, *25,* 366–376. (b)

Bloodstein O. *A handbook on stuttering.* Chicago: National Easter Seal Society for Crippled Children and Adults, 1975.

Boberg, E., Howie, P., & Woods, L. Maintenance of fluency: A review. *Journal of Fluency Disorders,* 1979, *4,* 93–116.

Brookshire, R. H., & Eveslage, R. H. Verbal punishment of disfluency following augmentation of disfluency by random delivery of aversive stimuli. *Journal of Speech and Hearing Research,* 1969, *12,* 383–388.

Brutten, E. J., & Shoemaker, D. J. *The modification of stuttering.* Englewood Cliffs, N.J.: Prentice-Hall, 1967.

Bryngelson, B. Sidedness as an etiological factor in stuttering. *Journal of Genetic Psychology,* 1935, *47,* 204–217.

Bryngelson, B. A study of laterality of stutterers and normal speakers. *Journal of Speech Disorders,* 1939, *4,* 231–234.

Bryngelson, B. Voluntary stuttering. In C. Van Riper (Ed.), *Speech therapy: A book of readings.* Englewood Cliffs, N.J.: Prentice-Hall, 1955.

Curlee, R. F., & Perkins, W. H. Conversational rate control therapy for stuttering. *Journal of Speech and Hearing Disorders,* 1969, *34,* 245–250.

Darley, F., Aronson, A., & Brown, J. *Motor speech disorders.* Philadelphia: W. B. Saunders, 1975.

Davis, D. M. The relation of repetitions in the speech of young children to certain measures of language maturity and situational factors, Part I. *Journal of Speech and Hearing Disorders,* 1939, *4,* 303–318.

Davis, D. M. The relation of repetitions in the speech of young children to certain measures of language maturity and situational factors, Parts II and III. *Journal of Speech and Hearing Disorders,* 1940, *5,* 235–246.

Dunlap, K. *Habits: Their making and unmaking.* New York: Liveright, 1932.

Egland, G. References. Cited in C. Van Riper, *Speech correction: Principles and methods.* Englewood Cliffs, N.J.: Prentice-Hall, 1954.

Flanagan, B., Goldiamond, I., & Azrin, N. Operant stuttering: The control of stuttering behavior through response-contingent consequences. *Journal of the Experimental Analysis of Behavior,* 1958, *1,* 173–177.

Glauber, I. P. The psychoanalysis of stuttering. In J. Eisenson (Ed.), *Stuttering: A symposium.* New York: Harper & Row, 1958.

Goldiamond, I. Stuttering and fluency as manipulable operant response classes. In L. Krasner & L. P. Ullmann (Eds.), *Research 7, in behavior modification.* New York: Holt, Rinehart & Winston, 1965.

Halvorson, J. A. The effects on stuttering frequency of pairing punishment (response cost) with reinforcement. *Journal of Speech and Hearing Research,* 1971, *14,* 356–364.

Hill, H. Stuttering: I. A critical review and evaluation of biochemical investigations. *Journal of Speech Disorders,* 1944, *9,* 245–261. (a)

Hill, H. Stuttering: II. A review and integration of physiological data. *Journal of Speech Disorders,* 1944, *9,* 289–324. (b)

Ingham, R. J. Operant methodology in stuttering. In J. Eisenson (Ed.), *Stuttering: A second symposium.* New York: Harper & Row, 1975.

Ingham, R. J., & Andrews, G. An analysis of a token economy in stuttering therapy. *Journal of Applied Behavior Analysis,* 1973, *6,* 219–229.

Johnson, W. An interpretation of stuttering. *Quarterly Journal of Speech,* 1933, *19,* 70–76.

Johnson, W. The role of evaluation in stuttering behavior. *Journal of Speech Disorders,* 1938, *3,* 85–89.

Johnson, W. A study of the onset and development of stuttering. *Journal of Speech Disorders,* 1942, *7,* 251–257.

Johnson, W. The Indians have no word for it, I. Stuttering in children. *Quarterly Journal of Speech,* 1944, *30,* 330–337.

Johnson, W. *Stuttering and what you can do about it.* Minneapolis: University of Minnesota Press, 1961.

Kasprisin-Burrelli, A., Egolf, D. B., & Shames, G. H. A comparison of parental verbal behavior with stuttering and nonstuttering children. *Journal of Communication Disorders,* 1972, *5,* 335–346.

Kidd, K. K. A genetic perspective on stuttering. *Journal of Fluency Disorders,* 1977, *2,* 259–269.

Lanyon, R. J. Bahvior change in stuttering through systematic desensitization. *Journal of Speech and Hearing Disorders,* 1969, *34,* 253–259.

Lenneberg, E. H. *Biological foundations of language.* New York: John Wiley, 1967.

Orton, S., & Travis, L. E. Studies in stuttering: IV. Studies of action currents in stutterers. *Archives of Neurology and Psychiatry,* 1929, *21,* 61–68.

Perkins, W. H. *Speech pathology: An applied behavioral science.* St. Louis: C. V. Mosby, 1971.

Perkins, W. H. Replacement of stuttering with normal speech, I. Rationale. *Journal of Speech and Hearing Disorders,* 1973, *38,* 283–294.

Perkins, W. H. Replacement of stuttering with normal speech, II. Clinical procedures. *Journal of Speech and Hearing Disorders,* 1973, *38,* 295–308. (b)

Perkins, W. H. Paper presented at Banff International Conference on Maintenance of Fluency, Banff, Canada, June 1979.

Perkins, W., Ruder, J., Johnson, L., & Michael, W. Stuttering: Discoordination of phonation with articulation and respiration. *Journal of Speech and Hearing Research,* 1976, *19,* 509–522.

Rubin, H., & Culatta, R. A point of view about fluency. *Journal of the American Speech and Hearing Assocation,* 1971, *13,* 380–387.

Ryan, B. P., & Van Kirk, B. The establishment, transfer and maintenance of fluent speech in 50 stutterers using DAF and operant procedures. *Journal of Speech and Hearing Disorders,* 1974, *38,* 3–10.

Saikorski, J. A. *Über das Stottern.* Berlin: Hirschweld, 1889.

Schwartz, M. The core of the stuttering block. *Journal of Speech and Hearing Disorders,* 1974, *39,* 169–177.

Schwartz, M. *Stuttering solved.* New York: McGraw-Hill, 1976.

Shames, G. H. *Pediatric clinics of North America.* Philadelphia: W. B. Saunders, 1968.

Shames, G. H. *Relapse in stuttering.* Paper presented at Banff International Conference on Maintenance of Fluency, Banff, Canada, June 1979.

Shames, G. H., & Egolf, D. B. *Experimental therapy for school-age children & their parents.* Final Report, Project No. 482130, Grant No. OEG-0-8-080080, Department of Health, Education and Welfare, U.S. Office of Education, June 1971.

Shames, G. H., & Egolf, D. B. *Operant conditioning: The management of stuttering.* Englewood Cliffs, N.J.: Prentice-Hall, 1976.

Shames, G. H., Egolf, D. B., & Rhodes, R. C. Experimental programs in stuttering therapy. *Journal of Speech and Hearing Disorders,* 1969, *34,* 38–47.

Shames, G. H., & Florance, C. L. *Stutter-free speech: A goal for therapy.* Columbus, Ohio: Charles E. Merrill, 1980.

Shames, G. H., & Sherrick, C. E., Jr. A discussion of nonfluency and stuttering as operant behavior. *Journal of Speech and Hearing Disorders,* 1963, *28,* 3–18.

Sheehan, J. G. Theory and treatment of stuttering as an approach-avoidance conflict. *Journal of Psychology,* 1953, *36,* 27–49.

Sheehan, J. G. Conflict theory of stuttering. In J. Eisenson (Ed.), *Stuttering: A symposium.* New York: Harper & Row, 1958. (a)

Sheehan, J. G. Prospective studies of stuttering. *Journal of Speech and Hearing Disorders,* 1958, *23,* 18–25. (b)

Sheehan, J. G. Conflict theory and avoidance reduction therapy. In J. Eisenson (Ed.), *Stuttering: A second symposium.* New York: Harper & Row, 1975.

Sheehan, J., & Martyn, M. M. Spontaneous recovery from stuttering. *Journal of Speech and Hearing Research,* 1966, *9,* 121–135.

Siegel, G. M. Punishment, stuttering and disfluency. *Journal of Speech and Hearing Research,* 1970, *13,* 677–714.

Strupp, H. Patient-doctor relationship: Psychotherapist in the therapeutic process. In W. J. Bachrach (Ed.), *Experimental foundations of clinical psychology.* New York: Basic Books, 1962.

Strupp, H. On the technology of psychotherapy. *Archives of General Psychiatry,* 1972, *26,* 270–278.

Travis, L. E. The unspeakable feeling of people with special reference to stuttering. In L. E. Travis (Ed.), *Handbook of speech pathology.* New York: Appleton-Century-Crofts, 1957.

Van Riper, C. *Speech correction: Principles and methods* (3rd ed.). Englewood Cliffs, N.J.: Prentice-Hall, 1954.

Van Riper, C. *The nature of stuttering.* Englewood Cliffs, N.J.: Prentice-Hall, 1971.

Webster, R. L. Evolution of a target-based behavioral therapy for stuttering. *Journal of Fluency Disorders,* 1980, *5,* 303–320.

West, R. An agnostic's speculations about stuttering. In J. Eisenson (Ed.), *Stuttering: A symposium.* New York: Harper & Row, 1958.

Williams, D. E. A point of view about stuttering. *Journal of Speech and Hearing Disorders*, 1957, *22*, 390–397.

Williams, D. E. A perspective on approaches to stuttering therapy. In H. Gregory (Ed.), *Controversies about stuttering therapy*. Baltimore: University Park Press, 1979.

Wingate, M. Calling attention to stuttering. *Journal of Speech and Hearing Research*, 1959, *2*, 326–335.

Wingate, M. Stuttering as phonetic transition defect. *Journal of Speech and Hearing Disorders*, 1969, *34*, 107–108.

Winitz, H. Repetitions in the vocalizations and speech of children in the first two years of life. *Journal of Speech and Hearing Disorders*, 1961, Monograph Supplement 7, 55–62.

Wischner, G. J. Stuttering behavior and learning: A preliminary theoretical formulation. *Journal of Speech and Hearing Disorders*, 1950, *15*, 324–335.

Wischner, G. J. Anxiety reduction as reinforcement in maladaptive behavior: Evidence in stutterers' representations of the moment of difficulty. *Journal of Abnormal Social Psychology*, 1952, *47*, 566–571. (a)

Wischner, G. J. An experimental approach to expectancy and anxiety in stuttering behavior. *Journal of Speech and Hearing Disorders*, 1952, *17*, 139–154. (b)

Wolpe, J. *Psychotherapy by reciprocal inhibition*. Stanford: Stanford University Press, 1958.

EARLY LANGUAGE DEVELOPMENT AND LANGUAGE DISORDERS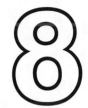

Laurence B. Leonard

Tony was first evaluated for speech and language difficulties at age 3 years, 1 month. At that time his parents reported that he produced only a few words. His most frequent communicative attempts involved gesturing, producing certain "favorite" syllables (such as "ba"), and whining. According to the parents' report, Tony seemed to understand much of what was said to him. They felt his hearing was normal, although at age 2 years he had received medication for a middle ear infection. Tony's motor development seemed to be within normal limits.

The initial speech and language evaluation confirmed the parents' impressions. Tony's performance on standardized language comprehension tests was approximately 6 months below that expected for his age. His speech, limited to single-word utterances, precluded the use of available standardized tests of language production. However, an analysis of a sample of his spontaneous speech revealed a level of usage seen in children at least a year younger. Audiometric testing was inconclusive. However, it appeared that Tony had normal hearing in at least one ear, at the frequencies most important for speech. Results from a performance scale of a standardized test of intelligence suggested a borderline level of intellectual functioning.

On the basis of the speech and language evaluation, it was recommended that Tony be enrolled in a daily preschool program emphasizing language learning activities. Along with the group language stimulation activities conducted in the preschool, Tony received daily individual therapy focusing on the production of functional multiword utterances. The individual therapy sessions were 30 minutes long. Following the individual session, Tony joined the other children in the group.

Testing conducted 9 months after Tony was enrolled in the preschool program revealed noticeable gains in the level of his linguistic functioning. His performance on standardized language comprehension tests was age-appropriate. Tony continued to have difficulties in language production. His performance on standardized language production tests reflected a level of functioning more like that of a child one year his junior. However, in absolute terms, Tony's language production gains were significant. Utterances three to five words in length were common. In addition, he asked questions frequently (for example, "Where Josh going?") and produced words and phrases in situations in which he previously exhibited a pattern of whining. Tony was more cooperative during this period, en-

abling a more complete assessment of his hearing. Results indicated hearing within normal limits.

You may now wish to listen to the speech sample accompanying this chapter, found on Audio Disc 1, Side 2 (sample #4).

Although most children seem to acquire their native language relatively easily, with no formal instruction, this critical task is very difficult for some children. These children need additional assistance, which is often provided by the speech-language pathologist. It has been estimated that language disordered children make up from 50% to 80% of the cases seen by speech-language pathologists who provide services to preschool children.

This chapter focuses on preschool-aged children, while the next covers the school-aged language disordered child.

Who are these young "language disordered" children? In general, we can say that children have a language disorder whenever their language abilities are below those expected for their age and their level of functioning. Obviously, this definition is quite broad and, we will see, allows us to consider children with widely varying characteristics as language disordered.

THE DIMENSIONS OF LANGUAGE

For a basic discussion of the components of language, review chapter 2.

The difficulties experienced by language disordered children vary considerably. Certain aspects of the language may prove troublesome for one child, while other aspects are difficult for another child. Many children have problems with more than one aspect of the language. In order to appreciate the types of linguistic difficulties that children have, let us review some of the major dimensions of language.

Lexicon

As anyone initially learning a second language can attest, if you don't understand it, speech seems like a run-together stream of sounds. Most young children work through this problem relatively quickly. However, for some children, the meaning of utterances such as "givedaddyahug" may remain a mystery for years. When these children do begin to segment the speech stream into meaningful components, the process is piecemeal, leaving much room for misunderstanding. For example, the child may begin to recognize that the sound sequence "daddy" is often used in association with her father. Thus, when she hears "give daddy a hug," the child may know that something is being done by her father or should be done to or for her father, but she might know little else. Of course, the fact that she can associate "daddy" with the father does not mean that she has full understanding of the word. She may associate this sound pattern with any adult male or any adult caregiver. These problems in identifying the words of the language and in learning their meanings are problems dealing with the **lexicon** of the language.

Phonology

When children do learn a word they have learned a correspondence between a sequence of sounds and a particular referent. This sound sequence may be altered in certain ways without changing the perceived meaning. (Consider your ability to recognize differences between the way a Southerner pronounces the word "bye" and the way this word is produced by a Northerner.) However, other types of changes in a sound sequence result in changes in the word perceived. For example, we would not regard "bee" and "bye" as the same word. Similarly, this little girl must recognize that when she hears "Give Daddy a tug" a response other than hugging is called for. Thus, children must learn which speech sound changes in the language are used to change meaning. This dimension is the **phonology** or sound system of the language.

Syntax

The child might also deal with **syntax,** the system used to organize and order words to form sentences. It is not sufficient to understand the individual words in an utterance such as "Dana hugged Mommy"; the child must also understand that the word preceding the action word usually refers to the person performing the action and that the word following the action word usually refers to the person or thing being acted upon.

Morphology

Knowledge of how words combine to form sentences will enable the child to interpret much of what he hears. However, a more complete understanding requires that the child have some command of the **morphology** of the language, that is, the structure of words and, importantly for our purposes, the ways suffixes and prefixes are added to words to provide greater specificity. For example, without knowledge that *-ed* is a suffix that indicates past tense, the child might interpret "Dana hugged Mommy" as an act that is taking place at the time of the utterance, much as we would interpret the sentence "Dana hugs Mommy."

Pragmatics

Along with an understanding of language, the child must learn how language is used. I recently observed an interaction that illustrates this point quite well. A speech-language pathologist came to the waiting room of a clinic to pick up a child with whom she was working. The child was seated next to his mother, eating a bag of popcorn. The speech-language pathologist sat down next to the child and, after a few introductory remarks, said, "Boy, I sure would like some popcorn." Although the child was generally responsive, he seemed to ignore this particular request. After a short delay, the mother said, "Jason, give her some popcorn." The child quickly complied. From what was known of the child's language comprehension skills, it appeared that he could comprehend the literal meaning of the speech-language pathologist's utterance. However, it was not clear that he understood that declarative sentences such as "I sure would like some popcorn" can also serve as requests in certain situations. This skill falls within the dimension of language called **pragmatics,** or the use of language in context.

We will not discuss phonological difficulties here because they have been discussed in chapter 5. However, do not infer that phonological problems are in addition to language disorders. These difficulties are an integral part of the condition (Leonard, 1979).

   Each of these dimensions of language—the lexicon, phonology, syntax, morphology, and pragmatics—can and does present difficulties for language disordered children. Although these dimensions represent different aspects of language, they interact continually. A child will rarely have problems with one dimension of language without having at least some difficulty with others (Bloom & Lahey, 1978). Following a brief overview of normal langue development, we will examine the kinds of difficulties young language disordered children have with these dimensions of language.

A SKETCH OF NORMAL LANGUAGE DEVELOPMENT

To better understand the nature of language disorders in children, let us look at a sketch of how young, normally developing children acquire language. Many investigators have found the study of normal children particularly useful in determining whether language disordered children show the same pattern of development as normal children but at a slower rate or whether language disordered children instead show a unique pattern of development.

Twelve to Eighteen Months

When the child is approximately 1 year old, he has achieved several important developmental milestones. He shows the ability to drink from a cup and has probably begun to walk. As noted by Piaget (1963), during this period, children's knowledge of the world comes chiefly from their own physical interactions with objects and persons in their immediate environment. In fact, Piaget refers to this general period of development as the *sensorimotor period,* which highlights the importance of physical experience at this age. For example, when given a new object, the child will experiment with new ways of using it. He will engage in searching activities to locate an object that has disappeared, suggesting that he has some understanding that objects have permanence. In addition, the child will attempt to imitate novel behaviors performed by other people.

At about the same time, he has usually begun to understand a few words that represent objects, people, or activities that appear quite frequently in his daily routine. Huttenlocher (1974) has traced this pattern of development. Initially, words are understood only if the referent is present. For example, if the child is asked, "Where's the blanket?" he may pick up the blanket if it has been placed in front of him along with several other objects. Within a couple of months, the child begins to show comprehension of these words even when the referent is absent. This comprehension usually reflects the child's knowledge of the typical locations of the objects. When asked "Where's the blanket?" the child will most likely go into the room where the blanket is usually kept. Not long after this stage, the child shows the ability to respond correctly even when the referent is not in its usual location. For example, when asked to get the blanket, the child may recall having left it in his sister's room and may retrieve it from there.

The examples provided in this chapter are written as an adult might pronounce them. However, young children often pronounce words in a simplified manner. These simplifications are not noted here only to better highlight those linguistic abilities on which we are focusing.

At the approximate age of 12 months, children also begin to produce their first words. For the next 6 months or so, as children compile a vocabulary of approximately 50 words, their speech is limited to single-word utterances. However, despite the limitation in the number of words they can produce in a single utterance, young children manage to express a variety of meanings. Their speech during this early period entails considerably more than labeling things in the environment (Greenfield & Smith, 1976). Some examples of these early meanings are presented in Table 8.1.

As you can see from the examples in Table 8.1, children at the single-word stage seem to talk about the disappearance of things, the locations of things, possessors of things, things acted on, the actions used on things, and of course, they name, request, and reject things. The fact that children usually talk about things that are or recently were in their presence is quite consistent with their cognitive development.

Although children's vocabularies are limited at this age, they nonetheless show some selectivity in what they say in particular situations. For example,

TABLE 8.1
Some Examples of Single-Word Utterances Used by Young Children.

Jill is inspecting an alphabet block while sitting on the floor. Upon hearing the door slam in the other room, Jill jumps up, drops the block, and runs to the other room. The block rolled under the couch near where Jill was sitting. When Jill returns, she looks at the area of the floor where she was playing.	gone
George is looking through a picture book when he sees his mother approaching with a cup of juice.	juice
After seeing that he will need to use both hands to hold the cup, George looks around and puts the book on a nearby chair.	chair
George then comes back to his mother and takes the cup.	
Kirsten is playing with an adult visitor. The adult rolls the ball past her. Upon retrieving the ball, Kirsten passes some slippers belonging to her mother. Kirsten points at the slippers, looking up at the visitor.	Mommy
Tanya is playing with a bead necklace when she sees the adult visitor's bag of toys. She looks in the bag and pulls out a cookie tin.	box
Tanya tugs the lid, having some difficulty removing it.	open
The adult visitor leans over and starts to help.	no

the work of Greenfield and Smith (1976) indicates that a child at this stage of development may name an object as he reaches for it ("cup"). Once it is in hand, however, the child is likely to say the name of the action to be performed on the object ("drink") rather than to say its name again. The selectivity seems to reflect a tendency to communicate about that aspect of the situation that may not already be known, rather than that aspect that is clear from what is being done or was just said.

During this period, children undergo rather dramatic changes in their comprehension skills. For every word the child produces, he comprehends another four. His comprehension vocabulary of object names is particularly large (Goldin-Meadow, Seligman, & Gelman, 1976). At the same time, the child shows an emerging ability to comprehend multiword utterances, provided that he knows the meaning of the individual words involved. For example, when asked to "kiss Andy," the child will often kiss the appropriate doll when two dolls are in front of him. When asked to "tickle Bambi", the child will pick up the second doll and perform the appropriate action (Sachs & Truswell, 1978).

Eighteen to Twenty-four Months

Between approximately 18 and 24 months of age, children begin to combine words in their speech. These two-word utterances are thought to reflect children's initial acquisition of syntax, as they must apply rules for combining words in order to convey particular meanings. As you can see from Table 8.2, the types of things children talk about during this two-word utterance period are not very different from the things they focused on during the earlier, single-word utterance period. Of course, children can be more precise once they begin to combine words. For example, "gone" conveys the idea that the child has noted the disappearance of something. The two-word utterance "shoe gone" tells us what it is that disappeared.

Children's two-word utterance usage shows the same sensitivity to what can be assumed from the context as did the earlier single-word utterance usage. At this stage, however, this sensitivity is usually reflected by stress or emphasis.

Several common types of two-word combinations used by young children are shown in Table 8.2. Other examples are presented by Bloom (1970), Bowerman (1973), and Brown (1973).

TABLE 8.2
Some Examples of Young Children's Two-Word Utterances.

Meaning	Example	Context
Pointing out or naming an object	that kitty	Child points to a picture of a cat.
Referring to another instance of an object or event	more fence	Child pulls out a section of a toy fence from a toy box after already having found two sections.
Specifying individual having privileged acces to object	Toddy bed	Child points to "litter box" used by the pet kitten, Toddy.
Counting or qualifying an object	big ring	Child holds up a loop earring he found on the floor.
Referring to movement where the goal of movement was a change in the location of the object	put box	Child puts a hand puppet into a shoe box.
Referring to movement by the actor	Nikki fall down	Child slips off her chair onto floor.
Referring to an object and its location, where no movement was involved	clock window	Child points to a wristwatch on the window ledge.
Specifying attention to an object or event	see doggie	Child watching a dog out the window.

For example, if the child were asked "Where's Bo?" he might say "Bo SCHOOL," with emphasis on the second word. However, if the question was "Who's at school?" the child might use a different pattern of emphasis, "BO school" (Wieman, 1976).

Two to Two and One-Half Years

As children approach their second birthday, they begin to enter into a different period of cognitive development, the preoperational period (Piaget, 1963). In this period, the child shows a tendency to find solutions to problems by mental means, rather than by acting first. For example, the child's searching behaviors appear to be thought out and are no longer dictated solely by where an object may have been last seen. The child begins to develop the ability to use symbols. The child is not dependent on things being immediately present, because he can create a mental substitute for them.

During this same stage, children often show a spurt in linguistic development. In a matter of months, they move from producing single- and two-word utterances to three- and four-word utterances. Many of these three- and four-word utterances are grammatically simple, affirmative, declarative sentences formed by combining content words such as nouns, verbs, and adjectives. Utterances such as "Put cup table," "Daddy want more milk," and "Mommy get coat" are common. However, on occasion, children produce utterances containing negatives, and questions are sometimes used. Utterances with negatives are initially produced with the negative word beginning the utterance, as in "No want that." When negatives appear in the proper position in the sentence, they often take a simplified form, as in "I no like that" and "Baby don't go now" (Klima & Bellugi, 1966). The questions used by children at this point in development are usually one of two types—they either request a yes or no answer or some piece of information. Yes-no questions are typically missing certain words that ordinarily indicate that a question is being asked, such as "You take me home?" for "Will you take me home?" Questions that request information are usually limited to a few forms that the child has probably heard a number of times. These questions serve important communicative functions for the child. Perhaps the most frequent are "What's that?" and "Where going?" (Klima & Bellugi, 1966).

At this age children are learning strategies for participating in conversations with those around them. Keenan (1974) has shed considerable light on the nature of these strategies. A first step in participating in dialogue, according to Keenan, is to learn when and how to take part in conversational turn taking. Initially, children seem to take their conversational turn by using only words used in the utterance which has just been spoken by the other person. For example, if the child's older sister said "Hey, kitty spilled the milk!" the child might respond with "Kitty spill milk." On occasion, the child may add a word, or change the intonation pattern, still preserving the basic meaning of the partner's initial utterance. For example, the child's response might have been "Naughty kitty spill milk" or "Kitty spill MILK." Before long, the child begins to show a greater capacity to add to the substance of the conversation. This is usually seen when he replaces one of the words in the initial utterance with another. For example, the child might respond to an utterance such as "Here's my new hat" with "Pretty hat."

Two and One-Half to Four Years

By approximately 2½ years of age, children's speech is no longer limited to content words. Function words such as "in" and "on" and suffixes such as *-ing* begin to emerge. Thus, the child may produce utterances such as "Oscar playing in water" where once he had said them as "Oscar play water." Within a few months, the child begins to use the articles "the" and "a," the possessive marker *-s,* and the past tense ending *-ed.* Not long after the child reaches the age of 3 years, considerable use of the verb "to be" is seen, as a main verb ("Chris is big") and as an auxiliary ("The bus is coming") (Brown, 1973; deVilliers & deVilliers, 1973). By this age the child uses a number of common pronouns, uses a greater variety of question forms, and may begin using the conjunction "and." Although short utterances may still be produced at this age, six- and seven-word utterances are not uncommon. The child's vocabulary at this point has grown to nearly 900 words.

The child's conversational abilities also become more sophisticated. For example, children of this age can not only take their conversational turn, but can use this turn to indicate to the partner that his or her initial utterance needs modification (Garvey, 1977). The use of "What?" in this role is common. If he didn't hear the utterance clearly, the child might say "What?" with rising intonation, indicating that the utterance should be repeated. If he heard the utterance, but wanted more details, "What?" might be produced with falling intonation.

> Older sister: I've got a surprise for you!
> Child: What? ↑
> Older sister: I've got a surprise for you.
> Child: What? ↓
> Older sister: A deadly bug!

Dore (1977) provides a number of examples of the various functions served by children's utterances.

Actually, the utterances produced by a 3-year-old can serve a variety of communicative functions. For example, in addition to serving declaring, requesting, and questioning functions, these children's utterances may serve functions of protesting, agreeing, joking, or qualifying.

It would be perfectly logical to assume that, when a child produces an appropriate, meaningful, and grammatical utterance, he or she has an understanding of that utterance comparable to that of an adult saying the same thing. However, this may not be the case, as the work of Chapman (1978) indicates. For example, 3-year-olds may use appropriate grammatical constructions when they describe the things that go on around them. However, their interpretation of utterances spoken to them is based as much on their knowledge of the world as it is on the grammatical construction being used. For example, when told "Put the block under the box," the child may put the block in the box—because blocks usually go inside boxes. A similar type of comprehension strategy is seen when the child answers questions. The answer "to the store" may be given whether the question is "When are we going?" "Why are we going?" or "Where are we going?"

Four to Five Years

When children reach 4 years of age, new milestones are reached. The child's average sentence length is five words, vocabulary exceeds 1,500 words, and new grammatical features appear. These include auxiliary verbs such as "can" and "may," reflexive pronouns such as "myself" and "yourself," pronouns such as "behind" and "beside," and conjunctions such as "but" and "if." The child's sentence constructions show greater complexity as well. Well-formed questions involving "when," "how," and "why" (for example, "How did you do that?") are the rule rather than the exception. Sentences with infinitives are used, as in "Debbie likes to tease me."

Children of this age also show new social skills. Perhaps the most notable of these is the child's emerging ability to take the listener's perspective or linguistic abilities into account. For example, 4-year-olds show a tendency to use shorter utterances, to speak more frequently in the present tense, and to use shorter utterances more frequently when talking to a baby or a doll than when speaking to their mothers (Sachs & Devin, 1976; Shatz & Gelman, 1973). This ability to modify speech style serves as the first indication that the child is moving beyond a strictly egocentric level of functioning. In fact, prior to studies of children's ability to adapt their speech style to the listener, it was commonly believed that egocentricity continued until children reached approximately age 7.

The strategies children use to interpret what is said to them also change somewhat by the time they pass their fourth birthday. One such strategy is seen when children interpret the meaning of a sentence strictly on the basis of its word order (Chapman, 1978). For example, children at this age interpret the two sentences "Walter is licked by the dog" and "Walter licks the dog" as if they had the same meaning, because the same words precede and follow the verb ("Walter" and "dog," respectively) in both sentences. In a short time, children will abondon this strategy in favor of a more adult-like interpretation of these sentences.

One of the most notable achievements during this stage is the ability to judge the suitability of utterances spoken by others. It appears to be one thing to comprehend an utterance and quite another to judge it as appropriate or not. For example, 3-year-olds who can comprehend and produce utterances such as "Get the block" have difficulty judging such utterances as appropriate while judging utterances such as "Block the get" as inappropriate (deVilliers & deVilliers, 1974). It is not until just past 4 years of age when children make this kind of judgment more consistently. Evidently, it is not until about this age that children learn to attend to the superficial form of speech independent of its meaning.

TYPES OF LANGUAGE DISORDERS

To many specialists in communication disorders, the term *language disordered children* calls to mind a particular group of children, but in fact many different types of children may have difficulties acquiring language. These include children with "specific language impairment," mentally retarded children, children with autistic-like characteristics, children with acquired aphasia, and hearing impaired children. Some of these groups of children have been the focus of scientific investigation and discussion for many years, while others have only recently been studied. For example, the earliest scientific journals included descriptions of mentally retarded children. Descriptions of children with specific language impairment and children with acquired aphasia did not appear until the 1800s. Reports of autistic children did not seem to appear until this century. The literature on each of these groups of children reveals a common trend. The earliest writings provided a general description of the disorder. Scientific articles and books soon followed, offering possible explanations for these disorders. Only in the last 20 years has there been a concerted effort to describe the language characteristics of each of these groups of children.

For discussion of children with hearing impairment, see chapter 10. Acquired aphasia, which occurs much more frequently in adults than in children, is covered in chapter 14.

The recent focus on language can be attributed in large measure to advances made in linguistics and the study of normal child language development. Advances in linguistics provided a methodology for looking at the language of these handicapped children, and the study of normal development provided us with an idea of what the most important characteristics of language in children might be. It is not difficult to find evidence of these influences. As the major focus of linguistics and the study of normal child language development has shifted, within a short time a similar shift has been seen in the characteristics of handicapped children's language that have received the greatest research attention. For example, in the past 20 years, there has been a shift from looking at the syntactic structures in children's utterances, to the types of meanings conveyed by these structures, to how these meanings and structures are put to use in a social context. This syntactic-to-semantic-to-pragmatic trend is now evident as well in the literature on language disordered children.

There are a few important differences in the language characteristics shown by the various groups of language disordered children. Because these differences suggest different treatment approaches for these children, we will discuss them here. However, remember that a number of the characteristics seen in one group can be seen in the other groups as well. In addition, the children in any one of these groups may differ from one another in certain ways. Therefore, we cannot assume that there is a single language pattern exhibited by, say, mentally retarded children, or that the language patterns of these children are unique to children with intellectual deficits.

Children with Specific Language Impairment

Children with specific language impairment have problems that seem, at least on first impression, to be confined to the area of language. (As we will see, this picture sometimes changes when more detailed testing is performed.) These children tend to perform within normal limits on tests of nonverbal intelligence. Their hearing is found to be adequate, and, except for their frustration in communicating, their emotional development seems unremarkable. Children with specific language impairment have been given various clinical labels, such as *language delayed, language deviant, language impaired, developmentally aphasic,* and *language disordered.* Some of these terms reflect a particular point of view about the nature of these children's linguistic difficulties. For instance, the label *language deviant* is sometimes used to suggest that the language of these children is somewhat different from that of younger, normally developing children. The label *developmentally apha-*

Chapter 9 discusses the many labels applied to these children when they reach school.

TABLE 8.3

Pattern of Development Shown by a Typical Language Impaired Child and a Normally Developing Child.

Child with Specific Language Impairment			Normally Developing Child		
Age	**Attainment**	**Example**	**Age**	**Attainment**	**Example**
27 months	First words	this, mama, bye bye, doggie	13 months	First words	here, mama, bye bye, kitty
38 months	50-word vocabulary		17 months	50-word vocabulary	
40 months	First two-word combinations	this doggie more apple this mama more play	18 months	First two-word combinations	more juice here ball more T.V. here kitty
48 months	Later two-word combinations	Mimi purse Daddy coat block chair dolly table	22 months	Later two-word combinations	Andy shoe Mommy ring cup floor keys chair
52 months	Mean sentence length of 2.00 words		24 months	Mean sentence length of 2.00 words	
55 months	First appearance of -ing	Mommy eating		First appearance of -ing	Andy sleeping
63 months	Mean sentence length of 3.10 words		30 months	Mean sentence length 3.10 words	
66 months	First appearance of "is"	The doggie's mad		First appearance of "is"	My car's gone!
73 months	Mean sentence length of 4.10 words		37 months	Mean sentence length 4.10 words	
79 months	Mean sentence length of 4.50 words			First appearance of indirect requests	Can I have some cookies?
	First appearance of indirect requests	Can I get the ball?	40 months	Mean sentence length of 4.50 words	

sic is typically used to suggest that the language problems are related to a neurological problem. But as we will see, the evidence for these points of view is not always strong. Therefore, we should not assume that children given these different clinical labels are necessarily quite different from one another.

The most notable feature of these children's language is that the large majority of the linguistic features reflected in their speech are slow to emerge and to develop. According to a recent review of the literature (Leonard, 1979), the particular linguistic features used by these children do not seem to differ from those seen in younger, normal children. However, because the linguistic features may differ from one another in their degree of delay, the relationship among these features in the speech of the child with specific language impairment may not always be the same as it is in normally developing children.

These points may become clearer if you examine the examples provided in Table 8.3.

We can see from Table 8.3 that linguistic features tend to be slower in emergence and development in language impaired children. For example, our sample language impaired child acquired her first words at a much later age than is seen in normal development. Similarly, two-word utterances and the use of forms such as *-ing* and *-s* were later to emerge than expected. Despite their late appearance, however, the features are not unlike those seen in a normal child's speech. The types of first words acquired are similar, and the meanings reflected in the two-word combinations are essentially the same. In addition, meanings such as recurrence (as in "more apple") precede those such as possession (as in "Mimi purse") in both children. Also, in both children, suffixes such as *-ing* appear before function words such as "is." However, the children are different in the relationships among these linguistic features in their speech. The suffix *-ing* shows up in the speech of the normal child at a time when her mean sentence length is 2.00 words. When the language impaired child has achieved the same mean sentence length, she does not yet use *-ing.* To cite another example, the normal child shows the ability to use question forms as an indirect request at a point when her mean sentence length is 4.10 words. However, the language impaired child appears to require a mean sentence length of 4.50 words before she uses indirect requests.

Mentally Retarded Children

Children described as *mentally retarded* are diagnosed according to two characteristics: (*a*) subaverage overall intellectual functioning and (*b*) personal independence and social responsibility that are below the level expected for the child's age and cultural group. However, language development, too, poses a problem for these children. Much of what we have said about the speech of children with specific language impairment can also be said about the speech of mentally retarded children. These children are slow to acquire most linguistic features, although the features themselves are usually the same as those seen in normal children (see, for example, Coggins, 1979). As with language impaired children, mentally retarded children may show more delay with certain features than others, resulting in a somewhat different relationship among these features than is typically seen in children who have no pronounced language-learning difficulties.

In mentally retarded children, the degree of language delay may depend in part on the severity of their overall developmental disability. Some children, for example, do not begin to use words until the age of 5; others may develop only through training programs allowing them to communicate by pointing to specially designed symbols; still others may be so severely involved as never to develop the ability to communicate. We do not yet know whether retarded children—particularly severely and profoundly retarded—learn in the same ways as normally developing children.

We do know, however, that the older a mentally retarded child is before he acquires a particular linguistic feature or ability, the less likely it is that his use of the feature or ability will resemble that of a younger, normal child. This factor of chronological age seems to be important for the study of the language of mentally retarded children (Greenwald & Leonard, 1979). It appears that the older the age of the child, the more likely he will acquire a linguistic feature by rote learning, and the less likely he will be to extend this feature in novel but appropriate ways. For example, children who learn the plural suffix -s at a late age may be more likely to try to learn which individual words take this suffix rather than to apply the suffix to a number of words as a general rule (Lovell & Bradbury, 1967). Thus, when faced with a nonsense word task such as "Look, here's a meeb. Oh, here comes another meeb. Now there are two _____," an older child may not be likely to apply the plural suffix.

Autistic Children

Language disorders are also prevalent in children described as autistic. *Autism* is a condition that we do not understand very well. It is defined according to the presence or absence of particular behaviors in the child. Among these are a failure to develop normal responsivity to other persons, a failure to use objects appropriately, and a generalized overreaction to certain sensory stimuli or a notable lack of response to other sensory stimuli. Another key ingredient in the definition of autism is the failure to develop normal verbal and nonverbal communication behaviors. Much of this atypical development rests in the fact that autistic children are slow to acquire communication skills. In this respect, they are similar to other language disordered children. However (as noted in a recent review by Baltaxe and Simmons, in press), several characteristics of their linguistic functioning set them apart from mentally retarded children and children with specific language impairment. These children often show high frequency of unsolicited imitative verbal behavior, called *echolalia*. Other groups of children, including normally developing children, show spontaneous imitations of the speech of others. But in the case of children with autistic-like characteristics, the imitations seem less intentional and communicative. For example, normal children are more likely to imitate new, unfamiliar words than familiar ones. When familiar words are imitated, they sometimes serve an acknowledgement function, much as an older child or adult might use "yes."

> Mother: Do you want some juice now?
> Child: Juice.

On the other hand, imitations like the following one are often observed in autistic children.

> Mother: Hi, Bobby.
> Bobby: Hi, Bobby.

Other characteristics reported in these children include confusions with pronoun distinctions such as "I" and "you," and a pronounced tendency to speak in a near-monotone. Another feature of autistic children's language that seems different from other groups of children is that their articulation skills, while not at age level, may often exceed their abilities in vocabulary, sentence structure, and social use of language. This is rarely the case with mentally retarded children or children with specific language impairment.

Children with Acquired Aphasia

The language disordered children described above have in common the fact that their language-learning difficulties are apparent from an early age. However, other children, after developing normally during the first years of life, lose their ability to function linguistically. This loss in linguistic ability is usually the result of some demonstrable brain damage arising from serious illness or trauma to the head. The most common term for this condition is *acquired aphasia*. According to Lenneberg (1967), if damage is confined to a single hemisphere of the brain and occurs before the age of 9 years, the child will often regain the lost abilities and will continue to develop normally thereafter. In more serious cases, residual problems may persist.

More detail on characteristics and treatment of aphasia appears in the chapter on adult aphasia, chapter 14.

The symptoms of the child's language difficulties depend upon the age at which the injury took place. The child who suffers injury before 3 years of age will often become temporarily mute and will show a general unresponsiveness to the speech of others. Significant and often rapid improvement in linguistic ability then occurs, with the child seemingly proceeding through the major stages of language development seen in children acquiring language for the first time.

In children suffering from injury after the age of 3, the symptoms are usually different. Verbal output and understanding are diminished but not absent altogether. However, word-finding problems may be seen, where the child seems unable to retrieve and say a word that he had used only moments before. For these children, recovery is somewhat slower, and residual problems are likely to be present in later years.

CAUSES AND CORRELATES OF CHILDHOOD LANGUAGE DISORDERS

As we have seen with other types of communication disorders, through the years there have been a number of theories of the causes of language disorders in children. Again, rather strong evidence is required before a factor or condition can be regarded as a cause of a language problem. In fact, only a few factors once thought to cause language disorders are presently viewed as likely or possible causes. More often, research has shown that the factors in question are related to language disorders in one or several groups of children, but not to the extent that they could be considered causes of the problem. In some instances, they, like the language deficits themselves, may be part of a more general problem. For the most part, the search for causes is a theoretical question.

Those factors most frequently associated with specific language impairment include (*a*) the perceptual ability of language impaired children, (*b*) their cognitive development, (*c*) their interaction with other people, and (*d*) brain damage. The perceptual ability that has recently received the greatest amount of investigative attention is the ability to discriminate among auditory signals that contain rapid acoustic changes (Tallal & Stark, 1980). This ability is necessary in order for us to perceive the difference between, say, the syllables "ba" and "da." A number of children with specific language impairment perform poorly on tasks in which they are required to discriminate between syllables like these. Quite possibly, their difficulties on these tasks are linked in some way to their difficulties with language. However, it does not seem likely that these difficulties are *causing* the language problems. Some of the children who perform poorly on these discrimination tasks have little difficulty using /b/ and /d/ appropriately in their speech. Some of the speech sounds with which they do have difficulty, however, such as /s/, are not easily characterized as sounds involving rapid acoustic changes.

It may seem paradoxical that cognitive ability has been implicated as a factor involved in specific language impairment. After all, children with this problem often perform within normal limits on nonverbal intelligence tests. Yet it is clear that there are an enormous number of higher order abilities that might be considered in our notion of a child's "intelligence." Children with specific language impairment may seem stronger in some of these abilities than others. Their relative strengths usully fall in areas such as using visual cues to match shapes and colors and to complete pictures—abilities assessed in several commonly used nonverbal intelligence tests. Some of their weaknesses can be seen on cognitive tasks designed around the theoretical framework developed by Piaget. For example, children with specific languge impairment have been found to have difficulties substituting one object for another in play, such as using a pencil as a fork to "feed" a doll. Another task proving troublesome is one in which the children have to blindly feel a geometric shape and then pick out the shape that they held on the basis of its visual form (Johnston, in press).

Findings ilke these suggest that the label *specific language impairment* may be misleading; these children's problems may not be confined to language. Some investigators have proposed that these difficulties with language may actually be due to certain types of cognitive deficits that cut across both nonlinguistic and linguistic skills. At this point, however, the nature of these deficits has not been described in adequate detail. Unless or until details have been provided, it would be premature to assume that the language difficulties of these children are other than linguistically based.

A third factor commonly associated with specific language impairment is the environment of the child, more specifically the nature of the interactions between the child and other family members, and the nature of their linguistic input. Through the years, a number of authors have raised the possibility that the linguistic environment of children with specific language impairment is deprived or, alternatively, that the parents of these children tend to talk for the children. These suspicions have been raised mainly because other possible causes, such as biological, intellectual, and emotional factors, have not proven to be valid. However, it has only been in recent years that systematic study of these children's environments has been conducted. The results of these studies tend to show that the environment of language impaired children is more directive and controlling than that of normal children of the same age. However, the direction of influence has not been clear. For example, although the mothers of the language impaired children studied engaged in fewer play and language activities with their children than did the mothers of the normal children, they also reported that their efforts in this direction had been consistently rebuffed by the children. Thus, the reluctance to interact seemed reciprocal, and we cannot assume that the mothers of language impaired children act differently from mothers in general.

See, for example, Wulbert, Inglis, Kriegsmann, and Mills, 1975.

These studies dealt with home environments that in most respects did not seem extraordinary. However, not all studies have focused on "typical" situations. During the early 1970s an unfortunate case of extreme parental neglect was reported in the literature, which served as a "natural" experiment on the importance of the environment for language development. Curtiss (1977) presents a detailed description of the child involved. From the age of 20 months to 13½ years, this child was principally kept alone in a single room, often harnessed to a chair by day and caged in a crib by night. She received little exposure to language. When the child was finally discovered and removed from her inhuman circumstances, she produced no speech and understood only a few words. Although medical records for this child at age 12 to 18 months suggest the possibility of problems in other aspects of development, it seems clear that the child's enforced isolation was a major factor in her failure to develop language. Once placed in a normal environment and provided with a great deal of language stimulation, she made significant gains in linguistic ability. Unfortunately, this case, while showing the benefits of language stimulation, does not shed much light on the relationship between what we might call "normally deprived environments" and language difficulties.

A number of authors have proposed that the difficulties experienced by children with specific language impairment are a consequence of brain damage. Damage to both hemispheres of the brain is often postulated, since the language development of these children is much slower than that of children suffering from acquired aphasia.

See, for example, Benton, 1964.

Children for whom there is the most clear-cut evidence of brain damage are those whose problems involve motor and sensory as well as language deficits. For children whose difficulties seem to rest principally in language, however, the evidence for brain damage is not particularly convincing. This may change with the advent of recent technological advances that let us assess brain functioning more precisely. However, there have been only a few cases reported in the literature where brain damage seems clearly implicated. In fact, in what may be the only case of language impairment subjected to examination after the death of the child, bilateral damage to the temporal lobes of the brain was found (Landau, Goldstein, & Kleffner, 1960).

As we noted earlier, the label *mental retardation* is reserved for children who perform significantly below their age level in intellectual functioning and personal independence and social functioning. The question of biological versus environmental causes here is quite controversial. In a number of children, the cause of mental retardation is suspected to be a chromosomal abnormality; for others, the suspected cause is brain injury suffered prenatally or during birth; for others, suspicions center on genetic inheritance. Among other medical factors cited by the American Association on Mental Deficiency are infections and intoxication, disorders of metabolism, prematurity, and gestational disorders (Grossman, 1977). These biological causes are usually associated with more severe retardation. In most other cases, particularly cases of mild retardation, the exact cause is unknown. However, borderline mental retardation has often been attributed to cultural and familial patterns. The majority of these children come from "culturally deprived or different backgrounds" (Dunn, 1968, 1980). They may be the victims of nutritional deficits or inadequate cultural and social stimulation (Brolin, 1976; Payne & Patton, 1981). The condition may be functional and reversible with adequate stimulation, or it may be permanent. It is also possible that mild retardation has a hereditary basis. A large-scale study of familial factors in mental ability in 1,490 families (close to 6,000 people) supports this view (DeFries, Ashton, Johnson, Kuse, McClearn, Mi, Rashad, Vanderberg, & Wilson, 1976).

Whatever the cause of the child's mental retardation, the fact that he or she is mentally retarded makes it very easy to conclude that the child's linguistic deficit is caused by the retardation. Yet the matter is not so simple. Many mentally retarded children's skills in language are considerably more depressed than their skills in areas such as motor, perceptual, and even intellectual development. Therefore, the statement that a mentally retarded child's deficits can be explained by the retardation is quite incorrect. Unfortunately, research has not yet uncovered explanations for why mentally retarded children's linguistic skills are often so low. Early studies of children whose level of functioning was low enough to lead to institutionalization showed that these children received only limited language stimulation. There is also some evidence that parents of some subgroups of mentally retarded children do not respond to their children in quite the same way as parents of normally developing children. However, as with the studies of children with specific language impairment, it is not clear that the parents' behavior is not simply a reaction to the lack of responsiveness of the child.

The cause of the language deficits exhibited by autistic children is also a mystery. Part of the problem is that we do not understand the root of their difficulty in relating to their environment. This question has provoked considerable controversy, and possible explanations have ranged from a reluctance to form interpersonal relationships to a malfunctioning of the child's neurophysiological system. To complicate matters further, many autistic children meet the standard criteria of mental retardation. The most promising studies to date suggest that autistic-like children may have an impairment in functioning of the left hemisphere of the brain. As the left hemisphere is usually thought to play a greater role in the processing of speech, this impairment may relate to these children's linguistic difficulty. However, at this point, this explanation must be regarded as sophisticated guesswork. Clearly, more research is needed.

The likely cause of acquired aphasia in children is, of course, much clearer than is the case for most other childhood language disorders. The fact that children with acquired aphasia were functioning normally prior to cerebral damage makes it probable that the injury is largely responsible for the ensuing language impairment. However, to date, we have not been able to find a close correspondence between a particular type or location of injury and a particular type of language deficit. Instead, a variety of injuries often lead to the same outcome—a mute child with comprehension difficulties. The reasons for this are not clear.

ASSESSMENT OF CHILDREN'S LINGUISTIC SKILLS

Testing

Before we say that a child has a language disorder, we must conduct a thorough examination of the child's linguistic skills. Usually two forms of assessment are used in the examination process. One form is the norm-referenced standardized test. Standardized language tests are available for both screening and diagnosis. Both types of standardized tests usually include normative data which indicate how children of various ages might be expected to perform on the test. Screening tests typically employ "cut-off" scores. If a child's perform-ance falls below the cut-off for his or her chronological age, further testing is warranted. Diagnostic tests usually provide percentile levels for each age level. Children who perform at a low percentile level, such as the 10th percentile, are generally suspected of having difficulties with the linguistic skills in question.

Certain other tests are "standardized" in the sense that they include items that should be passed by children at designated age levels, according to the research findings of the test developer or others. Percentiles are usually not available for these tests. Instead, the speech-language pathologist reports the specific items or developmental level of the items passed by the child. These tests might be called *descriptive.*

The tests available to speech-language pathologists for use with young children vary widely in terms of the specific dimensions of language tested, the theory behind the development of the tests, and importantly, how well they were standardized. A diagnostic test that is poorly standardized may provide less useful information than a well-designed screening or descriptive test.

Darley (1979) pro-vides a critical review of a number of tests for young children.

The second form of assessment used is the nonstandardized probe. Gen-erally, these probes are individually selected or devised for each child. They are often criterion-referenced. They are designed to examine some specific linguistic skill in considerable detail. Unlike the standardized test, no infor-mation is available concerning how a child of a particular age might be ex-pected to perform on the probe. The speech-language pathologist must instead rely on his or her knowledge of normal language development. The major contribution of nonstandardized probes is that they provide consider-ably more detail concerning the consistency of a child's problem with the linguistic feature and the contexts in which the problem is most notable (Leon-ard, Prutting, Perozzi, & Berkley, 1978). Another valuable aspect of nonstan-dardized probes is that they permit the speech-language pathologist to assess a number of pragmatic skills (for instance, conversational turn taking, under-standing indirect requests such as "Can you open the door?") that are not included in standardized tests.

Both standardized tests and nonstandardized probes use many of the same types of tasks. These tasks can be divided into receptive tasks, involving com-prehension, and expressive tasks, involving production.

Receptive Tasks

The most common form of receptive task involves identification or recogni-tion. In this task, the examiner produces a word or sentence and the child chooses the picture (from several alternatives) that represents an appropriate match for that picture. For example, the speech-language pathologist may place several pictures depicting actions in front of the child and say "Show me 'running.'" Some common tests which use this task are the *Test for Auditory Comprehension of Language* (Carrow, 1973) and the *Peabody Picture Vocabulary Test* (Dunn, 1965/1980). These tasks are especially useful in assessing lexicon and morphology.

Another receptive task is acting out. Typically, this task uses toys or objects that the child can manipulate. The examiner produces a sentence, and the child acts on the objects in a manner consistent with the sentence. For example, the speech-language pathologist might place a doll and a toy car in front of the child and say "Put the baby behind the car." The *Vocabulary Comprehension Scale* (Bangs, 1975) is an example of a test that uses an acting-out task. Acting-out can be used to assess vocabulary, morphology, syntax, and semantics.

The most difficult of the receptive tasks is the judgment task. Judgment tasks require the child to make a formal judgment of the suitabiilty of a word or sentence. A sentence is produced by the examiner, and the child is asked whether it was "right" or "wrong" or "silly" or "O.K." For example, the examiner might ask "Is this 'silly' or 'O.K.'—The is shining sun?" This task can be seen in several items of the *Bankson Language Screening Test* (Bankson, 1977). Again, it can be used to assess lexicon, morphology, syntax, and semantics.

It is essential that the speech-language pathologist be aware of the limitations involved in each of these tasks. The identification task allows the possibility that a child will appear to comprehend when actually his or her identification of the appropriate picture is based on a lucky guess. A child might also make a correct response on this test not because he or she knows the word or sentence, but because he knows enough about the alternative pictures to rule them out as possible selections. (Many of us have used a similar strategy when faced with multiple-choice tests.) Finally, identification tasks test a relatively superficial form of comprehension, that of recognition. Probably we have all had the experience of forgetting the melody or lyrics of a song that, when played for us, we recognize as the song in question. A similar process seems to be involved in identification tasks.

The chief precaution to take when administering an acting-out task is to insure that the child is not using a strategy that does not require full understanding of the material being presented. For example, young children may respond correctly to the sentence "The truck is pushing the car" not because they fully comprehend the sentence, but because their knowledge of the real world suggests that it is more likely for a truck to push a car than vice versa.

The major limitation of the judgment task is that it often proves too difficult for children under the age of 4 years. The apparent reason is that this task requires the child to think about the form of a word or sentence independent of its meaning. For example, young children seem to attend to the fact that two sentences such as "The boy runs down the street" and "The boy run down the street" have the same meaning. Not until they reach at least age 4 do they attend to the fact that one of these sentences is not constructed as well as it might be.

Expressive Tasks

One of the most commonly used tasks of linguistic expression is the elicited imitation task. In this task, the examiner produces a sentence, and the child is asked to repeat it. The assumption behind this task is that if a child does not use a particular linguistic feature properly, he or she is unlikely to use it in imitation—particularly if no undue attention is placed on the feature when it is presented by the speech-language pathologist. For example, a child who does not ordinarily use the article "the" in everyday speech is likely to imitate the sentence "Daddy put the ball on the table" as "Daddy put ball on table." The *Stephens Oral Language Screening Test* (Stephens, 1977) is one of several tests that employ elicited imitation. This task is helpful for assessing morphology, syntax, and semantics.

A somewhat similar procedure, used to assess the same skills, is the delayed imitation task. In this task, the child's response is further removed in time from the speech-language pathologist's production than is true for the elicited imitation task. Assume, for example, that a child's use of the plural *-s* is in question. The examiner might place two pictures in front of the child and say "The man sees the boy," "The man sees the boys"; then, pointing to one of the pictures, "Which one is this?" This task is used in the *Northwestern Syntax Screening Test* (Lee, 1971).

The carrier phrase task is another task of linguistic expression. A portion of a sentence is spoken by the examiner, and the child is asked to complete it. For instance, a child's use of the pronoun "she" might be tested by presenting three pictures of a particular girl performing different activities. The speech-language pathologist might describe the first two pictures for the child, and have the child describe the third. The following sequence might set the occasion for the child's use of a response that includes "she": "Look, here the girl is riding a bike, and here the girl is eating a cookie, and here (pointing to a picture of the girl throwing a ball) _____." This task can be seen, for example, in one of the subtests of the *Test of Language Development* (Newcomer & Hammill, 1977). It is especially useful in assessing morphology and syntax.

An expressive task that has certain features in common with the carrier phrase task is the parallel sentence production task. Typically, two pictures are placed in front of the child. The speech-language pathologist describes the first picture using a particular sentence pattern, and the child is asked to describe the second picture. It is assumed that the pattern used in the examiner's sentence will influence the type of sentence attempted by the child. For example, if a picture of a large ball and a picture of a small ball were used, the following interchange might be expected.

> Examiner: I'm going to talk about this picture (points to picture), and then you talk about that picture (points to other picture). Ready? (Points to first picture.) This is a big ball.
>
> Child: (Points to second picture.) This is a little ball.

The parallel sentence production task is quite useful in testing morphological and syntactic features that children might not otherwise attempt frequently.

A child's expressive language is often assessed by examining a sample of his or her spontaneous speech. If the child's utterances are to be truly spontaneous, of course, nothing in the questions or instructions should dictate how the child should respond. However, in order to increase the likelihood that the child will provide a sufficient number of utterances, or a sufficient number of utterances of a certain type, open-ended questions or requests are often presented (for example, "Tell me about this"). Thus, the utterances the child produces during these sampling situations are evoked or influenced to some degree by the speech-language pathologist. Collecting a sample of a child's speech is usually more time consuming than giving any one test of language. However, several studies have indicated that this inconvenience is offset by the fact that speech samples often yield more information about a child's linguistic skills than language tests. A portion of a speech sample obtained from a young child is presented in Table 8.4, along with examples of how the child's utterances might be analyzed for syntactic structure according to an adaptation of one of the more commonly used systems of analysis, *Language Sampling, Analysis, and Training* (Tyack & Gottsleben, 1974). If the speech-language pathologist sets up certain role-playing situations, spontaneous speech samples may help him assess the child's pragmatic skills.

TABLE 8.4
A Portion of a Speech Sample, Analyzed According to Syntactic Structure.

Child's Utterances	Gloss	Syntactic Description
1. That man buying gum.	That man is buying gum.	Dem + N + ~~Aux~~ + V + ing + N
2. I got a car.	I have a car.	Pro + V + Art + N
3. My mommy push the door.	My mommy pushed the door.	Poss + N + V + ~~Past~~ + Art + N
4. Santa Claus fat.	Santa Claus is fat.	N + ~~Cop~~ + Adj
5. Him not want ball.	He doesn't want the ball.	Pro* + Neg* + V + ~~Art~~ + N
6. Where the girl going?	Where is the girl going?	Wh + ~~Aux~~ + Art + N + V + ing
7. Her on big table!	She is on the big table.	Pro* + ~~Cop~~ + Prep + ~~Art~~ + Adj + N
⋮		
100. Gimme two car.	Give me two cars.	V + Pro + Quan + N + ~~Plural~~

Features in Error	Frequency Substituted	Frequency Omitted	Frequency Correct
Aux	4	12	5
Past	0	8	1
⋮			
Neg	5	0	3
Pro	10	0	9

Forms in Error	Frequency Substituted	Frequency Omitted	Frequency Correct
Aux—is	0	8	5
Aux—are	4	4	0
⋮			
Pro—her	3	0	1
Pro—them	1	0	1
Pro—him	6	0	7

Forms in Error	Construction—Correct (Frequency)	Construction—Error (Frequency)
Aux—is	N + Aux + V + ing (3) Art + N + Aux + V + ing (1) N + Aux + V + ing + Art + N (1)	Dem + N + Aux + V + ing + N (1) Wh + Aux + Art + N + V + ing (3) N + Aux + V + ing + Art + N (1) N + Aux + V + ing + Prep + Art + N (1) Art + N + Aux + V + ing + Art + N (1) Art + Adj + N + Aux + V + ing + Pro (1)
⋮		
Pro—him	N + V + Past + Pro (2) Dem + Cop + Pro (2) N + V + Pro + Art + N (2) Art + N + Aux + V + ing + Pro (1)	Pro + V + Art + N (2) Pro + Cop + Adj (1) Pro + V + Past (1) Pro + Neg + V + Art + N (1) Pro + Cop + Prep + Art + Adj + N (1)

Adj = Adjective	Dem = Demonstrative	Quan = Quantifier	
Art = Article	N = Noun	V = Verb	
Aux = Auxiliary	Poss = Possessive	Wh = "*Wh*-" word	
Cop = Copula	Pro = Pronoun		

As with receptive tasks, there are limitations to the use of expressive tasks. One risk involved in the use of imitation is that the child may have good auditory memory skills and repeat a sentence with greater accuracy than might be expected given his or her spontaneous speech characteristics. Carrier phrase tasks usually require only a one- or two-word response from the child. Therefore, even if a child produces a plural or past tense ending correctly, we do not know whether he can do so in a complete sentence. The greatest limitation of a spontaneous speech sample is that it may not include a number of linguistic features that infrequently occur. For example, the child may not attempt sentences in the passive voice such as "The car was hit by the train" or words that require the plural -*es* such as "dishes" in the speech sample. Yet the child might have difficulties with these linguistic features.

The Assessment Process

An example might be helpful in illustrating the assessment of a child who is suspected of having linguistic difficulties. Assume that a 4-year-old child is brought to a speech-language clinic with the parental complaint that he "doesn't seem to understand when we ask him to do things." Initial contact with the child in an informal rapport-building play activity suggests that the child's productions are limited to single- and two-word utterances. Because this level of linguistic expression is markedly delayed relative to his age, attention turns to whether or not this expressive problem might be due to limitations in comprehension.

After we have determined that the child's hearing sensitivity, based on audiometric testing, is within normal limits, we might give him a standardized comprehension test that includes both word comprehension and sentence comprehension. Assume that the child is found to perform slightly below average for his age level on the word comprehension section, and well below age level on the section dealing with sentence comprehension. Noting that the sentences on which the child had the greatest difficulty were not only the most grammatically complex but also the longest, we might administer another standardized comprehension test, one that tests the child's comprehension of increasingly longer sentences that have only limited grammatical complexity. Let us assume that on this test the child performs only slightly below age level.

See chapter 10.

If these two tests used the same type of task and were both standardized on children with cultural and socioeconomic backgrounds comparable to that of the child, we might assume that the child's problems rest mainly in comprehension difficulty with relatively complex grammatical constructions. Ordinarily, we should determine whether this apparent problem is caused by difficulty the child has with the type of task used in the standardized test. However, in this case we know that the child performed considerably better on the word comprehension section of the same test, which used the same task. Therefore, it seems reasonable to assume that the child's difficulty rests with the grammatical constructions themselves.

Actually, some standardized tests use a variety of tasks. When a child performs better on one section of the test than another, we cannot always tell whether the child has greater ability with the linguistic features assessed in the section or greater ability with the task used as the means of assessment.

At this point, nonstandardized probes would probably be selected. The probes would help us determine the degree of difficulty the child has with some of the grammatical constructions used in the standardized test. Typically, standardized tests cover a range of abilities falling within some fairly broad area of language such as receptive vocabulary or receptive grammar. Only a few test items are devoted to any particular type of word or grammatical construction. Without the use of probes, we would have evidence that the child is performing below age level on some area such as receptive grammar, but would be somewhat hard pressed to select a particular grammatical construction to teach the child.

In selecting particular grammatical constructions for detailed probing, we would examine the results of the standardized test and select those constructions the child found troublesome that are ordinarily acquired at the earliest ages. Alternatively, we might select from the test those constructions whose appearance in the everyday speech the child hears might well cause the kinds of comprehension problems noted by his parents. We might select two such grammatical constructions and design 10 probe items for each. The child's performance on these probes should provide more detailed information concerning the degree of difficulty he has with these constructions and the appropriateness of these constructions as a focus for language intervention than would be possible through an examination of the child's standardized test performance alone.

Instruction in the Assessment Process

An adequate evaluation of a child's linguistic skills should not be limited to the overall assessment of linguistic functioning and the identification of one or two linguistic features that might serve as initial targets for intervention. Some attempts should also be made to determine whether the child's comprehension or production of the feature seems amenable to instruction and, if so, which procedure seems most suitable. Generally, this process involves trying a sampling of plausible intervention procedures with the child until you find one or two that may be promising. These efforts usually take only a few minutes, as they are generally conducted during a diagnostic session that includes other activities important to the evaluation process—obtaining case history information, audiometric testing, the administration of language tests and probes, the assessment of the child's oral structure and functioning, and the assessment of other suspect aspects of the child's communicative functioning. However, the information obtained from these attempts at modifying the child's performance with these linguistic features can be invaluable to the process of designing intervention activities. Many of the procedures that might be appropriate to try during the diagnostic session are discussed in the section on intervention procedures presented below.

PROCEDURES FOR TEACHING SPECIFIC LINGUISTIC FEATURES

In certain respects, language intervention is not very different from articulation training, therapy directed toward increasing vocal control, or other treatment. Whenever approaching the task of modifying any behavior, the speech-language pathologist must keep certain principles in mind. For example, a careful specification of the desired or "terminal" behavior is needed, as well as a detailed description of the child's current or "entry" behavior. A carefully constructed sequence of steps in proceeding from the entry to the terminal behavior is also crucial. In addition, the criterion for moving from one step to the next must be spelled out. Within any given step, we should specify the verbal and/or visual stimuli used to evoke the child's response and describe the characteristics of the child's response that are needed for the response to be judged as accurate. Finally, the nature of the feedback the child receives for correct and incorrect responses must be detailed.

These principles do not dictate any specific procedure that must be used; and in fact, a number of language intervention procedures have been successfully employed. The particular procedures used are often based on the age and language abilities of the child and the theoretical orientation of the speech-language pathologist. Of course, trends can be seen in the language intervention procedures adopted. For example, there has been a recent trend toward procedures used in group settings that emphasize the social fuctions of language. Similarly, there has been a recent trend toward developing procedures for very young children. However, as long as children vary as widely as they do in the nature and severity of the linguistic difficulties and in the relative strengths they bring to language-learning tasks, there will always be a range of intervention procedures with which the speech-language pathologist should be familiar. We will discuss representative procedures, divided according to their major focus. These procedures can be used for work on morphological, syntactic, or semantic features. And by introducing new words as the child masters the use of the feature, the child's vocabulary can also be expanded.

Oral Language Production

Procedures Involving Direct Imitation

A significant number of intervention procedures use an imitation-based approach. Often imitation procedures employ visual stimuli such as pictures or enactments performed in the child's presence, verbal stimuli, such as a request or question asked of the child, and the use of an imitative prompt. For example, a procedure designed to teach the child the use of two-word utterances such as "push truck" and "throw ball" might include the following sequence at the outset.

See, for example, Gottsleben, Tyack, and Buschini, 1974; Gray and Ryan, 1973.

Speech-Language Pathologist: (Pushes a toy truck.) What am I doing? Say "push truck."
Child: Push truck.

These components are used to provide the child with maximum assistance during the initial stage of training, assistance that may be necessary because the child is being asked to attempt a linguistic feature that he or she has not used before. As the child becomes more proficient with the feature, the imitative prompt is removed.

Speech-Language Pathologist: (Tosses a ball.) What am I doing?
Child: Throw ball.

Other procedures using imitation appear to place fewer demands on the child. Some of these are an informal play format. A close inspection of these sessions often reveals considerably more than first meets the eye. Consider the following events. The setting is a preschool play/work room containing a number of toys such as blocks, toy silverware, dolls, wind up toys, a ball, and several toy cars. Three children attend the preschool sessions. Each produces speech limited for the most part to single-word utterances, although some

See, for example, Hart and Risley, 1975.

two-word utterances are heard. Some of the activities of one of these children are described below.

> (Child picks up a clear plastic box containing several toy cars. The child is unable to remove the lid of the box and looks up at the speech-language pathologist.)
> Child: Car.
> (Speech-language pathologist looks toward child, pauses.)
> Child: Car.
> Speech-language pathologist: What do you want?
> Child: Want car.
> Speech-language pathologist: Oh, let me help (opens box and child takes out a toy car).
>
> (A few minutes later the child joins the speech-language pathologist, who is playing with a doll. The pathologist "feeds" the doll using a toy fork.)
> Speech-language pathologist: Here, you play with the baby (gives child doll, continues to hold the fork, spoon, and cup). Maybe she wants a drink.
>
> (Child looks up at pathologist.)
> Child: Cup.
> (Speech-language pathologist looks toward the child, pauses,)
> Child: Want cup.
> Speech-language pathologist: (Hands the cup to the child) Here's the cup.
> (Several minutes later the child picks up the ball.)
> Speech-language pathologist: Oh, roll the ball over here. Roll the ball.
> (Child rolls the ball to pathologist, who then rolls it back.)
> Speech-language pathologist: Roll it again.
> (Child rolls ball to speech-language pathologist, who then pretends to attend to something else while still holding ball.)
> Child: Ball.
> (Speech-language pathologist looks toward child, pauses,)
> Child: Ball.
> Speech-language pathologist: Say "want ball."
> Child: Want ball.

The speech-language pathologist's goal for this session was to increase the child's use of certain highly functional two-word constructions, such as "want" combined with the name of the object or action desired ("want cookie," "want ball," "want go"). However, the procedure adopted requires the use of the target construction in a natural and situationally appropriate context. For this reason, the speech-language pathologist carefully selected the materials to be used in the session and determined beforehand the activities involving these materials that might set the occasion for the child's use of the target construction. Thus, the speech-language pathologist had placed some presumably desirable objects (toy cars) in a clear plastic container that she knew would be difficult for the child to open. Similarly, she deliberately withheld the cup when giving the child the doll and knowingly failed to roll the ball back to the child. Each of these was designed to result in a situation where the child had to make a request that could be expressed with the target construction.

The speech-language pathologist gave the desired assistance only when the child produced the request with this construction. As this was a new linguistic behavior for the child, however, "correct" requests could not be expected in each instance. Therefore, the speech-language pathologist planned the following strategy.

(1) Set the occasion for a request by the child.
(2) If the request is expressed in the target construction, give the child the assistance requested.
(3) If not, look at the child and pause. Give assistance if the target construction is used.
(4) If not, ask a question that contains one of the words the child should use in the request ("What do you want?") Give assistance if the target construction is used.
(5) If not, produce the request for the child to imitate. Give assistance if the imitation is accurate.

As you can see, additional clues are provided only when they seem necessary. With this procedure, it is assumed that when the child gains greater control of the target construction he will use it in his initial request, since this would enable him to obtain assistance most quickly.

Another type of imitation procedure begins at the nonverbal, motor level. *See, for example, Baer* This procedure is used with children who are not yet producing words and *and Sherman, 1964.* those whose imitative abilities are very limited. In the initial step of this procedure, the speech-language pathologist performs a gross motor act, such as raising her arms, and physically assists the child in imitating the act. After the child has been given this type of assistance for several times for several of these acts, the speech-language pathologist performs the acts and provides less physical assistance—for instance, by only touching the child's arms instead of lifting them for the child. When the child shows the ability to imitate these behaviors, the speech-language pathologist eliminates all assistance and presents only the behavior to be imitated.

During the next phase of training, the professional presents motor behaviors involving the facial area, most notably the mouth, lips, and teeth. For example, he might open and close his mouth in exaggerated fashion or stick out his tongue. The child is required to imitate these behaviors without physical assistance. Once the child shows a consistent tendency to imitate, the speech-language pathologist accompanies his motor behavior with a vocal behavior. For example, he might open and close his mouth while producing a vowel-like sound. The child would be required to produce both the motor behavior and the vowel-like sound. After the child develops increased ability to imitate vocalizations paired with motor behaviors, the speech-language pathologist begins to present vocalizations for the child to imitate with no accompanying motor act.

When the child shows an ability to imitate vocalizations, the speech-language pathologist begins to "shape" the vocalizations into productions that become more speech-like. For example, he might require the child to imitate productions such as "ahp" and "eem." Gradually, the child is required to imitate productions that have the potential to serve as words, such as "Mama" and "bye bye." Once the child consistently imitates these productions, the speech-language pathologist begins to teach the child their meanings. For example, the child will be asked to produce "Mama" in the presence of his mother or when shown a picture of the mother. "Bye bye" would be encouraged whenever someone leaves the room and when the child himself leaves for home.

A major advantage of imitation procedures is their effectiveness in evoking responses from the child that at least approximate the desired behavior. The intellectual and motor skills necessary to match the behavior of another person are intact in most children, provided that the particular behavior the child is asked to imitate does not greatly exceed his current skill level.

One of the limitations of imitation procedures is that they are somewhat awkward to use when attempting to teach pragmatics or linguistic features that are closely related to discourse. For example, children gradually develop an awareness that, when a question is asked of them, a response to the question is expected. In an imitation approach, the child must inhibit the tendency to respond to the question and instead attempt to produce the question himself.

> Speech-language pathologist: Say "Where am I going?"
> Child: Where am I going?

Procedures Involving Modeling

*See, for example,
Leonard, 1975.*

Several other language intervention procedures use a modeling approach. In this approach, the child observes someone else, usually the speech-language pathologist or a third participant, present examples of the linguistic feature serving as the focus of intervention. The child is not asked to imitate the modeled examples. Rather, the child is instructed that the model will be talking in a "special way" and that she should listen carefully, for she will soon be given a turn to speak. An example of a segment from a modeling session is presented below. In this session, a third participant is serving as the model. The focus of intervention is on the use of questions containing both "what" and the auxiliary verb "is."

> Speech-Language Pathologist: I have some pictures of some people doing some things and some animals doing some things. I'm not going to show you the pictures unless you ask me about them. But you have to ask in a special way. Bobby [the child], you listen to Julie [the model] first and then it will be your turn to ask questions. Ready? (Speech-language pathologist turns to model.) Ask me about the first picture. It shows a boy eating.
>
> Julie: What is the boy eating?
>
> Speech-language pathologist: The boy is eating an apple. See? (Shows picture.) That was a good question. This next picture shows a dog watching.
>
> Julie: What dog watching?
>
> Speech-language pathologist: You didn't ask very well.
>
> Julie: What *is* the dog watching?
>
> Speech-language pathologist: See? (Shows picture.) The dog is watching the goldfish. That was a

	good question. Try another. This shows the girl throwing.
Julie:	What is the girl throwing?
Speech-language pathologist:	(Shows picture.) An egg. I bet that will make a mess. That was a good question. O.K. Bobby, you ask some questions now. This picture shows a man cleaning.
Bobby:	What the man is cleaning?

As you can see, in a modeling procedure, the child does not attempt to immediately repeat the model's utterance. Instead, the child attempts to determine what form the utterance is expected to take by listening to the model and observing whether the speech-language pathologist regards the model's utterance as acceptable. Of course, this is a type of imitation, but it is a rule for combining and sequencing words that the child is imitating, not particular utterances that were spoken by the model. For example, the model had never produced the question "What is the man cleaning?" in the session described above, yet the child was asked to produce this question. (In our example, Bobby did not produce it with complete accuracy.) This approach can be helpful in working on pragmatics skills.

One language intervention approach that shares certain characteristics with this modeling approach might be called a *focused stimulation* approach. The approach of Lee, Koenigsknecht, and Mulhern (1975) seems to fall in this category. In this approach, the child is provided with concentrated exposure to particular linguistic features with which he has been found to have difficulty. In those instances where the child's expressive ability with these features is in question, he may be asked to produce the linguistic feature. However, compared with the modeling approach we have already described, focused stimulation involves a considerably higher degree of exposure for the number of responses required of the child.

A story-telling format is frequently used in this approach. The story told to the child contains two or three linguistic features proving troublesome for the child. Several examples of each feature appear in the story. For example, assume a child shows a tendency to produce "him" and "her" when "he" and "she," respectively, should be used ("Him flying a plane," "Her sleeping"), and uses the negative form "not" when "can't" should be used. The speech-language pathologist might devise several stories that include these features. Pictures might also be used to accompany the stories, in order to help the child understand the story.

> Here is a girl who likes to play games. *She* likes hide-and-seek and hop-scotch. *She* likes baseball too. The girl wants to learn new games. *She* wants to play football with her brothers. But the girl's father says no. "You *can't* play football," the father says. "You *can't* run fast and you will get hurt if they tackle you." "Then I'll tackle them," says the girl. "But you *can't* tackle them. They're too big," the father says. The girl is sad. But then *she* finds a new game—running.

Following the story, the speech-language pathologist may ask questions such as "What did the father say?" in order to give the child practice in producing the target linguistic features. Through the use of several stories containing these features, the child should acquire greater understanding of these features and how and where they are used in sentences. By being given the opportunity to respond verbally after each story, the child will gain greater control over his or her production of these features.

Procedures involving modeling seem well-suited for teaching children various linguistic features. Through the use of carefully selected examples produced by a model, the child is in a good position to learn how and where the linguistic feature is to be used. In addition, modeling seems somewhat less artificial than some approaches, making the transfer from use in the teaching environment to use in the child's natural environment more likely. However, the effectiveness of modeling depends upon the child's ability to pay attention. Unfortunately, a number of children do not demonstrate anything more than sporadic and fleeting attention to the speech of others. For these children, modeling procedures are probably not very effective.

Oral Language Comprehension

See, for example, Winitz, 1973.

Several language intervention procedures can be characterized as comprehension-based approaches. The assumption behind some of these procedures is that the child needs to understand particular linguistic features before he or she can be taught to produce them. Other procedures assume that if a child learns to comprehend these features, he will begin to produce them with little or no direct instruction in expression. Both types of procedures are similar in their methodology.

For example, assume that a child does not yet comprehend the double object construction used in utterances such as "She showed the boy the car" and "Daddy gave Mommy the baby." The speech-language pathologist may place three pictures in front of the child. One picture might depict a woman showing a boy a car, another might depict a boy showing a woman a car, and a third might depict a woman pointing to the boy while looking at the car (as if "showing" the boy to the car). The child would be asked, "Point to 'She showed the boy the car.' " If the child points to the wrong picture, the speech-language pathologist would indicate which picture was correct. This method would continue, using additional sets of pictures appropriate for other possible sentences involving the double object construction. Once the child consistently indicates comprehension, a production probe might be administered. For example, the speech-language pathologist may use a parallel sentence production task, where he describes a picture using the double object construction and asks the child to describe a second picture. The extent to which the child is able to use this construction will determine the extent to which the comprehension training facilitated the child's production abilities.

GENERALIZATION

As we have seen, we cannot discuss the issue of language intervention without also discussing generalization. Teaching a child to use a new linguistic feature is only half the battle. The other half comes in insuring that the child is able to construct his own utterances involving the new linguistic feature and that he is able to use these utterances in settings quite different from the setting in which the feature was first taught. Language consists of an infinite number of word combinations, and it is virtually impossible to provide a child with direct training on each of them. Similarly, the professional cannot accompany the child to every situation in which he might speak in order to insure that he has received training in every possible setting. Fortunately, generalization need not be left to chance. The speech-language pathologist can take active steps to increase its likelihood. We will describe some of these steps next.

Utterance Form Generalization

One type of generalization might be called *utterance form generalization* (Leonard, 1974). This type of generalization is essential for any language intervention procedure designed to teach some type of linguistic rule or construction. For example, assume that a child is taught the use of two-word utterances reflecting the "Action + Object" construction. Let us assume that these utterances were learned in the context of describing the speech-language pathologist's actions on the objects mentioned in the utterances. For example, the child learned to say "kick truck" when watching the speech-language pathologist kick a toy truck.

Some examples of these utterances appear in the first column of Table 8.5.

TABLE 8.5
Some Examples of Utterance Form Generalization.

	Untrained Examples Observed During Probes		
Trained Examples	**New Permutation**	**One New Element**	**Two New Elements**
throw ball throw truck kick truck	kick ball	roll truck	push block

There would certainly be little reason to believe that the child had acquired a linguistic rule if he or she did not also show untrained usage, like the examples in the second column of Table 8.5. In this column, the utterance listed involves both an action and object that was used during Action + Object training. However, during this training, the action was not performed on this particular object; other actions were used with the object. Yet, as this utterance represents only a recombination of trained material, it does not represent a significant extension of the trained behavior. However, as we move to the third and fourth columns of the table, the utterances reflect greater ability on the child's part to incorporate new words into the trained pattern. This usage seems to constitute evidence that the child has learned the rule. To cite an example, the child's use of "push block" reflects an ability to combine two words that were never used in Action + Object training. The fact that he could do this suggests that during training the child was learning a rule for combining words involved in an action-on-object relationship, not merely a series of particular word combinations. It is the speech-language pathologist's responsibility not only to teach the child a number of word combinations reflecting a particular construction or rule, but also to insure, through the use of untrained probes, that the child's usage reflects the rule rather than rote learning. If the child does not show rule application, the usual strategy is to provide additional examples of the rule in training. The assumption is that additional examples may tax the child's rote memory, leading him to look for more general principles that may provide cues as to how the words should be combined.

Position Generalization

Along with utterance form generalization, speech-language pathologists rely on *position generalization* (McReynolds & Engmann, 1974). Several linguistic features, such as the articles "a" and "the," adjectives, prepositions, and even certain verbs, can appear in different sentence positions. For example, "the" may appear in sentences such as "The knife is gone" as well as "Wanda saw the ghost." "Was" may appear in sentences such as "Hal was a singer" as well as "Was the man here?"

Position generalization may be promoted by providing the child with practice in using the trained linguistic feature in more than one sentence position. For example, the child might be taught the use of "the" in sentences such as "The ball rolled away" and "I took the ball from Jason." In the initial stage of this process, it might be helpful to the child if "the" preceded the same word ("ball") when its position in the sentence is changed. Subsequently, the words immediately following "the" could vary. Following this training, probes could be used to determine if the child is beginning to use "the" in still other sentence positions. For example, the child could be tested on sentences such as "He put it on the table."

Stimulus Generalization

See, for example, Mulac and Tomlinson, 1977.

One of the most exasperating experiences a speech-language pathologist can face is working with a child who shows good use of linguistic features in the clinic setting, but who shows little to no use of the features in everyday surroundings. Unfortunately, this problem is frequently encountered. The solution is to take active steps to facilitate stimulus generalization. A first step in promoting stimulus generalization is to note the differences between the stimulus conditions involved during language intervention activities and the conditions involved in the child's everyday speech. Minimally, these involve the physical setting in which the child's use of the trained linguistic feature may occur, the persons to whom the child may speak, thus using (or failing to use) the trained linguistic feature, and the particular utterances directed to the child that might lead him to respond with an utterance containing (or omitting) the trained linguistic feature. Once the child shows an ability to use the linguistic feature in one circumstance, the speech-language pathologist attempts to gradually modify the conditions surrounding this circumstance until it resembles the speaking situations in which the child ordinarily finds himself.

Another tactic for stimulus generalization is the use of transfer contracts, explained in chapter 7.

An example of the steps involved in facilitating stimulus generalization may be helpful. Assume that a child has been taught to use the past tense ending -ed when describing pictured activities for the speech-language pathologist in an assigned therapy room in a speech-language clinic. The procedure involves the speech-language pathologist presenting a picture and asking, "What just happened?" At this point, the clinician might perform activities himself and ask the child, "What just happened?" Subsequently, the parent could be asked to perform some act, and the speech-language pathologist could ask "What just happened?" In turn, the speech-language pathologist could perform the act, and the parent could ask the same question of the child. The next step might involve the speech-language pathologist performing some familiar act in a different setting, such as in the clinic's waiting room or by the front door. The parent could ask the usual "What just happened?" In the same setting, the parent might also ask the same question of the child when other people perform acts, such as the child's brother or sister. The next step would involve the parent asking the child this question when other family members perform various acts at home. During this period, the speech-language pathologist might expand the types of prompting questions asked of the child in the regular clinic setting, perhaps by asking the child to use the past tense ending in utterances serving as responses to questions such as "What did I just do?" "Tell me what you did." Eventually, the parent would be asked to use these questions in the home setting. Through the use of several prompting questions, different questioners, and different settings, the child should learn that his use of the past tense ending has general application and is not simply part of a "game" that is played whenever he goes to the speech-language clinic.

NONVOCAL COMMUNICATION

For some children, the acquisition of spoken language is not a realistic goal. The limited degree of physical control these children have over their speech mechanisms makes it unlikely that they would acquire the ability to produce recognizable speech. However, many of these children can acquire the ability to communicate if given alternative means. In recent years, a number of communication systems have been devised for these children. These systems allow the child to transmit messages without use of spoken language.

Many people with cerebral palsy have this problem; see chapter 13 for a parallel discussion.

Fristoe and Lloyd (1979) describe a number of these systems.

The particular nonvocal communication system selected will depend upon the motor abilities of the child and his or her level of intellectual functioning. The systems available range from one where the child nods when another person points to a picture representing a desired object to one where the child constructs a message on a specially designed typewriter whose output is displayed on a television monitor.

Let us look at an example of how a system of nonvocal communication might be taught to a child. Assume that a speech-language pathologist is working with a multiply handicapped child who is mentally retarded and has severe motor limitations which have prevented her from gaining any benefit from training in spoken language. The speech-language pathologist selects or designs a "communication board" to sit on the child's wheelchair arms. The board contains a number of pictures of common objects and activities arranged in rows and columns.

A major goal in this approach is to teach the child that her pointing at a particular picture serves as a request for the object or activity shown in that picture. However, she must also learn the picture that corresponds to each object or activity. The speech-language pathologist might initially place a single picture in front of the child. He would then place the child's finger on the picture and then present the corresponding object (for example, a radio) or have the child perform the corresponding activity (for example, drink some juice). Eventually, the child would be required to point to the picture without assistance from the speech-language pathologist, in order to receive the desired object or activity.

Once the child consistently points to the first object, the speech-language pathologist would introduce additional pictures corresponding to other objects and activities. Initially, the pictures would be presented singly in order to insure that the child has opportunity to learn the meanings of each one. Subsequently, two pictures would be presented at the same time, then three, and so on until the child shows the ability to point appropriately when the full complement of pictures is before her. As with other procedures, it is important to introduce new elements one at a time and to reinforce the child for gradually improving approximations of the correct response.

COUNSELING

Like other communication disorders, language disorders constitute a family problem, not simply a problem of the child. The family considerations involved can take a number of forms. First, we must determine whether the ways in which family members interact with the child might be contributing to the child's problem. Earlier in this chapter, we noted that the interactions between language disordered children and their parents are somewhat different from those between normally developing children and their parents. However, the reasons for this difference are unclear. The language disordered children are generally not very responsive to parents' attempts to communicate. Therefore, it would be unwise to assume that parents of language impaired children, even those who seem more directive than most parents, are the cause of their children's language problems.

At the same time, the speech-language pathologist must be on the lookout for extreme cases. For example, if a parent simply "gives up" and stops talking to the child, or talks to the child as if the child understood nothing that was said, the speech-language pathologist would have reason for concern. In these cases, it would be valuable to counsel the parents concerning the linguistic abilities the child does possess and the ways in which the parents might change their communications with the child. When parents of language impaired children are encouraged to increase their verbal commentary on their activities and supplement it with occasional questions directed to their child, significant increases in the child's linguistic skills may result (Whitehurst, Novak, & Zorn, 1972).

The literature on the interactions between parents and their normally developing children also offers a few suggestions concerning possible ways parents might interact with their language impaired children. For example, parents of normal children typically produce utterances that are shorter, grammatically and semantically simpler, more fluent, and more redundant when talking with less linguistically sophisticated children than when talking with more sophisticated children and adults. Their explicit corrective feedback seems limited to semantic inaccuracies in their children's utterances (Brown & Hanlon, 1970); corrections of grammatical inaccuracies are less frequent, and when they occur, they are rarely accompanied by words such as "no."

> Child: (Looking at picture in book.) See horsie, mom.
> Mother: No, that's a giraffe.
> Child: Waffe (looks at next picture). Sheeps. Look, a sheeps.
> Mother: Yes, sheep. They're eating some grass for dinner.

Parents might also be alerted to the possible influences that siblings may have on a child's linguistic development. Parents of language impaired children often express concern that older siblings may have a detrimental effect on their child's development because the older children understand the younger child's communicative intents and do not encourage the child to use his "best speech." However, research with normally developing children suggests that the age differential between older and younger child is a critical factor. When no more than 2 years separate the older and younger child, the linguistic development of the younger child actually seems to benefit, proceeding faster than that of only children and children with siblings who are considerably older (Nelson & Bonvillian, 1978).

Although parents of language impaired children may not be the cause of their child's difficulties with language, they may often feel that they are. Certainly many parents are concerned about whether their interactions with their child promote the child's linguistic development. However, other parents feel guilty—ranging from a feeling that they may have provided inadequate language stimulation for their child to acquire language properly to a feeling of guilt for not being able to "produce" a normal, healthy baby. The speech-language pathologist must determine the nature and degree of the parents' concerns. For those parents whose concerns are over providing the child with the most facilitative linguistic environment possible, counseling might include discussion of methods of providing the child with the most optimal linguistic input and the types of activities and interactions that might be most beneficial.

This is not to say that these parents have no needs of their own. One of my most vivid memories is of a mother who was faced with the problem of determining what to do about her son's tendency to get up in the middle of the night and explore electrical appliances, taste food kept in the refrigerator, and bend or break small household objects. Her decision, after considering the danger that might come to her son even with added precautions, was to lock him in his room once he went to sleep. The mother needed a great deal of support once this difficult decision was made. In some cases, counseling should be principally limited to the needs of the parents. These are the parents who may feel that they have caused or contributed in some way to their child's problem. These feelings may have been aggravated by other professionals (perhaps physicians or psychologists) who explicitly blame the parents for the young child's language delay. This is a particular concern with autism, which some feel to be basically an emotional problem. For parents such as these, efforts at instructing them in optimal language stimulation activities may simply confirm in their mind that they had been doing things "wrong" all along. The unwarranted guilt of these parents must be allayed before the focus turns to the linguistic needs of the child.

One of the chief counseling responsibilities of the speech-language pathologist is to inform parents when he feels the child would benefit from being seen by professionals in other fields. For example, a child's lack of motor coordination and poor attention span might justify an examination by a pediatric neurologist. A child's slow progress during language training, coupled with an apparent difficulty comprehending tasks whose instructions can be conveyed without the use of language, might warrant referral for psychological testing. It is important that the speech-language pathologist justify the referral. For example, a thorough neurological examination may result in the recommendation that the child do particular neuromotor exercises to improve coordination or that the child receive medication to improve his attention span. Psychological testing might suggest the need for instruction directed at other developmental skills in addition to language. It is not adequate to justify the economic and emotional expense of these referrals by simply telling parents that "more information would be helpful." The speech-language pathologist should clearly state what information can be gained and how it might be helpful.

Finally, it is important that speech-language pathologists provide parents with a reasonable estimate of what to expect for the future. We cannot and should not make detailed predictions of a child's future status. However, we can certainly provide parents with some general idea of the expected duration of treatment. Many language disordered children require years of treatment for their linguistic difficulties, and most experienced speech-language pathologists can identify these children by the initial severity of their problems and by their slow progress during the first several months of intervention. It would be unfair to convey a wait-and-see attitude to the parents of these children. They may need to make financial plans for a long period of receiving professional services, and they may need time to arrange their life-style to accommodate a long-term routine of transporting the child to the treatment facility.

See, for example, Weiner, 1974.

The speech-language pathologist must also assume one other responsibility. A number of long-term studies of language disordered children reveal that these children may have residual linguistic difficulties throughout childhood and into adolescence. Often these difficulties make the process of learning to read and write more problematic. Many of these children require extra help in reading and writing and may even be assigned to "special" classes to accomplish this end. The parents of children with more serious language problems should probably be alerted to this possibility and should be informed of some of the professionals in other fields who may provide useful guidance in this matter. The related problem of language disorders, as it affects school-aged children, is examined in depth in the next chapter.

SELECTED READINGS

Bloom, L., & Lahey, M. *Language development and language disorders.* New York: John Wiley, 1978.

Dale, P. *Language development.* New York: Holt, Rinehart & Winston, 1976.

deVilliers, J., & deVilliers, P. *Language acquisition.* Cambridge, Mass.: Harvard University Press, 1978.

McLean, J., & Snyder-McLean, L. *A transactional approach to early language training.* Columbus, Ohio: Charles E. Merrill, 1978.

Schiefelbusch, R. (Ed.). *Bases of language intervention.* Baltimore: University Park Press, 1978.

Schiefelbusch, R., & Lloyd, L. *Language perspectives: Acquisition, retardation and intervention.* Baltimore: University Park Press, 1974.

REFERENCES

Baer, D., & Sherman, J. Reinforcement control of generalized imitation in young children. *Journal of Experimental Child Psychology,* 1964, *1,* 37–49.

Baltaxe, C., & Simmons, J. Disorders of language in childhood psychosis: Current concepts and approaches. In J. Darby (Ed.), *Speech and language in medicine: From theory to practice.* New York: Grune & Stratton, in press.

Bangs, T. E. *Vocabulary Comprehension Scale.* Boston: Teaching Resources, 1975.

Bankson, N. W. *Bankson Language Screening Test.* Baltimore: University Park Press, 1977.

Benton, A. Developmental aphasia and brain damage. *Cortex,* 1964, *1,* 40–52.

Bloom, L. *Language development: Form and function in emerging grammars.* Cambridge, Mass.: MIT Press, 1970.

Bloom, L., & Lahey, M. *Language development and language disorders.* New York: John Wiley, 1978.

Bowerman, M. *Early syntactic development: A cross-linguistic study with special reference to Finnish.* New York: Cambridge University Press, 1973.

Brolin, D. D. *Vocational preparation of retarded citizens.* Columbus, Ohio: Charles E. Merrill, 1976.

Brown, R. *A first language: The early years.* Cambridge, Mass.: Harvard University Press, 1973.

Brown, R., & Hanlon, C. Derivational complexity and order of acquisition in child speech. In J. Hayes (Ed.), *Cognition and the development of language.* New York: John Wiley, 1970.

Carrow, E. *Test of Auditory Comprehension of Language, English/Spanish.* Boston: Teaching Resources, 1973.

Chapman, R. Comprehension strategies in children. In J. Kavanaugh & W. Strange (Eds.), *Speech and language in the laboratory, school, and clinic.* Cambridge, Mass.: MIT Press, 1978.

Coggins, T. Relational meaning encoded in the two-word utterances of Stage 1 Down's syndrome children. *Journal of Speech and Hearing Research,* 1979, *22,* 166–178.

Curtiss, S. *Genie: A psycholinguistic study of a modern-day "wild child."* New York: Academic Press, 1977.

Darley, F. (Ed.). *Evaluation of appraisal techniques in speech and language pathology.* Reading, Mass.: Addison-Wesley, 1979.

DeFries, J. C., Ashton, G. C., Johnson, R. C., Kuse, A. R., McClearn, G. E., Mi, M. P., Rashad, M. N., Vandenberg, S. G., & Wilson, J. R. Parent-offspring resemblance for specific cognitive abilities in two ethnic groups. *Nature,* 1976, *261,* 131–133.

deVilliers, J., & deVilliers, P. A cross-sectional study of the acquisition of grammatical morphemes in child speech. *Journal of Psycholinguistic Research,* 1973, *3,* 267–278.

deVilliers, J., & de Villiers, P. Competence and performance in child language: Are children really competent to judge. *Journal of Child Language,* 1974, *1,* 11–22.

Dore, J. Children's illocutionary acts. In R. Freedle (Ed.), *Discourse production and comprehension* (Vol. 1). Norwood, N. J.: Ablex, 1977.

Dunn, L. M. *Peabody Picture Vocabulary Test.* Circle Pines, Minn.: American Guidance Service, 1965; 1980.

Fristoe, M., & Lloyd, L. Non-speech communication. In N. Ellis (Ed.), *Handbook of mental deficiency.* New York: Lawrence Erlbaum Associates, 1979.

Garvey, C. The contingent query: A dependent act in conversation. In M. Lewis & L. Rosenblum (Eds.), *The origins of behavior: Communication and language.* New York: John Wiley, 1977.

Goldin-Meadow, S., Seligman, M., & Gelman, R. Language in the two-year old. *Cognition,* 1976, *4,* 189–202.

Gottsleben, R., Tyack, D., & Buschini, G. Linguistically-based training programs. *Journal of Learning Disabilities,* 1974, *7,* 197–203.

Gray, B., & Ryan, B. *A language program for the nonlanguage child.* Champaign, Ill.: Research Press, 1973.

Greenfield, P., & Smith, J. *The structure of communication in early language development.* New York: Academic Press, 1976.

Greenwald, C., & Leonard, L. Communicative and sensorimotor development of Down's syndrome children. *American Journal of Mental Deficiency,* 1979, *84,* 296–303.

Grossman, H. J. (Ed.). *Manual on terminology and classification in mental retardation.* Washington, D.C.: American Association on Mental Deficiency, 1977.

Hart, B., & Risley, T. Incidental teaching of language in the preschool. *Journal of Applied Behavior Analysis,* 1975, *8,* 411–420.

Huttenlocher, J. The origins of language comprehension. In R. Solso (Ed.), *Theories of cognitive psychology.* New York: Lawrence Erlbaum Associates, 1974.

Johnston, J. The language disordered child. In N. Lass, J. Northern, D. Yoder, & L. McReynolds (Eds.), *Speech, language and hearing.* Philadelphia: W. B. Saunders, in press.

Keenan, E. Conversational competence in children. *Journal of Child Language,* 1974, *1,* 163–183.

Klima, E., & Bellugi, U. Syntactic regularities in the speech of children. In J. Lyons & R. Wales (Eds.), *Psycholinguistics papers.* Edinburgh: Edinburgh University Press, 1966.

Landau, W., Goldstein, R., & Kleffner, F. Congenital aphasia: A clinicopathologic study. *Neurology,* 1960, *10,* 915–921.

Lee, L., Koenigsknecht, R., & Mulhern, S. *Interactive language development teaching.* Evanston, Ill.: Northwestern University Press, 1975.

Lenneberg, E. *Biological foundations of language.* New York: John Wiley, 1967.

Leonard, L. A preliminary review of generalization in language training. *Journal of Speech and Hearing Disorders,* 1974, *38,* 429–436.

Leonard, L. Modeling as a clinical procedure in language training. *Language, Speech and Hearing Services in Schools,* 1975, *6,* 72–85.

Leonard, L. Language impairment in children. *Merrill-Palmer Quarterly,* 1979, *25,* 205–232.

Leonard, L., Prutting, C., Perozzi, J., & Berkley, R. Nonstandardized approaches to the assessment of language behaviors. *Asha,* 1978, *20,* 371–379.

Lovell, K., & Bradbury, B. The learning of English morphology in educationally subnormal special school children. *American Journal of Mental Deficiency,* 1967, *71,* 609–615.

McReynolds, L., & Engmann, D. An experimental analysis of the relationship of subject and object noun phrases. In L. McReynolds (Ed.), Developing systematic procedures for training children's language. *ASHA Monograph,* 1974, *18.*

Mulac, A., & Tomlinson, C. Generalization of an operant remediation program for syntax with language-delayed children. *Journal of Communication Disorders,* 1977, *10,* 231–244.

Nelson, K. E., & Bonvillian, J. Early semantic development: Conceptual growth and related processes between 2 and 4½ years of age. In K. E. Nelson (Ed.), *Children's language* (Vol. 1). New York: Gardner Press, 1978.

Newcomer, P. L., & Hammill, D. D. *Test of Language Development,* Austin, Tex.: Pro-Ed, 1977.

Payne, J. S., & Patton, J. R. (Eds.). *Mental retardation.* Columbus, Ohio: Charles E. Merrill, 1981.

Piaget, J. *The origins of intelligence in children.* New York: W. W. Norton, 1963.

Sachs, J., & Devin, J. Young children's use of age-appropriate speech styles in social interaction and role-playing. *Journal of Child Language,* 1976, *3,* 81–98.

Sachs, J., & Truswell, L. Comprehension of two-word instructions by children in the one-word stage. *Journal of Child Language,* 1978, *5,* 17–24.

Shatz, M., & Gelman, R. The development of communication skills: Modification in the speech of young children as a function of the listener. *Monographs of the Society for Research in Child Development,* 1973, *38* (5, Serial No. 152).

Stephens, M. I. *Stephens Oral Language Screening Test.* Peninsula, Ohio: Interim Publishers, 1977.

Tallal, P., & Stark, R. Speech perception in language-delayed children. In G. Yeni-Komashian, J. Kavanaugh, & C. Ferguson (Eds.) *Child phonology, Vol. II: Perception, production, and deviation.* Cambridge, Mass.: MIT Press, 1980.

Tyack, D., & Gottsleben, R. *Language sampling, analysis, and training.* Palo Alto, Calif.: Consulting Psychologists Press, 1974.

Weiner, P. A language-delayed child at adolescence. *Journal of Speech and Hearing Disorders,* 1974, *39,* 202–212.

Whitehurst, G., Novak, G., & Zorn, G. Delayed speech studied in the home. *Developmental Psychology,* 1972, *7,* 169–177.

Wieman, L. Stress patterns of early child language. *Journal of Child Language,* 1976, *3,* 283–286.

Winitz, H. Problem solving and the delaying of speech as strategies in the teaching of language. *Asha,* 1973, *15,* 583–586.

Wulbert, M., Inglis, S., Kriegsmann, E., & Mills, B. Language delay and associated mother-child interactions. *Developmental Psychology,* 1975, *11,* 61–70.

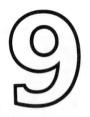

9

LANGUAGE DISABILITIES IN THE SCHOOL-AGE CHILD

Elisabeth H. Wiig

At 11 years of age, Jim was an active and physically attractive boy. He had completed the elementary grades in the regular classroom and was performing at or above grade level. He had, however, seen the school's speech-language pathologist for individual therapy for several periods during his elementary school years. Jim carried several diagnostic labels during his 11 years of life. He was called a child with articulation disorders, a child with a reverse swallowing pattern, a dysfluent child, and a child with delayed language acquisition. He narrowly escaped being labelled a child with a learning disability. The combined efforts of specialists, classroom teachers, and parents made it possible for Jim to achieve in the classroom.

Jim's early motor development was normal, and developmental milestones were reached before expected. His motor advantage is now evident in sports. Jim is a leader in ice hockey, football, and baseball. His speech and language development did not, however, conform to the normal pattern. When he was only 18 months old, he was referred by the pediatrician for an evaluation of his hearing and of his language acquisition. At 2½ years of age, Jim had not yet begun to talk. His intellectual ability was then evaluated with nonverbal tasks. All evaluations indicated performance within normal limits on all tasks but those requiring language expression. At about 3 years old, Jim finally uttered his first word or rather his first combination of three words. His spoken utterances were, however, unintelligible to anyone outside his family. At 4, Jim entered into a nursery school with a language stimulation class. His language development began to follow a normal pattern of growth but was still delayed. At 5, Jim entered the local public school in kindergarten. The teacher soon noticed that Jim had a poorer command of words than his classmates. He was still hard to understand when he spoke. He substituted sounds and articulated all speech sounds with his tongue too far forward in the mouth. During the year, Jim also became highly dysfluent. Sometimes his speech came to a complete halt in his efforts to say a word. During the spring term, Jim was referred to the speech-language pathologist for evaluation and intervention.

Speech therapy focused first on reducing the dysfluencies, primarily through parent counseling and teacher intervention. A second focus was on developing adequate vocabulary for entry into the first grade. Language intervention was continued through the summer and most of the first grade. Jim was then dismissed from therapy and future periodic assessment was recommended. At the beginning of the second grade, Jim was referred for more therapy. This time, the classroom teacher stressed that Jim had problems in spelling and oral reading. In the referral, the teacher stated that he felt Jim's articulation difficulties were interfering with his reading and spelling acquisition. Jim was enrolled for intensive articulation therapy. A reverse swallowing pattern was diagnosed, and articulation therapy was designed to account for this feature. After about a year and a half, Jim was again released from therapy.

By now, Jim's teachers were alerted to his potential language and learning disabilities. The school provided counseling and parent training sessions for Jim's parents, designed to alert them to Jim's needs for support at home and to train them to help Jim in his homework assignments. The classroom teachers monitored Jim to spot any developing learning problems. In the fifth grade yet another language-related problem emerged. Jim was not able to perform to expectation in language arts and written language assignments. This problem persisted throughout the fifth and sixth grades. Extra efforts were made in the classroom and in consultation with the speech-language pathologist to provide individual assistance for vocabulary development and written language formulation and expression. Jim's parents were again alerted to his new needs for support with homework.

Jim's future in junior high raises some questions in the minds of both his teachers and parents. Everyone expects that he may need assistance in Language Arts and English Composition, possibly in a resource room setting. It is also expected that he may run into problems in learning a foreign language, a requirement in his junior high school. Because of his abilities and involvement in sports and his good motivation and achievement in sciences, Jim is not expected to develop into a behavior or social adjustment problem in junior high. There is a general recognition by everyone involved that, without sustained speech and language intervention, Jim might not have reached his current level of achievement and personal adjustment.

You may now wish to listen to the speech sample accompanying this chapter, found on Audio Disc 1, Side 2 (sample #5).

In chapter 8 we looked at the kinds of difficulties some young children have as they develop language skills. Many of these children, even those who receive early speech-language intervention, continue to have language problems when they enter school. Other children have language problems that become evident only when they are faced with the academic challenges of school, or are compared with their classmates in terms of speech and language skills. These problems may seem to come and go, or to get better and worse, as the child advances to new academic levels. Furthermore, the changes we have all faced in growing up—particularly the stresses associated with adolescence—can be accompanied by "flare-ups" of language problems. In this chapter, we will examine the language problems commonly experienced by elementary and secondary school students and see what the speech-language pathologist can do to help them.

THE PROBLEM

See, for example, Froeschels (1918), Orton (1937), Goldstein (1948), Strauss and Kephart (1955), and Myklebust (1954).

Language and communication disorders are common among children with school learning problems. Some of these children are called *learning disabled;* some, *mentally retarded;* some, *learning handicapped;* some, *language disabled.* Whatever the label, these children have been the subject of concern for years, partially because the ability to use language is so critical in other academic skills. You cannot learn to read and write fluently if you cannot comprehend and produce your native language. And there are few subjects you can learn without reading (or understanding what is said to you), and few tests you can pass without writing (or expressing your knowledge somehow).

Language and communication disabilities in middle and late childhood may also result in inability to cope with increasing social demands. During preadolescence and adolescence, language disabilities may result in adjustment problems and widespread academic difficulties.

Speech-languge pathologists deal with students for whom language is the major problem, as well as with some for whom language delay is only a part of an overall learning delay.

Several relatively recent pieces of legislation have recognized that some school-aged children have handicaps attributable to *specific learning disabilities.* This group of children has been defined in *The Education for All Handicapped Children Act* (P.L. 94-142, 1975), as follows:

> Children with specific learning disabilities exhibit a disorder in one or more of the basic psychological processes involved in understanding or using spoken or written language. These may be manifested in writing, spelling, or arithmetic. They include conditions which have been referred to as perceptual handicaps, brain injury, brain dysfunction, dyslexia, developmental aphasia, etc. They do not include learning problems which are due primarily to visual, hearing, or motor handicaps, to mental retardation, or to environmental disadvantage. (p. 42478)

This definition is interesting but not very functional; that is, it does not describe the characteristics of these children or give precise criteria for deciding whether a given child fits the category. Most special educators appear to agree, however, on essential aspects of the definition (Johnson & Morasky, 1977).

(1) The child must have one or more significant delays or deficits in essential learning processes (perception, integration, verbal or nonverbal expression) and must require special education procedures for intervention or remediation.

(2) The significance of a delay or deficit in the essential learning processes must be determined by accepted diagnostic procedures in education, special education, and psychology.

(3) The child must show a discrepancy between expected performance, based on assessed intelligence, and actual achievement in one or more areas such as spoken, read, or written language, mathematics, and/or spatial orientation.

Thus a learning disabled child will have problems in *some but not all* academic skills. The learning disability may be reflected in the child's oral expression, listening comprehension, written expression, basic reading skill, reading comprehension, mathematics calculation, or mathematics reasoning (*Federal Register,* 42:250, December 29, 1977, p. 65083). Learning disabilities are not necessarily accompanied by delays in social skills or by emotional or behavioral problems.

In contrast, as we saw in the last chapter, a child who is mentally retarded must show "significantly subaverage general intellectual functioning existing concurrently with deficits in adaptive behavior" (Grossman, 1973, p 5). These children are likely to show delays in all academic areas.

Prevalence of Learning Disabilities and Mental Retardation

Estimates of the prevalence of learning disabilities among school-aged children reflect differences in the definitions or criteria used for inclusion in the group. Because we have no generally accepted operational definition or standardized evaluation procedures, estimates vary greatly, ranging from 1% to 30%. Some of these estimates are affected by practical constraints of finances and professional resources available. For example, several states say that from 1% to 3% of all school-aged children may demonstrate learning disabilities.

The prevalence of mental retardation in the population at large has been estimated at about 3%. Of these, the majority of the retarded, or about 2.5% of the population at large, fall within the category of borderline or mild mental retardation. Children with borderline mental retardation may be called *learning handicapped* or *mentally retarded,* depending upon individual patterns of strengths and weaknesses.

Mainstreaming refers to the process of placing children with handicaps in "the mainstream of education."

The language problems of more severely retarded children are handled, for the most part, according to "language age"; that is, like the younger child. See chapter 8 for specific information. A retarded child may have a hearing impairment or severe motor problems affecting speech. See chapters 10 and 13, respectively.

Today, many children with borderline mental retardation are integrated in school with the learning disabled in **mainstreaming** and special education service efforts. This combined group of children is often called *learning handicapped.* Not all of these children have significant difficulties with language. This is especially important to recognize when dealing with learning disabled students. Among mentally retarded children, there is a direct relationship between the degree of mental retardation and the degree of developmental language delay (Schiefelbusch, 1972). A similar relationship does not appear to exist among the learning disabled. This chapter focuses on the learning handicapped child—either learning disabled or mildly retarded—who *does* have a significant language problem.

Types of Learning Disabilities

We have identified at least three independent cluster of difficulties (**syndromes**) among children and adolescents with learning disabilities (Denckla, 1978; Erenberg, Mattis, & French, 1976; Mattis, French, & Rapin, 1975). The primary presenting syndrome is a language disorder syndrome. It is characterized by problems in language comprehension and expression, word-finding difficulties, and speech discrimination problems. The prevalence of the language disorder syndrome among the learning disabled ranges from about 40% to 60%.

The second syndrome is labeled an articulatory and *graphomotor dyscoordination* syndrome. It is characterized by articulatory and writing and drawing difficulties. The prevalence of this syndrome among the learning disabled ranges from about 10% to 40%.

Graphomotor dyscoordination refers to a problem of motor coordination which causes difficulties in performing the motor actions required for writing or drawing.

Visuospatial perceptual deficit refers to a problem of discriminating and differentiating similar visual stimuli such as letters and dealing with aspects of space.

The third syndrome is a *visuospatial perceptual deficit.* It is characterized by visual discrimination and visual memory problems. The reported prevalence among the learning disabled ranges from about 5% to 15%. Combinations of the language disorder and the graphomotor dyscoordination syndrome and of the language disorder and visuospatial perceptual deficit syndromes have also been reported.

Terms Used with Language Handicaps

In the evolution of the study of people with language problems, many different terms have been used to refer to various types of language problems. Some of them are widely used, while others are less common. But any of them may turn up in case histories or evaluation reports of the children seen by speech-language pathologists.

One common term is **dyslexia,** which refers to a condition involving the failure to master reading at a normal age level in the absence of a major debilitating disorder such as retardation, major brain injury, or severe emotional disturbance. Dyslexia is widely used to refer to a specific reading disability in school-aged children. The related term **alexia** refers to the acquired inability to perform all or some of the tasks involved in reading after the individual has learned to read. It is used for the reading disorders of adults with acquired brain damage.

Dysnomia is used here to refer to a developmental word-finding difficulty which interferes with a child's accuracy in finding intended names for persons, animals, objects, actions, or attributes. The related term **anomia** refers to an acquired word-finding difficulty due to brain damage. It is generally used for the world-finding difficulties associated with acquired aphasia in adults. **Aphasia** is a more general term, usually referring to any acquired language disorder caused by brain damage, resulting in partial or complete impairment of language comprehension, formulation, and use for communication. The term is generally used for acquired language disorders in adults who were once efficient speakers of the language.

Chapter 14 covers adult aphasia in depth.

A *language disorder syndrome* refers to a characteristic cluster of developmental (child) or acquired (adolescent or adult) language difficulties. It may encompass impairments of language comprehension and formulation, word-finding, and language use for interpersonal communication. It is more general than language disability, which is a developmental language disorder syndrome. Language disabilities are often mild enough to escape early detection but severe enough to interfere with the acquisition and use of language and communication skills in middle and late childhood. The developmental language disability syndrome associated with a diagnosed learning disability in a school-aged child is often called a **language-learning disability,** and the developmental delay in language acquisition associated with mental retardation is often called **language retardation.** However, the difference between language-learning disability and language retardation is more one of diagnosis than of intervention.

NORMAL LANGUAGE ACQUISITION DURING THE SCHOOL YEARS

Most learning disabled and mildly retarded children acquire the rules of language in the same order as normally developing children, although they show delays and often particular trouble spots. Before we look at the characteristic problems they have, we need to have a basic understanding of normal language acquisition patterns.

Development of Sentence Structure

School-aged children (5 to 7 years) with normal language development understand and produce sentences with structural (syntactic) characteristics much like those of adults. Young children learn to expand the subject, verb, and object into noun and verb phrase structures before they enter school. They also learn the basic rules for forming sentences which express negatives, yes/no and *wh-* questions, passives, and causal ("because"), conditional ("if"), and temporal ("when") relationships (Menyuk, 1977).

Even though the basic syntactic rules and structures have been acquired by this age, the children still use some immature sentence forms, and others remain to be acquired (Brown, 1971; Chomsky, 1969; Menyuk, 1969; Sheldon, 1974). Most children have trouble understanding sentences which feature expansions of the subject through either a subject complement (*"The possibility that my brother may visit* pleases me") or a subject relative ("The boy *who owns the dog* left for London") until the late elementary school years. These structures are not used in children's spontaneous speech till about 11 or 12 years of age; they are considered to reflect "syntactic maturity" (Hass & Wepman, 1974). Other sentence structures which are acquired in middle childhood include those with verbs such as "promise." This kind of verb causes a separation of the subject ("John") and its complement expansion ("to go"), as in "John promised Bill to go."

The ability to understand the alternative interpretations of sentences with **structural ambiguities** ("She told her baby stories"; "The duck is ready to eat") develops during the middle childhood and preadolescent years (Schultz & Pilon, 1973; Wiig, Gilbert, & Christian, 1978). The ability to deal with the alternative, nonliteral, figurative interpretations of idioms, similes, metaphors, and proverbs is also a development of the middle and late childhood years.

Complement *refers to a word, phrase, or clause used to complete the meaning of another term or phrase.* Relative *refers to a subordinated and dependent phrase or clause, introduced by a relative pronoun or adverb, referring to the main clause of a sentence.*

Structural ambiguity *refers to the characteristic of sentence structure that allows it to be interpreted in more than one way.*

Development of Word Meanings

As we saw in chapter 8, children with normally developing language have gone through several stages of vocabulary growth and concept acquisition by the time they begin school. The vocabulary of most 6-year-olds is about 2,500 words. Preschool children have a large vocabulary of symbols for human and other animate beings, inanimate objects, actions upon objects (transitive), and actions which do not involve objects (intransitive). They have acquired words to describe on-going events in the immediate environment or context. They also have words to refer to the past or the future, and they can express, among others, size, space, and time relationships among objects or events.

The early pattern of acquisition of words for agents and objects (nouns), actions (verbs), attributes and relationships (adjectives, prepositions) reflects the child's growing ability to differentiate distinctive properties of meaning (semantic features) (Clark, 1973). The pattern of acquisition seems to progress from generalization to specificity. Young children overgeneralize new words to inappropriate contexts because they have acquired only a partial meaning base for them. For example, they may use the word "dog" for all four-legged animals. Later in their development, children incorporate additional distinctive properties to form an expanded meaning base for the words they use. Words, as a result, acquire a broader and broader meaning base by the addition of semantic features. In return, words gain specificity; they become symbols for well-defined, circumscribed, and differentiated classes of objects, actions, or events. New words are also added, letting the children label more finely and differentiate better among members of a class.

In relation to the grammatical function of words and word classes, labels for agents-objects and actions are acquired first. Words which modify the agents-objects (size, color, shape, etc.) are acquired next. Words that describe relations of cause, condition, space, or time among agents-objects and actions are acquired last. Within each functional word class, the pattern of acquisition progresses at the same time from positive to negative, as in "big" before "little," and from relatively simple to relatively complex, as in "big" (+ space) to "tall" (+ space, + vertical) to "deep" (+ space, + vertical, + down) (Clark, 1971, 1972).

The positive, preferred, and usual reference in a pair of word opposites is called **unmarked;** *examples include "love," "full," and "friend." The negative, nonpreferred, unusual reference in the pair is called* **marked;** *examples include "hate," "empty," and "enemy."*

As children mature, they grow in the ability to differentiate meaning and to classify words by conceptual category using abstract meaning features (Anglin, 1970). This development results in ability to group words by their abstract meaning features, such as human, animate, inanimate, spatial-temporal relationships, and the like. The older children and young adolescents can think consciously about the meaning of words and use them for formal reasoning and problem solving.

Development of Interpersonal Communication Skills

As children with normal language development reach school age, they make significant gains in the effectiveness with which they communicate with others. For example, preschool children can communicate information to others about forms and shapes that have familiar names. They cannot, however, communicate effectively about abstract figures (Glucksberg, Krauss, & Weisberg, 1966). The ability to describe characteristics of abstract figures develops during the years from kindergarten through grade 5 (Krauss & Glucksberg, 1967).

We can observe similar growth in children's ability to adjust their language to the needs and communicative styles of others (Berko-Gleason, 1973; Flavell, Botkin, Fry, Wright, & Jarvis, 1968). At about 8 years of age, children can successfully adjust their language to all age levels. They develop the ability to take roles and to communicate effectively in role-playing activities during the preschool and middle childhood and adolescent years. During middle childhood and adolescence, they also learn to express a variety of types of intentions, increasingly using sarcasm, jokes, double-meaning expressions, and metaphoric language (Elkind, 1970; Gardner, 1973; Gardner, Kirchner, Winner, & Perkins, 1975; Schultz, 1974).

CHARACTERISTICS OF LANGUAGE DISABILITIES IN SCHOOL-AGE CHILDREN

Because every child develops a little differently, it can be difficult to differentiate between a child who is simply a little behind and one who has a language problem severe enough to warrant special intervention. Certain characteristics of language disabled children help the speech-language pathologist (and other members of a school assessment team) identify those children who need special language services, as well as those who might develop language problems along the way.

Early Language Delays

Clearly it would be helpful and cost-effective if we could identify children "at risk" for language disabilities on the basis of existing school records. Early language delays or early histories of speech or language problems are one important signal of potential language-learning disabilities. The importance of this signal has been reconfirmed recently by Ingram (1970) and Mason

(1976). They found that, among children with speech and language delays identified upon entry in the Edinburgh public schools, ⅓ showed reading and spelling retardation 2 years after starting school. This compared to figures of about 1 in 20 among children without early speech and language delays. The implications are that we should follow children with early speech or language delays and be alert to any persistent language disability which may cause learning problems.

Intellectual Functioning

Patterns of intellectual functioning may also help identify school-age children with potential language-learning disabilities. *The Wechsler Intelligence Scale for Children—Revised* (Wechsler, 1974), a widely used norm-referenced test, may provide evidence of discrepancies between verbal and performance intelligence that may identify children and adolescents at risk for language-learning disabilities. The *WISC-R* gives three scores—full scale IQ, verbal IQ, and performance IQ. Students with learning and language disabilities tend to obtain lower verbal than performance IQs, with discrepancies of 10 or more IQ points (Mattis, et al., 1975). This finding suggests that we should consider school-age children with significantly lower verbal than performance scale IQs to be at risk for language disabilities.

Academic Achievement

Academic under-achievement *refers to a discrepancy between the expected performance on an academic task based on estimates of intelligence and the actual observed performance.*

Profiles of academic underachievement in children with otherwise normal potential for learning may also be used to identify those who may have or may develop language disabilities. Many children with language-learning disabilities show one of two academic achievement test patterns (Rourke, 1975). The first pattern is one in which reading and spelling achievement are below grade level, while arithmetic achievement is at or above grade level expectations. The second pattern is one in which academic achievement in reading, spelling, and arithmetic are uniformly below grade and intellectual level expectations. Again, school-aged children who show either of these patterns of academic underachievement should be considered at risk for language disabilities.

Problems in Interpersonal Communication

Children with language-learning disabilities demonstrate their communication difficulties in everyday situations as well as in language-based school activities. Classroom teachers seem able to identify these children by their immature speech patterns, errors in verbal expressions, and difficulties in sentence comprehension and sentence formulation (Meier, 1971). These same children typically have difficulties in following oral directions in the classroom and in interpreting and answering *wh-* questions accurately (Chalfant & Foster, 1974; Lerner, 1976; Little, 1978; Schwartz & Murphy, 1975).

Other observations suggest that youngsters with language-learning disabilities may not be as capable as children with normal language development of adapting their language and communication styles to the listener's needs or to fit the interpersonal context (Bryan, 1978). These difficulties may contribute to the social interaction problems that we see among these students (Bryan, 1974, 1978; Bryan, Wheeler, Felcan, & Henek, 1976).

In verbal interactions with peers, children with learning disabilities make more "competitive" and "rejective" and fewer "helpful" and "considerate" statements than their peers. Parents, especially fathers, perceive differences in the

Communication competence refers to the successful use of language in a given context, achieved by applying the pragmatic rules and conventions that govern the use of language in

the specific context.
Register *refers to the range of word, phrase, sentence, and utterance choices and language styles available to allow a speaker to meet the language needs or expectations of a given listener.*

verbal abilities of their learning disabled and nonlearning disabled offspring (Owen, Adams, Forrest, Stolz, & Fisher, 1971). There is also evidence that children with learning disabilities are less able to communicate descriptive information about pictures to a listener then are their age peers with normal language development (Snyder, 1979). In combination, these observations suggest that children with learning disabilities may be delayed in achieving **communication competence** and mature styles and **register** in interpersonal communication.

Deficits in the Knowledge of Word Meanings (Semantics)

Investigations of the semantic abilities of school-aged children with language and learning disabilities show delays in the acquisition of the meaning of specific words or relationships among words. These delays follow patterns of normal language acquisition for the word categories or word relationships. These delays persist into adolescence if language intervention and remediation is not provided.

A performance on a language assessment which falls at or above the age which is 6 months below the child's chronological age is said to be within normal limits.

Students with learning disabilities (Johnson & Myklebust, 1967; Wiig & Semel, 1976) often earn vocabulary development scores within normal limits on picture vocabulary tests such as the *Peabody Picture Vocabulary Test* (Dunn, 1965/1980). In contrast, children and adolescents with borderline and mild mental retardation tend to experience general delays in vocabulary acquisition (Schiefelbusch, 1972).

Some children with language-learning disabilities present striking and specific lags in vocabulary knowledge and use. Analysis of their patterns of errors on vocabulary comprehension tasks frequently indicates islands of specific difficulties in acquiring adequate meanings for selected word categories. A given child may have difficulty with one or more categories such as multiple-meaning words, verbs, adjectives, adverbs, and prepositions.

When preadolescents with diagnosed learning and language disabilities were asked to interpret the alternative meanings of sentences with dual meaning words, a pattern emerged (Wiig, Semel, & Abele, 1981). First of all, these youngsters were significantly poorer at providing two interpretations for sentences such as "She wiped the glasses" and "He kept the watch" than their academically achieving age peers. Their performances proved, in fact, to be similar to those of a group of 7- and 8-year-old academic achievers. The quality of the first or only interpretations of the sentences of the learning disabled 12-year-old children gives us some insight into the variables that control their interpretations. The preferred interpretations of the dual meaning words could be related to their relatively high frequency of occurrence in the language, to multisensory (sensorimotor) experiences with the objects labeled by nouns, and to personal familiarity.

When children with language-learning disabilities are asked to follow directions or to answer questions after hearing a story, they often have problems in interpreting and remembering terms for space and time relationships, cause-effect relationships, and inclusion (all) or exclusion (none). Their difficulties encompass interpreting prepositional phrases of location, direction, or time ("before," "after"). They also encompass interpreting comparisons of size, speed, or other attributes in sentences with comparative and superlative adjectives. They have trouble interpreting sentences with terms of inclusion, such as "many," "some," or "several," or of exclusion, such as "none," "neither . . . nor," or combinations of these ("all . . . except"). They also have problems in interpreting sentences with cause-effect or conditional ("when . . . then,"

Table 9.1 summarizes selected problems in interpretation of words and concepts. Some of these problems will be "if . . . then") relationships and those with conjunction of clauses (LaPointe, 1976; Wiig, Lapointe, & Semel, 1977; Wiig & Semel, 1973, 1974, 1975).   *discussed in more detail below.*

TABLE 9.1
Word and Concept Comprehension Patterns among Children and Adolescents with Language and Learning Disabilities.

Error Pattern	Concept	Sample Interpretation
Misinterpretation of adjectives of space, time, and quality	The car is still <u>far</u> away. It is <u>early</u>.	The car is gone. It is morning.
Misinterpretation of adverbs	The man walked <u>proudly</u>.	The man was proud and he walked.
Misinterpretation of prepositions of location, direction, and time	The cat is <u>beside</u> the fireplace. He <u>crawled under</u> the wire. They go to Cape Cod <u>around</u> Memorial Day.	The cat is too close to the fireplace. He is right under that wire now. On Memorial Day they go to Cape Cod.
Misinterpretation of references for pronouns based on gender and number	<u>She</u> went to the store. <u>It is theirs</u>. They washed <u>themselves</u>.	He went to the store. It is hers/his. They washed the baby.
Misinterpretation of spatial relationships expressed by demonstratives	<u>That</u> is mine. <u>Those</u> are mine.	The one next to her/him is hers/his. The one that is close is hers/his.
Single (concrete and immediate) interpretations of multiple meaning words	He wiped the <u>glasses</u>. She did not <u>press the suit</u>.	It must be drinking glasses. The suit is wrinkled. She did not press it.
Literal interpretation of idioms, metaphors, and proverbs (figurative language)	He was about to <u>shoot his mouth off</u>. <u>She was as white as a sheet</u>. <u>Strike while the iron is hot</u>.	That's stupid. Who would shoot a bullet in his mouth? How come? Sheets aren't all white. You must use a hot iron to get the job done.

Deficits in the Knowledge of Word Formation Rules (Morphology)

Children with learning disabilities may ignore hard-to-hear parts of words, such as word endings, unstressed words, phrases, and parts of clauses, when listening to and interpreting spoken language (Golick, 1976). They may not perceive, abstract, or internalize the rules for applying and selecting words such as auxiliaries and modals, prepositions, conjunctions, and other function words that tend to receive low stress in speech. The word endings we use for **inflection** and **derivation** may cause special problems because they tend to be of relatively short duration and low intensity in running speech. These children tend instead to focus on and remember words in phrases, clauses, sentences, and paragraphs which stand out either because of stress or high information content. They may favor root words like nouns, primary verbs, and adjectives. The efficiency with which these children listen to and interpret running speech tends to be influenced by the context in which the utterances occur and the style, speed, intonation, and stress patterns used by the speaker.

Inflection refers to the expression of a grammatical function such as number (noun plural), tense (past tense of verbs), or comparison (comparative and superlative of adjectives) through addition of a word ending. Derivation refers to the formation of a new but related word from an already existing word in the language (e.g., "teach," "teacher").

In particular, school-aged children with language and learning disabilities may have difficulties interpreting and producing the distinctions of number (noun plural), case and gender (personal pronouns); tense, aspect, and mood (verbs); and comparison (adjectives). They may also have trouble interpreting the meaning and functions of derived nouns, adverbs, and the like and using them in sentences. Their problems suggest that they do not learn the word formation rules at the same rate and with the same consistency and degree of sophistication as children with normal language development. School-aged children with normal language development seem to acquire these rules incidentally and effortlessly and learn to apply them in speaking, reading, and writing.

Investigations of language-learning disabled and mentally retarded children indicate rather consistently that they may show delays in the acquisition of word formation rules (Golick, 1976; Johnston & Schery, 1976; Newfield & Schlanger, 1968; Vogel, 1974, 1977; Wiig, Semel, & Crouse, 1973). All these studies report that children with language-learning disabilities, dyslexia, reading retardation, mild mental retardation, and severe language disorders show significant delays in the acquisition of morphological rules when compared with their age peers with normal language development. They further report that the delays are quantitative and can be explained on the basis of the normal order of acquisition of the word formation rules.

Phonological condi-
tioning is the process
by which the choice
of inflectional word
endings is governed
by the nature of the
final speech sound in
the immediately pre-
ceding word.

The major difficulties experienced by all the children with learning disabilities occurred in acquiring the **phonological conditioning** rules for the -*ez* and -*ed* variations of the inflectional word endings. The studies show that the ability to use three word formation rule categories is most useful in identifying these children. They are the rules for forming noun plurals ending in /əz/, noun possessives singular ending in /əz/, and past tense of regular verbs ending in /əd/.

Deficits in the Knowledge of Sentence Formation Rules (Syntax)

Along with difficulties in semantics and morphology, language handicapped children may have significant problems in learning and using the rules for forming sentences. The nature and extent of these problems may vary. Disorders of formulation and syntax vary in nature and severity. In some instances the greatest problem is in **ideation** and productivity, while in others it is primarily syntactical. In the majority, however, both are present (Johnson & Myklebust, 1967, p. 228).

Ideation refers to the
process of forming
ideas, thoughts, or
images.

Again we see a remarkable consistency when the findings are compared across investigations. All studies of learning disabled children's use of syntactical rules showed that the delays in the acquisition of sentence structure and transformation rules follow a pattern of normal syntax acquisition. They also suggest that these children have trouble learning sentence transformations like the passive in which the usual order of presentation of agent-action-object is altered, interrupted, or reversed. These delays are reflected in both interpreting spoken language and formulating sentences. Again, the syntactic deficits persist into adolescence and young adulthood if they remain untreated (Wiig & Semel, 1976, 1980).

Many children with learning-language disabilities have increasing difficulty understanding, remembering, and using sentences as they become more and more structurally complex and involve syntactic compression. They may have problems in interpreting as well as in producing *wh*- questions, sentences with demonstrative pronouns ("this," "that," "these," "those"), passive sentences, sentences with indirect-direct object transformation, and sentences with embedded clauses such as noun complements and relative clauses. Let us look at their problems in more detail.

Embedded refers to
the quality of a word,
phrase, or clause
being placed within
an existing sentence
as in placing a relative
clause between the
subject and object of
an existing sentence.

When adolescents with language-learning disabilities were asked to repeat sentences with various complex structural features, a pattern of errors emerged. They were significantly poorer than their age peers who were academic achievers in recalling and repeating sentences with strings of modifying adjectives, as in "He has sold the long, heavy, grey, shiny car." They also had significant problems recalling sentences with embedded clauses, such as "The burglar that the police found escaped easily." Their greatest difficulties occurred, however, when sentences were syntactically well-formed but violated word selection rules, as in "Colorless green ideas sleep furiously," or when they contained a random word string, as in "Not in a tree to the lake ran with." The findings suggest that consistency and predictability of word meanings facilitate sentence recall, while inconsistencies or unexpected word choices present a barrier to the memory for sentence structure.

When language-learning disabled adolescents were asked to create sentences, they also showed syntactic delays. On a sentence formulation task which required them to use a given word in a sentence, they produced agrammatical and incomplete sentences. Their sentences tended to be simple, active, affirmative, and declarative. They used an agent-action-object sequence which is typical for younger children (age 7 to 8) and did not use sentence transformations used by academic achievers of their own age.

In a recent investigation, Wiig, Semel, and Abele (1981) evaluated the ability of 12-year-olds with learning disabilities to resolve sentences with two meanings caused by structural features. The results showed that these children

TABLE 9.2

Sentence Imitation Patterns among Children and Adolescents with Language Disorders or Learning Disabilities.

Error Pattern	Stimulus Sentence	Sample Repetition
Omission of words and phrases at the end, middle, and sometimes beginning of sentences	Jack likes hamburgers with relish, mustard, and ketchup.	Jack likes hamburgers. Jack likes hamburgers with ketchup.
Reversal of word sequences, often multiple	Jack likes hamburgers with ketchup.	Jack likes ketchup with hamburgers.
Omission of words in word sequences	The woman carried the twelve old, heavy brown books.	The woman carried twelve old books.
Substitution of related words in word sequences	Jack likes french fries and hamburgers with relish and ketchup.	Jack likes <u>hot-dogs</u> and hamburgers with <u>beans</u> and ketchup.
Omission of embedded clauses	The robber <u>that the police caught</u> escaped easily.	The robber escaped easily.
Reversals and omission of parts of a main clause when there is embedding	The robber that the police caught <u>escaped easily</u>.	That is the robber the police caught.
Omission of noun plural, possessive, and third person present tense word endings	Jack likes hamburgers with mustard and onions.	Jack like<u>_</u> hamburger<u>_</u> with mustard and onion<u>_</u>.
Substitution of function words and prepositions	Jack likes hamburgers with mustard and relish.	Jack likes hamburgers <u>and</u> mustard <u>or</u> relish.
Omission of unfamiliar words and word sequences	Pale luminous feelings blithely painted the ocean.	Pale is the ocean with . . . (I forgot).
Substitution of unfamiliar words and word sequences by familiar ones	The sky that the dream thought jumped cheaply.	The <u>cow</u> that the <u>man saw jumped</u> quickly.
Substitution of similar sounding words for unfamiliar ones	Pale luminous feelings blithely painted the ocean.	Pale <u>lucient failing</u> pilely licken.

performed significantly poorer than did their academically achieving age peers. When their performances on the task were compared to performances by 7- and 8- and 5- and 6-year old academic achievers, they were similar to those of the younger group. When the responses to the structurally ambiguous sentences such as "She told her baby stories" and "The duck is ready to eat" were analyzed, a pattern emerged. The adolescents' preferred or only interpretations of these sentences followed the rule that the first noun was the agent, followed by the action stated in the verb, and then followed by the

Tables 9.2, 9.3, and 9.4 present selected problems in imitating sen-

TABLE 9.3
Sentence Interpretation Patterns among Children and Adolescents with Learning Disabilities.

Error Pattern	Sentence Type	Sample Interpretation
Passives interpreted with the first noun as agent, verb as action, second noun as direct object (agent-action-object)	The train was hit by the car.	The train hit the car.
Indirect object followed by direct object is interpreted as direct and then indirect object	The mother showed the girl the baby.	The mother showed the girl to the baby.
In a noun-verb-noun-verb sequence, each noun interpreted as the agent of the action stated next	Jerry promised Susan to water the flowers.	Jerry promised and Susan was going to water the flowers.
The first noun in an ambiguous sentence is interpreted as the agent	The duck was ready to eat. Visiting relatives can be a nuisance.	The duck was about to eat. When relatives come to you, it can be a nuisance.

TABLE 9.4
Sentence Formulation Patterns among Children and Adolescents with Language Disorders and Learning Disabilities.

Error Pattern	Sample Utterance
Omission of articles	They came back into house. And then sheriff tries to calm her down.
Omission of subjects, objects, and verb phrases	The chair was broken, [. . .] went to their bedroom. Then she took [. . .] and went outside. Three little bears [. . .] in the house. And then her came back and she [. . .] turn.
Inconsistency in verb tenses	And then all she does is she drank the wine sauce. Yesterday I builded a plane and tomorrow I finished it.
Inconsistency in personal pronoun use (gender, case, number)	The needles made him feel tired and made him stomach feel so bad. And then the girl took his [her] hat and went home.
Inconsistency in forming reflexive pronouns	And then he washed hisself. The people saw theirselves.
Inconsistency in forming past tense of irregular verbs	And then he ringed the bell. The daddy wroted the teacher.
Inconsistency in selecting and forming relative pronouns	The boy which is my friend is at school. The girl whoses leg is broken is my friend.
Failure to complete a sentence, often with conjunction	After the ball game, you see [. . .]. If you go, you see. And before the boy, you see, we had turkey for Thanksgiving.

object (agent-action-object strategy). They had not as a group acquired an alternative strategy for interpreting sentences in which the first noun may function as either the agent or the object of an action, depending upon the meaning of the sentence.

tence structure, interpreting spoken sentences, and formulating spoken sentences, respectively.

Word-Finding Difficulties

Johnson and Myklebust (1967) first called attention to problems in word finding of children with learning disabilities. They named these difficulties *dysnomia* and described the problem as being "a deficit primarily in **reauditorization** and word selection" (p. 114). They also said that children with dysnomia understand and recognize the intended word, but they are unable to retrieve the intended word on command. These children may resort to gestures that can be highly descriptive and dramatic when they search for a word. In rapid conversation, the recurring search for specific words often results in characteristic speech patterns.

Reauditorization refers to the process of reconstructing or rehearsing digits, words, phrases, or sentences you have heard to yourself, as "in your head."

Table 9.5 summarizes some of these characteristics.

Recent studies have shown a renewed interest in the prevalence and characteristics of word-finding problems among children and adolescents with learning disabilities. Denckla and Rudel (1976) report evidence of dysnomia among children ranging in age from 8 to 10 years with diagnosed dyslexia. They analyzed and compared the word substitution errors and error categories and compared response delays of dyslexic and nondyslexic children. Children with dyslexia used **circumlocutions** in the form of descriptive definitions, such as calling a "stethoscope" a "thing which the doctor uses to listen to your heart," when they could not find a word. They also substituted words in picture naming. The word substitutions were predictable. They were related by association or by similarities in the speech sound or phonemic structure to the intended words. The word-finding problems seen in children with dyslexia and learning disabilities have also been seen among adolescents with untreated language-learning disabilities (Wiig, et al., 1977; Wiig & Semel, 1975). When adolescents with diagnosed learning disabilities were asked to name pictured objects, actions, and attributes on visual confrontation, they made word substitution errors. Their word substitutions were related to the intended word by association.

Circumlocution refers to a "round-about" way of speaking when a person cannot find a specific word for an object, action, event, or attribute, as in calling a brush "that thing you use to fix your hair with."

German (1979) explored the variables, word frequency, and stimulus context which influenced ease and difficulty of word finding in 8- to 11-year-old children with learning disabilities. Her findings indicate that a significant proportion of these children (43%) had word-finding difficulties with relatively low frequency words. Word-finding errors were prevalent on tasks involving open-ended questions and naming in response to verbal description. But with words of relatively high frequency, the learning disabled children performed similarly to academic achievers.

In a related study of the same children, German (in press) looked into the nature of the word-finding errors. The results showed that the children with learning disabilities used three significant word substitution patterns. The strongest pattern was one in which an intended word was substituted by a word of less complexity in meaning and with a greater range of application, as in calling a "rein" a "string." The second strongest pattern was one in which an intended word was substituted by a functionally descriptive word, as in calling a "shelf" a "bookholder." The third and weakest pattern was one in which the initial sounds of a word substitution were said and discarded, followed by accurate naming—as if to aid in the search. This pattern resulted in calling, for example, a "comb" a "br-, br-, comb."

TABLE 9.5

Idiosyncratic Language Expression Patterns among Learning Disabled Children and Adolescents. (From E. H. Wiig & E. M. Semel, *Language Assessment and Intervention for the Learning Disabled.* Columbus, Ohio: Charles E. Merrill, 1980. Copyright © 1980 by Bell & Howell Company. Used by permission.)

Error Pattern	Characteristic Expressions	Sample Utterances
Prolonged pauses	pause	I went to (pause) the store to buy (pause) some (pause) delicious (pause) something.
Semantically empty place holders	uh, uhm, err, ah, well . . .	I err ah went to err ah the uhm store to buy uh some err delicious well err something.
Stereotyped phrases	whatcha'ma call it, you know, you see . . .	You see, I went to the whatcha'ma call it store to buy that thing, you know.
Starters	and, then, and then, now, well, etc., used to begin sentences, phrases, and clauses	And then I went to the store and then I bought something well that was delicious.
Indefinites	this, that, something, somewhere . .	Somehow, I went to this place somewhere to buy something delicious.
Circumlocutions	descriptions rather than labels such as "things you can eat/drink/play with," etc.	I went to this place where you can buy things to eat and I bought something to eat that tasted delicious.
Words lacking specificity	thing, junk, stuff, place . . .	I went to this place to buy some stuff and I got some junk that tasted delicious.
Imprecise and restrictive verb use	got, made, put . . .	I got the fish. (caught) I made the dress. (sewed) I put the bulbs near the tree. (planted)
Borrowed word formations	invented or extended word use	I got volcano craters all over. (chicken pox)
Redundant repetitions of assertive phrases	I'm confident/positive/sure, He said so, He told me . . . , etc.	I'm confident, I'm sure he will come. He told me so. He said he will come.
Perseverative repetitions	repetitions of sounds, syllables, words, phrases, clauses, or ideas	I'm going to have cream, ice cream, vanilla ice cream.
Borrowing of words	use of words, often slang, which are appropriate in other contexts	The baby is all topsy turbie. (fell down)
Substitution of prefixes and suffixes	*dis-* for *un-*, *-ness* for *-ly*, *pro-* for *anti-* . . .	They did a lot of propollution demonstrations. (antipollution)

White (1979) explored the prevalence and characteristics of dysnomia in two groups of adolescents with reading retardation and with early, temporary delays in reading. Adolescents with dyslexia made three times as many verbal descriptions (circumlocutions) and word association errors on a picture-naming task than did academic achievers of the same age. A disorder syndrome emerged among adolescents with dyslexia. Dysnomia combined with sentence recall and repetition difficulties was observed in about half the group. Dysnomia in isolation existed in only one of the 25 adolescents with learning disabilities. Difficulties in sentence recall and repetition without associated dysnomia existed in about ¼ of the group.

Limited Fluency in Word Recall

The ease with which a person can produce several verbal responses varied in word, phrase, and sentence selections indicates the fluency and flexibility with which the person produces language. We can identify several abilities that contribute to facility and diversity in language use. Verbal fluency is a contributing ability. It is reflected in ready availability of a variety of words to describe any context or event. In educational and academic activities, verbal fluency in language formulation and production are rewarded in such subject areas as English composition, history, and social studies.

Language-learning disabled children often lack verbal fluency when asked to perform on selected language tasks (Bannatyne, 1971; Johnson & Myklebust, 1967; Lerner, 1971; Wiig & Semel, 1975, 1976, 1980). Their responses to word association tasks often show that they shift from one word group to another, almost randomly, in their efforts to find related words. They do not use efficient grouping or clustering strategies for word finding and production.

Language-learning disabled children use significantly fewer word associations on controlled association tasks for naming foods, animals, and toys than academic achievers of the same age and background. Their responses to the word association tasks indicate that they name foods and animals more or less at random; they do not name first one subcategory of foods or animals and then another in an effort to facilitate recall. These adolescents also gave immediate or delayed repetitions of already named foods or animals. In contrast, the academic achievers named foods, animals, and toys in obvious subgroups; and they did not repeat already named items within a category.

When asked to recall a list of words, children with learning disabilities seem to be unaffected by the original organization of words on the lists (Freston & Drew, 1974; Parker, Freston, & Drew, 1975). Instead, their recall of the words in the list is determined by the relative frequency of the words in ordinary use. Academic achievers, in contrast, recalled words in a list significantly better when the words were organized according to conceptual category, such as flowers, foods, and geometric forms. They took advantage of the previous organization of the input to aid their recall. Similar observations have been made of children and adolescents with borderline and mild to moderate mental retardation (Bilsky, Evans, & Gilbert, 1972; Evans, 1977; Spitz, 1966).

These limitations in verbal fluency may negatively influence both academic achievement and interpersonal interactions. Students with language handicaps may not be able to reflect their knowledge readily and adequately when asked. They may have problems communicating their feelings, attitudes, and intentions in social interactions. These limitations may present a barrier to full self-realization in educational and vocational achievement as well as in social and sexual interactions.

LANGUAGE PROBLEMS AND THE CURRICULUM

The demands of the traditional curriculum change considerably during the elementary and secondary school years. Early childhood curricula use teaching strategies which allow for multisensory experiences and emphasize language development and social-emotional growth in the child. The child is exposed to a variety of activities designed to develop academic readiness for reading and writing. The materials used in the classroom tend to be manipulative, three-dimensional, concrete, and already familiar to the child.

During the early elementary grades (K, 1, and 2), the focus of the curriculum shifts. It is now designed to provide opportunities for the child to develop basic skills in reading, spelling, writing, and arithmetic. The teaching materials now tend to feature pictures and more abstract, symbolic representations.

During the middle grades (3 and 4), the demands on language increase drastically. The emphasis in teaching shifts to include content areas such as social studies, beginning science, mathematics, and health education. The basic skills are reviewed, but they are no longer taught. Instead, the curriculum focuses on developing reasoning skills in the child. Towards the end of the middle grades, language becomes the major vehicle for teaching. Materials are more abstract and symbolic, and the child's performances are expected to reflect the ability to learn from read and spoken language input. There is also a heavier demand on the children to express themselves in written language. Children are asked to give spoken reports in the classroom. The reading materials feature vocabulary that is often unfamiliar, and the children must understand and learn new words on the basis of reading. The sentences in

FIGURE 9.1

Primary Emphasis on Basic Skills and Content Areas in the Traditional Curriculum. (From E. H. Wiig & E. M. Semel, *Language Assessment and Intervention for the Learning Disabled.* Columbus, Ohio: Charles E. Merrill, 1980. Copyright © 1980 by Bell & Howell Company. Used by permission.)

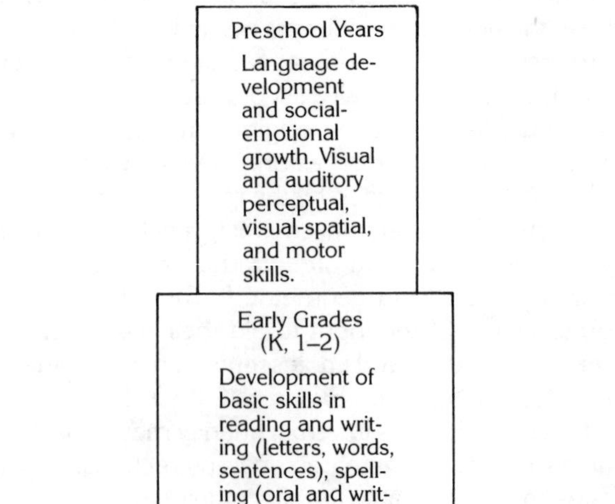

Preschool Years
Language development and social-emotional growth. Visual and auditory perceptual, visual-spatial, and motor skills.

Early Grades (K, 1–2)
Development of basic skills in reading and writing (letters, words, sentences), spelling (oral and written), and arithmetic

Middle Grades (3–4)
Review of basic skills and introduction of content areas such as English, social studies, mathematics, and science

Upper Grades (5–6)
Emphasis on acquisition of knowledge in content areas, including English, social studies, science, and mathematics

Junior and Senior High
Expansion of the content areas with emphasis on English (composition, literature, language arts, and study skills), social studies (American and world history, economics), foreign languages (French, Spanish, Latin), science (biology, chemistry, physics), mathematics (algebra, geometry), and vocational education

reading materials are also more complex and place demands on knowledge of sentence structure. Understanding and recall of meaning and of details becomes critical in reading, and the basic reading skills are assumed to have become automatic.

The traditional curriculum in the upper elementary grades (5 and 6) provides an even greater emphasis on language and on content. The youngsters are expected to be accurate and fluent in using basic academic skills and in remembering the content learned in the earlier grades. The curriculum now focuses on developing the strategies needed for more advanced problem solving. The language demands of the curriculum assume mature and efficient use of vocabulary and sentence structure and accurate and efficient formulation of language in speaking and writing.

The gradual change in the traditional curriculum from emphasizing basic skills during the preschool years and early grades to focussing on content areas in junior and senior high is illustrated in Figure 9.1.

Children with normal language development have all the prerequisites for a successful transfer of language skills from spoken language to the language of reading and writing. They also have the potential for rewarding communications with their peers and teachers in learning as well as in social settings. By comparison, children with language and communication delays or disorders show significant limitations in the language skills which are prerequisites for the traditional curriculum. We shall now take a look at the skills required for learning to read and spell.

Learning to Read and Spell

Reading is a complex skill. It requires the ability to recognize, recall, and differentiate letters and printed words as well as to match and remember the matches between written letters and letter sequences and their spoken sound or word counterparts. In addition, it requires the ability to relate a printed word or word sequence (sentences and paragraphs) to an accurate meaning base. As reading materials become more advanced, the ability to recognize and interpret various sentence forms and sentence transformations assumes an ever more important role.

As children learn to become proficient readers, they must interact with the reading materials. They cannot simply be passive. They must anticipate what is to follow and generate tentative hypotheses about what they are going to read next. These hypotheses must constantly be verified or rejected by comparison with the actual text.

The process of learning to read can be viewed as a process of learning to superimpose an already-known spoken language code on a new, secondary, visual symbol code. Proficiency in reading can only be acquired when the reader applies all of the normal knowledge of language and all of the normal language experiences to the process (Goodman, 1969).

Learning to spell can be viewed as a process of learning to superimpose the already-known code for speech sound and word meanings on the visual symbol system represented by printed letters and words (Chomsky, 1970). Spelling requires stable associations between printed letters and their speech sound counterparts. It also requires recognition and recall of variations of the expected correspondence between sounds and letters in words. Proficient spelling of words and word sequences depends on the ability to recognize and remember the spelling patterns for basic lexical units or words and to apply them to the various forms of a word in different contexts.

It should not be surprising that children with speech or language disorders may have trouble learning to read and spell. We can expect at least $\frac{1}{3}$ of all children with early speech and language delays to show reading and spelling difficulties in the early grades (Ingram, 1970; Mason, 1976). Among children with severe language and communication disorders and those who are non-verbal at age 3, the proportion of children with reading and spelling delays can be expected to be much larger.

CAUSES OF LANGUAGE-LEARNING DISABILITIES AND RETARDATION

In chapter 8 we looked at some of the possible causes of mental retardation and language disorders in young children. You may wish to review that discussion. At this point, we need only take a brief look at some more research on the causes of learning disabilities.

Language and learning disabilities are often implicitly assumed to be caused by neurological and physiological factors (Cruickshank, 1966; Kephart, 1971; Strauss & Lehtinen, 1947). This assumption is reflected in the various terms used to describe a learning disability, including *minimal brain dysfunction* (MBD) and *brain injury*. These terms imply that the learning disability results from organic causes. In particular, the term *brain injury* implies that an otherwise structurally normal brain has been damaged. This damage may occur before birth, during the birth process, or after birth. Pre-natal conditions that can cause brain damage in the fetus include poor nutrition, intoxication, other toxins (lead or mercury), and prenatal trauma. Early or prolonged labor causing **anoxia** and childhood diseases and head trauma may also cause brain damage.

Anoxia is a condition in which the oxygen supply to the brain is interrupted or inadequate.

Maturational or developmental lags which affect the development of essential functional areas or connecting pathways of the brain have also been cited as causes of learning disabilities (Bender, 1968). Recently, an in-depth post mortem study of the brain of a 20-year-old man with dyslexia received national attention (Galaburda & Kemper, 1979). The examining neurologists found distortions in the architecture of the left temporal lobe, which is the primary area for auditory language processing and association. They found "islands" of primitive and abnormally large *cortical* cells in clumps of misshapen layers of tissue. There was also an unusually high number of connecting fibers from the left temporal lobe. Finally, the primary language area in the left temporal lobe was of equal size to the corresponding area in the right temporal lobe, where the left temporal lobe is normally larger than the right. Thus, the possibility of structural-developmental causes of learning problems remains open.

Cortex is the outer layer of gray matter which covers most of the brain. Review chapter 4 for details on the parts of the brain.

Genetic and hereditary causes for language and learning disabilities must also be considered. The parent-offspring study of cognitive abilities cited in chapter 8 (DeFries, et al., 1976) suggests that verbal and spatial abilities follow a pattern of hereditability. Several studies of hereditary patterns among twins and among families of dyslexics and disabled readers also suggest that certain types of specific learning disabilities may be determined hereditarily (Finucci, Guthrie, Childs, Abbey, & Childs, 1976; Hallgren, 1950; Hermann, 1959; McGlannan, 1968; Owen, 1971).

Summarizing the studies of potential causes of language-learning disabilities, we must conclude that several causes are possible. In addition, several of the causal factors may combine. For instance, we can ask whether genetic or pre- or postnatal factors caused the structural abnormalities observed by Galaburda and Kemper (1979). We can also ask whether the familial patterns reported by McGlannan (1968) caused the disability or occurred together with structural deviations of the brain. As we saw in chapter 8, it is difficult to distinguish between causes and correlates of learning disabilities. However, there is enough evidence of a connection between learning disabilities and physical causes to suggest that the language-learning disabled youngster should be evaluated by medical specialists as part of an in-depth educational assessment.

ASSESSMENT OF LANGUAGE DISABILITIES

Language Screening

If possible, every child who enters the elementary grades should be screened for potential language disabilities. At the very least, all children suspected to be at risk for language disabilities or referred by teachers, parents, physicians, or other specialists should be screened. In addition, children who have problems in learning to read, spell, or write in the early grades should be referred for screening.

There are other critical stages in the educational process when children at risk for language disabilities should be evaluated at least briefly. Critical points in the educational process occur at the transitions from grade 3 to grade 4, from elementary school to junior high, and from junior high to senior high school.

One of several language screeing tests may be used to identify school-aged children with potential language disabilities (Bankson, 1977; Semel & Wiig, 1980b). The *Bankson Language Screening Test* (Bankson, 1977) probes language and visual processes or skill areas. The test contains 153 items grouped into five parts for semantic knowledge, morphological and syntactic rules, visual perception, and auditory perception.

The *Clinical Evaluation of Language Functions (CELF)* (Semel & Wiig, 1980b) *Screening Tests* were designed to probe aspects of language comprehension and expression at two grade ranges. The Elementary Level covers grades K to 5. It contains 48 items grouped in two sections on the basis of response mode. The first section of items uses a "Simon says . . ." format and requires motor action responses. The second section requires verbal responses to various requests. The Advanced Level covers grades 5 to 12. It contains 52 items in two sections. The first section uses a playing card identification format, and the second section requires verbal responses to various requests.

Diagnosis of Strengths and Weaknesses

Although the term *diagnosis* is somewhat imprecise, as we have seen, it most often refers to the process of identifying a child's strengths or weaknesses in a given ability or range of skills. It should also cover the youngster's own view of the language and communication problems and of his or her personal reactions and interaction styles. Another critical consideration is dialect; for example, what seem to be wide-ranging problems with using word endings may be dialectal variations. The second step in the diagnosis process, to obtain reliable, valid, objective, and measurable information about the youngster's language and communication abilities and behaviors, may be carried out by using formal language tests and informal test probes to determine the variables that control a specific language or communication behavior. Among variables of interest to the speech-language pathologist may be the relative level of complexity of the language input or language and communication responses required.

The approach used in the diagnosis of students' language disabilities will depend in part upon the diagnostician's views of the nature of language disabilities and of appropriate intervention approaches and strategies. We can identify several major approaches to the assessment of language and communication disorders in school-aged children. These approaches differ in the measures, procedures, and methods used to answer diagnostic questions as well as in their basic objectives. Four major approaches are commonly used:

(1) Diagnostic-prescriptive approaches (process or task analysis)
(2) Behavior-learning approaches
(3) Interactive-interpersonal (*pragmatic*) approaches
(4) Total environmental system approaches.

Diagnostic-Prescriptive Approaches

The diagnostic-prescriptive approaches to the assessment of language disabilities evaluate the language behavioral characteristics of either the child or the language inputs or tasks. That is, they identify a child's strength or weaknesses in a given language process, area, or skill. On the basis of the outcome of this evaluation, a decision is made whether or not the child needs language intervention or remediation and in which areas remediation is needed. Within the diagnostic-prescriptive approaches to language assessment, we can identify two different models: (*a*) a process or ability model and (*b*) a task-analysis model.

The Process or Ability Model   This model attempts to probe and differentiate functions and processes that are assumed to support or control the normal acquisition and use of language skills. The model is commonly applied in the assessment of language and learning disabilities in older children and adolescents. It is based on the assumption that a general or specific maturational or developmental lag or a neurological dysfunction will result in identifiable language disability syndromes or groups of deficits. The processes and functions that are sometimes evaluated include perceptual (auditory or visual), cognitive, memory, and neuropsychological or "psycholinguistic" processes or abilities. The evaluation may probe one or more of the abilities involved in perceiving and discriminating speech, interpreting spoken language, and formulating language for communication. The evaluation may be extended to include short- and long-term memory, verbal and nonverbal reasoning, word-finding and retrieval, and visual and motor processes involved in reading, speaking, and writing.

The Task Analysis Model   In this model, the characteristics of speech, language, and communication tasks (either stimuli or responses) are the focus of evaluation. The objective is to determine what kinds of tasks either facilitate or cause a breakdown of performances.

When this model is applied to an evaluation of language and communication disorders, the task analysis is often based on linguistic principles. The analysis often identifies the relative complexity and degree of difficulty of the spoken language stimuli and language responses. The analysis may consider the morphological structure, the syntactic structure, or the pragmatic functions.

Diagnostic Tests   Among diagnostic-prescriptive tests appropriate for school-aged children, we shall focus on commonly used test batteries. The *Illinois Test of Psycholinguistic Abilities (ITPA)* (Kirk, McCarthy, & Kirk, 1968) is based on a two-dimensional model of language and communication proposed by Osgood (1957). This model was expanded to form the basis for the *ITPA* to feature three rather than two dimensions. The three dimensions featured in the *ITPA* are (*a*) levels of organization (automatic or representational), (*b*) channels of communication (auditory vocal/motor or visual vocal/motor), and (*c*) psychological processes (reception, association, and expression). The *ITPA* contains 12 subtests, 7 of which evaluate various aspects of language such as sentence completion with appropriate word formations (morphology) and with associated words (auditory association). The remaining subtests probe visually based processes. The *ITPA* has been widely used in both educational and clinical settings and has been the object of a wide range of research. This research has related deficit patterns to diagnostic categories such as mental retardation and learning disabilities.

The *Detroit Tests of Learning Aptitude (DTLA)* (Baker & Leland, 1967) feature a modalities approach to the assessment of auditory and visual processes. Among auditory processes probed by subtests of the *DTLA* are auditory memory for words and sentences, word knowledge for antonyms, and knowledge of shared and different meanings of paired words. The *DTLA* has been widely used in educational settings. It has been standardized for age levels up to 19 years. Unfortunately, the age norms were gathered in the 1950s in urban Detroit, and they may not reflect today's youngsters.

The *Test of Language Development (TOLD)* (Newcomer & Hammill, 1977) features a linguistically based model for the evaluation of language abilities. It contains eight subtests. Two subtests each probe receptive and expressive language abilities at the levels of speech sounds (phonology), word formation (morphology), sentence structure (syntax), and word meaning (semantics).

The *Clinical Evaluation of Language Functions (CELF)* (Semel & Wiig, 1980a) is a relative newcomer to the field of language testing. It contains 11 major and 2 supplementary language subtests or probes. Three subtests feature controlled sentence structures and sentence transformations in comprehension, repetition, and sentence formulation tasks. Several of the subtests probe various aspects of word meanings, word relations, and word associations. Subtests are also included which probe rapid naming abilities and recall of oral directions and of details in spoken paragraphs. Each of the *CELF* subtests provides item-by-item analysis of the contents to allow identification of patterns in the error responses. Formal and informal methods and tasks for extension testing are also discussed for each subtest to allow the speech-language pathologist to identify the language variables which either facilitate or present a barrier to accurate responses. The *CELF* is criterion-referenced.

Behavior-Learning Approaches

The objectives of this approach are to identify the stimulus-response reinforcement relationships in language and communication behaviors and to determine the relative frequencies and probabilities of the occurrence of specific behaviors. It is often applied in evaluating the effects of word-finding difficulties on the spontaneous use of language. One objective of assessment within this context would be to obtain reliable measures of the frequency of word substitutions, pauses while searching for an intended word, functional

See Table 9.1.

descriptions rather than labels for nouns, and other characteristics of word-finding difficulties. A second objective might be to obtain reliable measures of the rate of speaking and the duration of pauses when word-finding difficulties occur during spontaneous speech. A third objective might be to determine the situations during which the word-finding difficulties either increase or decrease.

To obtain some of the behavioral measures, the speech-language pathologist may need to use electronic equipment. Equipment is available which provides a cumulative account of syllables and words spoken, duration of pauses, and elapsed speaking time. Different reading and speaking tasks may be assigned in order to determine if any changes occur in the frequency and time measures as a function of either tasks or communication contexts. The behavioral data obtained from the assessment may be used as a baseline for intervention and for future assessment of progress. With this approach, intervention will usually use the same techniques as assessment.

Interactive-Interpersonal (Pragmatic) Approaches

This approach seeks to assess aspects of the student's ability to communicate effectively in a variety of social and interpersonal communication contexts. The objective is to assess the relationships among spoken messages, the contexts in which they occur, and the interpreters of the messages (Morris, 1938). The focus is on identifying the child's existing strengths and weaknesses as a speaker.

The communicative competence of the child is judged in relation to his or her effectiveness in realizing one or more of the functions of language. These functions include (*a*) controlling (persuading, dissuading, justifying, and the like), (*b*) informing (questions, statements, justifications, and the like), (*c*) expressing (exclamation, approval, rejection, and the like), (*d*) ritualizing (greeting, calling, turn-taking), and (*e*) imagining (commentary, explaining, story-telling, and so on) (Wells, 1974).

A variety of formats may be used in interactive-interpersonal assessment of communication disorders. In one common format, called *descriptive communication* tasks (Glucksberg, et al., 1966), the child describes objects, pictures, or events. Informal and formal discourse may also be used in assessment. The objectives may be to evaluate whether the child knows the rules for conversation and responds appropriately to *wh-* question probes. Role playing may also be used to assess how effective the child is in informing, controlling, ritualizing, or expressing feelings or in shifting style to meet the needs of various listeners (such as peers, adults, and younger children). The child may also be assessed in a structured activity such as telling a story.

Methods of analyses to meet these objectives in language evaluation have been discussed by, among others, Hymes (1972), Labov (1972), Sabsay (1979), and Ure and Ellis (1977).

Total Environmental System Approach

The total environmental system approach to language evaluation for the school-aged child may combine the process, task analysis, and interpersonal-interactive approaches. It also seeks to assess what happens when the child with a language disability applies his or her oral language abilities to the academic processes of reading, spelling, writing, and gaining information from classroom and textbook instruction. It evaluates and considers the student's needs for adaptation and enhancement of language components of the curriculum and instruction. It integrates an evaluation of verbal language skills with an appraisal of nonverbal communication skills. This approach also takes into account the child's feelings and adaptive or nonadaptive reactions to language-based formal tasks and to interpersonal and social communication contexts, and determines the need for counseling at various stages of development. Finally, it considers the quality of the reactions of other significant individuals—parents, siblings, peers, and teachers—to the child's language and communication efforts in order to assess counseling needs.

The total environmental system approach to language evaluation can only be implemented by team effort. It requires the contributions of a variety of specialists, such as reading and math specialists, vocational counselors, guidance counselors, and psychologists. To be successful, all members of the team must be conscious of the contributions of language to academic achievement and formal learning and to psychosocial adjustment and growth.

Extension Testing

Extension testing, which often follows formal diagnosis, explores in more depth the variables which seem to be primary in contributing to the child's errors. Errors in either responding to spoken language or formulating messages may result from a single variable or combination of variables such as the complexity of the task, directions, instructions, contents, or the mode of the response. By systematically varying tasks, contents, or responses required, the speech-language pathologist can evaluate the child's performances to observe when a breakdown occurs. The speech-language pathologist can (a) reduce the complexity of an oral command, (b) reduce the number of words, phrases, or clauses in spoken sentences, (c) increase the familiarity of the word choices in spoken sentences, (d) change the sentence structure, (e) ask for a pointing rather than a spoken response, and (f) change from a spoken sentence input to a printed sentence input, to mention only a few examples.

In effect, extension testing is used to establish a baseline at which the youngster can respond correctly. It also helps identify the required adaptations of language demands and the possible ways in which language can be enhanced to facilitate classroom success.

Intervention-Based Assessment

Once we have a clear picture of the child's baseline performance, it is time to set goals and choose targets for intervention. As the intervention program proceeds, it is important to monitor the child's progress regularly. If the child's language performances do not improve in response to intervention, it is difficult to justify the use of specific strategies or materials. When the student does not show definite improvement, the speech-language pathologist may have to consider a change of therapists, intervention objectives, sequences, strategies, or materials or a change to develop compensatory strategies which will minimize the effects of the language disability.

LANGUAGE INTERVENTION AND REMEDIATION

Approaches to the intervention and remediation of language disabilities fall into the same categories as the approaches to language assessment. In most cases, the speech-language pathologist will use intervention techniques that correspond to the assessment techniques chosen.

Process (Ability) and Task Analysis Approaches

One of the objectives of the process (ability) approaches to language intervention may be to strengthen and normalize processes that are considered basic to normal language acquisition and use. Auditory perception, auditory memory, verbal association, and sentence formulation for verbal expression are among the possible targets of the remediation objectives.

Remediation objectives may be directed towards strengthening the child's language comprehension and use in various activities such as speaking, reading, and writing. The objectives may focus on increasing the level of complexity in meaning, structure, or communicative function (pragmatics). Intervention procedures for these last objectives are often based primarily on linguistic models. Still other approaches to language intervention combine cognitive, linguistic, and other process-oriented approaches (Muma, 1978; Wiig & Semel, 1976, 1980).

Process or task analysis approaches or combinations of the two have been applied widely in educational and clinical settings. We can outline some commonly used principles for intervention in this approach. Although these guidelines exemplify process (ability) and task analysis approaches, some of the principles emphasize behavior-learning principles.

(1) Follow normal developmental sequences and schedules.
   (a) Teach unfamiliar vocabulary and language concepts (semantics) in the order in which they normally develop.
   (b) Teach word formation and sentence structure and transformation rules (morphology and syntax) in the order in which they are normally acquired.
   (c) Emphasize the communication functions (informing, controlling, feeling, ritualizing, and imagining) relevant to the youngster's development and educational and social setting.
   (d) Teach levels of the functions in the order in which they are normally acquired.

(2) Consider principles of learning and reinforcement in carrying out the intervention objectives.

*In **distributed** practice, time intervals intervene between training sessions; in **massed** practice, training sessions are presented with no intervening time between.*

   (a) Provide **distributed** rather than **massed** practice to facilitate retention.
   (b) Provide opportunities for generalization and transfer of acquired skills to curriculum tasks and social contexts.
   (c) Provide positive reinforcement and select appropriate rewards and reward schedules to accelerate learning and facilitate retention.

(3) Arrange early personal success for the student.
   (a) Teach words, sentence structures and transformations, and communication functions that are most important for the child and contribute most to his success in academic or vocational settings or in social and interpersonal interactions.
   (b) Begin with the words, sentence structures and transformations, and communication functions that are easiest to learn on the basis of either length, complexity, or frequency.
   (c) Begin with the words, sentence structures and transformations, and communication functions that are emerging or that the child uses correctly some or most of the time.

(4) Consider the impact of specific language and communication deficits on learning potential, acceptance by others, psychosocial development and adjustment, communication effectiveness, and self-realization.

(a) Begin with vocabulary and language concepts and sentence structures and transformations which contribute the most to the youngster's learning potential and communication effectiveness.
(b) Emphasize the communication functions and levels of the functions which contribute the most to the youngster's acceptance in interactions with peers and adults and contribute the most to overall communicative effectiveness.

Behavior-Learning and Performance-Oriented Approaches

The objectives of behavior- and performance-oriented approaches to language and communication intervention are to modify, decrease, or increase existing language behaviors within a variety of contexts. The modifications are brought about by applying operant conditioning procedures (Hewitt, 1967; Mowrer, 1978).

See page 109 for a definition of operant conditioning.

The emphasis in intervention here is on overt, observable, disordered language and communication behaviors which can be reliably measured. One objective of intervention may be to **extinguish** a specific language or communication behavior considered to be disordered or deviant. In that case, putting the child in a situation where he receives no stimulation or withholding a positive reinforcer after an undesired response may be used to decrease the probability that the response will occur again. Another objective may be to increase the probability that the child will use normal and desirable behaviors that he already uses occasionally. In that case, the speech-language pathologist would reward the child when he performs the desirable language behaviors. Yet another objective might be to modify existing language and communication behaviors to develop an age-appropriate form. In that case, the clinician would shape the desired behavior by reinforcing the child for responses which resemble the target skill. As the child masters an approximation of the target, he is required to move to a closer approximation before he is reinforced again. The speech-language pathologist continues to reinforce successive approximations until the child is able to perform the final target behavior.

Imitation and modeling, as discussed in chapter 8, are techniques often used to get the child to begin to make appropriate responses.

Operant conditioning procedures are often a component of linguistically based language intervention programs. They are also used to modify or extinguish habitual patterns in the spontaneous speech of youngsters with word-finding difficulties. These procedures can be used to modify unacceptable and sometimes maladaptive interpersonal communication behaviors as well. For example, these procedures have been successfully used to modify the negative, aggressive, and rejective language often used by language-learning disabled adolescents.

Interpersonal-Interactive Approaches

The objectives of interpersonal-interactive approaches to language intervention are to strengthen pragmatic abilities and develop communicative competence. Communicative competence has already been discussed in the context of normal language acquisition. A specific objective may be to help the child learn to interpret contextual cues which may modify the meaning of verbal expressions, as in the case of indirect requests such as "Can you open the door?" Other objectives may be to strengthen role-taking and role-playing abilities, develop nonverbal social perception, expand the social register, and increase the range of verbal and nonverbal communication styles available.

Strategies and procedures relevant to an interactive-interpersonal approach to language mediation have been discussed by, among others, Muma (1978), Rees (1978), and Wiig and Semel (1976, 1980).

Total Environmental Systems Approaches

The objective of a total environmental systems approach to language intervention may be to set up events and situations which will set the stage for new language and communication experiences from which communication strategies can be acquired. Like assessment, intervention in this approach assumes the involvement of a team of professionals, all oriented towards language and communication goals. This approach considers the characteristics of the child, the task, the context, and the listener—and the dynamic interactions among them. It also considers the effects which result from differences from child-to-child, listener-to-listener, and context-to-context. This comprehensive approach to language intervention accounts for each individual child's needs for adaptations of language input for learning and interpersonal interactions. It also accounts for the child's strength and potential for compensation for inadequate abilities. Advocates of this approach seek to strengthen adaptive communication strategies to develop insight into the the child's compensatory and coping strategies, and to develop awareness of the dynamics of interpersonal interactions. The ultimate objective is to establish everyday communicative competence to support the child's potential for vocational or professional achievement and for psychosocial and sexual adjustment.

Adaptations refers to the process of changing the characteristics of the language content, structure, or task to match the child's existing abilities or language needs.

Compensation refers to the process of calling adequate abilities or strengths into play to substitute for inadequate abilities or weaknesses.

Counseling issues for the language disabled school-aged child are the focus of the next section.

A total environmental systems approach to language intervention may have to be approached through process or task analysis, behavioral, or interactive-interpersonal language intervention or through an integration of these techniques. An essential component of this approach is counseling of the youngster and of parents, siblings, and other significant individuals.

The choice of any one approach to language intervention and remediation will be determined by several factors. One determining factor is the relative severity and extent of the language and/or learning handicap. Another determining factor is the availability of a team of specialists and the facilities required to implement a given approach. A third factor considered is the motivation of the student and of significant other people in the environment. Any one approach should be chosen not only for its inherent qualities, but also in relation to the people involved.

COUNSELING THE LANGUAGE-LEARNING DISABLED

Children with language and learning disabilities are often recognized by their parents as being "different" (Brutten, Richardson, & Mangel, 1973). The perception of a child as different may result in subtle changes in parent-child interactions and may reduce the quality of the youngster's up-bringing. We can identify common reactions associated with language-learning disabilities. Kindergarten children with learning disabilities have been reported to be immature, poorly socially adjusted, and impulsive. A look at the behavioral and personality problems of learning disabled children in the primary grades reveals a pattern. Among the maladaptive characteristics which have been attributed to these children are aggression, lack of responsibility, poor interpersonal relationships, and disinterested, angry, and hostile reactions and behaviors (Keogh, Tchir, & Windeguth-Behn, 1974).

Clinical observations suggest that the problems of learning disabled youngsters in interpersonal relations and adaptive social behaviors are intensified during puberty and adolescence. The critical contributing factor seems to relate to the increased desire and expectations for social and personal interactions with members of the opposite sex. Learning disabled adolescents may enter into this stage of life with conflicting feelings about themselves. Counseling in association with other approaches to intervention and remediation may help language-learning disabled youngsters learn to accept themselves.

Experiences with counseling learning disabled adolescents and young adults suggest that insight into the nature and implications of verbal and nonverbal language and communication difficulties may have several benefits. It may improve motivation for intervention and mediation. It may also facilitate compensation for specific difficulties and result in the development of adaptive coping strategies. Counseling often relieves the anxieties associated with the remediation process and modifies the secondary emotional reactions to the frustrations of having limitations.

In counseling the language-learning disabled, it is important to allow the youngster to express his feelings—positive or negative— about himself and others. The speech-language pathologist must help the child gradually develop insight into the nature of the disability, the effects of his limitations, and his personal reactions to his difficulties. The counseling process should usually be nondirective. This is not to say that counseling cannot take a directive approach at times. In the directive approach, the specialist would share professional knowledge and experiences with the youngster. The timing of directive counseling is important. Questions should not be anticipated or answered before the child is ready to deal with the professional's views.

Parental and family counseling is also an important means to facilitate personal adjustment and growth of self-esteem in the language-learning disabled. No parent is prepared to raise a child with a disability. Most parents have high expectations when their children enter school, and having to accept the fact that your child does not meet your expectations is not easy. As with other communication disorders, parents frequently feel guilty about the possibility of having caused the disability, either through negligence, heredity, or other involvements. The burden of guilt can be especially grave in families with a history of learning disabilities. Parents of the language-learning disabled may need nondirective counseling to learn to accept and deal with their own feelings, to become aware of their nonsupportive reactions, and to adopt supportive roles in their interactions with their child. Brothers and sisters may have similar guilt feelings and may reject or, at the least, not support the learning disabled child. They may need counseling to gain insight into the nature of the disability and to develop awareness and tolerance of coping strategies so that they can be supportive.

To pull this all together, let us now take a look at the intervention procedures used with an adolescent who was diagnosed rather late to have language-learning disabilities.

Bob—Educational and Clinical Management

When Bob was referred for an in-depth language evaluation, he was 14 years old and in the 8th grade in a suburban public school. His parents were concerned about his academic achievement. His grades in English, reading, and social studies had declined from B's to low C's and D's over a period of about 3½ years. At the time of his referral, Bob's performance on a test of academic achievement placed him about three grades below his actual grade level in reading and spelling. Bob's teachers had recently commented on his classroom performances in rather negative terms. They called his performances "weak," "inconsistent," and "confused," and commented on his learning as a "roller coaster" process. Bob's parents had begun to consider the possibility that Bob's language skills might not be adequate for the academic tasks he faced in his classroom.

The first question that arose in preparation for the language evaluation was whether Bob had received speech or language therapy or special assistance in the early grades, and he had not. Bob's early developmental milestones in motor, speech and language, and social development were reported to have occurred within the expected age ranges. The second question which arose concerned whether estimates of Bob's verbal and nonverbal intellectual capacities and potential indicated performances within the normal range. The results of an assessment of intelligence using the *WISC-R* (Wechsler, 1974) placed Bob's verbal IQ in the average range and his performance IQ in the high average-bright range. His full-scale IQ fell in the average range. More importantly, however, the school psychologist reported a discrepancy of 18 IQ points between the verbal and performance IQs. Areas of relative weaknesses were observed on verbal tasks which probed the recall of general information, stored knowledge, and word knowledge. On a picture completion task, Bob named some missing parts incorrectly and failed to identify some of them, indicating an area of relative weakness.

Several formal tests of language ability were given to Bob. Among them were the *Peabody Picture Vocabulary Test* (Dunn, 1965) and selected subtests of the *Illinois Test of Psycholinguistic Abilities* (Kirk, McCarthy, & Kirk, 1968) and the *Detroit Tests of Learning Aptitude* (Baker & Leland, 1967). These tests were complemented by informal testing of specific language functions and tasks. Silent reading and listening comprehension were assessed using subtests of the *Durrell Analysis of Reading Difficulty* (Durrell, 1955). A spontaneous language sample was obtained and analyzed.

On tests of word knowledge, Bob's ability to perform depended upon the task requirements. When he was asked to match words with pictures (*PPVT*), his performance was only 6 months below age level, within normal limits. When he was asked to tell how two words were alike and then how they were different (*DTLA*), his performance level fell about 2 years below age expectations. When Bob was asked to define words (*DTLA*), his performance level fell about 3½ years below age level. When asked to name word opposites (*DTLA*), the performance level was about 3 years below age level. More importantly, however, Bob's verbal responses to test items provided insight into the quality of his knowledge of components of word meanings. He was better able to tell about shared features or components of meaning in two related words than to tell about nonshared meaning features. When he told how two words differed in meaning, he named either a functional use or an obvious visual difference such as size or color. Bob named essential meaning features only when the words were related to objects or events with which he had great familiarity or experience.

Several subtests were administered to probe Bob's ability to recall spoken words, sentences, and oral directions. The performances on all tests fell well below age-level expectations. Bob's ability to repeat sentences proved relatively best among the performances. His performances fell about 3 years below age level. When asked to repeat a series of unrelated words, Bob's performance was relatively lower, with a 6-year discrepancy between performance age and chronological age. Bob's ability to follow spoken directions also fell about 6 years below age-level expectations. The error patterns on all of the tests of recall of spoken words, sentences, and directions were revealing. In all instances, associative, antonym, or synonym word substitutions appeared to present a barrier to performance. For example, Bob substituted "east" for "south," "nice" for "good," "millions" for "thousands," and "comes" for "passing" when repeating words and sentences. When Bob performed actions in response to oral directions, he consistently substituted spatial and directional words. For example, he substituted "under" for "over," "first" for "last," and "left" for "right." Based on the error pattern, it appeared that Bob had significant word substitution problems on listening tasks and that these problems may be interfering with his performance in school. Informal tests of sentence structure indicated that Bob had acquired the structural rules for complex sentence transformations. Complex sentence transformations were also used in his spontaneous speech sample.

In this case, the most pressing delay seemed to involve the acquisition of adequate word meanings. Bob had a second difficulty in recalling and retrieving words accurately on both formal tasks and in spontaneous speech. These two problems seemed related. On this basis, one of the priority objectives for direct language intervention was to expand Bob's knowledge of meaning components and features for familiar and unfamiliar words. A second objective was to establish an appropriate and consistent meaning base for words relating to space, direction, and time. A third objective was to facilitate accuracy in word recall and word retrieval and in spontaneous speech production.

Several approaches were used in intervention. They included process and task analysis approaches to develop Bob's word knowledge and strengthen his semantic abilities and a process approach to develop word-finding strategies and self-cueing techniques to facilitate speed and accuracy in word finding. Behavior modification was used to modify the now-habitual effects of earlier word-finding problems on his spontaneous speech. Bob was also given descriptive communication and role-playing tasks to improve his communicative competence in a variety of contexts. The carry-over effects to oral and silent reading, reading comprehension, and writing were monitored.

The direct language intervention resulted in gains of about 3 years on tasks of word knowledge after 1 year of intervention. On tasks which required recall of words, sentences, and oral directions, the gains were relatively greater— about 4 years of developmental age equivalence. After a year, Bob was able to use strategies for word finding and self-cueing techniques except when he was under stress in the classroom or when he was interacting with girls. Some but not all of the habitual patterns which had resulted from his word-finding problems were extinguished in his spontaneous speech, but language intervention was continued to reach the objectives in this area. Carry-over to academic tasks was noticed during the year, reflected in improvements in Bob's grades.

The direct language intervention was combined with consultation with the classroom teacher so that she could adapt and enhance the language of the curriculum to meet Bob's needs. It was also combined with counseling for Bob and his parents. The parental counseling revealed that they had a strong pattern of denying Bob's problems. Counseling for both Bob and his parents was continued to deal with the attitudes and behaviors of rejection.

CONCLUSION

In sum, it is never too late to intervene with children with language-learning disabilities. Even if an adolescent has been through a successful course of language intervention as a child, new problems may crop up as the demands for language sophistication increase. The effects of problems on school performance and social interactions can be so wide-ranging that we must be prepared to intervene whenever necessary.

SELECTED READINGS

Benton, A. L., & Pearl, D. *Dyslexia: An appraisal of current knowledge.* New York: Oxford University Press, 1978.

Bryan, T. H., & Bryan, J. H. *Understanding learning disabilities* (2nd ed.). Sherman Oakes, Calif.: Alfred Publishing, 1978.

Haring, N. G., & Bateman, B. *Teaching the learning disabled child.* Englewood Cliffs, N.J.: Prentice-Hall, 1977.

Johnson, D. J., & Myklebust, H. R. *Learning disabilities: Educational principles and practices.* New York: Grune & Stratton, 1967.

MacMillan, D. J. *Mental retardation in school and society.* Boston: Little, Brown, 1977.

Mercer, C. D. *Children and adolescents with learning disabilities.* Columbus, Ohio: Charles E. Merrill, 1979.

Muma, J. R. *Language handbook: Concepts, assessment, intervention.* Englewood Cliffs, N.J.: Prentice-Hall, 1978.

Neisworth, J. T., & Smith, R. M. *Retardation: Issues, assessment, and intervention.* New York: McGraw-Hill, 1978.

Payne, J. S., & Patton, J. R. *Mental retardation.* Columbus, Ohio: Charles E. Merrill, 1981.

Smith, R. M. *An introduction to mental retardation.* New York: McGraw-Hill, 1971.

Wiig, E. H., & Semel, E. M. *Language disabilities in children and adolescents.* Columbus, Ohio: Charles E. Merrill, 1976.

Wiig, E. H., & Semel, E. M. *Language assessment and intervention for the learning disabled.* Columbus, Ohio: Charles E. Merrill, 1980.

REFERENCES

Anglin, J. *The growth of word meaning.* Cambridge, Mass.: MIT Press, 1970.

Baker, H., & Leland, B. *Detroit Tests of Learning Aptitude.* Indianapolis: Bobbs-Merrill, 1967.

Bankson, N. W. *Bankson Language Screening Test.* Baltimore: University Park Press, 1977.

Bannatyne, A. *Language, reading, and learning disabilities.* Springfield, Ill.: Charles C Thomas, 1971.

Bender, L. Neuropsychiatric disturbances in dyslexia. In A. H. Keeney & V. T. Keeney (Eds.), *Dyslexia.* St. Louis: C. V. Mosby, 1968.

Berko-Gleason, J. Code switching in children's language. In T. Moore (Ed.), *Cognitive development and the acquisition of language.* New York: Academic Press, 1973.

Bilsky, L. H., Evans, R. A., & Gilbert, L. Generalization of associative clustering in mentally retarded adolescents: Effects of novel stimuli. *Journal of Mental Deficiency,* 1972, *77,* 77–84.

Brown, H. D. Children's comprehension of relativized English sentences. *Child Development,* 1971, *42,* 1923–1936.

Brutten, M., Richardson, S.O., & Mangel, C. *Something is wrong with my child.* New York: Harcourt Brace Jovanovich, 1973.

Bryan, T. H. An observational analysis of classroom behaviors of children with learning disabilities. *Journal of Learning Disabilities,* 1974, *7,* 26–34.

Bryan, T. H. Social relationships and verbal interactions of learning disabled children. *Journal of Learning Disabilities,* 1978, *11,* 107–115.

Bryan, T. H., Wheeler, R., Felcan, J., & Henek, T. "Come on dummy": An observational study of children's communications. *Journal of Learning Disabilities,* 1976, *9,* 661–669.

Chalfant, J. C., & Foster, G. E. Identifying learning disabilities in the classroom. *Slow Learning Child,* 1974, *21,* 3–14.

Chomsky, C. *The acquisition of syntax in children from 5 to 10.* Cambridge, Mass.: MIT Press, 1969.

Chomsky, C. Reading, writing, and phonology. *Harvard Educational Review,* 1970, *40,* 287–309.

Clark, E. V. On the acquisition of the meaning of "before" and "after." *Journal of Verbal Learning and Verbal Behavior,* 1971, *10,* 266–275.

Clark, E. V. On the child's acquisition of antonyms in two semantic fields. *Journal of Verbal Learning and Verbal Behavior,* 1972, *11,* 750–758.

Clark, E. V. What's in a word. In T. Moore (Ed.), *Cognitive development and the acquisition of language.* New York: Academic Press, 1973.

Cruickshank, W. M.(Ed). *The teacher of brain-injured children.* Syracuse: Syracuse University Press, 1966.

DeFries, J. C., Ashton, G. C., Johnson, R. C., Kuse, A. R., McClearn, G. E., Mi, M. P., Rashad, M. N., Vandenberg, S. G., & Wilson, J. R. Parent-offspring resemblance for specific cognitive abilities in two ethnic groups. *Nature,* 1976, *261,* 131–133.

Denckla, M. B. Retrospective study of dyslexic children (1975). Reported in A. L. Benton & D. Pearl (Eds.), *Dyslexia: An appraisal of current knowledge.* New York: Oxford University Press, 1978.

Denckla, M. B., & Rudel, R. G. Naming of object-drawings by dyslexic and other learning disabled children. *Brain and Langauge,* 1976, *3,* 1–15.

Dunn, L. M. *Peabody Picture Vocabulary Test.* Circle Pines, Minn.: American Guidance Service, 1965, 1980.

Durrell, D. D. *Durrell Analysis of Reading Difficulty.* New York: Harcourt Brace Jovanovich, 1955.

Elkind, D. *Children and adolescents.* New York: Oxford University Press, 1970.

Erenberg, G., Mattis, S., & French, J. H. *Four hundred children referred to an urban ghetto developmental disabilities clinic: Computer assisted analysis of demographic psychological, social, and medical data.* Unpublished manuscript, 1976.

Evans, R. A. Transfer of associative clustering tendencies in borderline mentally retarded adolescents. *American Journal of Mental Deficiency,* 1977, *81,* 482–485.

Finucci, J. M., Guthrie, J. T., Childs, A. L. Abbey, H., & Childs, B. The genetics of specific reading disability. *Annals of Human Genetics,* 1976, *40,* 1–23.

Flavell, J. H., Botkin, P. T., Fry, C. L., Wright, J. C., & Jarvis, P. E. *The development of role-taking and communication skills in children.* New York: John Wiley, 1968.

Freston, C. W., & Drew, C. J. Verbal performance of learning disabled children as a function of input organization. *Journal of Learning Disabilities,* 1974, *7,* 424–428.

Froeschels, E. *Kindersprache and Aphasia.* Berlin: Verlag von S. Karger, 1918.

Galaburda, A. M., & Kemper, T. L. Cytoarchitectonic abnormalities in developmental dyslexia: A case study. *Annals of Neurology,* 1979, *6,* 94–100.

Gardner, H. *The arts and human development.* New York: John Wiley, 1973.

Gardner, H., Kircher, M., Winner, E., & Perkins, D. Children's metaphoric productions and preferences. *Journal of Child Language,* 1975, *2,* 125–141.

German, D. J. N. Word-finding skills in children with learning disabilities. *Journal of Learning Disabilities,* 1979, *12,* 176–181.

German, D. J. N. Word-finding substitutions in children with learning disabilities. *Journal of Language, Speech, and Hearing Services in the Schools,* in press.

Glucksberg, S., Krauss, R. M., & Weisberg, R. Referential communication in school children: Method and some preliminary findings. *Journal of Experimental Child Psychology,* 1966, *3,* 333–342.

Goldstein, K. *Language and language disorders.* New York: Grune & Stratton, 1948.

Golick, M. *Language disorders in children: A linguistic investigation.* Unpublished doctoral dissertation, McGill University, 1976.

Goodman, K. Analysis of oral reading miscues: Applied psycholinguistics, *Reading Research Quarterly,* 1969, *4,* 9–30.

Grossman, H. J. (Ed.). *Manual on terminology and classification in mental retardation.* Washington, D.C.: American Association on Mental Deficiency (Special Publication Series No. 2), 1973.

Hallgren, B. Specific dyslexia ("congenital word blindness"): A clinical study. *Acta Psychiatrica et Neurologica Scandinavica,* 1950, Supplement No. 65.

Hass, W. A., & Wepman, J. M. Dimensions of individual difference in the spoken syntax of school children. *Journal of Speech and Hearing Research,* 1974, *17,* 455–469.

Hermann, K. *Reading disability: A medical study of word-blindness and related handicaps.* Copenhagen: Munksgaard, 1959.

Hewitt, F. Educational engineering with emotionally disturbed children. *Exceptional Children,* 1967, *33,* 459–467.

Hymes, D. On communication competence. In J. B. Pride & J. Holmes (Eds.), *Sociolinguistics.* New York: Penguin Books, 1972.

Ingram, T. T. S. The nature of dyslexia. In F. A. Young & D. B. Lindsey (Eds.), *Early experience and visual information processing in perceptual and reading disorders.* Washington, D.C.: National Academy of Sciences, 1970.

Johnson, D. J., & Myklebust, H. R. *Learning disabilities: Educational principles and practices.* New York: Grune & Stratton, 1967.

Johnson, S. W., & Morasky, R. L. *Learning disabilities.* Boston: Allyn & Bacon, 1977.

Johnston, J., & Schery, T. K. The use of grammatical morphemes by children with communication disorders. In D. Morehead & A. Morehead (Eds.), *Normal and deficient child language.* Baltimore: University Park Press, 1976.

Keogh, B. K., Tchir, C., & Windeguth-Behn, A. A teacher's perception of educationally high risk children. *Journal of Learning Disabilities,* 1974, *7,* 367–374.

Kephart, N. *The slow learner in the classroom* (2nd ed.). Columbus, Ohio: Charles E. Merrill, 1971.

Kirk, S. A., McCarthy, J. J., & Kirk, W. D. *Illinois Test of Psycholinguistic Ability* (Rev. ed.). Urbana: University of Illinois Press, 1968.

Krauss, R. M., & Glucksberg, S. The development of communication competence as a function of age. *Child Development,* 1967, *4,* 255–260.

Labov, W. *Sociolinguistic patterns.* Philadelphia: University of Pennsylvania Press, 1972.

Lapointe, C. Token test performances by learning disabled and academically achieving adolescents. *British Journal of Disorders of Communication,* 1976, *11,* 121–133.

Lerner, J. W. *Children with learning disabilities* (2nd ed.). Boston: Houghton Mifflin, 1976.

Little, L. J. The learning disabled. In E. Meyen (Ed.), *Exceptional children and youth.* Denver: Love, 1978.

Mason. A. W. Specific (developmental) dyslexia. *Developmental Medicine and Child Neurology,* 1976, *9,* 183–190.

Mattis, S., French, J. H., & Rapin, I. Dyslexia in children and young adults: Three independent neuropsychological syndromes. *Developmental Medicine and Child Neurology,* 1975, *17,* 150–163.

McGlannan, F. K. Familial characteristics of genetic dyslexia: Preliminary report of a pilot study. *Journal of Learning Disabilities,* 1968, *1,* 32–38.

Meier, J. H. Prevalence and characteristics of learning disabilities found in second grade children. *Journal of Learning Disabilities,* 1971, *4,* 1–16.

Menyuk, P. *Sentences children use.* Cambridge, Mass.: MIT Press, 1969.

Menyuk, P. *Language and maturation.* Cambridge, Mass.: MIT Press, 1977.

Morris, C. W. Foundations of the theory of signs. *Interactional encyclopedia of unified science, 1.* (No. 2). Chicago: University of Chicago Press, 1938.

Mowrer, D. E. *Methods of modifying speech behaviors.* Columbus, Ohio: Charles E. Merrill, 1978.

Muma, J. R. *Language handbook: Concepts, assessments, intervention.* Englewood Cliffs, N.J.: Prentice-Hall, 1978.

Myklebust, H. R. *Auditory disorders in children: A manual for differential diagnosis.* New York: Grune & Stratton, 1954.

Newcomer, P., & Hammill, D. D. *Test of Language Development.* Austin, Tex.: Pro-Ed, 1977.

Newfield, M. U., & Schlanger, B. B. The acquisition of morphology by normal and mentally retarded children. *Journal of Speech and Hearing Research,* 1968, *4,* 693–706.

Orton, S. T. *Reading, writing and speech problems in children.* New York: W. W. Norton, 1937.

Osgood, C. A behavioristic analysis of perception and language as cognitive phenomena. In *Contempoary approaches to cognition.* Cambridge, Mass.: Harvard University Press, 1957.

Owen, F. W., Adams, P. A., Forrest, T., Stolz, L. M., & Fisher, S. Learning disorders in children: Sibling studies. *Monographs of the Society for Research in Child Development,* 1971, *36*(4, Serial No. 144).

Parker, T. B., Freston, C. W., & Drew, C. J. Comparison of verbal performance of normal and learning disabled children as a function of input organization. *Journal of Learning Disabilities,* 1975, *8,* 386–392.

Rees, N. S. Pragmatics of language application to normal and disordered language development. In R. L. Schiefelbusch (Ed.), *Bases of language intervention.* Baltimore: University Park Press, 1978.

Rourke, B. P. Brain-behavior relationships in children with learning disabilities. *American Psychologist,* 1975, *30,* 911–920.

Sabsay, S. *Communication competence in Downs' syndrome adults.* Ann Arbor, Mich.: University Microfilms International, 1979.

Schiefelbusch, R. Language disabilities of cognitively involved children. In J. V. Irwin & M. Marge (Eds.), *Principles of childhood language disabilities.* New York: Appleton-Century-Crofts, 1972.

Schultz, T. Development of the appreciation of riddles. *Child Development,* 1974, *45,* 100–105.

Schultz, T. R., & Pilon, R. Development of the ability to detect linguistic ambiguity. *Child Development,* 1973, *44,* 728–733.

Scwartz, A. H., & Murphy, M. W. Cues for screening language disorders in preschool children. *Pediatrics,* 1975, *55,* 717–722.

Semel, E. M., & Wiig, E. H. Comprehension of syntactic structures and critical verbal elements by children with learning disabilities. *Journal of Learning Disabilities,* 1975, *8,* 53–58.

Semel, E. M., & Wiig, E. H. *Clinical Evaluation of Language Functions.* Columbus, Ohio: Charles E. Merrill, 1980. (a)

Semel, E. M., & Wiig, E. H. *CELF Screening Tests: Elementary and Advanced Levels.* Columbus, Ohio: Charles E. Merrill, 1980. (b)

Sheldon, A. *The acquisition of relative clauses in English.* Indiana University Linguistics Club Papers, Bloomington, Indiana, 1974.

Snyder, L. *Pragmatic abilities of children with learning disabilities.* Paper presented at the Language Disorder Symposium, University of Denver, Colorado, 1979.

Spitz, H. H. The role of input organization in the learning and memory of mental retardates. In N. R. Ellis (Ed.), *International review of research in mental retardation* (Vol. 2). New York: Academic Press, 1966.

Strauss, A. A., & Kephart, N. C. *Psychopathology and the education of the brain-injured child.* New York: Grune & Stratton, 1955.

Strauss, A. A., & Lehtinen, L. E. *Psychopathology and education of the brain-injured child* (Vol. 1). New York: Grune & Stratton, 1947.

Ure, J., & Ellis, J. Register in descriptive linguistics and linguistic sociology. In O. Uribe-Villegas (Ed.), *Issues in sociolinguistics.* The Hague: Mouton, 1977.

Vogel, S. A. Syntactic abilities of normal and dyslectic children. *Journal of Learning Disabilities,* 1974, *7,* 47–53.

Vogel, S. A. Morphological ability in normal and dyslexic children. *Journal of Learning Disabilities,* 1977, *10,* 35–43.

Wechsler, D. *Wechsler Intelligence Scale for Children–Revised.* New York: Psychological Corporation, 1974.

Wells, G. Learning to code experience through language. *Journal of Child Language,* 1974, *1,* 243–269.

White, E. J. *Dysnomia in the adolescent dyslexic and the developmentally delayed adolescent.* Unpublished doctoral dissertation, Boston University, 1979.

Wiig, E. H., Gilbert, M. F., & Christian, S. H. Developmental sequences in the perception and interpretation of lexical and syntactic ambiguities. *Perceptual and Motor Skills,* 1978, *46,* 959–969.

Wiig, E. H., Lapointe, C., & Semel, E. M. Relationships among language processing and production abilities of learning disabled adolescents. *Journal of Learning Disabilities,* 1977, *10,* 292–299.

Wiig, E. H., & Semel, E. M. Comprehension of linguistic concepts requiring logical operations by learning disabled children. *Journal of Speech and Hearing Research,* 1973, *16,* 627–636.

Wiig, E. H., & Semel, E. M. Logico-grammatical sentence comprehension by learning disabled adolescents. *Perceptual and Motor Skills,* 1974, *38,* 1331–1334.

Wiig, E. H., & Semel, E. M. Productive language abilities in learning disabled adolescents. *Journal of Learning Disabilities,* 1975, *8,* 578–586.

Wiig, E. H., & Semel, E. M. *Language disabilities in children and adolescents.* Columbus, Ohio: Charles E. Merrill, 1976.

Wiig, E. H., & Semel, E. M. *Language assessment and intervention for the learning disabled.* Columbus, Ohio: Charles E. Merrill, 1980.

Wiig, E. H., Semel, E. M., & Abele, E. Perception and interpretation of ambiguous sentences by learning disabled twelve-year-olds. *Learning Disabilities Quarterly,* 1981, *4,* 3–12.

Wiig, E. H., Semel, E. M., & Crouse, M. A. B. The use of morphology by high-risk and learning disabled children. *Journal of Learning Disabilities,* 1973, *6,* 457–465.

part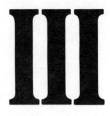

Communication Disorders of Special Populations

EDITORS' COMMENTS

Leonard L. LaPointe contributed to these editorial comments.

Since the dawn of humanity, when terrified primates huddled in dark caves wondering what to do next, the acts of eating and breathing have come automatically and instinctively. With the gradual evolution of the human brain, sequences of peculiar noises could be generated with the lungs and the mouth. When it was realized that others reacted to these noises, people became aware of the power and utility of oral communiation. The shadow of prehistory does not record in any detail the emergence of this singularly human trait. The cave drawings contain no clue as to what the first words might have been, although there is good reason to believe that the first word probably was neither *soufflé* nor *wiener.* Perhaps it was a gutteral grunt that approximated the oral equivalent of "No!" or "Not at the moment!"

We can assume that as long as humans have possessed oral communication we have run the risk of its impairment or loss. No doubt early man did not incur head injury from hang gliders, skateboards, or running a motorcycle over a canyon edge, but a variety of traumatic causes of nervous system damage impaired the speech of the Cro-Magnon. Falls from trees, tribal wars, rock slides, a dominant male's club to the skull of a would-be-suitor, claw wounds from an enraged pterodactyl, clumsily getting in line of fire during the stoning of a mammoth—all had the potential to inflict massive brain injury and compromise speech. All of these, plus the unseen miniature explosions that could take place within the head, underscored the dependence of speech on the integrity of the nervous system.

Egyptologists have uncovered early pictorial evidence of awareness of the connection between the brain and speech in the hieroglyphics of the tombs. Greek physicians wrote of speech loss after wounds to the head. Medieval artists and scholars busied themselves painting ceilings and drawing body parts, but paid little attention to the brain or to speech.

Then, in the 1800s, interest in the speech-brain connection mushroomed. European physicians of this period described in exquisite detail the baffling array of nonsense that emerged from the mouths of their brain-injured patients. Most of these early clinical case reports described disturbances in speech, understanding, reading, and writing that later came to be known as variants of the disorder aphasia. But even at this same time, some careful observers were beginning to express the caution that not all brain-related affectations of speech were necessarily linked to a twisted appreciation of language symbols. Other explanations could account for the less-than-perfect communication noticed after brain damage, but sometimes sorting out the reason for a specific speech symptom could be difficult. Controversy erupted about the relationship of language (the symbol system agreed upon and used by a community) to speech (the process of orally producing that symbol system) and about specific portions of the brain responsible for each. Some of that controversy continues today, though we have come a long way, particularly in the last 20 years, toward the goal of a better understanding of the brain's role in communication.

In Part II of this text we focused on the major categories of disorders of human communication, likening each of these disorders to individual rooms in a mansion. We entered each room to perceive its unique features and qualities. But it soon became apparent that, while we entered a new room with each transition to a new disorder, the demarcation between rooms became blurred. Issues and characteristics often overlap. A cause that you may initially have thought was unique to a disorder may have been mentioned as the potential origin for several of the disorders. The complexity of the disorders of human communication and of their impact on people's lives blends into a pattern.

In Part I, the all-encompassing responsibility of the human brain and the central nervous system pervaded our discussion of the anatomical and physiological systems involved in using language. The brain and central nervous system are responsible for controlling and integrating movements and patterns of movements, and parts of the brain are responsible for correlating and integrating pieces of information from within our bodies and from the world around us. They are also implicated in deciding on and executing a plan of action on the basis of that information. Other parts of the brain are implicated in making sense out of what we hear and of what people say to us. In Part II, the role of the brain and central nervous system in interpreting spoken language, formulating our ideas into a language code, and expressing our thoughts, ideas, and feelings through speech is referred to again and again. Part III will focus even more closely on the communication effects of deficits in or injury to the body—especially the brain and central nervous system—on human communication. Separate chapters cover impairments of hearing and birth defects related to cleft lip and palate. Impairments of the ability to plan, coordinate, and execute the motor movement patterns for speech are the focus of the chapters on neurogenic disorders of speech and cerebral palsy. Impairments of the ability to interpret, formulate, and produce spoken language in adults who were once efficient language users are the focus of the chapter on aphasia in adults.

The last chapter of Part III, "The Clinical Process and the Speech-Language Pathologist," occupies a unique position in this text. It deals with our involvement in, and contributions to, the clinical process as speech-language pathologists. The chapter for some of us represents a "looking back" at our professional lives. It gives us an opportunity to assess our past growth, as well as our successes and failures as individuals and as helping professionals. It touches on the essence of the profession of speech-language pathology and for some of us renews our commitments.

For you, this chapter should provide a glimpse of the potential of your future. It should allow you to gain new insights into yourself as a unique individual with a unique dedication and promise. It should point out your best feature (as well as your worst). It will give you hope for growth in spite of your limitations as a single person. It will bring about a stronger commitment to a future in speech-language pathology in some of you; it may suggest other directions for self-realization to others of you. It is meant to open you up to yourselves and your potential. It is meant to help you open yourselves to others who contribute to your professional growth—teachers, supervisors and, last but not least, the child, adolescent, or adult with a communication disorder.

HEARING AND AUDITORY DISORDERS 10

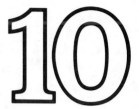

J. L. Northern
M. Lemme

Shauna's responses to sound were inconsistent by the age of 5 months, so her mother observed her carefully over the next 3 months. Finally convinced that her daughter had hearing problems, the mother took Shauna to several doctors, all of whom felt that Shauna probably had normal hearing. Undaunted, the mother continued seeking confirmation of her suspicions. Finally, when Shauna was 11 months old, her hearing loss was confirmed by an audiologist in a major medical center hospital, and she was fitted with hearing aids.

Shauna was the result of a normal delivery and has one normal-hearing older sister. The best medical guess of the cause of her hearing loss is that the mother was exposed to measles during pregnancy. Shauna's motor development was within normal age milestones. She was initially diagnosed to have severe bilateral conductive type hearing loss due to a congenital problem.

Although fitted early with hearing aids, by the age of 2 years, 5 months, Shauna's speech and language had developed only to the 15-month level. With extensive speech and language stimulation treatment, Shauna progressed in her use of receptive and expressive language. By the age of 3 years, 5 months, her overall language abilities were commensurate with her chronological age, but she still was delayed in auditory perception tasks. At the age of 4 years, 4 months, she demonstrated a great deal of spontaneous speech and language, but some difficulty was experienced in attempting to understand her vocalizations.

Shauna continued to receive special speech therapy sessions throughout her preschool years and obtained good auditory performance with her hearing aids. Her kindergarten report described her as a "delightful, outgoing, friendly child whose speech is 90% intelligible, and her language level seems normal for her age." On the Peabody Picture Vocabulary Test, *her single word receptive vocabulary age score was 5-7 when she was 5-6 in chronological age.*

Continued audiologic examinations which became more precise as Shauna grew older indicated a severe bilateral mixed-type hearing loss by the age of 7½ years. At this time her body-type hearing aids were replaced with ear-level type hearing aids. Her composite score on the Illinois Test of Psycholinguistic Abilities *was 9-0 years, well above her 7½-year-old chronological age. However, her speech patterns were described as "markedly slovenly," and she continued to need special speech therapy.*

By the age of 8 years, 8 months, Shauna was in third grade and doing well academically. Her ITPA scores were within age limits, except for the test areas of auditory association and grammatic closure. At the age of 9 years, 9 months, her speech was described as "markedly improved" with good control of the "th" and "ch" sounds.

Shauna still wears bilateral behind-the-ear hearing aids and is a most personable, out-going youngster who wants to be a "teacher for deaf children" when she grows up. Her speech, which appears on the enclosed recording, was made while she was 11 years old.

You may now wish to listen to the speech sample accompanying this chapter, found on Audio Disc 2, Side 3 (sample #6).

Hearing loss is one of the most common health-handicapping conditions among children and adults. Although precise statistics are difficult to obtain, it is estimated that nearly 15,000,000 Americans have partial hearing impairments that interfere with communication. Each year some 3,000 to 4,000 profoundly deaf babies are born in the United States; an additional 45,000 children currently have hearing impairments that require special education in schools and classes for the deaf. No doubt untold numbers of children have significant hearing loss that has yet to be identified.

The main problem for these children and adults is not the hearing loss *per se,* but that the hearing sense is the cornerstone upon which our unique human communication system is built. In infants, normal hearing is prerequisite to the normal development of speech and language. The identification of individuals with hearing impairment and their subsequent habilitation (in the case of infants and young children) or rehabilitation (in the case of adults) lies within the province of the professional field known as *audiology.*

Audiology is the science of hearing, and those professionals trained in this area of expertise are known as *audiologists.* Audiology is a relatively new discipline, developed after World War II to help veterans with combat-inflicted hearing impairments. It is a field that combines the specialty interests of many other areas, including physics, psychology, medicine, education, and sociology. The audiologist is trained to assess the hearing handicap of children and adults in order to help them overcome their handicap by means other than medicine or surgery. The audiologist may work in a wide variety of settings— from medical facilities to public schools to schools for the hearing handicapped to private practice. Audiologists work with a wide variety of other professionals, as well as patients and/or clients. They are also well versed in the fundamental principles of selecting, fitting, and evaluating patient performance with all types of hearing aids.

Audiologists perform a wide variety of functions. They work with physicians to perform special hearing tests to aid in the diagnosis of hearing disorders which can be medically or surgically treated. They perform therapy for individuals with hearing loss to help them use amplification with hearing aids for maximum educational, social, or vocational benefit. They help parents understand, accept, and manage their hearing-impaired child and the child's speech and language problems. They differentiate between peripheral hearing loss and central auditory processing disorders in a child who is having difficulties in school. They work with older people, in whom hearing loss is very common, to maintain a full, satisfying communication life.

The evaluation of hearing is not simple. The precipitating causes of auditory disorders may be intermittent or permanent, and the resulting hearing loss may be progressive, transient, or variable. The testing techniques involve expensive electronic equipment, careful selection of appropriate test materials, and knowledge of human development and behavior. The whole person must be considered during testing, and the results may be significantly influenced by illness, apathy, inattentiveness, low motivation to cooperate, emotional problems, mental retardation, neurological disease, and so on and so forth. Accurate test findings, however, are extremely important; and the audiologist is continually challenged to achieve valid and reliable hearing test results. To understand and evaluate hearing impairment, we must first look at the process of "normal" hearing.

ANATOMY AND PHYSIOLOGY OF THE HEARING MECHANISM

The phenomenon of hearing is the result of a complex series of events. Sound energy, originating as vibration and transmitted through the air, is captured by the outer ear, which funnels it inside. There it strikes the tympanic membrane, causing it to vibrate. These vibrations are transmitted across the middle ear space to the inner ear by three small bones (or ossicles), known as the *malleus, incus,* and *stapes.* In addition to serving as a conductor for sound energy, the tympanic membrane and middle ear ossicles amplify the sound by two simple mechanical principles: (*a*) level action of the ossicles and (*b*) the surface relationship between the vibrating area of the tympanic membrane with the funneling of sound energy onto the smaller surface area of the footplate of the stapes. This middle ear amplification amounts to approximately

These parts of the ear are pictured in Figure 10.1.

FIGURE 10.1
Cross-Section of the Hearing Mechanisms.

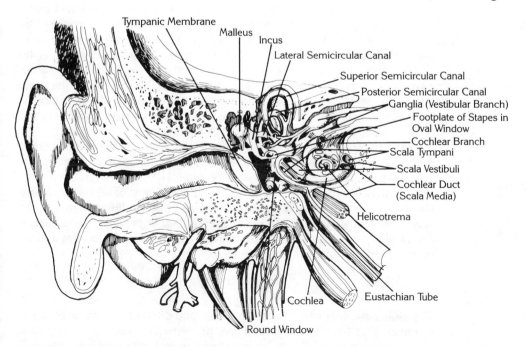

Tympanic Membrane
Malleus
Incus
Lateral Semicircular Canal
Superior Semicircular Canal
Posterior Semicircular Canal
Ganglia (Vestibular Branch)
Footplate of Stapes in Oval Window
Cochlear Branch
Scala Tympani
Scala Vestibuli
Cochlear Duct (Scala Media)
Helicotrema
Eustachian Tube
Cochlea
Round Window

Decibels (dB) are the units used to measure loudness of sound. The decibel scale is explained in detail below.

30 **decibels** (dB) and may be lost when defects or diseases inhibit either or both of the amplifying mechanisms.

The vibration transmitted by the stapes induces motion in the fluids of the cochlea, which is the seat of hearing in the inner ear. Within the cochlea, fluid fills two ducts known as the *scala vestibuli* and the *scala tympani*. These parallel scalae communicate with each other at the helicotrema, in the apical tip of the cochlear coils. When sound vibration displaces the stapes into the scala vestibuli, a simultaneous outward motion occurs in the scala tympani at the round window membrane.

The vibratory fluid motion ultimately causes a nerve impulse, with the cochlear sensory end organs (or hair cells) acting as mechanical transducers. Some 16,800 hair cells are arranged in the cochlea in one inner row and three to five outer rows resting on supporting cells. These supporting cells in turn rest on the basilar membrane to compose the structure known as the *organ of Corti*. The organ of Corti is contained in a third fluid-filled cochlear duct, known as the *scala media* or *cochlear duct*. This third duct fits between the scala vestibuli and scala tympani throughout the entire 2½ turns of the cochlea. The hair cells have a very orderly arrangement related to sound frequency.

Recall that one hertz (Hz) equals one cycle per second; this is the unit used to measure sound frequency.

Hair cells that respond to high frequency sounds (above 2,000 Hz) are located in the basal turn of the cochlea, while hair cells that respond to frequencies below 2,000 Hz are found in the middle and apical cochlear coils.

The fluid motion in the scala tympani displaces the basilar membrane in a traveling wave pattern, producing a sheering effect on the hair-like processes of the cell. This in turn results in a mechanical-chemical change which stimulates nerve impulses. Thus, the vibratory energy initiated by the tympanic membrane is transformed into hydraulic energy in the cochlea and then into neural impulses in the auditory nerve.

The Auditory Nerve

The nerve fibers that innervate the hair cells in the cochlea collect as the cochlear branch of the eighth cranial nerve. Just outside the cochlea, the vestibular branch of the eighth cranial nerve coming from the three semicircular canals joins the cochlear branch. These two branches of the eighth cranial nerve, also known as the *auditory nerve,* wind together like a rope and pass through the internal auditory meatus toward the medulla in the brainstem. Before it reaches the medulla, the eighth nerve divides into two branches, which go to the cochlear nuclei in the brainstem, where second-order afferent auditory neuron cell bodies are located.

Impulses are transmitted to the brain by chains of neurons, linked to other neurons at junction points to several levels. First-order neurons are the first link in the chain from the sensory organ (here, the ear) to the brain. Second-order neurons constitute the second link in the chain, and so on.

Experimenters have found that fibers in the eighth nerve are "tuned" or most responsive to certain frequencies or a specific range of frequencies. The threshold of a fiber is most sensitive at its "tuned" frequency—which can then be used to name the fiber, such as "7,000 Hz fiber." Most of the auditory nerve fibers are high frequency units, usually above 1,000 Hz. It is remarkable that only a few fibers of the eighth nerve are required to preserve good hearing. The auditory nerve must be cut more than half way through to have a measurable effect on hearing.

Brainstem Pathways

The higher auditory pathways are complex and often escape significance for students, who tend only to memorize the names of the relay stations and major neuronal paths. It is important to realize that, although first-order neurons from the cochlea reach the brainstem in the cochlear nuclei, most of the activity that ultimately reaches the cortex of the brain is by way of fourth-order neurons. This seemingly too complex system seldom breaks down because there are numerous alternate paths to the cerebral cortex.

There are two pairs of cochlear nuclei, a *dorsal* and a *ventral* cochlear nucleus, on each side of the medulla. They are referred to collectively as the *cochlear nuclei of the medulla.* Although some of the neurons of the cochlear nuclei ascend on the same side of the system, most cross over to the opposite side in the trapezoid body. Auditory units in the cochlear nuclei are also sensitive to specific frequencies. The number of discharges from a single cochlear nucleus unit is related to the intensity of the acoustic stimulus. Inhibitory units have also been reported in the cochlear nuclei. Under certain circumstances, they inhibit response rather than excite the unit.

The principal terminations of second-order afferent auditory neurons are in the nuclei of the trapezoid body and the superior olivary nucleus. The superior olive is the first structure in the medulla which receives fibers from both ears. It may play a role in the localization of sound. From here, neurons course upward in the loosely compacted neurons of the lateral lemniscus to another principal relay station, the nucleus of the inferior colliculus. Collaterals of second- and third-order neurons are given off to the reticular formation, which provides an indirect, diffuse, second sensory pathway to the cerebral cortex. The reticular formation is closely related to arousal and attention during sleep, so that a crying baby may wake only its mother, or so that you can sleep soundly through a barrage of noise but wake suddenly upon hearing a soft familiar voice.

Most of the fibers in the lateral lemniscus pathway terminate in the inferior colliculus, but some bypass it and end in the next relay station, the medial geniculate body. So far as we know, all direct projections to the auditory cortex are relayed in the medial geniculate body.

The auditory cortex is responsible for the fine discrimination that is necessary in understanding speech. Attempts to map the cortical responses to auditory stimuli have identified the temporal lobe as the responsive area, sometimes further localized as Brodmann's areas 41 and 42. The cortex has at least two frequency map projections which are the reverse of each other. As early as 1943, Kryter and Ades showed that, under appropriate conditions, cortical lesions have no appreciable effect on the absolute thresholds of pure tone stimuli. This is true even when there are extensive bilateral cortical lesions. Thus, the ability to respond by pure tones does not depend upon the cerebral cortex. These same investigators reported that removal of the inferior colliculi created a loss of approximately 15 dB in pure tone sensitivity; destruction of the entire auditory system from the midbrain to the cortex created a pure tone loss of about 40 dB. Thus, the most important aspect of auditory sensitivity to pure tones is due to intact neurons below the inferior colliculi, and a person with a loss of 75% of the neurons of the auditory nerve may have a nearly normal range of hearing.

See Figure 4.30.

Pure tone *is a single-frequencied, or very simple, sound.*

ACOUSTIC ASPECTS OF HEARING AND SOUND

Nature of Sound

The dual nature of sound was pointed out in the early 1700s, when a British philosopher asked if a falling tree makes noise when no one is nearby to hear the sound. A psychological view considers *sound* the quality that gives rise to the sensation of hearing. For the physicist, a propagating disturbance in the air may be considered a physical quantity or sound wave. Acoustics is the branch of physics dealing with the generation, transmission, and modification of sound waves. We must know about sound waves in general to understand the production and reception of speech.

Sound waves in the air are an example of physical phenomena that involve wave motion. A wave motion is produced by the vibration of certain matter; for sound waves, it is air particles which are set into vibration. Any description of sound must include consideration of frequency and intensity, as well as spectrum.

Frequency

Objects that can be set in motion vibrate most easily at a specific rate, referred to as **resonant frequency.** The vibrating movements of an object alternately increase (compression) and decrease (rarefaction) the density of surrounding air molecules. Thus, the pattern of movement of the vibrator is imprinted upon the air in the form of sound waves. The number of complete cycles about its rest position that take place in one second is the frequency of the sound wave; again, this is expressed in Hz.

Frequency is the primary determinant of the pitch of a tone. Thus, pitch refers to the psychological perception of the frequency of a stimulus. Humans can normally hear sound waves whose frequencies lie between 20 and 20,000 Hz. The range most often used in conversational speech is 500 to 2,000 Hz.

Intensity

The dynamic range of human hearing is impressive. The ratio of the faintest audible sound to the most intense tolerable sound is approximately 10,000,000 to one. To deal conveniently with such a range of values, we use a logarithmic system, the decibel scale, to describe sound intensity.

The decibel is an arbitrary unit that expresses the ratio of a measured power or pressure to a reference value. Since it is not an absolute measure, it has no meaning unless the reference value is specified. The usual reference value for

Pa is the abbreviation for Pascals.

sound pressure is 20_mPa, and the value is referred to as a dB SPL (sound pressure level). For conversational speech, the average pressure level of the voice at 5 feet is 60 dB SPL. Because of the logarithmic nature of the decibel scale, every 10 dB increase represents a ten-fold multiplication of sound. Thus, 50 dB is 10 times louder than 40 dB; 100 dB is a million times stronger than 40 dB. Futhermore, the 10 dB difference between 110 and 120 dB is

Table 10.1 shows the dB levels of several ordinary sounds.

much greater than the 10 dB difference between 40 and 50 dB.

The decibel notation used in clinical applications is based on the absolute threshold intensity for human hearing, which varies from frequency to frequency. This measurement is called dB HL (hearing level). It differs by frequency so that the normal ear can just detect a tone of 0 dB HL. Thus, the decibel scale used to describe environmental noise (dB SPL) has a different reference level than the decibel scale used to describe a hearing impairment (dB HL).

Just as pitch represents the psychological perception of frequency, loudness represents the psychological perception of intensity.

Spectrum

You may wish to review parts of chapter

Tuning forks vibrate as a whole, producing a corresponding simple sound wave. Vocal cords vibrate in segments, each vibrating at a different rate, and generate highly complex sound waves. Most of the daily sounds we hear are complex sounds comprised of two or more different frequencies. To help us deal with the great variety of complex sound waves, they can be divided into their simple component parts by electroacoustic or mathematic analysis. The resulting representation of signal amplitude as a function of frequency is called the sound *spectrum.*

6, which describes the physical properties of speech sounds in depth. You may also wish to check back to chapter 4's discussion of how the vocal cords work.

TABLE 10.1
Noise Levels of Common Sounds.

Source	Perception/Hearing	Sound Level in dB
Whisper	Just audible	10
Rustle of leaves		30
Normal conversation	Comfortable	50
Auto traffic		60
Window air-conditioner	Loud	80
Snowmobile/Motorcycle		95
Power lawnmower	Very loud	100
Pneumatic jackhammer/Chain saw		110
Rock music		115
Oxygen torch	Uncomfortably loud	120

A pure tone spectrum is shown by a single vertical line, while a periodic complex tone spectrum is a series of vertical lines, representing each of its component frequencies. For periodic waves, each frequency component or harmonic is a multiple of the fundamental or lowest frequency. The speech sound /ə/ has a periodic waveshape. Aperiodic wave-forms, which can have components at all frequencies, have corresponding spectra which consist of continuous rather than discrete line spectra. The speech sound /ʃ/ has an aperiodic waveshape. The sound spectrograph is a convenient instrument that can measure and display the continually changing spectrum of speech.

Acoustic Characteristics of Speech Sounds

To review a bit, the General American English speech sounds are described frequently in terms of the way they are produced. In traditional articulatory phonetics, the main divisions are (*a*) voicing, related to vocal fold vibration, e.g., voiced or voiceless; (*b*) place, related to articulators used to constrict the vocal tract, e.g., tongue or lips; and (*c*) manner, related to degree of nasal, oral, or pharyngeal cavity construction, e.g., plosives, fricatives, nasals. Thus /b/ in the word *be* is a voiced bilabial plosive. In contrast, acoustic phonetics identifies speech sounds in terms of acoustic parameters—frequency composition, relative intensities, and durational changes.

A thorough discussion of speech acoustics is presented by Minifie (1973).

Vowels are characterized by periodicity produced by vocal fold vibration. Vowel quality is determined by energy in several frequency regions, called *formants,* whose center frequency depends on the shape of the vocal tract. The first three formants are the most important for correct recognition of English vowels. Vowels are usually more intense and relatively longer than consonants. As we have seen, the glides /w, j/ and semivowels /r, l/ resemble vowels.

Fricative consonants are characterized by aperiodic noise, and may be voiced or voiceless. They are frequently classified in voiced–unvoiced cognate pairs. Each member of the pair is articulated in the same way and has similar acoustic characteristics except for the presence or absence of voicing. The frequency regions differentiate consonant pairs; for example the /ʒ, ʃ/ pair has

Figure 10.2 shows the

frequency and inten-
sity of selected
English sounds and
everyday noises.

energy between 2,500 and 4,500 Hz, while the /z, s/ pair has energy in the frequency region of 3,500 through 8,000 Hz. The /h, f/, and /ə/ are less intense than the rest of the fricatives.

Plosive consonants or stop consonants are produced when air pressure is built up to the point of complete closure in the vocal tract and is then released

FIGURE 10.2

Frequency and Intensity of English Language and Other Sounds. (From J. Northern & M. Downs, *Hearing in Children* (2nd ed.). Baltimore: The Williams & Wilkins Co., 1978. Copyright © 1978 by The Williams & Wilkins Co. Used by permission.)

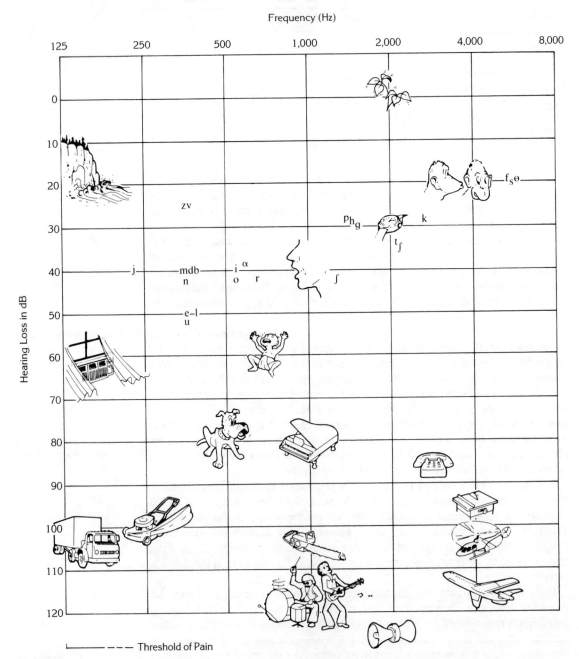

abruptly, causing a burst of air. A silent period followed by a burst of air is distinctive in plosives and identifies them as different from other consonants. The unvoiced plosives are characterized by an aspiration period prior to the onset of the succeeding voiced vowel; the voiced plosives are characterized by the burst of air immediately preceeding the onset of the succeeding vowel. Acoustic cues for differentiation among the various plosives are the frequency of the released burst and the second formant transitions; that is, changes in the center frequency of energy in the burst of /b/ and /p/ are relatively low frequency; of /d/ and /t/ are relatively high frequency; and /k/ varies with the adjacent vowel.

Nasal consonants are sustained voiced sounds in which sound radiates from the nose instead of the mouth. As with the plosive consonants, second formant transitions are important in distinguishing nasal consonants.

Duration of a segment of a wave can distinguish plosives from fricatives (for example, /t/ and /s/) and enable listeners to identify two sounds with identical formants as different vowels. In addition, the duration of the vowel segments in words determines the stressed syllable.

Variation in Acoustic Parameters of Speech Sounds

Skinner (1978) has suggested that infants would recognize speech sounds with relative ease if they were not spoken in rapid succession and if their acoustic features were constant. However, as we have seen, speech sound acoustic cues vary (*a*) each time an individual speaker produces a speech sound, (*b*) from speaker to speaker, and (*c*) with changes in phonetic context as they are modified by adjacent speech sounds and stress patterns.

Most children and adults recognize the ambiguous, sometimes even distorted, acoustic cues provided in everyday conversation with remarkable ease. While there are multiple acoustic cues for recognizing speech sounds, other cues include the general speech situation or context, our previous experience and expectations, and most importantly, our knowledge of the language. Speech recognition partially depends upon the acoustic signal and partially upon the listener's language experience. Through extensive listening experiences, the infant learns where the boundaries of speech sounds and words occur in connected speech. This process is called **segmentation.**

In different listening environments over a period of time, the average intensity of speech varies between 50 and 65 dB SPL. Ordinary background noise varies between approximately 35 and 68 dB SPL. For normal hearing adults, the situation where noise is 10 to 15 dB below the level of speech does not create difficulty in listening, since they can fill in missing acoustic cues. In contrast, the linguistically unsophisticated infant cannot fill in the missing acoustic details, and speech energy needs to be 30 dB louder than the background masking noise.

Suprasegmentals

Connected speech carries suprasegmental information, which depends on rhythm of speech and consists of stress and intonation patterns as well as durational characteristics. Stressed speech sounds or words are longer in duration, more intense, and higher in fundamental frequency than unstressed speech sounds. Change in the fundamental frequency of voiced sounds contribute to intonation, which helps us identify sentence type. There is little definitive information about the specific role of suprasegmental parameters;

but within broad limits, they can be specified for various grammatical configurations (Lieberman, 1967).

HEARING AND HEARING LOSS

Sound is such a common part of everyday life that it is easy to take hearing for granted. We hear most sounds because they are transmitted to us by air conduction. As we have seen, sound waves travel to the tympanic membrane and across the middle ear ossicles. As the ossicles vibrate, fluid waves are created in the cochlea. These waves mechanicaly bend the sensory hairs in the organ of Corti.

For a cross-section of the hearing mechanism showing the bone conduction pathways, see Figure 10.3.

The fluids of the inner ear can also be set into motion by vibrations carried through the skull. Since the inner ear system is completely encased in the temporal bone, sound may be transmitted directly by bone conduction, without need for the tympanic membrane or middle ear ossicles. The perception of a pure tone sounds exactly the same to a listener whether it is transmitted by air conduction or by bone conduction, since the same physiological events occur in the inner ear. We hear our own voices both by bone conduction and air conduction. That is one of the reasons why your own voice sounds unusual when you hear it from a tape recorder; that is one of the few instances in life when you hear your own voice primarily if not entirely by air conduction.

FIGURE 10.3
Bone Conduction and Air Conduction Pathways in Hearing.

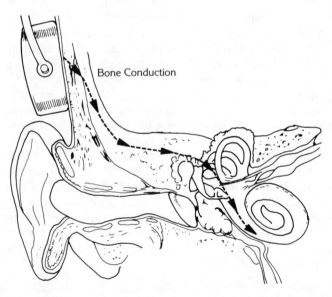

Bone Conduction

Nature of Hearing Loss

A conductive loss involves the mechanical transmission of sound, while a sensorineural loss involves the neural transmission of sound impulses.

Hearing losses are generally identified as **conductive** or **sensorineural**. When a combination of both types of hearing loss occurs, we speak of a *mixed* hearing loss. When a person displays auditory dysfunction, yet his or her peripheral hearing mechanisms are functioning within normal limits, the loss is called a *central auditory defect.*

Conductive hearing loss occurs when there is interference of any sort in the transmission of sound from the external auditory canal to the inner ear. The inner ear, in such cases, is capable of normal function, but the sound vibration is not able to reach the cochlea through the normal air conduction pathway. With a conductive loss, there is a peripheral hearing loss for air-conducted sounds, while sounds conducted to the inner ear by bone conduction are heard normally. Most conductive hearing losses can be corrected through medical treatment or surgery.

Causes of conductive hearing loss include foreign objects or debris in the external auditory canal, **otitis media,** problems associated with tympanic membrane movement such as perforation, **middle ear effusion,** and congenital abnormalities of the ear canal, middle ear, or external ear. If a conductive hearing loss is identified early, the underlying disease process can often be resolved during its initial stages.

Otitis media is inflammation of the middle ear; middle ear effusion is accumulation of fluid behind the tympanic membrane.

Mild conductive hearing loss may be a cause of speech and language problems in children (Holm & Kunze, 1969). Some of these children are inadvertently labeled *learning disabled* or develop behavior problems as a result of their hearing problem. A number of research studies have confirmed that some children with recurrent conductive hearing loss may show severe delays in developing reading, arithmetic, and language skills. Medical treatment is the first line of defense against the negative effects of mild conductive hearing loss. Northern and Downs (1978) suggest that careful use of hearing aid amplification and supplemental home speech and language stimulation programs may help alleviate the problems of minimal auditory deficit. However, the best means to avoid educational problems is to use careful hearing testing techniques to identify children with mild hearing impairments as early as possible.

Sensorineural hearing loss occurs when there has been damage to the hair cells of the cochlea or to the auditory nerve fibers. Damage to the hair cells is not easily differentiated from neuronal damage, so the resultant hearing loss is called *sensorineural.* New testing techniques, such as electrocochleography, offer promise as objective means of differentiating between sensory and neural hearing impairment.

In sensorineural hearing loss, the air and bone conductive hearing thresholds are the same. Sensorineural hearing loss may easily be overlooked during a physical examination, since both the external auditory canal and tympanic membrane appear normal. Unfortunately, sensorineural hearing loss is generally irreversible. Common causes include viral and bacterial infections, drug toxicity, excessive noise exposure, congenital abnormality, and head trauma. Young children who have severe sensorineural hearing loss before they learn to talk have difficulty developing normal speech and language. Treatment for sensorineural hearing loss consists of auditory training in the use of hearing aids and special education techniques to develop speech and language.

Central auditory dysfunction manifests itself in decreased auditory comprehension. For example, a child may have a normal range of hearing ability and show a normal audiogram, but be unable to recognize or interpret speech. Central auditory dysfunction is a complex problem and is discussed more fully later in this chapter.

Degree and Severity of Hearing Loss

An important consideration with any hearing loss is the degree of impairment. Common descriptive terms used to identify degree of hearing loss include *mild* hearing loss (loss of 15 to 40 dB), *moderate* hearing loss (41 to 65 dB), *severe* hearing loss (66 to 89 dB), *profound* hearing loss (90 to 110 dB), and

Figure 10.4 shows an audiogram of a child with a moderate hearing loss, as well as the usual ranges of hearing loss.

anacusis or total hearing loss. Sometimes borderline categories of hearing impairment are described with a combination of terms, such as *moderately severe* hearing loss. We graph an individual's hearing loss on an audiogram, which shows both frequency and dB ranges.

The handicap caused by a hearing loss is also a function of whether the loss is unilateral or bilateral. For instance, people with a totally deaf ear on one side but with normal hearing on the other side may function quite well in most situations. However, they often have difficulty localizing sounds and separating the target signal from a noisy background.

FIGURE 10.4

Audiogram Showing Levels of Hearing Loss.

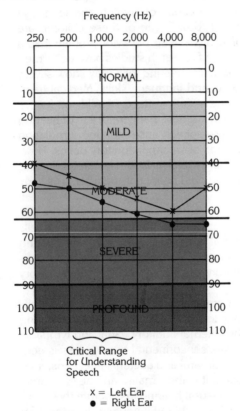

THE ROLE OF HEARING IN COMMUNICATION

Hearing in Speech and Language Development

Rooted in biologic development, the unique human ability to use language and to speak depends on a brain that transforms experience to symbols. The innate capacity to learn speech and language is related to the maturation of the brain (Lenneberg, 1967). It is through hearing that speech and language are organized most efficiently in the brain.

Chapter 8 details early language development in the normal child.

Normal hearing and the experience of listening to speech are prerequisite to normal speech development and later language formulation. This auditory-linked acquisition of speech and language is a function locked to early periods in the infant's life. With 2 to 3 years of listening experience, children learn to glean meaning from speech sounds and to abstract the rules of language. The longer auditory language stimulation is delayed, the less efficient will be the language facility. If the child has no language stimulation for the first 3 years of life, he is not likely to reach his full language potential. The same auditory processes that operate in the initial learning of language continue to control speech and language function through later life.

Conversely, the child who loses her hearing after the age of 3 can retain her language skills and even her speech with appropriate management.

Development of Infant Auditory Perception and Auditory Comprehension

Research on prenatal hearing indicates responses to sound appear during the fifth month of gestation; thus the newborn has been hearing for at least 4 months. Newborns can discriminate all the acoustic parameters of an auditory stimulus. They discriminate on the basis of frequency, intensity, and stimulus dimensions. Low frequency sounds tend to have a soothing effect, while high frequency sounds can produce distress. Speech-like signals are particularly effective in producing responses in newborns and are even more potent for the older infant (Eisenberg, 1976).

Data from infant speech perception studies have provided evidence that infants can make distinctions similar to those made by adults between some acoustic speech sound features. Eimas and his associates (Eimas, Siqueland, Jusczyk, & Vigorita, 1971), using conditioned sucking rates, have demonstrated that 1-month-old infants can differentiate the onset time distinction between the speech sounds "pah" and "bah." Eilers and colleagues (Eilers, Wilson, & Moore, 1977) have demonstrated that 6-month-old infants can recognize speech sounds despite variations caused by different speakers and phonetic context.

Around the age of 10 months, babies begin to demonstrate the rudiments of auditory comprehension, responding to a few words such as their names or the word *no*. It is usually assumed that comprehension begins before the child starts to use verbal expression and continues to exceed our expressive abilities throughout life. The 2-year-old follows simple directions and points to body parts on command. Gradual increments in comprehension of syntax are noted from 3 to 8 years of age (Lee, 1971). People continue to improve comprehension of complex and tricky syntax and to add lexical terms throughout life.

Effect of Peripheral Hearing Loss on Speech and Language

Reduced or defective hearing sensitivity does not cause one specific kind of communication problem. The effects of a peripheral hearing loss depend primarily on its degree, configuration, stability, and the age of onset. In the hearing impaired child, language development is also influenced by the extent and type of early training; the type and timing of amplification; visual, emotional, and intellectual factors; and family attitude. As we have seen, age of onset of the hearing loss is an especially important factor in language development. A child who sustains significant hearing loss after he has acquired language (3 or 4 years of age) will have a less severe linguistic deficit than the child whose hearing loss is present at birth or develops within the first few months of life.

*The first type is called **postlingual** hearing loss; the second, **prelingual**.*

The major effect of a peripheral hearing loss is the loss of audibility for some or all of the important acoustic speech cues. Traditionally, there has been disagreement as to how different degrees of hearing loss should be categorized. The term **hearing impaired** generally includes a broad range of hearing ability from profoundly deaf to mildly hard of hearing. **Deaf** is defined as a hearing loss of at least 70 dB HL, which precludes the understanding of speech through audition. **Hard of hearing** is defined as a loss of 35 to 69 dB HL, which makes the understanding of speech through audition difficult, but not impossible. An individual with a loss of greater than 70 dB HL is likely to have the speech and language problems we usually associate with deafness.

Mild Hearing Loss (15–40 dB HL)

A 15 to 25 dB loss will have mild impact on communication and language learning. Vowel sounds are heard clearly, but voiceless consonants may be missed. In children with a 25 to 40 dB HL hearing loss, auditory learning dysfunction after the first year results in inattention, mild language delay, and mild speech problems. The child hears only the louder, voiced speech sounds. The short unstressed words and less intense speech sounds (like voiceless stops and fricatives) are inaudible. The acoustic cues of speech that are audible may be perceived differently by a child with a conductive loss than a child with a sensorineural hearing loss.

Moderate Hearing Loss (41–65 dB HL)

These children miss almost all of the speech sounds at conversational level, but they can learn language with the help of hearing aid amplification. They may show inattention, language retardation, speech problems, and learning problems. Children with moderate hearing losses often have difficulty learning abstraction in the meaning of words and the grammatical rules of language, because they cannot hear some of the speech sounds and they hear others inaccurately. They hear vowels better than consonants. Short, unstressed words such as prepositions and relational words, as well as word endings (-s, -ed), are particularly difficult to hear. This reduction of information can lead to confusion among speech sounds and word meaning, limited vocabulary, difficulty with multiple meanings of words, difficulty in developing object classes, confusion of grammatical rules, errors in word placement in sentences, and omission of articles, conjunctions, and prepositions. The speech articulation of the child with moderate hearing loss shows omitted and distorted consonants and consonants substituted for other consonants which sound the same to the child. Strangers may have difficulty understanding the speech of the child with moderate hearing loss.

Severe Hearing Loss (66–89 dB HL)

Language and speech will not develop spontaneously, but with early special education and amplification with hearing aids, these children may eventually function as well as hard of hearing persons. Without amplification, they cannot hear sounds or normal conversation. They can hear their own vocalizations, loud environmental sounds, and only the most intense speech when spoken loudly at close range. With hearing aids, they can discern vowel sounds and differences in manner of consonant articulation. This degree of hearing loss generally results in severe language retardation, speech problems, and learning dysfunction.

Profound Hearing Loss (90 dB HL or Greater)

Language and speech must be learned by intensive special education. Without amplification through hearing aids, these children are unable to hear any sounds. With amplification, they may hear the rhythm patterns of speech, their own vocalizations, and loud environmental sounds. Profound hearing loss results in severe language retardation, speech problems, and learning dysfunction.

Deaf children commonly have voice, articulation, resonance, and prosody problems. Their vocal pitch is frequently higher than that of normal hearing people, and the prosodic features of intonation and stress are lost, giving their voices a monotonous quality. The speech of the deaf is characterized by (*a*) slow temporal patterning, (*b*) inefficient use of the breath stream, (*c*) prolongation of vowels, (*d*) distortion of vowels, (*e*) abnormal rhythm, (*f*) excessive nasality, and (*g*) addition of an undifferentiated neutral vowel between abutting consonants. The articulation of the severe to profoundly hearing impaired has been observed to have excessive mandibular movement, lack of tongue movement, posterior tongue positioning, voiced-voiceless confusions for consonants, problems with coarticulation, substitution of visible sounds for those difficult to see, better articulation for initial speech sounds than for medial or final speech sounds, stop/plosive confusion, and the intrusion of an undifferentiated neutral vowel between abutting consonants. Studies of speech intelligibility indicate that, at best, naive listeners understand 20% to 25% of deaf speech. Deaf people tend to use concrete rather than abstract words and poor syntactic constructions.

Central Auditory Processing Disorders

Auditory processing of spoken language is a complex, highly dynamic act which appears to involve a number of "stages" of analysis and synthesis— selection, recognition, and interpretation. Auditory processing depends upon the ability to establish relationships between internally generated expectations and received acoustic signals. Involved in the processing of auditory stimuli are the cognitive processes of attention, memory, perception, and comprehension (Lemme & Daves, 1981). There is a lack of concensus concerning the structures, processes, and strategies that are used to process spoken language. The growing interest in auditory processing disorders (often called *auditory-perceptual deficits*) has yet to clarify the definition and description of symptoms in these disorders.

Central auditory disorders often exist in the presence of normal hearing sensitivity, although they may appear along with peripheral hearing loss. The ability to process auditory information accurately is essential to the acquisition of language and to subsequent academic skills. Frequently, the deaf child and the child with central disorders seem similar in that neither shows the normal milestones of prespeech and prelinguistic skills.

Auditory Language/Learning Disorders

Auditory processing skills develop as children grow older and are believed to stablilize in the 7th or 8th year of life. Children who have problems in processing auditory material may be referred to by professionals from a variety of disciplines, depending upon the presenting symptoms. The problem may initially appear as an inability to acquire language in the normal developmental sequence. More subtle problems may not be identified until the child is in school and has difficulty with reading, writing, or spelling. Due to the broad spectrum of symptoms, these children may be called *learning disabled* or *language disordered.*

Central auditory processing disorder is a symptom without a disease. While the language and learning problems appear to stem mainly from an inability to use auditory input effectively, no one has been able to find the cause or

Chapter 9 has discussed the language problems of learning disabled children in depth.

specific nature of the breakdown. While etiology is of utmost significance in any consideration of auditory language/learning problems, it is difficult to identify a single cause; different etiological factors may show up in similar behavioral symptoms. Auditory processing difficulties may stem from reduced auditory acuity, from specific damage to the central nervous system, from environmental or psychological causes, or from cognitive dysfunction.

The difficulty in a central auditory processing disorder is not in the ability to receive sound, but in the ability to code and integrate an auditory message into meaningful information. This requires intact processing at relatively high perceptual and conceptual levels. The most prevalent view today is that these disorders result from a dysfunction of a specific auditory skill or set of skills. While we can identify major components of auditory procesing, it is hard to accept the concept of a set of discrete auditory skills, since each skill consti- tutes only one facet of a complex process (Sanders, 1977). Rees (1973), after reviewing studies which suggested that auditory processing disorders (dis- orders in auditory memory, auditory sequencing, auditory closure, and so on) are responsible for language disorders, concluded that instead of an auditory perception problem the children in those studies had language disorders. In addition, she emphasizes that the importance of any given subskill to speech and language acquisition remains to be proven. Recent research supports the notion that efficient auditory language processing takes place simultaneously at all levels of analysis and places demands upon attention and memory as well as auditory skills.

In recent years, there has been growing concern for the group of children who, despite adequate sensory, motor, and intellectual functioning, have dif- ficulty learning. Among the problems these "learning disabled" children some- times exhibit are those associated with auditory learning. The most prevalent specific learning disabilities are those in which language abilities are impaired. The language problems of these youngsters are "multifaceted, defying unitary description," and their linguistic deficits are often related to reading retardation and reductions in mathematics skills (Wiig & Semel, 1976, 1980).

Auditory Processing Dysfunction Subsequent to Brain Injury

See chapter 14.

While the normal adult has no difficulty under ordinary circumstances, most of us have some problems when an auditory message is rapid, linguistically complex, or frequently interrupted. These factors can create serious problems for adults with mild auditory processing deficits. At the extreme end of the continuum of auditory processing deficits is the aphasic adult. Aphasia is a language problem resulting from acquired brain damage. It is characterized by difficulties in listening, reading, speaking, and writing. This reduction or loss of capacity to interpret and formulate language symbols is not the result of sensory, motor, or intellectual dysfunction.

There is almost always demonstrable impairment of auditory processing in aphasia, probably because of the great dependence of language on the auditory system. However, these auditory disorders are not all alike; they range in severity and have different characteristics and patterns. Some aphasic adults have trouble understanding word meanings; others may have little or no difficulty in recognizing words, but have difficulties when high-level analysis of speech is required. For example, the aphasic adult may be unable to retain and understand spoken messages which are long and contain a great deal of information. In general, there is no universal impairment of auditory per- ceptual and temporal sequencing abilities that can explain these problems.

In therapy, the speech-language pathologist must observe and analyze problems encountered by aphasic adults as they respond to spoken language. Undoubtedly, among the various processes responsible for control over language function, auditory processes are the most important in relationship to the aphasia.

EVALUATION OF HEARING IN CHILDREN

There are few handicaps more serious in the development of a young child than impairment of hearing. Identifying hearing loss in children is not an easy task, and the hearing impaired child often presents a confusing clinical picture. Delays in the identification of children with hearing loss are not uncommon, and each misadventure in accurate diagnosis of hearing loss causes an irretrievable loss of time for the habilitation of the child's hearing and language problems.

Accurate quantification and evaluation of a child's hearing impairment is important to the medical diagnosis and management of the problem. An experienced audiologist must determine the degree of hearing impairment in the young child. The difficult-to-test child may have to be referred to an audiology center for additional evaluation. The determination of hearing loss in many children is an on-going process and may require more than one test session. Although we prefer to evaluate happy, cooperative children, unfortunately they do not all fit this description. The two main tenets of evaluating hearing in children are: (*a*) no child is too young for hearing testing, and (*b*) the earlier and more accurate the identification of hearing impairment, the better the prognosis for alleviating the handicap.

Evaluation of the difficult-to-test child is described in the next section of this chapter.

Hodgson (1978) suggests several factors which can help the audiologist test the young child and explain possible test difficulties. The child's mental age will establish which responses are reflexively present and which responses can be learned. Chronological age provides a standard by which to compare the child's responses with the normal population. The child must have the motor and perceptual ability to make the required reponses. The child's willingness to perform depends upon the youngster's motivation, fears, and rapport with the audiologist. Typically, prior experience with auditory testing makes the child less apprehensive. The test environment should be appealing and flexible. The child who appears initially cooperative may give a false impression of being able to perform at a given level, so the audiologist must be ready to resort quickly to a simpler technique for testing hearing if necessary. There is no substitute for experience when attempting to evaluate hearing in infants and young children.

Infant High-Risk Register for Hearing Loss

The concept of high risk assumes that we can identify a small group of children whose history or physical condition identifies them as having a high chance of having the target handicap. The high-risk register for hearing impairment will involve 6% to 7% of a general nursery population; from this group, the yield of deafness can be expected to be about 1 in 67 babies (Downs, 1978).

The following are the "ABCD's" of the most common factors associated with deafness:

(A) *Affected family*—The presence of a hearing loss (other than the hearing loss that occurs in old age) in a family member markedly increases the likelihood that the infant will have a form of deafness.

(B) *Bilirubin levels too high*—Hyperbilirubinema due to mother-child blood group incompatibility can cause mild to profound hearing loss.

(C) *Congenital rubella syndrome*—Rubella at any time during pregnancy may produce hearing loss in the child. The hearing loss can be the sole symptom or one of many defects.

(D) *Defects involving the ears, nose, or throat*—Malformed, low-set, or absent external ears; cleft lip or palate (including submucous cleft); or any other anatomic abnormalities of the otorhinolaryngeal system are often present along with hearing handicap.

(S) *Small at birth*—Infants weighing less than 1,500g (3lb, 5 oz) at birth have an appreciably greater risk of having hearing defects.

Auditory Maturation

Every normal child undergoes an identifiable sequence of auditory development behavior. Knowledge of this developmental sequence is fundamental to the hearing testing of infants and children.

The test of choice for a baby between 2 months and 24 months is production of an orienting response using noisemakers. The testing is done in a sound-treated room in which noise and visual distractions are kept to a minimum. The failure of a child to localize properly to an auditory signal does not indicate that the child is deaf or hard of hearing. The lack of response may be due to low interest in the sound, delayed auditory maturation, or mental or other physical impairment. The use of noisemakers to stimulate the expected auditory responses is intended to be a screening technique only. Additional work and intensive evaluation by an experienced audiologist is in order for any baby who repeatedly fails to produce an appropriate orienting response.

The most common neonatal response to sudden sound is the auropalpebral reflex (APR). In the awake infant, the APR is a quick, roving movement of the eyes, a definite eye-blink, or obvious eye-widening. If the baby is asleep, the APR may be seen as a sudden tightening of the eyelids. Other behavioral responses seen in young babies, less than 3 months of age, include **Moro's startle response,** cessation of on-going activity, limb movement, facial grimacing, sucking, arousal, breathing change, or rudimentary localization of the eyes toward the sound source.

See Figure 10.5.

The normal development pattern of infant responses to sound, presented in a quiet environment, is as follows.

Birth to 4 Months

Eye-widening, eye-blink, startle, or arousal from sleep are easily noted in a very quiet environment with a normal hearing baby. A beginning primitive effort to turn the head toward the sound may be seen by age 4 months.

4 Months to 7 Months

A horizontal plane head turn toward the sound source is the expected response. At 4 months, the head turn is slow and labored; but by 6 months of age, the head turn should be definite and brisk.

7 Months to 9 Months

At 7 months, the baby should be able to seek a sound source on a lower plane. The child will initially look toward the side and then down below the

FIGURE 10.5

Maturation of the Auditory Response. (From J. Northern & M. Downs, *Hearing in Children* (2nd ed.). Baltimore: The Williams & Wilkins Co., 1978. Copyright © 1978 by The Williams & Wilkins Co. Used by permission.)

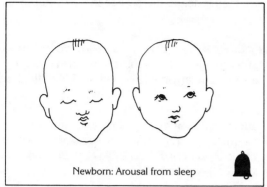

Newborn: Arousal from sleep

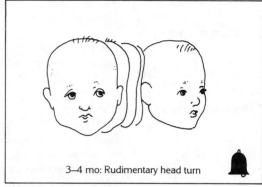

3–4 mo: Rudimentary head turn

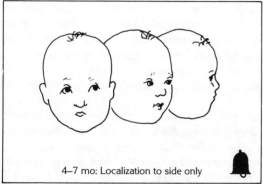

4–7 mo: Localization to side only

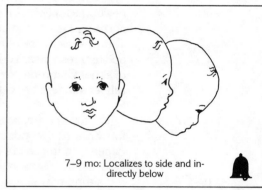

7–9 mo: Localizes to side and in- directly below

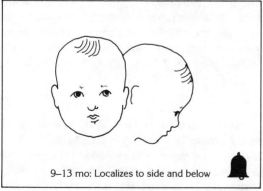

9–13 mo: Localizes to side and below

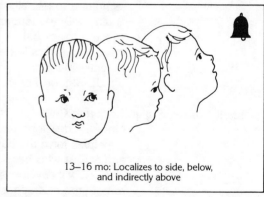

13–16 mo: Localizes to side, below, and indirectly above

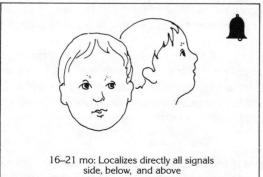

16–21 mo: Localizes directly all signals side, below, and above

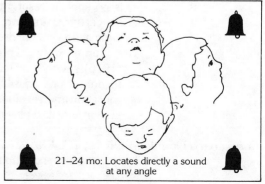

21–24 mo: Locates directly a sound at any angle

horizontal plane. He may not be able to find a sound source presented above and to the side of his head. By the age of 9 months, the baby should be mature enough to seek out the higher sound source in a two-step head turn.

9 Months to 24 Months

At 9 months of age, the indirect higher plane localization becomes a direct, brisk orienting response. By the age of 12 months, the normal hearing child should be able to localize sounds in any plane on either side of the body.

Behavioral Observation Audiometry

Behavioral observation audiometry (BOA) relies on responses of a young child to various acoustic stimuli presented through speakers. The speakers are usually placed at an angle to the child. Responses are defined relative to the auditory maturation level of the child.

Northern and Downs (1978) recommend the use of toy noisemakers with newborns for BOA. The testing should be conducted in a sound-treated room, and a period of absolute silence should preceed each stimulus presentation. Two observers are often used to increase the reliability of confirming each auditory response. The sound output of each toy should be measured ahead of time. Common toy noisemakers include a small bell, a plastic rattle, a rubber squeeze toy, cellophane tissue paper, and a loud bell or loud squeeze toy.

The toy noisemakers are held motionless within 3 inches of the infant's ear for some 10 seconds before initiating the sound. The expected response will depend on the child's auditory maturational level. Again, failure of the infant to locate the sound does not necessarily indicate hearing loss. The particular test sound may simply not be interesting to the infant. Accordingly, it is good technique to use all of the toy noisemakers, beginning with the softest and ending with the loudest. In fact, the last toy noisemaker should be the loud squeeze toy or bell. At all ages, the child should show a startle response to these "loud" toys if they are presented properly. The normal infant will blink violently, jump, or sometimes even cry if he suddenly hears the loud sound (75 dB SPL or more).

Evaluation of Hearing in the Young Child

Once the development of auditory and speech functions is understood, these principles form the basis for evaluating hearing in infants and children. The audiologist who has substantial experience in evaluating hearing in normal children will develop the clinical insight and keen observation skills required to note the discrepant responses of children with auditory handicaps. There is no specific testing technique to fit all children all the time. Flexibility, patience, understanding, and persistence are the watchwords of successful hearing testing with children.

Numerous testing techniques are possible with children. Jerger and Hayes (1976) say that difficult-to-test children should be evaluated with as many techniques as possible for accurate cross-checking of test results. The two most common evaluation techniques are conditioned orientation reflex (COR) audiometry and play conditioning audiometry.

Conditioned Orientation Reflex (COR) Audiometry

When a visual or auditory stimulus is presented to an infant or a young child, she will reflexively turn her head toward the source of the stimulus in an orienting response. Also known as "visual reinforcement audiometry," the technique uses classical conditioning practices to condition the orientation response. A light (or a lighted transparent toy) is flashed at the same time that a sound-field auditory signal is presented. After a few trials, presentation of only the auditory stimulus should cause the child to orient toward the sound source, a response which is recorded by illuminating the toy or flashing the light. Threshold response levels (lowest levels at which the response can be aroused) can be established with soundfield warble tone signals, **narrow-band noise,** or speech signals.

Narrow-band noise *is filtered noise presented in certain frequencies at near-equal intensities.*

The COR technique has many advantages. It is particularly useful for children between 12 months and 3 years of age. The testing procedure is relatively simple and quick, usually accomplished in 10 minutes or less. According to Suzuki and Ogiba (1961), the test is reliable in over 80% of children. However, some children do not condition well, especially children with severe hearing loss who have not learned to localize sound. Obviously, this sound field technique really only tests the child's better hearing ear.

Behavioral Play Audiometry

The best technique for 3- to 4-year old children is "play conditioning," in which some motivational activity such as putting rings on a tower, dropping blocks in a can, or building a pegboard fence with pegs is used to hold the youngster's interest. With earphones on the child's ears, the audiologist teaches the child to perform the required activity each time he hears a pure tone. For example, the youngster holds a block above a box until a loud tone is presented. The child is taught to drop the block immediately, and the action is appropriately rewarded by the audiologist. When the child is able to perform the activity without help, the entire hearing test can be given, for both air conduction and bone conduction.

Speech Audiometry

A cooperative youngster of 3 or older will follow simple commands, identify body parts, and point out common toys. Using these tasks with the sound-field system or under earphones, the speech reception threshold can be established for each ear. Many young children are too shy to repeat words verbally, but they will follow simple speech identification tasks. Some audiologists prefer to begin children's hearing evaluations using speech audiometry to estimate the hearing levels for each ear.

The 4- or 5-year-old youngster with adequate speech and language patterns may cooperate with tests of speech discrimination. If the child will repeat words, the audiologist can use available special children's word lists. Closed-set pictures presented on cards are also used for children to point out the appropriate object representing the perceived word.

Specific Audiological Techniques

Hearing tests cover a wide range of purposes and techniques, beginning with simple pure tone screening, to diagnostic tests designed to identify the specific site of pathology in the auditory system, to advanced physiological procedures that require special skills and expensive equipment.

Hearing Screening

The goal of a hearing screening program is to distinguish those people who probably have some hearing problem from those who probably do not. People who "fail" the screening tests may or may not have ear problems and are thus tagged for additional testing to determine the cause of the screening failure. Virtually every state has an active hearing screening program, and for nearly 40 years hearing screening has proven to be one of the most acceptable screening procedures among a multitude of health detection programs.

Hearing screening should be administered to all preschool children, kindergarteners, and primary school children. The utility of screening in the early grades is evident from reports indicating that 63% of all ultimate hearing losses will be identified by screening in kindergarten and 85% by screening at the third grade level.

The basic instrument needed for hearing screening is the portable screening audiometer. Portable audiometers are manufactured by numerous special instrument companies and are relatively inexpensive. However, they must be recalibrated at regular intervals. The screening levels recommended by ASHA are 20 dB at 1,000, 2,000, and 4,000 Hz. If the 20 dB tone is not heard at 4,000 Hz, a 25 dB screening tone can be used. Hearing screening tests should be conducted by someone who has had appropriate training and should be done in a quiet room away from street noises, foot traffic, visual distractions, and other disturbances, which may result in an inaccurate or unreliable hearing test.

The child should be comfortably seated to one side and slightly behind the audiometer, with the chair at a 45° angle to it. The child should be in a position where the tester can see his or her face during the test. The child should not be able to see the other children or the operation of the audiometer dials. The audiometer headset must be placed carefully and snugly over the ears, with the red receiver on the right ear and the blue receiver on the left ear. The receiver openings should be lined up directly with the canal openings of the ears. The child's hair must be pushed back so it is not between the ear and the receiver. Glasses should be removed.

The child is told to listen for faint sounds or "beeps" and is instructed to indicate when he or she hears the tone by raising one hand when the tone is present and dropping it when the tone ceases. Younger children can be taught to respond to the tone by dropping a colored stick into a box or by similar techniques that convert the test into a game. Missed tones should be retested several times.

Threshold Audiometry

People who have a possible hearing loss detected by screening should be referred for a more thorough hearing test. Many factors must be taken into consideration to obtain reliable audiometric test results. The location of the testing room is important, since environmental noise may obscure auditory thresholds. The audiometer must be in good operating condition and must be calibrated at least every 6 months. The audiologist must know how to instruct the child or adult about the test procedures. Positioning of the headset, earphones, and bone oscillator is important, since poor placement can produce incorrect threshold measurements. The person must feel comfortable during the test; factors such as the test chair, the temperature, the time of day, the interactions with the tester, and motivation will affect the reliability of the test. Other important factors include age, intelligence, reaction time, and previous experience with hearing tests. The techniques of manipulating the audiometer are simple, but the techniques of evaluating hearing in frightened or sick children can be difficult.

Air Conduction   Basic audiometry generally includes pure tone air conduction and speech tests, as well as pure tone bone conduction tests. *Air conduction* refers to the measurement of audiometric thresholds with signals heard through earphones mounted on a headset. The ear with the best hearing is always tested first.

Several psychophysical procedures can be used to arrive at the threshold measurement. The best technique is an ascending method, in which the threshold is measured by progressively increasing the intensity of the stimulus sound from inaudibility to audibility. The stimulus is increased in 10 dB steps until the person hears the tone; the stimulus is then decreased in 5 dB steps until the person no longer perceives it. The threshold is "bracketed" until the audiologist finds a level at which the tone is heard 50% of the time.

With a typical child or adult who understands instructions easily, the air conduction test begins with a sample pure tone stimulus of 40 or 50 dB (or even louder if necessary), which can be heard easily. Once the person has been oriented to the tone and the testing procedure, the signal is reduced to a low level (0 dB), and the ascending approach is begun. The first frequency to test is 1,000 Hz, because it is the easiest of the test tones to hear. Following 1,000 Hz, most audiologists test 2,000, 4,000, 8,000, 500, and 250 Hz, in sequence, for each ear. Any time the tester wishes to check on reliability, the threshold at 1,000 Hz can be reestablished quickly.

Bone Conduction   With the use of the headband, the bone vibrator from the audiometer is placed on the mastoid behind the test ear, without touching the pinna and with the test ear not covered by an earphone. Thresholds for pure tones are determined for air conduction measurements. Bone conduction test frequencies range from 250 to 4,000 Hz; the intensity output is limited to 60 or 70 dB.

Bone conduction measurements are somewhat more difficult than air conduction measurements because vibrations are transmitted to the entire skull, including both cochleas; therefore, it is not always clear which ear is hearing the sound. The audiologist must keep in mind that, in certain situations, the signals presented to one ear are actually perceived in the nontest ear. Unless he or she is constantly on the lookout for these cases, it is easy to measure and record erroneous findings. The audiologist controls which ear is being tested by bone conduction by **masking** the opposite ear with an air conduction earphone.

Masking

Masking is a technique in which a sound is presented to the nontest ear to remove it from the test procedure. The preferred masking sound is narrowband noise. In air conduction measurements, masking must always be considered when the threshold of the test ear is 40 to 50 dB different from the possible cochlear (bone conduction) response of the opposite ear. The primary mode for lateralization, or cross-hearing, of the test tone is through bone conduction. Therefore, during air conduction measurement, if there is a difference of 40 dB or more between the unmasked air conduction threshold of one ear and the bone conduction threshold of the opposite ear, the better ear must be masked when testing the poorer ear.

Since it is difficult to know which cochlea is being stimulated by the bone-conducted test signal, many audiologists mask as a matter of course. Several techniques are available for determining how much masking should be used.

Use of the correct masking level is important, since too little masking or too much masking may affect the results.

Evaluation of Hearing in the Older Child

Figure 10.6 shows a youngster undergoing a pure tone audiological test.

By 5 or 6 years of age, the child of normal intelligence can cooperate in the traditional technique of raising a finger each time he or she hears a pure tone. With some children, additional praise, encouragement, and reinforcement are necessary to maintain full interest in the task. Speech audiometry, including determining the speech reception threshold and speech discrimination, are especially easy with the older child.

The audiologist must be careful, however, with results obtained from children who show exaggerated behavior or who seem to try to be unsuccessful in hearing the sound. Other "red flags" include inconsistent results between testing sessions, poor agreement between pure tone and speech audiometry, or easy understanding of conversational speech while claiming a "severe hearing loss." Special care must be taken in evaluating the hearing of these children, and a thorough discussion with the parents is in order.

FIGURE 10.6
Child Raising Hand in Response to Hearing a Pure Tone.

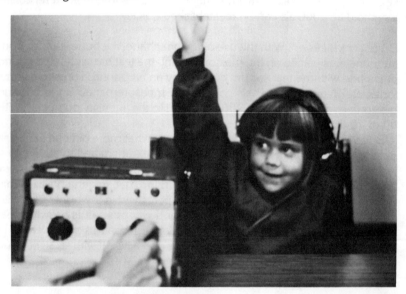

HEARING EVALUATIONS IN SPECIAL POPULATIONS

The evaluation of hearing with difficult-to-test children poses substantial problems. Some normal children turn out to be difficult to test, but in general this term is reserved for those children with mental retardation, multiple handicaps, deaf-blindness, and cerebral palsy. Also worth special mention are certain groups of children who have a high incidence of hearing loss or middle ear disease.

The Mentally Retarded

The retarded child is often not sufficiently mature neurologically to show reflexive auditory awareness or localization tasks. Obviously, many retarded children do not condition well to pure tone audiometry because they learn slowly or because they are either too hyperactive to cooperate or too lethargic to respond. Testing of the severely or profoundly retarded child can be further complicated by the physical handicaps and behavior disorders these children often have. Brain damage in some of these children makes physiological responses unreliable. Yet accurate assessment of their hearing function or their middle ears may be critical for educational placement or medical or surgical treatment. In many cases, mentally retarded children considered to be untrainable have been shown to have hearing loss, fitted with amplification, and placed in more normalized education environments.

These conditions can be aggravated by medications for other problems such as seizures.

The incidence of defective hearing in the mentally retarded is several times greater than in normal children (Lloyd & Reid, 1966). Even a mild degree of hearing loss may have disproportionate impact on the mentally retarded child because he is less capable of compensating easily and quickly with the aid of his other senses.

Down's Syndrome

*Down's syndrome was once known as **mongolism** because of the characteristic appearance of the eyes.*

Down's syndrome is the result of a chromosomal abnormality. It is well known to most audiologists because it occurs frequently (1 in 770 births). It is characterized by a list of nearly 50 features which appear with varying strength. Moderate to severe mental retardation is almost universal in Down's syndrome children. Ear symptoms commonly associated with Down's syndrome include small, narrow external auditory canals, abnormal external ear configuration, and a strong tendency for middle ear effusion.

There is some evidence that children with Down's syndrome have a higher than normal incidence of hearing loss, but there is little unanimity regarding the incidence or nature of the hearing problem. No doubt much of the confusion in the literature regarding the incidence and types of Down's syndrome hearing loss results from the difficulty of evaluating hearing in this population.

An extensive research effort was conducted at the University of Colorado Medical Center to evaluate the incidence and type of hearing problem in 107 Down's syndrome children. The project has resulted in reliable pure tone and speech audiometry for 90% of 107 children with Down's syndrome older than 5 years of age. Only 15% of the group had bilaterally normal hearing, 50% had significant bilateral conductive loss, 15% had sensorineural hearing loss, and 9% showed mixed hearing impairment (Downs, 1980).

The Deaf-Blind Child

Evaluation of the deaf-blind child may be the most formidable task facing the audiologist. The task is even more difficult because many deaf-blind children are retarded as well. In these children, the audiometric evaluation may be limited to observation of the primitive behavioral auditory orientation responses, the acoustic startle reflex, or quieting behavior to the brief introduction of various interesting sound stimuli. When severe visual, motor, or other neurological deficits are present, the basic reflexive auditory responses may be inhibited or absent. These children should be referred to a facility with audiologists experienced in the evaluation of deaf-blind children.

Cleft Lip and Palate Children

See also chapter 11.

Deformities of the lip and palate are among the most common major congenital malformations, occurring in 1 in 900 newborns. The incidence of recurrent otitis media in children with oral cleft has been reported in various studies as between 10% and 90%, depending on the criteria selected for definition of hearing impairment (Paradise & Bluestone, 1974). There is no question, however, that children with cleft lip and palate have a higher incidence of hearing loss than normal children. Jarvis (1976) gives an excellent summary of hearing problems in 350 children with cleft palate. His study shows that the presence of hearing loss in these children rises steadily to a maximum at about 6 years of age and then declines somewhat. The incidence remains stable from age 9.

Craniofacial/Skeletal Disorders

Children with craniofacial and/or skeletal disorders often have congenital conductive or sensorineural hearing loss. Middle ear anomalies are of major importance, because they are frequently correctable by modern microsurgery. Accurate diagnosis of the particular middle ear problem can aid in making surgical decisions.

Cerebral Palsy

See chapter 13.

The communication problems associated with cerebral palsy frequently include impaired hearing. While figures vary considerably, prevalence of hearing loss in the cerebral palsied population is substantially higher than in the normal population. Some estimates run as high as 41% (Nober, 1966). This is not surprising, since the same events which cause cerebral palsy can also be responsible for peripheral hearing loss and central auditory disorders.

Hearing disorders of every variety and degree have been reported among the cerebral palsied population. They most typically include conductive losses, high frequency sensorineural losses, intermittent losses, and central processing disorders. In these children, hearing problems can be complicated by their other physical disabilities as well as by their frequently restricted environmental experience. When auditory problems are not detected and treated, the child may find it unrewarding to listen, which may influence the development and production of spoken language.

MANAGEMENT OF THE HEARING IMPAIRED

Once a youngster has been identified as having a hearing handicap, and all considerations have been given to medical and surgical treatment, the additional management is a long-term process. The function of hearing is not isolated, and many specialists will be involved in the ultimate management of each hearing impaired child. These specialists may include a primary care physician (perhaps a pediatrician), an otolaryngologist, an audiologist, an ophthalmologist, a speech-language pathologist, a social worker, a hearing aid specialist, and a teacher of the deaf. These professionals would monitor the child's hearing problem, advise the family, and judge the child's potential in relation to his educational program. After the initial diagnosis is confirmed, the young child should be reevaluated every 6 months until age 5 or 6, and once a year thereafter.

For an overview of the handicapping effects of an untreated hearing loss, see Table 10.2.

Amplification and Auditory Training

Figure 10.7 shows child wearing hearing aid.

As we have already seen, most hearing impaired people are not deaf; they retain some **residual hearing.** The first step in the management program is to determine if the hearing impaired person is a candidate for a hearing aid. If so, the audiologist prescribes one to amplify sounds to the wearer's threshold

TABLE 10.2
Handicapping Effects of Hearing Loss.

Average Hearing 500-2,000 (ANSI)	Description	Possible Condition	What Can be Heard Without Amplification	Handicapping Effects (If not Treated in 1st Year of Life)	Probable Needs
0-15 dB	Normal range	Conductive hearing losses	All speech sounds	None	None
15-25 dB	Slight hearing loss	Conductive hearing losses, some sensorineural hearing losses	Vowel sounds heard clearly; may miss unvoiced consonant sounds	Mild auditory dysfunction in language learning	Consideration of need for hearing aid; speech-reading, auditory training, speech therapy, preferential seating
25-40 dB	Mild hearing loss	Conductive or sensorineural hearing losses	Only some of speech sounds, the louder voiced sounds	Auditory learning dysfunction, mild language retardation, mild speech problems, inattention	Hearing aid, speechreading, auditory training, speech therapy
40-65 dB	Moderate hearing loss	Conductive hearing loss from chronic middle ear disorders; sensorineural hearing losses	Almost no speech sounds at normal conversational level	Speech problems, language retardation, learning dysfunction, inattention	All of the above, plus consideration of special classroom situation
65-95 dB	Severe hearing loss	Sensorineural or mixed losses due to a combination of middle ear disease and sensorineural involvement	No speech sounds of normal conversations	Severe speech problems, language retardation, learning dysfunction, inattention	All of the above; probable assignment to special classes
95 dB+	Profound hearing loss	Sensorineural or mixed losses due to a combination of middle ear disease and sensorineural involvement	No speech or other sounds	Severe speech problems, language retardation, learning dysfunction, inattention	All of the above; probable assignment to special classes

of hearing. However, wearing a hearing aid is not enough to help hearing impaired people make the best of their residual hearing. Consequently, most programs include **auditory training** designed to help the hard of hearing use their residual hearing.

The extent of the auditory training program will depend on the individual's hearing loss. Most programs involve increasing the person's awareness of both environmental and speech sounds, ability to localize sound, sound discrimination abilities, and finally word recognition abilities (Heward & Orlansky, 1980). Auditory training may be carried out by speech-language pathologists and/or special educators.

FIGURE 10.7
Child Wearing a Hearing Aid.

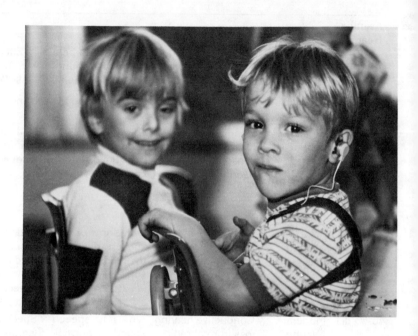

Speechreading

Along with learning to use their ears (and hearing aids) to the maximum extent possible, most hearing impaired people use their eyes to receive messages from other people. One useful skill is speechreading, or discerning what words are being spoken by watching the lips, jaws, and expressions of the speaker. Most people who lose their hearing after they have mastered language skills learn to use speechreading to some extent on their own. In children who are born deaf or who develop a severe hearing impairment before they learn to talk, speechreading can be taught. Unfortunately, speechreading has limited use because many phonemes which sound different look the same. For example, voiced and unvoiced cognates cannot be distinguished by lip movements. To test this out, go to a mirror and watch yourself say "fairy" and "very." It has been estimated that only 20% to 30% of conversational speech can be perceived by speechreading.

Approaches to Communication Skills

As we've seen throughout this book, everyone wants and needs to communicate with other people. Not being able to express yourself easily and clearly is frustrating and can lead to all kinds of negative feelings. Adults who lose their hearing already have full language skills. For them, speech is not too great a problem; although if the loss is severe, they may eventually need to work with a speech-language pathologist on maintaining precise articulation. Without the feedback that comes with hearing your own speech, articulation skills tend to deteriorate over time.

See chapter 5.

A common problem that comes with the hearing loss that accompanies aging is a change in the loudness of speech; remember your grandfather or Aunt Helen who talked louder and louder as he or she became "deafer and deafer." If either the elderly person or the family feels that this loudness (or excessive softness) is a problem worth attending to, it can often be remedied with simple voice exercises.

See chapter 6.

Unfortunately, the young child's problem of expressing himself is not so easily managed, and even the question of what kinds of skills to teach is quite controversial. In the United States today, there are at least three common approaches to language skills for severely hearing impaired children: the manual approach, the oral approach, and total communication. Even though language skills are usually taught by the special educator, speech-language pathologists and audiologists should be aware of the differences between these approaches to better serve their students.

The Manual Approach

The manual approach involves teaching hearing impaired people to use their hands and bodies to communicate. Fingerspelling is a technique in which each letter of the alphabet is represented by a unique hand position. Each word is spelled out letter by letter. While this may sound tedious, people do become quite proficient at it. It has the advantage of using the same elements (letters, words, syntax) that are used in written communication.

A second manual technique is sign language. American Sign Language (ASL) is one system used widely by deaf adults. It involves using the hands, body, and trunk in gestures that symbolize whole words or even more complex concepts. Fingerspelling is used for words such as proper names that have no special signs. The advantage of sign language is that it seems to be fairly easy to learn; it gives the child some way to express himself. A disadvantage is that each sign language has its own symbols, syntax, and word order, which are not necessarily the same as those of "normal" English. For example, ASL is based on French language rules for word order and syntax. Some experts feel that learning two languages at the same time (which is, in essence, what the deaf child learning to read and to use sign languge is doing) is too demanding and confusing, expecially for a child who may be having trouble with the basic idea of language. Furthermore, only those people who know the particular sign language can communicate with the hearing impaired person.

The Oral Approach

The oral approach stresses the use of speech in communication. Auditory training and speechreading are especially critical here, along with on-going work on articulation, intonation, and stress. Children are taught to monitor their own speech by becoming aware of how it feels to make each speech sound (called **kinesthetic feedback**) (Lowenbraun & Scroggs, 1978). In some oral programs, the students are prohibited from using any signs or gestures at all; they are, in effect, forced to learn to talk. And many hearing impaired children—even those with profound losses—do learn to have "normal" speech. The advantages of this approach are the opportunities it gives the hearing impaired to interact with anyone with normal hearing. In addition, it obviously relates directly to the development of reading, writing, and other language skills.

Total Communication

Total communication involves using any and all means of communication—including auditory training, speechreading, fingerspelling, sign language, and speech. The goal is to develop language skills by all available methods rather than one specific technique. Because hearing impaired children continue to have difficulty mastering both basic and advanced concepts of language, total communication, which is the newest approach to educating the hearing impaired, is becoming more and more widely used.

CONCLUSION

Working with the hearing impaired is one of the stiffest challenges a language professional meets—with the new mainstreaming laws, one that may be appearing more frequently in the case loads of those who work in the public schools. Whether you are an audiologist testing a toddler, a speech-language pathologist helping a child learn to articulate /b/ and /p/, or a special education teacher teaching the rules for making plurals, you face an enormous obstacle in the language deficiencies of people who cannot learn language by hearing it. Unfortunately, even with improved hearing aids, microsurgery, and new educational approaches, we are less than successful with the overall language development of hearing impaired children. And, of course, oral language acquisition affects other important skills, including reading and concept acquisition. The audiologist who evaluates the degree of hearing loss and the speech-language pathologist and teacher who help overcome it must work closely with the child and the family, so that the potential achievements as well as the problems of the hearing impaired are clearly understood. The language professional must also continue to work with all the other professionals involved to follow the child's progress and modify the program as often as necessary.

SELECTED READINGS

Connor, L. E. *Speech for the deaf child: Knowledge and use.* Washington, D.C.: Alexander Graham Bell Association for the Deaf, 1971.

Davis, H., & Silverman, S. R. (Eds.). *Hearing and deafness.* New York: Holt, Rinehart & Winston, 1970.

Eisenberg, R. B. *Auditory competence in early life.* Baltimore: University Park Press, 1976.

Martin, F. N. *Introduction to audiology.* Englewood Cliffs, N.J.: Prentice-Hall, 1975.

Minifie, F. D., Huion, T. J., & Williams, F. (Eds.). *Normal aspects of speech, hearing and language.* Englewood Cliffs, N.J.: Prentice-Hall, 1973.

Northern, J. L. (Ed.). *Hearing disorders.* Boston: Little, Brown, 1976.

REFERENCES

Downs, M. P. Auditory screening. *Otolaryngology Clinics of North America, 1978, 11,* (3), 611–629.

Downs, M. P. (Ed.). Communicative disorders in Down's syndrome. *Seminars in Speech, Language, and Hearing.* New York: Brian C. Decker, 1980.

Eilers, R. E., Wilson, W. R., & Moore, J. M. Developmental changes in speech discrimination in infants. *Journal of Speech and Hearing Research, 1977, 20,* 766–780.

Eimas, P. D., Siqueland, E. R., Jusczyk, P., & Vigorita, J. Speech perception in infants. *Science, 1971, 171,* 303–306.

Eisenberg, R. B. *Auditory competence in early life.* Baltimore: University Park Press, 1976.

Heward, W. L., & Orlansky, M. *Exceptional children.* Columbus, Ohio: Charles E. Merrill, 1980.

Hodgson, W. Testing infants and young children. In J. Katz (Ed.), *Handbook of clinical audiology.* Baltimore: Williams and Wilkins, 1978.

Holm, V. A., & Kunze, L. H. Effect of chronic otitis media in language and speech development. *Pediatrics,* 1969, *43,* 833–839.

Jarvis, J. R. Audiologic status of children with cleft palate: A review of 350 cases. *Audiology,* 1976, *15,* 242–248.

Jerger, J., & Hayes, D. The cross-check principle in pediatric audiometry. *Archives of Otolaryngology,* 1976, *102,* 614–620.

Kryter, K. D., & Ades, H. W. Studies on the function of the higher acoustic nervous centers in the cat. *American Journal of Psychology,* 1943, *56,* 501–536.

Lee, L. *Northwestern Syntax Screening Test.* Evanston, Ill.: Northwestern University Press, 1971.

Lemme, M. L., & Daves, N. H. Models of auditory linguistic processing. In N. J. Lass, J. L. Northern, D. E. Yoder, & L. V. McReynolds (Eds.), *Speech, language, and hearing.* Philadelphia: W. B. Saunders, 1981.

Lenneberg, E. *Biological foundations of language.* New York: John Wiley, 1967.

Lieberman, P. *Intonation, perception and language. (Research Monograph No. 38).* Cambridge, Mass.: MIT Press, 1967.

Lloyd, L., & Reid, M. J.: The incidence of hearing impairment in an institutionalized mentally retarded population. *American Journal of Mental Deficiency,* 1966, *71,* 746–763.

Lowenbraun, S., & Scroggs, C. The hearing handicapped. In N. G. Haring (Ed.), *Behavior of exceptional children* (2nd ed.). Columbus, Ohio: Charles E. Merrill, 1978.

Minifie, F. D. Speech acoustics. In F. D. Minifie, T. J. Huion, & F. Williams (Eds.), *Normal aspects of speech, hearing and language.* Englewood Cliffs, N.J.: Prentice-Hall, 1973.

Nober, E. Hearing problems associated with cerebral palsy. In W. Cruickshank & G. Raus (Eds.), *Cerebral palsy.* Syracuse: Syracuse University Press, 1966.

Northern, J. L., & Downs, M. P. *Hearing in children* (2nd ed.). Baltimore: Williams and Wilkins, 1978.

Paradise, J. L., & Bluestone, C. D. Early treatment of the universal otitis media of infants with cleft palate. *Pediatrics,* 1974, *53,* 48–54.

Rees, N. S. Auditory processing factors in language disorders: The view from procrustes bed. *Journal of Speech and Hearing Disorders,* 1973, *38,* 304–315.

Sanders, D. A. *Auditory perception of speech.* Englewood Cliffs, N.J.: Prentice-Hall, 1977.

Skinner, M. W. The hearing of speech during language acquisition. *Otolaryngology Clinics of North America,* 1978, *11,* 631–650.

Suzuki, T., & Ogiba, Y. Conditioned orientation audiometry. *Archives of Otolaryngology,* 1961, 74, 192–198.

Wiig, E. H., & Semel, E. M. *Language disabilities in children and adolescents.* Columbus, Ohio: Charles E. Merrill, 1976.

Wiig, E. H., & Semel, E. M. *Language assessment and intervention for the learning disabled.* Columbus, Ohio: Charles E. Merrill, 1980.

11

CLEFT
PALATE

Betty Jane McWilliams

When referred to the Cleft Palate Center, Martha was a 10-year-old girl who had been born with an isolated cleft of the soft palate. The defect had been repaired by a plastic surgeon when she was 18 months of age, and no additional surgery had been undertaken since. Martha had a history of otitis media which had been controlled at least partially by repeated myringotomies with the insertion of polyethylene tubes from the age of 3 months. She had a very mild hearing impairment which was not thought to be of significance to speech but indicated the need for continued ear care.

While she had not had a cleft involving the maxillary arch, she none-theless had a severe anterior crossbite. Martha was awaiting orthodontic intervention at approximately age 11. Otherwise, this little girl had excellent dental health.

Her receptive language abilities had always appeared to be within normal limits, but she had used no expressive language until 4 months after the palate was repaired. During the preschool years, she showed slight reductions on all subtests of the Illinois Test of Psycholinguistic Abilities. By age 8, she tested within normal limits on the ITPA. Her mental abilities had developed much as her linguistic abilities had. During the preschool years, Martha had a verbal IQ on the Wechsler Intelligence Scale for Children of 99 and a performance IQ of 100. Thus, there was no difference between the two scales, and she appeared to have average mental ability. However, by age 8, her Wechsler verbal IQ had increased to 120 and her performance IQ to 117. She then tested in the "bright normal" classification of children.

Martha was referred to the Cleft Palate Center by a school speech-language pathologist who asked for suggestions for speech therapy. Speech examination revealed that she had moderate, visible, bilateral, consistent nasal emission. Her hypernasality was rated as severe, and she was slightly hoarse. The intelligibility of her speech was severely impaired, primarily because of many articulation errors including omissions, pharyngeal fricatives, and glottal stops. These gross articulation errors made it difficult to assess her intraoral pressure. However, she could produce both /p/ and /b/, but these phonemes were reduced in intraoral pressure. The speech examination suggested that this child was suffering from velopharyngeal incompetence and that speech therapy by itself would not be helpful to her. It was, therefore, decided to evaluate the velopharyngeal valve.

Warren pressure flow studies revealed evidence of greater resistance in the right nostril than in the left, but the resistance was not great enough to eliminate air flow through the nasal passages. Multiview videofluoro-scopy showed a short soft palate with good mobility. However, in lateral projection, the soft palate never made contact with the posterior pharyn-geal wall. The frontal projection showed that there was about 50% lateral pharyngeal wall movement and that it occurred at the expected level of the velar eminence. The basal view was consistent with the lateral and frontal views. The instrumental findings were consistent with the speech symptoms and indicated the need for further physical management. In this case, a pharyngeal flap was recommended and carried out.

Following the pharyngeal flap surgery, both multiview videofluoro-scopy and pressure flow evaluations revealed a mechanism capable of achieving velopharyngeal closure. It was possible for Martha to completely eliminate the flow of air through the nostrils during the production of selected speech tasks, primarily /p/ and /b/, but it was impossible to predict what she would do with other consonants which she could not at that time produce. Speech therapy was recommended for the elimination of gross articulation errors. She was treated as an articulation problem and profited well from therapy designed to establish new patterns of consonant production. Her speech was eventually normal except for sibilant errors related to her dental crossbite. Speech therapy was discontinued until the completion of orthodontic work, after which her speech patterns were reassessed to determine the need for continued speech therapy. No addi-tional speech therapy was necessary since the sibilant production had been self-corrected.

You may now wish to listen to the speech sample accompanying this chapter, found on Audio Disc 2, Side 3 (sample #7).

The second special group we will look at is people with cleft palates and related disorders. These birth defects will seriously affect speech if left un-treated. While we now have surgical techniques to repair some defective struc-tures, the surgery may not be totally effective. In addition, some people have less obvious defects which go untreated. Thus children and adults with cleft palates, including those who have had surgery, are often referred for speech-language intervention. The speech difficulties of people with cleft palates are caused by problems involving the coupling of the oral and nasal cavities. Under these circumstances, the system cannot be closed in order to create the pressure inside the mouth that is necessary first for sucking and swallow-ing and then for production of speech sounds. As we have seen, correct articulation of the nasal sounds /m, n, ŋ/ depends upon the ability to open the velopharyngeal valve, thus connecting the oral and nasal cavities, and precise articulation of the other consonants and all vowels requires that critical valve to be completely closed.

Speech-language pathologists should be aware that conditions other than clefts can affect the ability to separate the oral and nasal cavities and to create sufficient intraoral pressure. These conditions include malfunction or mal-arrangement of palatal and pharyngeal muscles, short palate, deep pharynx, and sudden loss of the adenoidal mass. The speech of a person with any of

These structures were identified in chapter 4.

these problems is complicated and requires extensive study if it is to be well managed. This chapter will discuss these related conditions as well as cleft palate and lip.

BASIC CONCEPTS

Why Clefts Occur

*Recall that the **maxilla** is the upper jaw; the **mandible** is the lower jaw.*

The human face develops complexly and rapidly during the first 10 weeks of gestation. If there is a disruption at some point between the 6th and 10th weeks, a cleft may result. Simply stated, if the medial nasal process and the right and left maxillary processes fail to move toward each other so that fusion can occur around the 7th week, some form of cleft lip will be present when the child is born. The formation of the hard palate occurs slightly later, when the palatal shelves, which also have their origin in the maxillary processes, unite with the nasal septum. The tongue is developing along with these other structures, and it drops down as mandibular growth provides the space. This lowering of the tongue permits the palatal shelves to move together. Fusion takes place from the front to the back of the mouth (anterior to posterior). Any disruption in this process will result in a palatal cleft. The earlier the interruption occurs, the more extensive the cleft will be.

It is easier to describe *what* happens (or fails to happen) to cause a cleft than it is to explain *why*. Parents are usually concerned about the why, and professionals who work with them and their children must be sensitive to their questions and anxieties. In some cases, superstition will influence the parents' behavior to the detriment of the child. As one mother said, "This is my cross to bear. I am being punished by God for 'something' I did." And another, "When I was seven-months pregnant, I saw a woman shoot herself in the head. The blood ran down her lip, right where my baby's cleft is. It 'marked' my child." Or, "People will know it's because I tried to abort my baby and failed." These real statements reflect guilt and fear and no understanding about the origins of clefts.

The developmental failures that cause clefts cannot be attributed to the moral shortcomings of mothers and fathers. Clefts are probably related to many genetic factors coming together under adverse environmental conditions. This means that the genetic programming of the developing infant predisposes it to some alteration in the growth pattern and that the environment also contributes to the disruption. For example, a tongue may be genetically "programmed" to drop down into the mandible on the late side of normal and may then be delayed further by some environmental factor such as radiation, a minor tranquilizing or anticonvulsant drug, or a virus. Thus the genetic makeup of the child interacts with the environment to create the cleft. In some cases, particularly in a number of the more than 100 syndromes associated with clefting (Cohen, 1978), the cause appears to be purely genetic.

Clefts vary in their occurrence rate from one racial group to another. Orientals have the highest rate of about one in 500 births. Caucasians are some place in the middle of the frequency scale, with estimates ranging from one in 750 to one in 1,000 births. Blacks are least likely to have clefts, and estimates for them range between one in 1,900 to one in 3,000 births. Just why this racial difference is present is not clearly understood, but it is another point in support of a genetic theory of causation.

Clefts also affect more boys than girls. A cleft is usually the only congenital abnormality present, but approximately 25% of all children born with clefts will have some other defect as well. Clefts sometimes appear as part of certain clinical syndromes that include other specific abnormalities.

While the literature suggests that clefts involve both the lip and palate about twice as often as the palate by itself, this conclusion may now be open to question. In the past 10 years, the Cleft Palate Center at the University of Pittsburgh has had an average caseload of 1,000 children and adults. In that period, nearly half of those seen with palatal clefts had no lip impairment. This shift in statistics, at least for this population, is of concern because the isolated cleft is more likely to be associated with other birth defects and with clinical syndromes than is the complete cleft lip and palate. We need to conduct further study of this population because the risk of recurrence within the family may be notably increased in some cases.

The fact that family background plays an important role in clefting means that families of infants born with clefts should have careful genetic workups in order to give them the best possible advice and guidance. Speech-language pathologists are interested in this issue because anxious parents cannot provide the most adequate linguistic environment for their children. In addition, parents will ask questions of any professional person with whom they feel comfortable. If necessary, the untrained speech-language pathologist should refer these inquiries to other professionals who are competent to handle these emotionally loaded questions. Genetics, embryology, anatomy, and growth and development of the face are fields that are growing in relationship to speech pathology and audiology, and increasing numbers of students are delving into these related subjects.

These topics can provide excellent material for a term project or special report. A starting place for additional reading would be the first six chapters in Grabb, Rosenstein, and Bzoch (1971).

The Nature of Clefts

Clefts may be of a number of different types and may range from minimal to severe defects. Cleft lip may be a simple notch or a more complete cleft on

FIGURE 11.1

(a) Infant with a Left Incomplete Cleft Lip. (b) The Same Infant after Lip Repair.

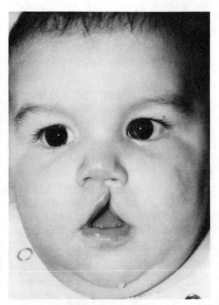
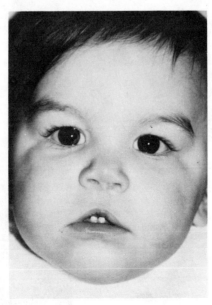

See Figures 11.1 through 11.5.

only one side (see Figure 11.1), or it may be very extensive, involving both sides of the lip and extending into the nostril (see Figure 11.2). We refer to these clefts as *unilateral* or *bilateral.* Those that occur unilaterally are usually on the left side for some reason that we do not clearly understand. A cleft palate may be a complete cleft that extends all the way through the soft and hard palate and alveolar or dental ridge on one or both sides. Figure 11.4 shows a classification of the various types of clefts (Kernahan & Stark, 1958). Some clefts extend through portions of the face, as is shown in Figure 11.5.

Of special interest to the speech-language pathologist is the submucous cleft palate. This is a true muscular cleft, but it is covered with a thin mucous membrane that makes it likely that the defect will be overlooked—often until a speech problem persists into childhood and fails to respond to intervention. Not all submucous clefts cause speech problems, but those that do require the care provided for overt clefts. The submucous cleft can often be seen by a careful examiner. The uvula may be bifid, or look as if it is double. In reality, it has a small cleft. There may be a bluish line through the middle of the soft palate where the muscles underlying the mucosa are separated, and there may be a notch in the posterior border of the hard palate that can be palpated or felt. Speech-language pathologists are often the observers who discover these anatomical variations and realize that the person needs the help of others before speech is likely to improve.

FIGURE 11.2

(a) Infant with Bilateral Complete Lip and Palate. (b) The Same Infant after Repair.

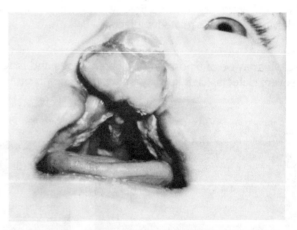

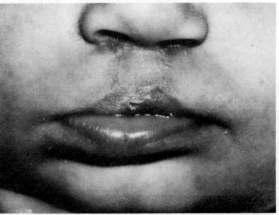

FIGURE 11.3

(a) Infant with Left Unilateral Cleft Lip and Palate. (b) The Same Infant Following Lip Repair. Note widely spaced eyes and flattened nasal bridge.

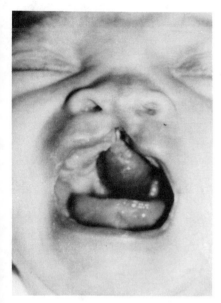 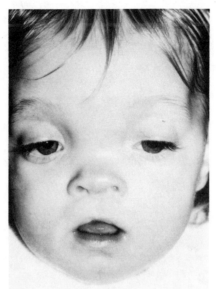

Other Structural Palatal Deviations

The overt or submucous cleft palate is not difficult to diagnose. However, there are other structural problems that pose more serious problems, even of description. Kaplan, Jobe, and Chase (1969) have described and illustrated some of these conditions. They include a deep nasopharynx, which means that the space between the soft palate and the throat is enlarged because the rear wall of the throat is deeper than usual. Thus the soft palate, while capable of normal movement, cannot compensate for this added distance. The hard palate may also be somewhat short, so that the soft palate is carried too far forward in the oral cavity to be effective; or the soft palate itself may be too short. This latter condition is often associated with soft palate musculature that is malpositioned and has its insertion in the hard palate instead of properly in the posterior part of the soft palate.

Other deviations include palatal immobility, inconsistent movement, or movement that is not synchronized with speech. These problems may result from neurological impairment and require careful study. *See chapter 12.*

Craniofacial abnormalities are defects of the head and face, and they often include palatal abnormalities as well. These problems have a variety of forms, and they were once thought to be untreatable because of their extent and complexity. Tessier (1971) revolutionized the surgical approach to these children, and it is now not uncommon for them to undergo massive procedures designed to correct or minimize their deformities (Christiansen & Evans, 1975). Since speech-language pathologists are finding many new and challenging opportunities to work with these children, it is appropriate to mention them briefly here. Let us look at an example to illustrate the problems encountered.

When we first saw him, Peter was a 5-year-old boy with Apert syndrome, which is known also as *acrocephalosyndactylia*. He had a unique appearance similar to that of other children with the same diagnosis. His forehead *See Figure 11.6.*

FIGURE 11.4

Cleft Classification Proposed by Kernahan and Stark (1958) and Adopted by the International Confederation for Plastic Surgery in 1967. (From D. A. Kernahan & R. B. Stark, "A New Classification for Cleft Lip and Cleft Palate," Plastic and Reconstructive Surgery, *1958, 22, 435. Used by permission.)*

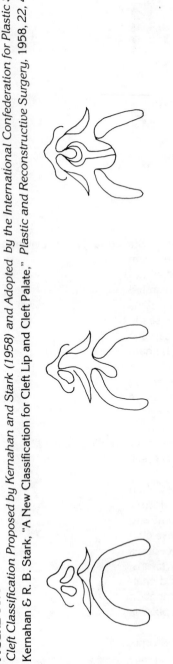

1. Unilateral, Subtotal Cleft of Primary Palate

2. Unilateral, Total Cleft of Primary Palate

3. Bilateral, Total Cleft of Primary Palate

4. Subtotal Cleft of Secondary Palate

5. Total Cleft of Secondary Palate

6. Unilateral, Subtotal Clefts of Primary and Secondary Palates

7. Unilateral, Total Cleft of Primary and Secondary Palates

8. Bilateral, Total Cleft of Primary and Secondary Palates

was bulbous or *bossed,* his nose was somewhat beaked, and his eyes were too far apart. His midface was small, and he had a *very* high-arched palate with a proliferation of tissue in the maxilla. This latter condition, while not a true cleft, resembled one and had been so diagnosed—even though his speech was hyponasal (too *little* nasal component in speech rather than too much). His hands and feet were mittenlike. Peter had average mental abilities, but his appearance had led everyone to underestimate his capacities. He was

FIGURE 11.5

(a) Infant with Left Lateral Facial Cleft. (b) The Same Child after Repair.

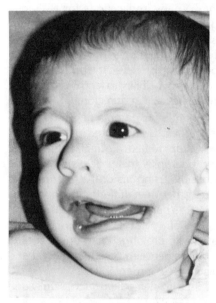
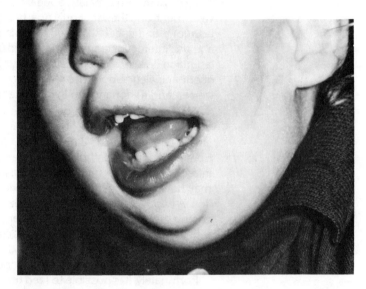

FIGURE 11.6

(a) Boy with Apert Syndrome. (b) Hand Deformity Associated with Apert Syndrome.

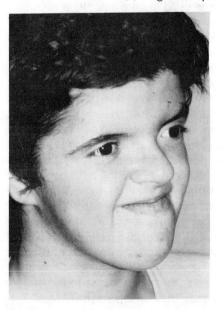
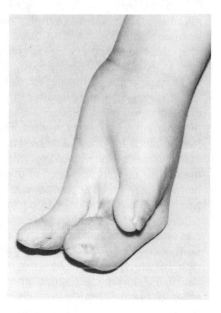

socially underdeveloped for his age, and his mother had removed him from nursery school when other children asked questions about his appearance and called him a "bad monster." His expressive language was at age level. Peter required extensive plastic surgery followed by intensive language intervention in a social setting. Apert syndrome is just one example of many conditions about which we can now do something to bring some improvement. Speech-language pathologists are finding new professional opportunities working with these children (Peterson-Falzone, 1973).

Development of the Child with Cleft Palate

The opening in the palate appears to have many implications for early development, and these are only now being recognized as they affect subsequent language and speech. In fact, there is still a great deal that we do not know, and the interactions among several different problems as they may relate to language development are still largely speculative. However, the primitive state of our knowledge does not relieve us of the responsibility to learn as much as we can and to continue to investigate the issues still in question.

Feeding problems are usually the first hurdle for parents and infant, and these are reflected in protracted feeding times. Uninstructed parents often struggle for as long as 2 hours to get their infant to take 4 ounces of formula. Speech-language pathologists are eager to simplify this process so that the infant may have as much success as possible using his oral structures and may have a rewarding feeding experience rather than suffering from frustration. A happy feeding time also encourages the parent in the quiet talking and cooing that are the natural accompaniments of a pleasant experience shared with the infant. The frustrations associated with prolonged and unsuccessful feeding create tensions that disrupt the bonds between parent and child and thus can affect the early stages of linguistic development.

Fortunately, it is possible to feed the infant with cleft palate successfully and thus to lay a portion of the foundation necessary for future verbal behavior. A simple compressible bottle lets the parent apply light pressure to the plastic bag and ease the formula gently through a cross-cut nipple while the infant is held in a sitting position. This helps the child to take a bottle in about 20 minutes and provides a simple means of assuring success. The speech-language pathologist with a basic concern for solving feeding problems is often the one to instruct the parents and to follow the baby's progress, along with a pediatrician. This type of intervention represents the earliest speech and language programming for cleft infants (Paradise & McWiliams, 1974).

Ear disease is present from birth in *all* infants with cleft palate (Paradise, Bluestone, & Felder, 1969; Stool & Randall, 1967), but there is no increased risk when only cleft lip is present. The ear disease seems to be related to the malfunctioning of the Eustachian tube, caused at least in part by an alteration in the action of the tensor veli palatini muscles. There is no question about the middle ear effusion seen in these children or about the mild conductive hearing losses that accompany it. Left untreated, the otitis media may get worse and lead eventually to permanent handicapping hearing loss. Theoretically, even these early mild hearing losses could slow down both language and articulatory development. While children with palatal clefts do lag behind normal children in these abilities, there are many possible explanations for the delay, of which hearing loss is but one. The precise role of these mild hearing deficits is far from clear at this time. However, there is no question but that we strive for normal hearing in all children at as early an age as possible.

Recall from the last chapter the long-lasting effects of early hearing loss.

The goal, then, is not in question, but the method for achieving it is. We know that ear disease improves in most cleft children as they get older, as it does in all children generally, and that there is often dramatic change following the surgical repair of the soft palate. A few children retain persistent and recurring middle ear disease into their teens and adulthood. Some writers (Paradise & Bluestone, 1969) advocate routine myringotomies with tubes in the first 2 or 3 months of life, with careful follow-up and repeated procedures as these are needed. However, there is no clear evidence that that approach is any more successful than a more conservative system of doing myringotomies and inserting aeration tubes at the first evidence of discomfort, active infection, or marked increase in the amount of fluid present. Most babies who are watched carefully and for whom the more conservative treatment is used will require myringotomy some time after 6 months of age and prior to the first birthday. The speech-language pathologist must always be alert to the possibility of hearing loss in children with palatal clefts and of the need for frequent air- and bone-conduction audiometric testing.

A myringotomy is a small surgical incision through the tympanic membrane to allow drainage of fluid from the middle ear; drainage tubes are sometimes left in place to allow continued aeration of the ear.

Psychosocial problems can also influence the way in which language and speech emerge. This is true for all children, but the baby with a cleft is undoubtedly at increased risk in this regard. The parents must come to terms with the defect and all that that entails and accept the less-than-perfect child about whom they have no doubt dreamed. Parents are understandably disappointed, shocked, and in a sense, grief-stricken (Tisza & Gumpertz, 1962). Yet most of the research done to date shows that parents are, for the most part, realists who quickly accept their baby, the cleft, and themselves. Individual parents will vary in their ability to deal with this kind of problem just as they vary in other regards (McWilliams, 1970). Some will do beautifully from the beginning, and a few will never accommodate to what they view as a disaster. The speech-language pathologist must be very sensitive to parents and the ways in which they interact with their children. A perceptive mother or father can accomplish miracles with a child and can encourage and foster communicative skills better than a clinician ever could, while another parent may be destructive to everyone's efforts to make communication skills functional.

To pursue this topic further, see Graham, 1978.

As for the children themselves, there is no strong evidence to suggest that they are any more or less likely to be emotionally disturbed than are children who do not have clefts. This is not to imply that cleft children are not emotionally disturbed. Some are, and the implications for language and speech can be overwhelming. The mother who punished her child when he tried to say a few simple words before his palate had been surgically repaired is a case in point. She believed that her little boy would talk better later on if she consistently silenced him as long as the palate remained open. She exemplifies the parent in desperate need of extensive counseling, with special emphasis on handling the early stages of verbal development. The speech-language pathologist is frequently involved in guidance programs like this, and must also be alert to the clues of more serious problems requiring the intervention of a psychiatrist, psychologist, or social worker.

While children with palatal clefts generally show adequate psychosocial development, they are subject to some unique problems inposed upon them by a society that tends to penalize people for their differences. This may be especially true during the school years. These children often do not participate in classroom activities to the extent of their abilities, they are teased because of their facial disfigurement or speech, and they may feel less "popular" than their peers. They also seem to be slightly immature socially and to prefer the

For more complete coverage of the psychosocial issues of cleft palate, see McWilliams and Smith (1973).

company of somewhat younger children. The speech-language pathologist has an important role in helping these children develop and use conversational skills, in orienting teachers to ways of minimizing the handicap in the classroom, and in working to alter negative attitudes in all students. There is far more to helping people learn to communicate than stressing only the mechanics of speech.

Mental development is still another aspect of growth that has worried speech-language pathologists. The ranges in IQ reported for children with clefts have often been lower than for control populations (Clifford, 1979; Goodstein, 1961; Lamb, Wilson, & Leeper, 1972; McWilliams, 1973; Ruess, 1965). Mean IQ, while within the normal range, has also been found to be significantly lower than for noncleft controls. Goodstein (1961) suggests that these findings might be explained by the presence in the study groups of children with isolated palatal clefts. These clefts are often associated with other congenital abnormalities and with an increased occurrence of mental retardation. McWilliams and Matthews (1979) report no reduction in mean IQ for children with unilateral or isolated palatal clefts except when *either* had other birth defects. The unilaterals, however, appeared to be slightly superior to those with isolated clefts; and both of these groups had higher mean IQs than did the unilaterals with other congenital problems. The latter group, however, was superior to those with isolated clefts associated with other problems. A cleft that occurs by itself does not seem to be a predictor of problems with mental development as it is when other malformations are also present.

More recent studies seem to be reporting less evidence of problems in the cleft population than was noted earlier. Since both retarded and gifted children are found in all classifications of clefts, we must not draw any conclusions about anyone without the benefit of close observation and careful testing (Richman, 1976). This is especially important; Richman (1978) found that teachers underestimated the abilities of bright children with facial disfigurement and overestimated the capabilities of less able children.

Speech-language pathologists must always be aware that intelligence is one important factor in language and speech development, but that it interacts with many other aspects of development as well. Thus, it is possible for a very bright but psychologically impaired child to be less efficient as a communicator than a slow child who feels comfortable as a person. This subtle interplay among many different characteristics is not as well understood as we hope it will be in the future. All that we can say now is that we should recognize the complex nature of problems associated with cleft palate and take them into account in the clinical management of these children.

Another finding reported many times in the literature is that verbal IQ is usually significantly lower than performance IQ in children with cleft palate (Lamb, et al., 1972; Ruess, 1965). However, these studies did not take into account the nature of the speech skills of the children being studied, so it is difficult to interpret the findings. McWilliams and Musgrave (1972) did not find superior verbal or performance IQ when children were grouped on the basis of speech competency. Whether speech was normal or seriously impaired, verbal IQ was as likely to be superior to performance as the other way around. In a later study (McWilliams & Matthews, 1979), there were again no significant differences between performance and verbal IQs in children whose speech ranged from normal to moderately defective. None had evidence of severe cleft-related speech disorders. Again, it appears that, as additional evidence is accumulated on children treated by modern methods, indications of problems with overall mental development and with verbal intelligence in particular grow less compelling.

The exception to this is in the *early* development of children with cleft palate. A number of studies have shown that infants with palatal clefts are a bit more erratic in the first 2 years of life and a bit behind other children in development (Fox, Lynch, & Brookshire, 1978). These are not serious deficits, and they have not been very well explained. No one knows, for example, whether they are the result of hearing loss, altered parent-child interactions, the cleft itself, early feeding problems, or a combination of all of these factors. We do know that not all children experience this delay and that it can be minimized by good parental counseling (Brookshire, Lynch, & Fox, 1980). No baby with a cleft should automatically be described as "slow," even if he shows early developmental variations. Many will be quite precocious later on. There are significant gains made in test scores in the early years of life unless marked mental retardation is present (Musgrave, McWilliams, & Matthews, 1975).

Again, the precise cause or causes of these early developmental delays and of subsequent catch-up development are not known. A young child with a cleft has many more less-than-desirable experiences early in life than are usual in babies with no special problems. There maybe countless clinical evaluations, several surgical procedures, separation from parents, initial feeding problems, ear disease, and often increased parental anxiety and concern. Any one of these factors could conceivably make the business of learning to live in the world just a bit difficult and slow down the process. The speech-language pathologist is concerned with these problems because parents need assistance in understanding what is happening and in learning how to provide the best possible environment to insure optimal development when the children are older. It is always tempting to stress speech and language because we are most intimately concerned with communication. However, in the early years of a child's life, we must be willing and able to assist with general development, since language and speech are expressions of a totally integrated person and never emerge in isolation. A speech-language pathologist is a developmental specialist who must be well qualified in this aspect of our specialty.

Influenced by all of these variables, language generally develops more slowly in children with clefts than in those without special problems. These differences can be recognized in early infancy and account for many of the variations in early mental development we have just discussed.

When a child's first words do not emerge until between 18 and 24 months, the whole developmental sequence is moved back in time, and major landmarks are reached at later ages. This is one reason that nursery school seems to be especially helpful to these children. The emphasis upon the normal sequencing of development allows cleft children to have stimulation and encouragement in a properly arranged time frame. This indirectly encourages language behavior appropriate to the level on which the child is functioning and sets the stage for purposeful interaction with other children, with communication playing an important role. While we do not expect the average 3-year-old with a cleft to compete on an equal verbal footing with her peers, we do expect, under optimal circumstances, that these deficits will be largely overcome by school age. In fact, many children with clefts are superior in language skills by the time they go to first grade. Interestingly, those who do

You may wish to review the sequence of normal development presented in chapter 8.

best seem to be the children who are encouraged to talk and who have good reason to believe that what they have to say is important and that the way they say it is acceptable.

The early language problems seen in children with clefts become less marked as they get older (Musgrave, et al., 1975; Shames & Rubin, 1971), but the evidence suggests strongly that the mean sentence length remains somewhat shorter than it is for peers, even though the longest sentences used are quite appropriate for the children's chronological age. For reasons still not completely explained, many children with clefts do less talking than other children. Since this reduction in the quantity of verbal output cuts across the entire population, regardless of speech ability, the most reasonable explanation lies in some aspect of self-esteem or in the way in which many people respond to other people who have defects in appearance or speech proficiency.

Again, the speech-language pathologist should always remember that we talk about children with clefts as a group and that group data cannot be applied to individuals, who may not conform at all to group trends. Careful assessment of each individual is, therefore, essential.

Articulation development is frequently slow in children with clefts or with velopharyngeal closure problems from other causes. This observation has been made repeatedly (Bzoch, 1959; Philips & Harrison, 1969; Van Demark, 1966; Van Demark, Morris, & Vandehaar, 1979). These delays are complicated, and the explanation for them is not clear. A part of the reason may lie in the fact that these children cannot impound sufficient intraoral pressure for consonant sound production. Even early babbling is less rich than it is in unimpaired children. After surgery, if the sphincteric velopharyngeal valve is successfully constructed so that separation between the two cavities is possible, articulation, while slow for chronological age, often becomes normal even as early as age 5 or 6. As noted earlier, we have seen many children begin first grade with articulation superior to that of their peers. However, if the valve is not competent, if the child uses it inefficiently, if coexisting dental problems are influential, or if learning is not complete, articulation development continues to lag, often seriously and well into the teens (Van Demark, et al., 1979).

Other possible causes for articulation problems include hearing deficits and psychosocial immaturity. It is clear that these causes may be directly or indirectly related to the cleft. It is always important to distinguish those errors that are caused by the cleft and those that are secondary to it, or the treatment plan may be faulty. An example of this is a 9-year-old who had no consonant content in his speech pattern. He was *assumed* to have velopharyngeal incompetence and was referred for that problem. However, during the assessment, he produced in words all of the consonants except /s/, and that was in error because of dental distortion. He responded well to speech intervention and never required any additional surgery to improve his velopharyngeal closure. Unfortunately, the clinical error is more likely to be to continue speech therapy when the problem lies with the valve or the teeth or some other underlying condition that requires change before therapy can succeed.

The Cleft Palate Team

Clearly, no speech-language pathologist, regardless of training and skill, could successfully manage all of the needs of a child with a cleft. Yet these associated problems are so entwined with each other that treatment for one may influence or be influenced by treatment for another. Communication among specialists and joint participation in planning is thus highly desirable. Recognizing this, more than 50 years ago, pioneers in this field began to meet together in teams to examine and treat patients who had previously seen a surgeon in one place, a dentist in another, and so on. This team approach to management is popular today, and there are many such groups regularly established to handle cleft palate and related disorders. The professional interaction in clinics led to the establishment of what is now known as the American Cleft Palate Association, an interdisciplinary organization whose membership of about 1,500 is comprised of nearly ⅓ physicians, ⅓ dentists, and ⅓ speech-language pathologists and other behavioral scientists. The Association welcomes students to a membership category especially for them and encourages them to attend annual scientific meetings. The organization's official publication is *The Cleft Palate Journal,* which caries the designation "An International Journal of Craniofacial Anomalies." This reflects the growing interest in the many other birth defects affecting the head and face with which members are concerned.

Even speech-language pathologists working outside of clinical settings may want to become extended members of cleft palate teams serving in their communities. No one should ever work alone with these complicated problems that require the combined thinking of many different individuals. The speech-language pathologist on the cleft palate team needs and appreciates the opportunity of working with field clinicians in order to coordinate their efforts.

SPEECH DISORDERS

The goal of any surgery to close a palatal cleft or to improve velopharyngeal closure is to make normal or socially acceptable speech possible. Fortunately, this result is achieved quite often. Statistics vary from one series of cases to another. The highest success rate, 91%, was reported by Morley (1967) for a series of patients whose surgery was performed by Fenton Braithwaite. But for those people who do not develop speech at this level of proficiency, there are several basic concepts that underlie all diagnosis and treatment.

First, children with clefts of the lip rarely have speech disorders traceable to that problem. Although there is reference in the literature to speech disorders caused by cleft lip, that is almost never the case.

Second, children with all types of clefts are candidates for all of the major speech problems just as other children are, and they may have disordered communication not even remotely associated with the birth defect. "The wed wabbits wun" freely through the speech of these children just as they do in the speech of all children.

Third, if palatal clefts are not repaired so that intraoral pressure may be satisfactorily created, speech disorders will result from this problem, which we call *faulty velopharyngeal closure.* We shall emphasize these disorders in the discussion below. In addition, we will look at those difficulties that are traceable to other oral and dental problems which are a part of the cleft condition and which also influence speech patterns.

As we have mentioned before, the process of diagnosis begins with the speech-language pathologist gaining control over a very important instrument—his or her own ear. "The ultimate measure of the adequacy of speech is always its effect on listeners, and it is here that the speech pathologist must

For a program designed to teach listening skills as they relate to velopharyngeal incompetence

and associated disorders, see the Audio Seminar in Velopharyngeal Incompetence *(McWilliams & Philips, 1979).*

begin" (McWilliams, 1980). It is the ear that will suggest what avenues should be explored and what instruments should be used in further evaluations. It is the ear that will determine the extent to which remedial procedures are indicated and when they have succeeded or failed. For these reasons, speech-language pathologists must learn to be competent listeners.

Language Disorders

It is never wise to stress speech production if the underlying problem has to do with linguistic competence or with expressive language usage. Thus, cleft children, who are particularly prone to early language delay, should be carefully followed from birth, and appropriate stimulation programs should be recommended as needed (Brookshire, et al., 1980). However, we must remember that language deficits seen in preschool children tend to be less apparent in later childhood. Of course, any child who retains either receptive or expressive language deficits should be examined and treated as any other language-impaired child. A word of warning is appropriate here. Sometimes children with clefts speak poorly, and they may elect to talk as little as possible in order to protect themselves against the social stigma that may be attached to their poor speech patterns. It would be a mistake to treat those youngsters as language-impaired rather than as speech-impaired. It is quite important to discern the difference between the two.

Again, chapters 8 and 9 on language disorders give more complete discussion of approaches to these problems.

Speech Characteristics

As we have seen, children with clefts or other problems which lead to similar speech patterns suffer primarily from velopharyngeal incompetence, or the inability to separate the oral from the nasal cavity. The reason for the incompetence may be that the palate is too short to contact the posterior pharyngeal wall (the back of the throat) or the wall may be too deep. There may be too little movement in the lateral pharyngeal walls to permit them to make their contribution to the sphincteric closure. There may be too little or too inconsistent movement in the soft palate or in the posterior pharyngeal walls. The palate may be unable to adapt to the dramatic new space created suddenly when the adenoids are removed. Recently Warren (1979) has reported a case in which webbing tied down the palate and restricted its movement. All of these conditions prevent the successful separation of the oral from the nasal cavity during the speech tasks that demand closure. Thus, air important to articulation is lost through the nose. The speech problems that result may be quite simple, or they may be complex, multifaceted, and difficult to sort out.

Visible nasal escape is the most minimal of all the speech symptoms in these cases. It may be seen on sounds other than the nasals when a mirror is placed beneath the nostrils, even when speech sounds normal in every way. That would indicate a valve of reduced efficiency, but no one would recommend intervention of any sort if that were the only symptom. However, visible nasal escape may exist as a part of a more extensive group of disorders, which we discuss below. It is important to remember that nasal escape may be mild or severe, consistent or inconsistent. It is most likely to occur on /s/, a consonant that is voiceless, requires relatively high intraoral pressure, and is a continuant. This type of consonant demands the maintenance of air pressure in the mouth over time and so is relatively difficult to produce when there is even a small loss of air through the velopharyngeal portal. In order of difficulty, the consonants most likely to be affected are sibilants, other fricatives, affricates, and plosives. Thus, it is possible to have air loss on /s/ and /z/ but none on plosives, because they demand less of the valving mechanism. In other words, a plosive can be produced satisfactorily with a greater velopharyngeal gap than is true for a sibilant. In the vowel family, the most demanding sounds are /i/ and /u/, with other vowels being less difficult when velopharyngeal incompetence is present.

Nasal escape is a red flag that the valving mechanism is less than adequate. However, if there is no nasal escape, we cannot conclude that the mechanism is adequate. There may be resistance in the nasal airway—a blockage of some type—that prevents the exit of air through the nose even though the portal is not obliterated during speech. Thus nasal escape is an important symptom, but its absence is not proof of velopharyngeal competency.

Audible nasal escape is air that comes inappropriately through a faulty velopharyngeal valve and encounters enough nasal resistance to cause a slight noise that can be heard during speech. You can produce a sound like this by exhaling forcibly through your nostrils. In other words, the airstream is greater than the space through which it must circulate, and there is a slight noise that can be heard along with the speech sounds. This is distracting and is a more serious symptom pointing to velopharyngeal incompetency than is the simple audible nasal escape.

Nasal turbulence is simply a more severe form of audible nasal escape. It occurs when there is marked resistance to the stream of air so that a highly turbulent noise accompanies the production of speech sounds. This is most likely to occur on continuants such as /s/, and the noise may sometimes be close to a snort. Air escape accompanied by turbulence is extremely damaging to the speech signal and is distracting for the listener. This symptom may exist alone or may be accompanied by some of the more severe problems which we will be discussing as we move through this chapter. Whether it exists by itself or in combination with other problems, it alone is of sufficient importance to warrant attention. Differential diagnosis is necessary because this speech symptom is usually accompanied by both velopharyngeal incompetence and increased resistance in the nasal airway. Speech intervention is not recommended without complete study of the valve, and it becomes a diagnostic problem for the entire cleft palate team.

Hypernasality, ranging from very mild to very severe, is the speech symptom which speech-language pathologists are most familiar with and are most likely to be knowledgeable about. It is associated for the most part with velopharyngeal incompetence and is considered to have its greatest influence on changing the characteristics of vowels. Interestingly, however, the vowels, although marked by increased nasal characteristics, remain identifiable so that intelligibility is not greatly impaired. The recorded speech samples which accompany this chapter will help you recognize that. The speech *sounds* defective to the listener because there is too great a nasal component, but it can be understood unless the velopharyngeal incompetence is so great that it also destroys some of the major characteristics of the consonants. Thus, even though hypernasality *per se* is vowel phenomenon, the factor that contributes most to a reduction in speech intelligibility is the change that occurs on pressure consonants. We will discuss this more in detail later.

Because hypernasality may be very mild and inconsistent, may be somewhat more severe so that we would describe it as moderate, or may be extremely severe, we need some method for objectifying the impression which we have when we hear speech. Many researchers and most clinicians have found a scaling technique to be useful for assessing the degree of hyper-

*Recall that **hypernasality** is that quality of speech produced by too much nasal resonance.*

nasality that is present, often using a five-point or a seven-point scale. On the scale, a 1 would represent normal nasal elements in the speech pattern. That would mean that there is no undue hypernasality and that the only consonants showing appropriate nasal characteristics are /m/, /n/, and /ŋ/. Where 2 would represent very slight, almost imperceptible hypernasality, 3 and 4 would represent degrees of mild hypernasality. Scores of 5 and 6 would be moderate, and 7 would be very severe hypernasality. The problem with using such scales is that they must be reliable. This means that one speech-language pathologist listening to a given speech sample and rating it at 7 should agree with other similarly trained speech-language pathologists. It would never do to use a scale unreliably. It is very difficult to develop this high level of agreement, and usually speech-languge pathologists working within a given setting must listen to many speech samples and rate them together in an effort to arrive at consistent agreement. Agreement between raters should be above 90% wherever possible. The speech-language pathologist should be able to rate single words, an easier task than the additional requirement of rating connected discourse. The average of the ratings of many listeners is generally more accurate than are the ratings of one or two. However, specific training helps to make speech-language pathologists more accurate.

More severe degrees of hypernasality are associated with other speech problems that we will discuss as we go along. The greater the degree of hypernasality, the greater the evidence of decreased ability to impound intraoral pressure, that great necessity for adequate speech production and correct consonants. We will be saying many times in this chapter that speech intervention is rarely the answer to problems that are anatomically and physiologically determined.

If you will return in your thoughts for a minute to the section on nasal escape, you will realize that a reduction in intraoral pressure is generally associated with nasal escape. Always remember that nasal escape is nothing more than the air which is lost through the velopharyngeal portal and sent under pressure through the nostrils to the outside. However, again, if increased nasal resistance partially or completely blocks that passageway, the nasal escape will not occur; and you may hear hypernasality or some variation of it without the nasal escape that your common sense tells you should be present. When faced with that dilemma, it is quite possible that /m/, /n/, and /ŋ/, which should be accompanied by nasal escape, will not be, and you can check those sounds as an added means of evaluation. Another simple task which clinicians can use is simply to see whether or not the individual can exhale through the nostrils. This is sometimes not possible through either nostril or may occur through one nostril and not the other. If the exhaled airstream is not circulated in the usual way, certainly there will be no nasal escape during speech.

Hypernasality is the outstanding speech characteristic associated with velopharyngeal incompetence. Thus, when many speech-language pathologists hear hypernasality, they automatically believe that velopharyngeal incompetence is present. Most of the time they will be right. However, there are other problems associated with clefting that may also contribute to the general impression of hypernasality. One of these is the oronasal fistula, which is an opening between the oral cavity and the nasal cavity. Not all oronasal fistulae are symptomatic. However, when one is located behind the maxillary central incisors, for example, it may be highly symptomatic, and the person may produce an /s/ sound by placing his tongue against the fistula and forcing the air through the channel, thus forcing the air into the nose. This individual would get nasal escape and would have what might sound like hypernasality, but it would not necessarily be associated with velopharyngeal valving deficits. This is one reason that a good oral examination is always essential; we need to find any collateral problems that may be influential. Incidentally, if there is a question of this kind of involvement, it is possible to close these fistulae with dental wax, chewing gum, or a temporary prosthesis (Bless, Ewanowski, & Dibbell, 1980) and determine how the speech changes with the little makeshift appliance in place. It is even possible to run air studies under the two conditions. We will discuss more about that a little later.

A prosthesis is an artificial replacement for a missing or undeveloped part of the body.

Anterior fistulae are one of several conditions that may cause confusion for speech-language pathologists and interfere with their ability to assess hypernasality easily and accurately. Even the use of scales can be complicated by the presence of other difficulties that make it somewhat difficult to hear the hypernasality. The beginning speech-language pathologist should not be discouraged by this; time and experience will aid in creating new skills and improving old ones.

Hyponasality is another characteristic that must be discussed in association with problems of velopharyngeal valving. As we have pointed out, hypernasality is the most consistent clinical finding when the valve does not close appropriately, but it is not unheard of to hear hyponasality as well. This is likely to occur when the nasal passageways or the entry to them is almost totally blocked, as in the case of enlarged adenoids or blockage within the passages themselves. Under those circumstances, the speech may sound hyponasal, and /m/, /n/, and /ŋ/ will have insufficient nasalization. Speech-language pathologists are often puzzled by that characteristic and assume that velopharyngeal valving must be intact if hyponasality exists. However, this is not necessarily the case, because the extra tissue simply impedes the passage of air which would go through the faulty valve into the nasal airway if it were capable of doing so. It is very important to learn that simple lesson. Removing the adenoidal mass or opening up the nasal airways under these circumstances will lead immediately to hypernasality because of the inadequacy of the velopharyngeal valve. It is important for beginning speech-language pathologists particularly not to be embarrassed if they think they hear hyponasality in an individual who more reasonably would be expected to have hypernasality.

The speech of individuals with palatal clefts and related disorders sometimes has a muffled quality that makes it much less distinct than it is if it were hyper- or hyponasal. This muffled sound, called *cul-de-sac resonance,* occurs when there is velopharyngeal incompetence accompanied by anterior blockage of the nasal airway. The air passes through the faulty valve into the nasal passages, where it cannot exit because of the increased resistance. If you will hold your nostrils together and then attempt to talk through your nose, you will hear a similar sound. Try the sentence "Sissy sees the sun in the sky." Then release the nostrils and hear the hypernasality on the sentence when you leave your palate relaxed as you speak through your nose. Next, speak normally, so that you may detect the changes in your own speech. You can see that any alteration in the velopharyngeal valve or in the nasal airway changes the characteristics of the speech and that we must be alert to how these varying conditions affect the speech pattern that we are hearing and trying to assess.

I have watched numerous students as they have attempted to evaluate speech. First they would write on their evaluational chart that the speech was hypernasal. Then they would erase the hypernasality and write that it was hyponsasal, and then they would be in utter confusion. The reason is that hypo- and hypernasality may exist together in some speakers with velopharyngeal incompetence. This is a rare phenomenon, but it does occur; and we must be prepared to deal with it. It is an unusual speech pattern, and it occurs for many of the same reasons that cul-de-sac resonance occurs. The velopharyngeal valve is incompetent, and air that should be going through the oral cavity passes into the nasal cavity where it is trapped by a *partial* obstruction in the nasal passages. The quality of vowels is changed, and there is likely to be nasal escape on high pressure consonants, particularly /s/, the most demanding of all of the consonants. It is a little less likely to find escape under these circumstances on the less-demanding plosives. The problem with the nasals occurs because the obstruction is so great that it does not permit enough air to escape for /m/, /n/, and /ŋ/, and those sounds are altered. It is important to recognize that /m/, /n/, and /ŋ/ do not become /b/, /d/, and /g/. They approach those sounds but do not match them specifically because there is still a limited amount of nasal resonance present. They are simply changed so that they become nonstandard consonants.

Articulation Disorders

Articulation disorders constitute the most devastating aspect of velopharyngeal valving problems. You will recall that we said that hypernasality was the most outstanding characteristic of velopharyngeal incompetence, but that the damage to consonants is the variable that interferes most with intelligibility.

When thinking about articulation disorders, it is necessary to keep in mind that differential diagnosis to discover the cause of these disorders is extremely important. We have mentioned the role of maturation in both language and speech development. You will remember that children with clefts develop their articulation skills more slowly than do children without clefts (Bzoch, 1959; Philips & Harrison, 1969). However, the speech-language pathologist must be certain that the articulation disorders that are being heard are maturational in nature. For example, a 5-year-old child might well say "/wed/ (red), /free/ (three), /lello/ (yellow)." Those errors have none of the components which would suggest organic causes of the type associated with palatal clefting or velopharyngeal incompetence from other causes. They do, instead, reflect a developmental stage in a young child, and you would assess them that way.

There will also be the occasional child with an unusual pattern of articulation that is easy to associate with velopharyngeal incompetence. One 5-year-old boy had well-developed consonants in all contexts except that he substituted a nasal snort for /s/. This sound was accompanied by massive nasal escape which did not appear anywhere else except where it was appropriate on /m/, /n/, and /ŋ/. He had all of the other fricatives and was highly stimulable for /s/. In short, he had a peculiar articulation error with an overall speech pattern that was not consistent with velopharyngeal incompetence. He responded quickly to articulation therapy. We might refer to such a problem as pseudovelopharyngeal incompetence.

Another similar situation exists with a few children who substitute glottal stops for plosives but have perfect fricative articulation. Since the fricatives demand more of the velopharyngeal valve than do the plosives, it is not logical for a faulty mechanism to be associated with defects on easier but not on harder phonemes. Thus it would be logical to attempt articulation intervention in such a case.

It is quite probable that the early hearing losses we have talked about may play a role in the slow development of articulatory skills. A study by Holm and Kunze (1969), while being far from conclusive, did point to the possibility of an increase in articulation errors in children with histories of repeated middle ear disease. This is yet another reason for watching the ears very carefully and for attempting to minimize ear disease whenever possible. Since the Holm and Kunze study, there have been other studies that have suggested the influence of early ear disease on several aspects of development (Needleman, 1977). Ventry (1980), in an assessment of the research that has been done to date, points to its shortcomings; and we want to make a strong plea here for keeping an open mind and continuing to evaluate the influences of early otitis media on the language and speech development of all children, especially those with problems of velopharyngeal valving. The needed data are simply not available at this time. We may be over- or underemphasizing the seriousness of this early disease as it relates to language and speech.

In a child who has a cleft or other condition which causes velopharyngeal valving problems, we may also find other, related structural deviations which affect consonant articulation. One of the outstanding of these is defects in dentition. The cleft frequently affects the alveolar arch, causing arch collapse on the side of the cleft, and there may be missing teeth that change the architecture of the mouth. Spaces of this type frequently result in the child's closing that anterior opening by pushing his tongue into the space during consonant articulation, particularly on tongue-tip sounds. These kinds of errors are cleft-related to the extent that the dental problems are a part of the cleft picture. However, they are not articulation errors that relate to poor velopharyngeal valving, although that may also be present. In our experience, when there is faulty dentition, there is almost always resultant sibilant articulation difficulties and sometimes distortion of /t/ and /d/ as well. This is so very common in these children that we have come to expect to hear and see it.

Figure 11.7 illustrates such a problem.

FIGURE 11.7
Tongue Posture Associated with Midfacial Deficiency with Disruption of Relationships Between the Maxilla and the Mandible.

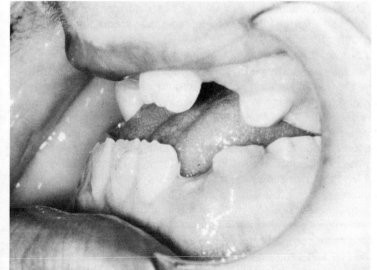

The evaluation must involve both listening and watching to determine how the sounds are being produced. In many instances, it may be the only speech problem which an individual has. We cannot stress enough the importance of distinguishing these problems from those that relate to velopharyngeal incompetency. The record for correcting these dentally determined errors through speech intervention has not been promising. We usually prefer to wait to institute speech therapy until after any anatomical defects have been corrected. Otherwise, the long period of intervention can be extremely discouraging to the child or adult client, frustrating to the speech-language pathologist, and prohibitively expensive.

The articulation disorders that we worry most about are those that are associated with velopharyngeal incompetence, which we shall discuss next. Articulation disorders associated with velopharyngeal incompetence appear to increase in severity as the velopharyngeal opening during speech becomes greater. This is not a one-to-one relationship, but we know that mild openings affect articulation to a lesser extent than do broad openings. Velopharyngeal competence is undoubtedly necessary for normal speech production (Morris, 1968; Shelton, Morris, & McWilliams, 1973a, 1973b). However, it is possible for a person to have very slight velopharyngeal incompetence, such as would be present with simple air escape without any articulatory deterioration. The opening can only be very minimal or the signs will become more apparent. Many different studies have shown that the first consonant to deteriorate in the presence of velopharyngeal incompetence will be the voiceless continuant /s/. As we mentioned earlier, the sounds then follow through the sibilant family to affricates, then to other fricatives, and finally through the plosives. Therefore, if you hear an error on a plosive sound, the velopharyngeal incompetency is probably greater than in those cases where you hear errors only on the consonant /s/. For these reasons, /s/ is the most frequently misarticulated of all consonant sounds among people who have velopharyngeal incompetence, and it will be defective if the incompetence is marginal, borderline, mild, moderate, or severe. Plosives are more likely to become defective when the opening is moderate or severe. The first symptom that will be noted in articulation, and the simplest one, is a reduction in intraoral pressure. In other words, the sounds are accurately articulated, they sound close to normal, but the intraoral pressure is not quite enough for a completely adequate production. The wider the opening, the more sounds that will be involved; and the presence of plosive errors heralds a wider gap (Subtelny & Subtelny, 1959).

We do not understand why some speakers with velopharyngeal incompetence accept the loss of intraoral pressure and the escape of air through the nasal airway and go on talking in spite of these variations, without attempting to compensate for the loss of pressure. When a speaker is able to do that, intelligibility can be quite high. However, many speakers find it either unacceptable or too difficult to keep up a conversational stream with so little air pressure in the oral cavity for consonant production. These speakers take steps (of which they themselves are not consciously aware) to make up for the losses in pressure by producing sounds in other ways. We refer to this as *compensatory articulation,* and much of it contributes to a decrease in intelligibility and makes the clearing up of articulatory errors more difficult because they are more complex.

One of the first and simplest compensations which a speaker may make on his own is to produce sibilants in a linguapalatal manner. This means that, instead of producing an /s/ with the tongue-tip against the rugae, the produc-

Recall that the rugae

tion is moved just a little bit behind the dental arch, and the blade instead of the tip of the tongue articulates with the most anterior part of the hard palate. This creates a less distinct /s/ sound, and the difference in production can be readily heard. Other speakers, probably those with less competence, produce sounds like /s/ even further back in the mouth and may actually use the posterior part of the tongue elevated against the posterior margin of the hard palate. Other speakers constrict the pharynx for the production of /s/ and create what we call a *pharyngeal fricative*. These pharyngeal fricatives have a sibilant-like character but obviously are produced in quite the wrong part of the mouth in an effort to have access to as much air as possible for production. They are gross errors of articulation and can contribute markedly to a reduction in intelligibility.

When the velopharyngeal incompetence is great enough to affect plosive sounds, speakers may resort to still other techniques. They may do fairly well with /p/ and /b/ because they can trap some buccal air behind the lips and make a plosive-like sound that is recognizable. The /t/ and /d/ become a little bit harder, and they may move these back and produce them more lingua-palatally. The /k/ and /g/ may constitute real difficulties, and some people produce them glotally so that the **glottal stop** is substituted for /k/ and /g/.

In any attempt to outline the kinds of compensations that people use, it is almost inevitable that we will overlook some or that a new one will be heard that has never been heard before. This is why it is so important to try to discern what an individual is doing when he produces the various sounds of our language. An example of this is one child who sniffed instead of attempting an intraoral /s/. The sniff gave a sibilant-like characteristic and avoided the necessity for high intraoral pressure, which was not available.

The beginning speech-language pathologist should be aware that the articulation errors which we refer to as *gross* are rarely accompanied by nasal escape. The reason for this is that the critical velopharyngeal valve is bypassed, and velopharyngeal closure is not required. Thus the worst speakers may demonstrate very little in the way of nasal escape, and you may be foooled into thinking that the mechanism is competent and that speech intervention could change the articulation patterns. This is only rarely the case.

Gross errors in articulation constitute a subsystem of the English language. This subsystem incorporates nonstandard English sounds that can be produced by people who have velopharyngeal competency. In fact, in some sections of the country, glottal stops are used in certain combinations as a part of standard English. An example is the New England glottal substitution in the word "bottle" instead of the standard American "bottle." However, the New Englander who does that has complete competency to produce /t/ and /d/ when they are demanded. This is not usually true of the person who uses glottal stops throughout his speech pattern to compensate for velopharyngeal incompetence. The problem with these gross errors is that, even after the velopharyngeal valve has been corrected, the system of communication that has been developed will remain, and speech intervention will be necessary to teach the individual to function up to the potential of the new valve. If the person does not have these gross articulation errors and has only reduced intraoral pressure, sometimes improving the valve improves the speech to the extent that no further intervention is required. Once again, it is clear that differential diagnosis is extremely important in understanding the nature of articulation errors, the potential for intervention, and the results once intervention has been instituted.

are the ridges behind the dental arch.

Recall that the glottal stop is a clicking-like sound, a plosive that is produced by expelling air quickly through the approximated vocal cords. Although it is not a phoneme of standard English, it is a variation used in some American dialects and is a phoneme of some other languages, including Danish.

It is extremely important for speech-language pathologists who are going to be handling children with clefts and other problems causing velopharyngeal incompetence to be highly alert to the probability that gross articulation errors, including glottal stops and pharyngeal fricatives, are strong indicators of velopharyngeal incompetence. No speech-language pathologist should try to correct these errors without giving the child the benefit of a comprehensive diagnostic workup. While it is true that there will not be complete services available for all children throughout the United States, no child should be denied the opportunity to have the best physical mechanism possible. Once that has been created or it has been determined that nothing further can be done, the speech-language pathologist can begin the long, slow process of attempting to change the gross errors to errors that are less devastating to intelligibility. This is a very difficult task for both the child and the professional, and progress is almost always very slow.

Voice Disorders

Voice disorders also occur in association with velopharyngeal incompetence. The hypernasality associated with this phenomenon is sometimes referred to as a voice disorder; but as we saw in chapter 6, it is more accurately a disorder of resonance since its origins are not in the vocal tract but in the resonating cavities. When an individual struggles to be less hypernasal than his velopharyngeal valving mechanism dictates, he will sometimes try to control the air stream below the level of the larynx and increase vocal tension. We have seen children literally struggle to keep air from being sent forth with vocalization. If you try this for yourself, bearing down on the diaphragm, you will hear the hard tense voice that results. These added strains on the larynx will sometimes lead to hoarseness. This is one more sign that we are dealing with a vocal mechanism or tract that is an interactive system and that it is impossible to modify it at one level without influencing what occurs elsewhere. Thus, changes in the phonatory patterns are not surprising when you realize that the larynx is the first valve in a series of valves in the vocal tract.

The tense speech that occurs in this pattern is vocally abusive. Sometimes the speech is totally or periodically aphonic. It can be extremely hoarse and difficult for the speaker and listener alike. The intriguing thing about these phonatory disorders is that they may not be associated with other evidences of velopharyngeal incompetence, and so the basic problem may not be suspected. Any child with a cleft or other sign of potential velopharyngeal incompetence should be suspected of having this problem if he becomes hoarse or periodically aphonic.

The hoarseness that is heard in children with clefts is very frequently accompanied by bilateral vocal cord nodules (McWilliams, Bluestone, & Musgrave, 1969; McWilliams, Lavorato, & Bluestone, 1973), and the velopharyngeal valving mechanism is likely to be of only borderline efficiency. The vocal cord nodules tend to be retained in cleft children longer than they are in children who do not have clefts but who also suffer from vocal abuse for other reasons. Improving the velopharyngeal valve seems to be more effective in changing the voice quality than either speech intervention or surgical removal of the vocal cord nodules.

There are other vocal considerations that must also be taken into account in these children. We have dubbed one of these the "soft-voice syndrome." Because there is such a tremendous loss of air through the velopharyngeal portal, children and adults too will sometimes resort to speaking very quietly so that they do not have to initiate as much subglottal air pressure in order to create voice. Since they are using less air, there is not quite so much available to be lost through the nasal passages. Of course, there is not very much available in the oral cavity either, so that the relationships remain quite similar. Sometimes asking an individual to speak more loudly will reveal the presence of hypernasality. However, it is not always easy to get these speakers to increase volume. They can have real difficulty speaking louder (Bernthal & Beukelman, 1977).

It should be clear by this time that the speech problems associated with all types of velopharyngeal incompetence are complex and that careful diagnostic studies are extremely important before a decision is made to intervene in any way to help the individual speak more efficiently.

Intelligibility

When speech is being assessed in order to determine the severity of a problem and what should be done about it, it is always necessary to make an overall judgment about the degree of defect and the extent to which intelligibility is impaired. A given person can have a marked alteration in the way he speaks which is readily recognized by the casual listener as aberrant even though it is completely understandable or intelligible. On the other hand, defective speech may be understood not at all or at varying degrees along a continuum. This factor may be assessed by using a variety of rating scales that would place completely intelligible speech at a number 1 and completely unintelligible speech at a number 5 or perhaps a number 7. Again, speech-language pathologists must develop rater reliability in the use of these scales, but they are helpful in determining overall how handicapping a particular problem is. If speech is slightly defective but is generally intelligible and socially acceptable, treatment might be less aggressive than if speech were socially unacceptable and unintelligible.

ASSESSMENT

As we have seen, assessment begins with the speech-language pathologist using his ear for differential listening. It will be the speech pattern that will ultimately help decide what additional steps should be taken. No final decisions can be made from the use of the ear alone, but no final decisions can be made from other techniques which exclude the ear. Thus, the diagnostic examination should begin with the speech-language pathologist listening in a highly critical and sophisticated manner to the nature of the individual's speech. Remembering the kinds of characteristics that are associated with velopharyngeal valving problems will indicate whether or not that is a probable cause of the disordered speech patterns.

Articulation Assessment

Chapter 5 discussed formal articulation tests.

The assessment process then moves very quickly to more formal testing. Formal articulation tests are as relevant to the diagnostic procedures used with these cases as they are for children with articulatory disorders. In dealing with cleft palates and related disorders, however, the articulation test must go beyond the judgment that a given sound is either in error or not. We are now talking about differential diagnostic articulation testing, and that means that each error found must be described as completely as possible, so that we understand as much as we can about the manner of production and the intricacies of the disorder. This information will help us make the ultimate decision as to whether the error conforms to the dynamics of articulation deficits resulting from velopharyngeal incompetence.

It is always important in evaluating articulation to do stimulability testing. We want to know how much better an individual can speak than he habitually does in conversation. Thus we like to learn something of the discrepancies between articulation produced during conversation and during a formal articulation test and various stimulability tests, We cannot assume that, because an individual can produce a given consonant in some context, she can "learn" to produce it in conversational speech. Keep in mind that velopharyngeal valving is something a person with borderline abilities can sometimes struggle to achieve in the production of an isolated sound or of a single word but cannot achieve during the rapid-fire muscular demands of free-flowing speech. However, doing stimulability testing gives us some idea of the depth of the problem. If a person is capable of producing most of the sounds but cannot do so in conversation, it may well be that intervention would be effective—*after* we have determined that the velopharyngeal valve is adequate to the task. On the other hand, it may be that a borderline valving mechanism can meet the demands of one situation but cannot achieve what is necessary under more complex conditions.

The articulation testing should be carried out using a small dental mirror to determine whether or not there is nasal escape present on the various sounds or, of course, if the nature of the errors is such that nasal escape would not be present. The speech-langauge pathologist will also test for the freedom of the nasal airway.

The evaluation should include an assessment of the nature of nasality, rating it at least on a five-point scale ranging from normal to severely hypernasal. Hyponasality can be marked as present or absent, as can hypo-hypernasality and cul-de-sac resonance. The other characteristics such as nasal turbulence should also be recorded in association with the articulation test and in relation to the sounds on which the extra noise occurs.

Oral Examination

An oral examination usually follows the articulation evaluation, although it may not be particularly helpful in cases of suspected velopharyngeal incompetence because that all-important valve cannot be visualized by looking into the mouth. Traditionally, the speech-language pathologist asks the individual to open the mouth and say "ah," while looking at the movement of the palate. We may determine that the palate does move or does not move under that particular condition, but that is about all that this study can do. The valve itself is higher in the nasopharynx and is concealed from the eye. Do not ever believe that you can look into the mouth and make a decision about whether or not velopharyngeal closure is being achieved. However, the examination of the oral cavity can give clues to unusual structure or function. Earlier in the chapter we described the submucous cleft palate, which can often be seen. This is very important in cases with undetermined evidence of velopharyngeal valving problems in speech. Another bit of information that can be gained is whether or not the person has a gag reflex. If a gag reflex is not present, we would suspect some lack of motor integrity that might be causing some of the problems. During the oral examination, we can also look for oronasal fistulae and for dental problems that appear to be related to the speech pattern.

In sum, the oral examination provides clues but does not permit the making of decisions in the absence of other diagnostic data.

Hearing Evaluation

A hearing evaluation should be a part of every clinical workup on a child with a cleft or other type of velopharyngeal incompetence. The careful audiological study should include **tympanometry.** The tympanometry is done to be sure that there is no fluid in the middle ear even though the person's hearing may be within essentially normal limits. If there is middle ear fluid, there is usually a mild to moderate air-bone gap, so the audiological evaluation should include both air- and bone-conduction testing. Speech reception thresholds provide information about how well the individual is using the hearing that he has. These tests are precautionary in nature and should be used for making referrals if there is any suggestion at all that the hearing is not what it should be. There is never a justification for undertaking language or speech intervention in the presence of a treatable hearing loss without first seeing that something is done to bring the hearing up to the best level possible.

Tympanometry is a measurement of the resistance to the flow of sound energy at the tympanic membrane during various pressure changes.

Evaluation of Velopharyngeal Competence

This assessment is undertaken when the preliminary studies suggest that there is a problem with valving. Table 11.1 summarizes the speech symptoms which are, in general, associated with varying degrees of velopharyngeal competence and incompetence. Many approaches have been tried, and we will discuss them briefly here. We have previously noted that velopharyngeal valving incompetence leads to a reduction in intraoral pressure and an increase in air flow through the nostrils on sounds other than /m, n/, and /ŋ/. Thus a simple technique for evaluating the velopharyngeal valve is to hold a mirror beneath the nostrils to see if it steams on inappropriate sounds.

A long time ago, great stress was placed upon determining whether or not an individual could blow up a paper bag, blow out candles, blow ping pong balls up inclined planes, and perform many other similar kinds of tasks. However, no objective information is derived from activities of that type, and we now know that there is no direct relationship between the ability to blow and the ability to speak well (McWilliams & Bradley, 1965; Shprintzen, McCall, & Skolnik, 1975). Therefore, it makes little sense to use blowing activities for diagnosis. Blowing has other difficulties inherent in it. Respiratory effort influences pressures of air flow and can mislead the observer into believing that the velopharyngeal valve is functioning efficiently when, in reality, the change has to do only with the management of greater or lesser amounts of air. The individual may be capable of making certain adjustments in the oral tract that may also influence what happens during blowing, so that the data derived are misleading and difficult to interpret. Fox and Johns (1970) speculate that, if you anchored the tongue outside the mouth and then had the person puff out his cheeks, the person would not be able to use the tongue humping that sometimes controls the velopharyngeal valve. The ability to puff out the cheeks was then assumed to be an indicator of velopharyngeal valving integrity. However, the evidence is not strong that this technique provides enough information to make final treatment decisions. Some professionals have attempted to measure the amount of air that is lost through the nostrils, but this technique has proved unsatisfactory because of the alterations in nasal resistance that might result in no nasal air flow even in the presence of an inadequate velopharyngeal valve. In addition, respiratory effort, as mentioned

*Various
Air Flow
Studies*

above, will influence the amount of air that goes through any available passage, so that the severity of the air escape is not a very good indicator of the size of the velopharyngeal gap.

TABLE 11.1
Speech Characteristics Associated with Varying Degrees of Velopharyngeal Competence and Incompetence.

Speech Characteristic	Velopharyngeal Valving
Normal	Competent
Anterior sibilant errors	Competent
Nasal escape or hoarseness	Borderline
Mild hypernasality or mild hypo-hypernasality	Borderline to borderline incompetent
Moderate or severe hypernasality, nasal escape or turbulence, sibilant and/or plosive distortions caused by reduced intraoral pressure	Incompetent
Very severe hypernasality, nasal escape or turbulence, pharyngeal and/or laryngeal sibilants and plosives	Grossly incompetent

Tests using blowing or nasal escape have never been very satisfactory. A group at the University of Iowa attempted to change that by developing the Hunter Oral Manometer (Morris, 1966). This is a device through which the individual blows with nostrils open and then with nostrils occluded. The difference between the recorded pressures taken under the two conditions supposedly measures velopharyngeal competence or incompetence. If the two measures are the same, the mechanism is assumed to be incompetent. However, a recent study (McWilliams, Glaser, Philips, Lawrence, Lavorato, Beery, & Skolnick, submitted) found this instrumentation to be highly unreliable in predicting the competency of the velopharyngeal valve. We do not recommend that beginning speech-language pathologists use this device to assess the competency of closure. Scores achieved during sucking are somewhat better predictors than are scores achieved during blowing (McWilliams, et al., submitted; Moore & Sommers, 1974; Weinberg & Shanks, 1971). Noll, Hawkins, and Weinberg (1977) also questioned the adequacy of the Hunter Oral Manometer and suggest that it not be used as the "sole method for evaluating velopharyngeal closure." We worry about using it at all, since the data derived from it appear to be quite erratic and unpredictable. However, at the time of its original development, it represented an important milestone in attempting to objectify our observations.

Warren and DuBois (1964) made a remarkable contribution to the assessment of velopharyngeal valving when they successfully acquired measurements of intraoral pressure and of nasal air flow taken during speech. These measurements are mathematically translated into an equation, and an estimate of the size of the velopharyngeal orifice area is determined. This technique is still widely used and has been simplified recently for the average speech-language pathologist with the development of Perci instrumentation (Warren, 1979). The Perci is a small instrument, readily portable, which can provide evidence about the adequacy of velopharyngeal closure during speech (based upon the earlier theories of Warren and DuBois). This instrument remains to be validated against other methods of assessment. Its advantage is that the measurements are taken during speech rather than during an activity like blowing, which is different from the speech task and differs in its requirements for velopharyngeal closure. Warren has suggested that orifice areas large than 20mm^2 are always associated with defective speech. However, this does not mean that defective speech does not occur at openings below that size. McWilliams and coworkers (submitted) found that any orifice area greater than 5mm^2 almost invariably had some characteristics suggesting velopharyngeal valving problems.

The technique developed by Warren and DuBois provides information about air flow through the nasal passages and about intraoral pressure. It does not provide any information about the location of the deficit in space, about the contour of the gap, or about the way in which the mechanism works. The speech-language pathologist is responsible for relating these data to speech. Another advantage is that the technique does not "invade" the body, and many clinicians find it useful when its limitations are kept in mind.

Radiology

Radiological techniques have long been used to visualize the velopharyngeal valve and its various components. The first technique used was still X-rays, taken in the lateral dimension and showing the mechanism only in profile. It was not possible to look at the sphincter itself. Still X-rays were filled with shortcomings. Speech is a dynamic event, and these studies were done during the production of a single sound—often the undemanding /a/. No one was quite sure where in the sound production the picture was taken. Therefore, we could not be certain that any failure to close was because of a defect or simply a matter of timing, or whether any closure that was observed was possible under the more complex demands of connected discourse. Yet some speech-language pathologists still persist in using these films, which we call *cephalometrics,* without appropriate reservations.

Cinefluoroscopy, or X-ray recorded on motion picture film, was developed next. This technique has a decided advantage over the old still studies. Cinefluoroscopy also permits a lateral projection, but at least a part of the mechanism can be seen in action. Again, the view is in profile, and sometimes what appears to be competence is not, because closure is not being obtained in the lateral parts of the valve that can not be seen. In addition, exposure to radiation is a factor to be considered when using this approach—as it must be with any method using X-ray.

McWilliams and Girdany (1964) first used videofluoroscopy, X-ray data recorded on video tape, for speech studies. This approach has the advantage of reducing radiation and permitting longer speech samples for study. These examinations, although in motion, are still done in lateral projection, and there is no way that the total valve can be visualized. They improved the technique somewhat by doing the lateral studies with the head in extension. This very slight deepening of the nasopharynx does, in borderline cases, unmask velopharyngeal incompetency that is not seen in the true lateral position (McWilliams, Musgrave, & Crozier, 1968). An advantage of both cine- and videofluoroscopy over still X-ray studies and over aerodynamic studies is that both provide information about the consistency of palatal and pharyngeal wall movement, its timing in relationship to speech production, and the patterning of the movements. These factors are relevant because some speakers sound as if they have velopharyngeal incompetency when they do not have that precise problem. Instead, they have motor difficulties that relate to the way in which the palate and pharyngeal structures are used for speech, and it is

FIGURE 11.8

Cephalometric X-ray with Two Tracings, One Showing a Normal /s/ and the Other an /s/ Produced with a Velopharyngeal Opening.

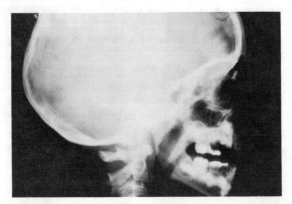

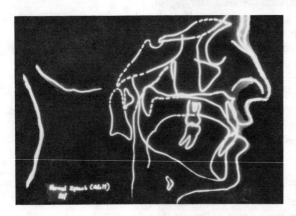 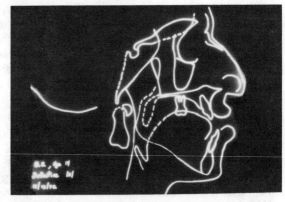

Figure 11.8 shows a cephalometric X-ray and two tracings—one of closure achieved on a normal /s/ and the other of the opening seen on an abnormal /s/.

necessary to determine that that is the case. A disadvantage of cine- and videofluoroscopy is that they do not provide information about the size and shape of the orifice and about its location. However, the techniques remain clinically useful, are widely used, and yield acceptable clinical data in a large percentage of cases.

Skolnick (1970) further developed videofluoroscopic methodology by introducing a technique called *multiview videofluoroscopy*. This approach uses the lateral projection in motion as did the earlier methods, but adds a frontal projection so that the movement of the lateral pharyngeal walls can also be observed. This frontal view shows the sides of the throat in motion as they would look if you could remove the tongue and soft palate and view these structures directly. The base view, which is a view of the sphincter itself taken while the patient is in a sphinx-like position, actually shows the velopharyngeal orifice with the soft palate and the posterior and the lateral pharyngeal walls. Much more information about velopharyngeal closure than was previously available can be derived from multiview videofluoroscopy, but the speech-language pathologist must evaluate the data from all three views and synthesize it in order to draw conclusions. Figure 11.9 is a sketch of the lateral, frontal, and base views. The lateral view looks much like the illustrations shown in Figure 11.7. The key to these studies, however, is that they are dynamic rather than static.

FIGURE 11.9

Schematic Representation of the Three Views Used in Multiview Videofluoroscopy. (From M. L. Skolnick, G. N. McCall, & M. Barnes, "The Sphincteric Mechanism of Velopharyngeal Closure," *Cleft Palate Journal,* 1973, *10,* 287. Used by permission.)

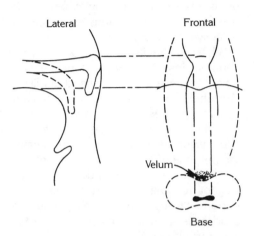

Lateral   Frontal

Velum

Base

The advantages of multiview videofluoroscopy are that it shows the presence or absence of an opening between the nasal and oral cavities during speech; it provides reliable information about the size of the opening; it identifies to some extent the location where the observation is being made, but falls short of directly locating the vertical position of the sphincter. This latter information has to be arrived at by synthesizing data from the three views—lateral, frontal, and basal. Multiview videofluoroscopy also lets us evaluate the reliability of the examiners, and it can delineate the contour of the opening and reveal the nature of velar and pharyngeal movements. These criteria were suggested by Morris, Shelton, and McWilliams (1973) and have been expanded slightly (McWilliams & Philips, 1979). To the extent that these criteria are acceptable to the average clinician and researcher, multiview videofluoroscopy offers the best means for studying this valve yet available to us.

Other Techniques

Another technique that has considerable clinical promise at this time is the nasoendoscope. This is an instrument that incorporates a fiberoptic bundle that is passed through the nasal airway and manipulated to reflect the velopharyngeal orifice as the speech-language pathologist watches and examines the orifice through an external viewing device. It is being used with increasing frequency, but does require a well-trained person to administer the examination. Electromyography (Fritzell, 1969) and ultrasound (Minifie, Hixon, Kelsey, & Woodhouse, 1970; Skolnick, Zagzebski, & Watkin, 1975) are also in use but remain in the fairly early stages of development. They are of limited applicability and are not available to the average speech-language pathologist working in the field. Their research potential is being increasingly recognized, however.

Choosing Assessment Techniques

The best information that we have about various techniques of assessing velopharyngeal closure tells us that it is quite important to use some type of instrumental approach in diagnostic evaluations. The speech-language pathologist's ear and sophisticated examination procedures reveal the need to study the valve.

Again, Table 11.1 summarizes the speech symptoms associated with various degrees of velopharyngeal competence and incompetence.

McWilliams and Philips (1979) have shown that the listener's perceptions of speech problems related to faulty velopharyngeal valving can be reliable predictors of what is likely to be found when the valve is evaluated. They developed a rating system to aid speech-language pathologists in making objective decisions.

When the relationship between speech and probable valving deficit is apparent, instrumentation should be used. It is discouraging to realize that we do not yet have a single device that will provide all of the information required. Our choice is to use multiview videofluoroscopy in combination with aerodynamic studies of the type developed by Warren and DuBois (1964). This combination of data, together with reliable speech assessments, provides the information necessary for making treatment decisions. And, after all, that is the purpose of assessment. We want to know what the person's problem is, why it exists, what we can do about it, and what the prognosis is likely to be. It is not possible at this time to avoid the diagnostic step of assessing the all-important velopharyngeal valve. To ignore it is to be guilty of malpractice and of administering speech therapy that may be inappropriate and even harmful and thus unethical.

CLINICAL MANAGEMENT

The purpose of all assessment is to help speech-language pathologists plan the most satisfactory management so that the affected individual may have the best opportunity to realize his full potential in whatever area is involved. Thus, the communication specialist wants to find an approach to care that will make it likely that the person with disordered speech will be able to communicate as effectively and efficiently as our modern knowledge and technology permits. In dealing with cleft palates and related problems, several types of intervention approaches are available.

Improving Velopharyngeal Valving

It is almost never possible, except in rare and unusual cases, to improve velopharyngeal valving through speech intervention alone. For this reason, speech-language pathologists need to work in concert with plastic surgeons and dental specialists in order to improve the potential for the velopharyngeal valve to work effectively.

One procedure frequently used today is known as the *pharyngeal flap operation*. This is surgery that elevates a flap of tissue from the posterior pharyngeal wall, brings it forward, and attaches it to the soft palate. The procedure often makes it possible for the lateral pharyngeal walls to close around the palato-flap structure and, probably, for the soft palate to be lengthened somewhat. Results from pharyngeal flap surgery have been promising and have often made normal speech possible for people who were previously seriously defective. Like any other surgery, the success rate is not 100%, and it varies from one series of reported cases to another. But we have never seen a patient made worse for having had this procedure, and most improve noticeably, many eventually acquiring normal speech.

The pharyngeal flap procedure usually leads to a certain amount of mouth breathing and to frequent snoring at night. Sometimes speech may be hyponasal following the surgery, but in some cases this lasts only until the swelling from surgery subsides and healing is complete. The pharyngeal flap operation can do a great deal to reduce hypernasality. However, it will not change the gross articulation errors which we talked about earlier, and speech therapy will be necessary to do that.

A second approach to the correction of velopharyngeal incompetency is to do something to build out the posterior pharyngeal wall. Various types of implants have been used, including teflon (Bluestone, Musgrave, McWilliams, & Crozier, 1968; Bluestone, Musgrave, & McWilliams, 1968). This type of procedure is most successful in individuals who have very slight velopharyngeal incompetence. It is not possible to inject enough material into the posterior pharyngeal wall to take care of large openings. We prefer to use the teflon implant with people who already achieve a light touch contact between the soft palate and the posterior pharyngeal wall during a lateral videofluoroscopic study but who lose that contact when the head is hyperextended. Teflon implants have their highest rates of success with people with those characteristics. They may show a small midcentral gap on basal view videofluoroscopy and small amounts of nasal air flow on pressure flow studies. When the only characteristic of the speech is a reduction in intraoral pressure, the implant, like the pharyngeal flap, is likely to make immediate and amazing changes in speech production. Where there are gross articulatory errors, intervention through speech therapy will be necessary.

In some instances, we need to correct velopharyngeal incompetency through the use of a prosthetic speech aid or a palatal lift. The prosthetic speech aid is a dental appliance with a bulb to close off the air passage between the mouth and the nasal cavity. The palatal lift, on the other hand, is designed to elevate a soft palate which moves poorly and to give it an opportunity to make contact with the posterior and lateral pharyngeal walls. Prosthetic speech aids are not used as frequently as they once were, but they are still valuable aids in the treatment of people with the velopharyngeal in-

FIGURE 11.10

Prosthetic Speech Aids—One with Dentures; the Other Without. Note the posterior bulb that fills space and provides a contact for lateral and posterior pharyngeal wall movement.

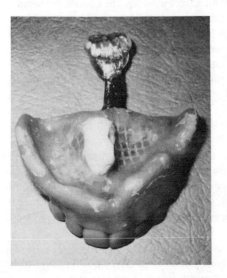 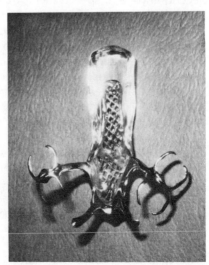

competence and should be seriously considered if surgery is contraindicated for any reason. Figure 11.10 shows prosthetic speech aids with the bulb attachment; one includes a denture while the other does not.

These prosthetic speech aids are usually fitted in the presence of the speech-language pathologist, who can assist in determining proper placement and size of the bulb. In this situation, air pressure studies are of great help, as is auditory evidence of a reduction in nasal flow and of increase in intraoral pressure.

Correcting Dental Problems

Sometimes, as we have already seen, speech problems are related to the presence of dental problems that can be completely or partially corrected. These problems include missing teeth, maxillary collapses on the side or sides of the cleft, midfacial defiency, narrow maxilla, and restricted size of the oral cavity. These are difficult anatomical deficits to overcome in speech production or through speech therapy. Although some people are able to manage adequately and automatically without any speech therapy, few accomplish this task. Many wind up in therapeutic programs to which they respond poorly. Therefore, we recommend that, wherever possible, dental needs be taken care of before speech therapy is begun. This means that the speech-language pathologist will work in close conjunction with the dental specialists so that dental treatment can be timed very closely with the initiation or resumption of speech therapy, after a period of rest.

More and more, when people have midfacial deficiency, surgical intervention is used to move the midface forward and bring it into better alignment with the mandible. If you stop to think about it for a minute, you will realize that having your jaws in proper alignment provides oral architecture capable of housing the tongue in a way that it can accurately be used for speech. Before these procedures are carried out, the tongue rests between the extruded mandible and the retracted maxilla, so that it is difficult if not impossible to produce the tongue-tip sounds accurately, even after a great deal of speech therapy.

The intent of this section has been to tell you of some of the techniques other than speech therapy that should be considered seriously before subjecting anyone to speech therapy based upon inadequate or inaccurate diagnostic information. Very often, the best speech clinician will be the plastic surgeon or the dentist. The speech-language pathologist must be wise enough and well-trained enough to recognize when a mechanism is functioning at its maximum and when additional speech therapy will not be beneficial. It takes a sophisticated and confident speech-language pathologist to recognize that speech therapy is not for everyone who has a communication problem.

Speech Therapy

You may already have gathered that we are not particularly impressed with the results of speech therapy for problems related to cleft lip and palate and to velopharyngeal incompetency. However, there are certain aspects of speech therapy which should be understood, some of which the speech-language pathologist should be prepared to become involved in.

Work on Language

The child who is born with cleft lip and palate or cleft palate usually does experience mild delays in early development. For this reason, it is important to instruct parents early in good positive methods of stimulation which they can use at home. Talking to babies, reading to them, describing activities that are going on in the household, parallel talking as the child plays—these are all techniques which parents use almost automatically but in which they can be encouraged and reinforced to good advantage.

As the child develops, small informal play groups are often indicated, particularly if the child is isolated from other children. This kind of experience can often be accomplished informally in neighborhoods or more formally in a cleft palate center or in regular nursery schools, which we prefer. We have also had experience using creative dramatics as a technique for naturally encouraging the verbal output of children with clefts. It is interesting to note that the children began by being almost nonverbal, but quickly initiated spoken language and expressed many of their innermost feelings. This experience was fun for the children and did not suggest to them that something was wrong—only that there was an interesting activity available to them once each week (Irwin & McWilliams, 1974; Tisza, Irwin, & Zabarenko, 1969).

Brookshire and colleagues (1980), as mentioned earlier, have formalized suggestions for dealing with these early developmental problems, and many clinics are engaged in parent counseling and early childhood stimulation to eliminate the lag in language performance. Results have been promising, and we encourage you to keep this type of approach in mind.

It cannot be stated too often that the informal way is effective for most children. However, for many, the language disorder is a true form of disordered development and will require management of the type recommended for young children with language disabilities. The fact that the child has a cleft or some other problem that may influence velopharyngeal valving may complicate language therapy but will not change it.

You may wish to review chapter 8; remember that what is written there applies equally to children with birth defects.

Articulation Therapy

When children have articulation errors that are either unrelated to velopharyngeal valving or are related to valving problems that have been corrected, intensive programs of articulation therapy should be undertaken. Again, it is not necessary to describe the therapy for children with clefts. Their needs are very similar to those of children with articulation disorders in general. It is always discouraging when speech-language pathologists believe that a cleft or related problem somehow takes the child out of the mainstream of articulation therapy and demands something of a different nature. This is not the case, and we urge you to work with these problems from the point of view of consonant articulation.

See chapter 5.

Therapy to Accomplish Velopharyngeal Closure

In 1968, Shelton, Hahn, and Morris reviewed the literature concerning speech training and therapeutic exercises as they influence velopharyngeal closure. They found no evidence to indicate that motor exercises do anything to improve velopharyngeal competence. But this is not to say that some professionals do not continue to try all sorts of approaches to handling velopharyngeal incompetence through speech therapy. We shall discuss a few of them here.

It was once thought that articulation training might have an influence on velopharyngeal closure. In other words, if an individual learned to produce significant consonant sounds more effectively, that person would also probably handle the velopharyngeal valve somewhat better. However, Shelton, et al. (1969) did not find this to be the case. The exception to that might be with an individual who has the ability to close the velopharyngeal portal but does so inconsistently. Articulation therapy might then be influential in helping him use the mechanism more appropriately. There are no very good data available on this issue, but it is a therapeutic approach that is often successfully used for this type of problem.

Exercises and training of various types have also been suggested for improving function in the velopharyngeal valve. Again, the overwhelming burden of research evidence fails to support the claim that such exercises are useful. Cole (1971) suggests that, if exercises are going to be effective, changes will occur within 3 months. We would suspect that, when this is the case, velopharyngeal incompetency *per se* is not being dealt with. Again, the individual who has ability to close off the velopharyngeal portal but does not habitually do so may be a candidate for this type of approach. Shelton, et al. (1973a) concluded a discussion of this issue by suggesting that these methods are still experimental and essentially unproven. Additional experimental work is needed before speech-language pathologists attempt to correct real velopharyngeal incompetency through programs of special exercise.

Bulb-reduction therapy was suggested by Blakely and Porter (1971). It is interesting to note that the boy on whom they reported had palatal paralysis and weakness in the muscles of the pharynx. They made an appliance in order to help him achieve velopharyngeal closure. For 3 years he wore the appliance and had some speech therapy. His speech improved, and hypernasality was essentially eliminated. As the program proceeded, it was possible to reduce the size of the speech bulb very gradually and finally to discontinue its use entirely. The authors claim that the boy continued to have "satisfactory" speech, even though lateral cephalometrics (whose shortcomings have already been discussed) showed a sizeable opening between the soft palate and the pharyngeal wall during speech. Weiss (1971) also attempted bulb-reduction therapy and felt that he had success with 20 patients who were carefully followed. These patients all had "good palatal pharyngeal compensation ability." The information that is missing from this report is definite data regarding the nature of the velopharyngeal closure at the beginning of therapy.

There is no adequate proof that bulb-reduction therapy (Shelton, Lindquist, Arndt, Elbert, & Youngstrom, 1971) is effective and, if it is, the conditions under which it can be expected to succeed. Until such data are forthcoming, we cannot specify those children who might profit from this kind of management. Since appliances are expensive and the program is time-consuming, it is not recommended as the first choice at this time.

Tongue posturing of a faulty nature was pointed out by McDonald and Koepp-Baker (1951). As we mentioned above, some individuals with velopharyngeal incompetency appear to hump the posterior portion of the tongue in an effort to compensate for the faulty valve. This obviously places the tongue in a negative position so far as speech is concerned. It is difficult to produce anterior tongue sounds, and the size of the oral cavity is reduced so that the relationship between the air that enters the mouth and that which enters the nasal cavities is further upset, leading to an increase in the hypernasality. This undoubtedly occurs, but the conclusion that speech therapy to change tongue posture is the answer to the problem is probably erroneous; the tongue humping is itself a compensatory behavior in response to a faulty valve. Therapy designed to lower the tongue in the oral cavity may somewhat reduce the severity of the hypernasality, but is not likely to eliminate it. This would be a possible approach only if no other possibilities existed and if the high posterior tongue carriage continued after secondary surgical procedures to improve the velopharyngeal valving.

The whistling-blowing approach described by Shprintzen, et al. (1975) is one that should be well understood by all speech-language pathologists dealing with velopharyngeal incompetency. On videofluoroscopic studies, these authors saw that some people achieved velopharyngeal closure during whistling or blowing, but that they did not use the observed closure during speech activities. We do know, however, that speech is much more demanding than blowing and requires many more minute and complicated gestures. In addition, a number of the subjects in the study did achieve velopharyngeal closure on some speech task or had had secondary surgical procedures designed to improve velopharyngeal closure. This latter group had failed to make the expected improvements in speech. For these types of cases, the whistling-blowing approach appears to be sensible and worth trying.

Shprintzen and colleagues have outlined a very detailed system of therapy that is designed to use whistling or blowing as precursors to vocalization so that the closure obtained on one task may be incorporated into speech. These wise investigators make no claims that this system of therapy is effective for any degree of velopharyngeal incompetence. They have attempted to specify the conditions under which it may be expected to be effective, and this is the kind of work that is necessary for any therapy that is designed to improve velopharyngeal valving. Since the approach seems to work in only limited cases, it is obvious that an assessment of the velopharyngeal valve and its ability to close effectively under certain conditions, preferably on speech tasks, is an essential preliminary step to the planning of speech therapy.

CONCLUSION

We have been trying throughout this chapter to help you understand that the speech problems associated with clefts and related disorders are often very complicated and require the assistance of many specialists in addition to the speech-language pathologist. Unfortunately, there are still too many children in this country who have been in speech therapy for many years for the purpose of correcting velopharyngeal incompetence, without having any diagnostic studies to help the speech-language pathologist understand the nature of the problem being treated. If it is your best judgment that you cannot be helpful to a particular child or if you need diagnostic consultation, then you have an obligation to make this clear to the school authorities and to the parents and to help arrange for additional assistance as close to the child's home as possible. There are certain types of human problems that cannot be well or successfully managed in every small community throughout the country. When those problems strike, it is necessary to seek help elsewhere, even if it involves traveling a great many miles. The child's family has the right to know that making that trip might change their child's life by helping him become a more effective communicator. They should have the opportunity to decide for themselves and with their child just how important speech is and to understand the limitations of speech therapy. Finding extra help for a child may well be a speech-language pathologist's major contribution to better speech.

SELECTED READINGS

Grabb, W. C., Rosenstein, S. W., & Bzoch, K. R. (Eds.). *Cleft lip and palate*. Boston: Little, Brown, 1971.

McWilliams, B. J. (Ed.). *ASHA Reports No. 9*. Washington, D.C.: American Speech and Hearing Association, 1973.

McWilliams, B. J., & Philips, B. J. *Audio seminar in velopharyngeal incompetence*. Philadelphia: W. B. Saunders, 1979.

Paradise, J. L., & Bluestone, C. D. Diagnosis and management of ear disease in cleft palate infants. *Transactions of the American Academy of Ophthalmology and Otolaryngology*, 1969, *73*, 709–714.

Paradise, J. L., Bluestone, C. D., & Felder, H. The universality of otitis media in 50 infants with cleft palate. *Pediatrics*, 1969, *44*, 35–42.

Shames, G. H., & Rubin, H. Psycholinguistic measures of language and speech. In W.C. Grabb, S. W. Rosenstein, & K. R. Bzoch (Eds.), *Cleft lip and palate*. Boston: Little, Brown, 1971.

Skolnick, M. L. Videofluoroscopic examination of the velopharyngeal portal during phonation in lateral and base projections: A new technique for studying the mechanics of closure. *Cleft Palate Journal*, 1970, *7*, 803–816.

Warren, D. W., & DuBois, A. B. A pressure-flow technique for measuring velopharyngeal orifice area during continuous speech. *Cleft Palate Journal*, 1964, *1*, 52–71.

REFERENCES

Bernthal, J. E., & Beukelman, D. R. The effect of changes in velopharyngeal orifice area on vocal intensity. *Cleft Palate Journal*, 1977, *14*, 1.

Blakeley, R. W., & Porter, D. R. Unexpected reduction and removal of an obturator in a patient with palate paralysis. *British Journal of Communication*, 1971, *6*, 33–36.

Bless, D., Ewanowski, S. J., & Dibbell, D. G. Clinical note: A technique for temporary obturation of fistulae. *Cleft Palate Journal*, 1980, *16*, 297–300.

Bluestone, C. D., Musgrave, R. H., McWilliams, B. J., & Crozier, P. A. Teflon injection pharyngoplasty. *Cleft Palate Journal*, 1968, *5*, 19–22.

Bluestone, C. D., Musgrave, R. H., & McWilliams, B. J. Teflon injection pharyngoplasty—Status 1968. *The Laryngoscope*, 1968, *78*, 558–564.

Brooksire, B. L., Lynch, J. I., & Fox, D. R. *A parent-child cleft palate curriculum, developing speech and language*. Tigard, Ore.: C. C. Publications, 1980.

Bzoch, K. R. A study of the speech of a group of preschool cleft palate children. *Cleft Palate Bulletin*, 1959, *9*, 2–3.

Christiansen, R. L., & Evans, C. A. Habilitation of severe craniofacial anomalies—The challenge of new surgical procedures: An NIDR Workshop. *Cleft Palate Journal*, 1975, *12*, 167–176.

Clifford, E. Psychological aspects of cleft lip and palate. In K. Bzoch (Ed.), *Communication disorders related to cleft lip and palate* (2nd ed.). Boston: Little, Brown, 1979.

Cohen, M. M., Jr. Syndromes with cleft lip and cleft palate. *Cleft Palate Journal*, 1978, *15*, 306–328.

Cole, R. M. Patterns of orofacial growth and development. IN H. L. Morris (Ed.), *Patterns of orofacial growth and development, Proceedings of the conference, ASHA Reports No. 6*. Washington, D.C.: American Speech and Hearing Association, 1971.

Fox, D., & Johns, D., Predicting velopharyngeal closure with a modified tongue-anchor technique. *Journal of Speech and Hearing Disorders,* 1970, *35,* 248–251.

Fox, D., Lynch, J., & Brookshire, B. L. Selected developmental factors of cleft palate children between two and thirty-three months of age. *Cleft Palate Journal,* 1978, *15,* 239–245.

Fritzell, B. The velopharyngeal muscles in speech: An electromyographic and cineradiographic study. *Acta Oto-Laryngologica,* 1969, Supplementum 250, 1–81.

Goodstein, L. D. Intellectual impairment in children with cleft palates. *Journal of Speech and Hearing Research,* 1961, *4,* 287–294.

Grabb, W. C., Rosenstein, S. W., & Bzoch, K. R. (Eds.). *Cleft lip and palate.* Boston: Little, Brown, 1971.

Graham, M. (Ed.). *Cleft palate: Middle ear disease and hearing loss.* Springfield, Ill.: Charles C Thomas, 1978.

Holm, V. A., & Kunze, L. H. Effect of chronic otitis media in language and speech development. *Pediatrics,* 1969, *43,* 833–839.

Irwin, E. C., & McWilliams, B. J. Play therapy for children with cleft palates. *Children Today,* 1974, *3,* 18–22.

Kaplan, E. N., Jobe, R. P., & Chase, R. A. Flexibility in surgical planning for velopharyngeal incompetence. *Cleft Palate Journal,* 1969, *6,* 166–174.

Kernahan, D. A., & Stark, R. B. A new classification for cleft lip and cleft palate. *Plastic and Reconstructive Surgery,* 1958, *22,* 435–441.

Lamb, M., Wilson, F., & Leeper, H. A comparison of selected cleft palate children on the variables of intelligence, hearing loss, visual-perceptual-motor abilities. *Cleft Palate Journal,* 1972, *9,* 218–228.

Lamb, M., Wilson, F., & Leeper, H. The intellectual function of cleft palate children compared on the basis of cleft type and sex. *Cleft Palate Journal,* 1972, *10,* 367–377.

McDonald, E. T., & Koepp-Baker, H. Cleft palate speech: An integration of research and clinical observation. *Journal of Speech and Hearing Disorders,* 1951, *16,* 9–20.

McWilliams, B. J. Psychological development and modification. *ASHA Reports No. 5.* Washington, D.C.: American Speech and Hearing Association, 1970.

McWilliams, B. J. (Ed.). *ASHA Reports No. 9.* Washington, D.C.: American Speech and Hearing Association, 1973.

McWilliams. B. J. (Ed.). Communication problems associated with cleft palate. In R. J. Van Hattum (Ed.), *Communication disorders.* New York: Macmillan, 1980.

McWilliams, B. J., Bluestone, C. D., & Musgrave, R. H. Diagnostic implications of vocal cord nodules in children with cleft palate. *The Laryngoscope,* 1969, *79,* 2072–2080.

McWilliams, B. J., & Bradley, D. P. Ratings of velopharyngeal closure during blowing and speech. *Cleft Palate Journal,* 1965, *2,* 46–55.

McWilliams, B. J., & Girdany, B. The use of televex in cleft palate research. *Cleft Palate Journal,* 1964, *1,* 398–401.

McWilliams, B. J., Glaser, E. R., Philips, B. J., Lawrence, C., Lavorato, A. S., Beery, Q. C., & Skolnick, M. L. *A comparative study of four methods of evaluating velopharyngeal adequacy.* Submitted for publication, 1980.

McWilliams, B. J., Lavorato, A. S., & Bluestone, C. D. Vocal cord abnormalities in children with velopharyngeal valving problems. *The Laryngoscope,* 1973, *83,* 1745–1753.

McWilliams, B. J., & Matthews, H. A comparison of intelligence and social maturity in children with unilateral complete clefts and those with isolated cleft palates. *Cleft Palate Journal,* 1979, *16,* 363–372.

McWilliams, B. J., & Musgrave, R. H. Psychological implications of articulation disorders in cleft palate children. *Cleft Palate Journal,* 1972, *9,* 294–303.

McWilliams, B. J., Musgrave, R. H., & Crozier, P. A. The influence of head position upon velopharyngeal closure. *Cleft Palate Journal,* 1968, *5,* 117–124.

McWilliams, B. J., & Philips, B. J. *Audio seminar in velopharyngeal incompetence.* Philadelphia: W. B. Saunders, 1979.

McWilliams, B. J., & Smith, R. M. Psychosocial considerations. In B. J. McWilliams (Ed.), *ASHA Reports No. 9.* Washington, D.C.: American Speech and Hearing Association, 1973.

Minifie, F. D., Hixon, T. J., Kelsey, C. A., & Woodhouse, R. J. Lateral pharyngeal wall movement during speech production. *Journal of Speech and Hearing Research,* 1970, *13,* 584–594.

Moore, W., & Sommers, R. Oral manometer ratios, some clinical and research implications. *Cleft Palate Journal,* 1974, *11,* 50–61.

Morley, M. *Cleft palate and speech* (6th ed.). Baltimore: Williams and Wilkins, 1967.

Morris, H. L. The oral manometer as a diagnostic tool in clinical speech pathology. *Journal of Speech and Hearing Disorders,* 1966, *31,* 362–369.

Morris, H. L. Etiological bases for speech problems. In D.C. Spriestersbach & D. Sherman (Eds.), *Cleft palate and communication.* New York: Academic Press, 1968.

Morris, H. L., Shelton, R. L., & McWilliams, B. J. Assessment of speech. In B. J. McWilliams (Ed.), *ASHA Reports No. 9.* Washington, D.C.: American Speech and Hearing Association, 1973.

Musgrave, R. H., McWilliams, B. J., & Matthews, H. P. A review of the results of two different surgical procedures for the repair of clefts of the soft palate only. *Cleft Palate Journal,* 1975, *12,* 281–290.

Needleman, H. Effects of hearing loss from early recurrent otitis media on speech and language development. In B. Jaffe (Ed.), *Hearing loss in children.* Baltimore: University Park Press, 1977.

Noll, J., Hawkins, M., & Weinberg, B. Performance of normal six- and seven-year-old males on Oral Manometer tasks. *Cleft Palate Journal,* 1977, *14,* 200–205.

Paradise, J. L., & Bluestone, C. D. Diagnosis and management of ear disease in cleft palate infants. *Transactions of the American Academy of Ophthalmology and Otolaryngology,* 1969, *73,* 709–714.

Paradise, J. L., Bluestone, C. D., & Felder, H. The universality of otitis media in 50 infants with cleft palate. *Pediatrics,* 1969, *44,* 35–42.

Paradise, J. L., & McWilliams, B. J. Simplified feeder for infants with cleft palate. *Pediatrics,* 1974, *53,* 566–568.

Peterson-Falzone, S. J. Speech pathology in craniofacial malformations other than cleft lip and palate. *ASHA Reports No. 8.* Washington, D.C.: American Speech and Hearing Association, 1973.

Philips, B. J., & Harrison, R. J. Articulation patterns of preschool cleft palate children. *Cleft Palate Journal,* 1969, *6,* 245–253.

Richman, L. C. Behavior and achievement of cleft palate children. *Cleft Palate Journal,* 1976, *13,* 4–10.

Richman, L. C. The effects of facial disfigurement on teachers' perception of ability in cleft palate children. *Cleft Palate Journal,* 1978, *15,* 155–160.

Ruess, A. L. A comparative study of cleft palate children and their siblings. *Journal of Clinical Psychology,* 1965, *21,* 354–360.

Shames, G. H., & Rubin, H. Psycholinguistic measures of language and speech. In W.C. Grabb, S. W. Rosenstein, & K. R. Bzoch (Eds.), *Cleft lip and palate.* Boston: Little, Brown, 1971.

Shelton, R. L., Chisum, L., Youngstrom, K. A., Arndt, W. B., & Elbert, M. Effect of articulation therapy on palatopharyngeal closure, movement of the pharyngeal wall, and tongue posture. *Cleft Palate Journal,* 1969, *6,* 440–448.

Shelton, R. L., Hahn, E., & Morris, H. L. Diagnosis and therapy. In D. C. Spriestersbach & D. Sherman (Eds.), *Cleft palate and communication.* New York: Academic Press, 1968.

Shelton, R. L., Lindquist, A. F., Arndt, W. B., Elbert, M., & Youngstrom, K. A. Effect of speech bulb reduction on movement of the posterior wall of the pharynx and posture of the tongue. *Cleft Palate Journal,* 1971, *8,* 10–17.

Shelton, R. L., Morris, H. L., & McWilliams, B. J. Nonsurgical management of cleft palate speech problems. In B. J. McWilliams (Ed.), *ASHA Reports No. 9.* Washington, D.C.: American Speech and Hearing Association, 1973. (a)

Shelton, R. L., Morris, H. L., & McWilliams, B. J. Anatomical and physiological requirements for speech. In B. J. McWilliams (Ed.), *ASHA Report No. 9.* Washington, D.C.: American Speech and Hearing Association, 1973. (b)

Shprintzen, R. J., McCall, G. N., & Skolnick, M. L. A new therapeutic technique for the treatment of velopharyngeal incompetence. *Journal of Speech and Hearing Disorders,* 1975, *40,* 69–83.

Skolnick, M. L. Videofluoroscopic examination of the velopharyngeal portal during phonation in lateral and base projections: A new technique for studying the mechanics of closure. *Cleft Palate Journal,* 1970, *7,* 803–816.

Skolnick, M. L., Zagzebski, J. A., & Watkin, K. L. Two dimensional ultrasonic demonstrations of lateral pharyngeal wall movement in real time—A preliminary report. *Cleft Palate Journal,* 1975, *12,* 299–303.

Starr, P., Chinsky, R., Canter, H., & Meier, J. Mental, motor, and social behavior of infants with cleft lip and/or palate. *Cleft Palate Journal,* 1977, *14,* 140–147.

Stool, S. E., & Randall, P. Unexpected ear disease in infants with cleft palate. *Cleft Palate Journal,* 1967, *4,* 99.

Subtelny, J., & Subtelny, J. D. Intelligibility and associated physiological factors of cleft palate speakers *Journal of Speech and Hearing Research,* 1959, *2,* 353–360.

Tessier, P. The definitive plastic surgical treatment of the severe facial deformities of craniofacial dysostosis. *Plastic and Reconstructive Surgery,* 1971, *48,* 419.

Tisza, V., & Gumpertz, E. The parents' reaction to the birth and early care of children with cleft palate. *Pediatrics,* 1962, *30,* 86–90.

Tisza, V., Irwin, E., & Zabarenko, L. A psychiatric interpretation of children's creative dramatics stories. *Cleft Palate Journal,* 1969, *6,* 228–234.

Van Demark, D. R. A factor analysis of the speech of children with cleft palate. *Cleft Palate Journal,* 1966, *3,* 159–170.

Van Demark, D. R., Morris, H. L., & Vandehaar, C. Patterns of articulation abilities in speakers with cleft palate. *Cleft Palate Journal,* 1979, *16,* 230–239.

Ventry, I. Effects of conductive hearing loss: Fact or fiction. *Journal of Speech and Hearing Disorders,* 1980, *45,* 143–156.

Warren, D. W. Perci: A method for rating palatal efficiency. *Cleft Palate Journal,* 1979, *16,* 279–285.

Warren, D. W., & DuBois, A. B. A pressure-flow technique for measuring velopharyngeal orifice area during continuous speech. *Cleft Palate Journal,* 1964, *1,* 52–71.

Weinberg, B., & Shanks, J. C. The relationship between three oral breath pressure ratios and ratings of severity of nasality for talkers with cleft palate. *Cleft Palate Journal,* 1971, *8,* 251–256.

Weiss, C. E. Success of an obturator reduction program. *Cleft Palate Journal,* 1971, *8,* 291–297.

12 NEUROGENIC DISORDERS OF SPEECH

Leonard L. LaPointe

Jack was a 75-year-old gentleman from Booth Bay, Maine, who presumably suffered a brainstem stroke. He and his wife, desiring a change to a warmer climate and another opinion regarding prognosis and treatment of his speech impairment, sought our services at a Florida Veterans Administration Medical Center. Presenting signs included paralysis of all limbs, impaired swallowing with no speech output, but intact awareness and intact auditory comprehension.

Mr. Dickerson was a tall, muscular gentleman who looked 15 years younger than his age. He was alert, very intelligent, and looked the part of one who has spent an active outdoor life engaged in stimulating jobs and adventure. Most of his life had been spent on the sea. He had been a frigate officer in the Coast Guard in WWII, and had worked as a yacht broker, shipyard manager, marine surveyor, and, in the words of his wife, "knew tons about sailing, rigging, and navigation and was one of the finest racing helmsmen on the East Coast." In 1958 he ran the Race Committee for the New York Yacht Club for the America's Cup Races. Jack is the type of rugged, knowledgeable and self-reliant person that you encounter in fiction but seldom have the opportunity to meet in real life.

He was initially treated at a large medical center where he received physical therapy and treatment for his motor speech disorder. He was able to ambulate with the aid of a wheelchair and walker but he was left with some residual paralysis.

We used a standardized protocol to preserve his responses on both audio and video tape recordings and evaluated his speech output by careful listening and by observing his responses to a series of speech and nonspeech tasks. He showed intact comprehension of both written and spoken language and at no time did we suspect anything other than completely intact language and mental status. His motor speech system, however, was ravaged, and he presented a severe flaccid dysarthria characterized by reduced range, direction, and velocity of movements involving respiration, the velum, the tongue and lips, and to a lesser extent the larynx.

Jack's speech was unintelligible, except for isolated single words. Further evaluation assessed levels of word and sentence intelligibility as well as the quality of his articulation of vowel and consonant combinations by word position.

He and his wife were advised not to expect a return of recovery to the speech skills he had before his stroke and that the best speech treatment could hope to offer would be improvement of some of the parameters of the motor speech system and perhaps some limited and compensated speech to aid in the expression of daily needs, as well as the possibility of learning to use some nonverbal, alternate methods of communication.

Jack's wife is as interesting and self-reliant as her husband. She is a nurse who is knowledgeable, questioning, and tenacious. She proved to be an assertive, independent, and highly motivated spouse who demanded an active role in her husband's rehabilitation. We agreed to a 6-week treatment program of 2 to 3 sessions per week. Throughout the program Mrs. Dickerson worked with her husband on selected speech tasks that were compatible with our treatment goals.

During treatment, careful charting and plotting of baserate performance and progress on all tasks was documented, and progress was noted on nearly all of the specific treatment objectives. Jack also was provided a Canon Communicator (a pocket-sized, keyboard operated electronic device with a ticker-tape printout) and was instructed in its use. He expressed the desire to use it only in crisis situations or when he was unable to intelligibly convey a message. Throughout treatment, his wife maintained an active role, not only in carrying out tasks at home, but frequently by contributing ideas for tasks.

Overall intelligibility on words and syllables increased from 4% and 36% respectively on April 3 to 12% and 67% on May 16. These gains were modest and the result of an intensive cooperative effort between clinic and spouse, yet they were reported by both Jack and his wife to be worth the effort.

At the end of May, they returned to Maine for the summer with the resolve to continue daily work on some of the objectives we had outlined and with the promise that they would call on us again when the snow flies and the water freezes. Winter indeed returned to Maine, and 8 months later I received another call informing me that Jack and his wife were returning to Florida and wanted to stop in for a week of re-evaluation, more specific suggestions for home treatment, and renewal of our acquaintance.

Jack's speech had responded remarkably to the direction and persistence of his home program, and he had regained enough compensated, functional communication to make his daily needs and wants known and even communicate by telephone. Word intelligibility was now in the 60% to 80% range.

You may now wish to listen to the speech sample accompanying this chapter, found on Audio Disc 2, Side 3 (sample #8).

Lurking in the damp recesses of the private thoughts of many of us is the fear that if ever we should suffer brain damage we would end up either insane or mentally retarded. As is evident from previous chapters in this book, sanity and intellectual function are but two of the wonders regulated by the human nervous system. The human nervous system is usually divided into two major parts: the central nervous system (CNS), including the brain and spinal cord; and the peripheral nervous system (PNS), including the cranial nerves and spinal nerves. This division is shown in Figure 12.1. This complex system, the center of which is an unassuming, squishy, three-pound, pinkish-white mass,

FIGURE 12.1
Central Nervous System (CNS) and Peripheral Nervous System (PNS) of Humans.

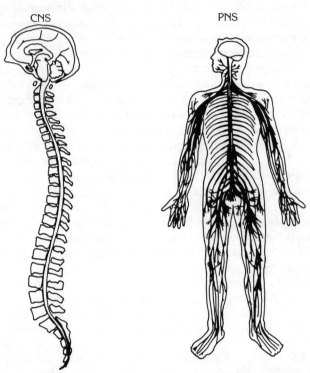

CNS   PNS

See Figure 12.2.

has evolved into the primary director of human behavior. Unlike that of the striped bass and other lower animals, the human nervous system has added features and functions that allow behaviors far more complex than treading water or devouring a minnow. As we have seen, in addition to centers of language and memory, certain regions are associated with hearing, vision, smell, touch, taste, and other senses. Other areas are associated with regu-

FIGURE 12.2
Brain of Man and of Striped Bass. (Man on the right.)

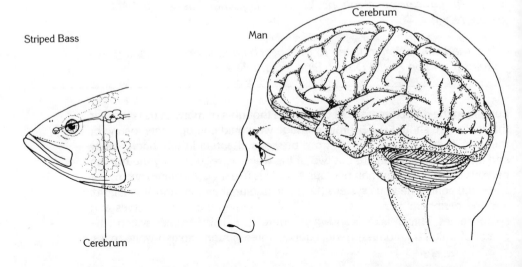

Cerebrum

Striped Bass   Man

Cerebrum

lating the vital functions of the body such as automatic breathing, maintaining blood pressure and heart rate, and digesting food. Still other centers and systems are responsible for movement and patterns of movement, from a simple movement such as pinching the nostrils to indicate reaction to a referee's judgment, to the complex series of moves of a gymnast's full twisting dismount from the parallel bars. Other regions of the brain are responsible for correlating and integrating many tiny bits of information to make plans or programs of action.

Impairment of the planning, coordination, and timed execution of the movement patterns that result in the curious act we know as speech is the subject of this chapter. No human movement patterns are as intricate or as complex or as intertwined with all the human activities of learning, loving, and living. Far more area of the brain is devoted to the control of the tiny muscular adjustments of the tongue, lips, vocal folds, and other speech articulators than to those muscle groups needed for walking upright. Far more coordination and synchrony is needed for speech than for riding a unicycle, threading a needle, rolling a log, or removing a thorn from the foot. The amazing thing is that the act of speech becomes so automatic that we hardly think about it— until something goes wrong.

CLASSIFICATIONS AND DEFINITIONS

The area of **neurogenic** impairment of speech has been a fertile ground for controversy and desk-pounding argument over the years. Some of this disagreement can be traced to the unbridled proliferation of terms and labels for speech disorders. This growing pool of unclearly defined terms has spawned argument and misunderstanding, particularly in the branch of speech-language pathology that has been so closely related to the medical environment. No standardized terminology or classification system has emerged, and labels have been assigned seemingly at the whim of the labeler. Most labels have been generated to serve the particular interest or specific point of view of a group or a discipline. By contrast, the familiar blind men and the elephant seem remarkably astute. Different goals and different jargon can create very real barriers to crossdisciplinary cooperation. Fortunately, some of these problems have diminished in recent years.

> *Neurogenic simply means arising from the nervous system.*

Neurologically based disturbances in the selection, sequencing, and coordinated production of speech sounds have been labeled *oral apraxia, verbal apraxia, phonemic paraphasia, literal paraphasia, oral-verbal apraxia, anarthria, dysarthria, apraxic-dysarthria, cortical dysarthria, phonetic disintegration,* and a score of other terms. Though we still do not have a standard set of terms, some of the less frequently used and esoteric labels are falling by the wayside, and some labels seem to be gaining acceptance through the frequency of their appearance in the literature. A few writers, notably Darley (1967), have long advocated a more precise and consistent system of terminology. Perhaps the next decade will see the adoption of more precise and reliable systems of describing the dimensions of speech that are apt to go awry after brain damage.

In addition to widely varying use of specific descriptive terms, classification of disturbed oral communication can be problematic. The borderline between speech and language is sometimes unclear, as is the decision as to whether or not a specific disturbed speech event is the result of an error in articulatory timing or speech sound selection. Communication is a unitary process in the sense that it is the product of a complex, interrelated system requiring co-ordination of several components of the body. At the same time, the act of communication loses some of its relevance if the environment and its context are ignored. The damage that disturbs this delicate sequence of sensory-muscular-integrative events therefore can affect the function of the respiratory mechanism, the tone-producing mechanism, the resonance system, and the system of articulation that shapes and molds the air or sound stream into recognizable words.

It is wise to bear in mind the holistic nature of communication; it is an act that truly is greater than the sum of its parts. For the sake of understanding, though, we can analyze this integrated system. Disorders of *voice* are ade-quately covered in other chapters of this book, as will be the syndrome called *cerebral palsy* and its effects on communication and the linguistic-symbolic disorders of *language* (aphasia). This chapter focuses on the output trans-missive disorders of *speech* that are shattered by damage to the nervous system. These include the neurogenic phonological selection and sequencing disorders (apraxia of speech) and the dysarthrias. These disorders can occur in adults or in children, but we will focus on the problem in adults.

See chapters 6, 13, and 14 respectively.

Dysarthria

Current use of the term **dysarthria** is somewhat more precise than earlier concepts of the disorder. If you were to consult a dictionary or several of the dozens of textbooks in the medical field of clinical neurology, you might get the impression that dysarthria is simply a disturbance of articulation caused by nervous system damage. Colorful though not very precise adjectives are used to describe the resultant articulation defect. "Slurred" and "scanning speech" are typical of the speech descriptions of the dysarthric person.

Current definitions are more inclusive than those of the past, and dysarthria now refers to a *group* of related speech disorders resulting from disturbed muscular control over the speech mechanism. Clinical research at the Mayo Clinic (Darley, Aronson, & Brown, 1975) has nurtured a concept of the disorder that includes impairment in the coexisting motor processes of respiration, phonation, articulation, resonance, and prosody.

Underlying the condition of dysarthria is a fundamental disturbance of movement or motoric function caused by damage to the nervous system. The motions and synchrony of the components of the speech system may be impaired in range, velocity, direction, force, or timing. Negative signs, such as slowness or inadequate range of movement, are frequently the outcome. However, in some types of dysarthria, depending upon the areas of the nervous system affected, the movement disorder is overlaid with positive character-istics, such as excessively fast or involuntary movements or movement overshoot due to uninhibited activity of intact parts of the nervous system.

Motor impairment of the articulators, including the lips, tongue, jaw, and soft palate, tends to produce a greater effect on the intelligibility of speech

Table 12.1 lists some of these colorful, though inexact, per-ceptual terms gleaned from past writings on dysarthria.

People with cerebral palsy are more likely to have dysarthria than other neurogenic speech problems; see the next chapter.

TABLE 12.1
Colorful, if Inexact, Early Perceptual Descriptors of Dysarthric Speech.

Slurred	Unclear	Scanning	Mush mouth
Thick	Staccato	Clumsy	Hot potato speech
Jerky	Explosive	Cerebral-palsied	Foreign body mouth
Indistinct	Squirrel tongue	Slobbery	Wobbly words

than do disturbances of the laryngeal or respiratory systems. The most prominent features that affect intelligibility are those that result from distorted consonant sounds, repeated or prolonged sounds, distorted vowels, or irregular articulatory breakdown.

Apraxia of Speech

The other disorder to be discussed in this chapter is the neurogenic phonologic selection and sequencing problem that we will call **apraxia** of speech. Arguments over this disorder have existed for a century or more, and the disagreements seemed to have reached a rolling boil in the mid-1970s (LaPointe, 1975). Nearly everyone can find common ground of agreement on some of the speech characteristics exhibited by those who have the disturbance, but there have been objections as to what to call it (Kertesz, 1979; Martin, 1974). The term *apraxia* of speech appears to be gaining favor in the literature and that is the label we will use.

Apraxia of speech is a neurogenic phonologic disorder resulting from sensorimotor impairment of the capacity to select, program, and/or execute, in coordinated and normally timed sequences, the positioning of the speech muscles for the volitional production of speech sounds. The loss or impairment of the phonologic rules of the native language is not adequate to explain the observed pattern of deviant speech, nor is the disturbance attributable to weakened or slowed actions of specific muscle groups. Prosodic alteration, that is, changes in speech stress, intonation, or rhythm, may be associated with the articulatory problem either as a primary part of the condition or in compensation for it. One of the remarkable characteristics of the disorder is the demonstration of moments of error-free production during automatic or emotional utterances ("WHY can't I say the word *telephone* when I want to!"), compared to disturbed volitional attempts at uttering the same word or words ("fela . . . tef . . Stella! . . felaphone.")

TABLE 12.2

Characteristic Features of Dysarthria and Speech Apraxia.

Dysarthrias	Apraxia of Speech
Very little difference in articulatory accuracy between automatic-reactive and volitional purposive speech (no error-free production).	Articulatory accuracy is better for automatic-reactive speech than for volitional-purposive speech (moments of error-free production).
Substitution errors are infrequent. Speech is characterized more by phonetic distortions and omissions.	Substitution errors are more frequent than other error types.
Except occasionally in hypokinetic dysarthria, no difficulty with initiation of speech.	Initiation difficulty is frequent; characterized by pauses, restarts, repetition of initial sounds, syllables, or words.
Consonant clusters are frequently simplified; speech sound additions are rare.	Consonant clusters may be simplified but more frequently the intrusive schwa /ə/ is inserted within clusters ("puh-lease" for "please").
Audible and silent groping of the articulators to locate target articulatory placements is rare or nonexistent.	Audible or silent groping and articulatory posturing to locate target articulatory placements is common.
Quality of production and error type is consistent when asked to repeat the same utterance; some improvement may be noted under conditions of extreme effort or motivation.	Variability in production of repeated utterances is common. Error type may change or production may very off and on target, particularly on repeated utterances of polysyllabic words.

Table 12.2 lists some of the contrasting features of the dysarthrias and apraxia of speech. These differentiating features will vary in usefulness, depending on the severity of the presenting signs and symptoms of each patient, but they can be used as general guidelines for differentiating the dysarthrias from apraxia of speech in most patients.

Table 12.3 lists some of the possible ways of classifying the motor speech disorders.

Certain classification systems have come in and out of favor over the years. Today systems that combine perceptual features with speech processes and the functions of the speech valves seem to be preferred by many clinicians and researchers. This contemporary method of viewing and classifying motor speech disorders will be developed in the following section.

TABLE 12.3
Possible Ways to Classify Motor Speech Disorders.

Age	Congenital, developmental, acquired.
Cause	Stroke, head trauma, disease, etc.
Site of lesion	Brainstem, cerebellar, etc.
Level of lesion	Peripheral, central
Speech processes	Respiration, phonation, articulation, resonance, prosody
Speech valves	1, 2, 3, 4, 5, 6, 7*
Speech events	Neural, muscular, structural, aerodynamic
Perceptual features	Pitch, loudness, voice quality, intelligibility, bizarreness

*See point-place discussion.

BASIC CONCEPTS

As we mentioned briefly earlier, underlying the speech disturbances of dysarthria and apraxia is motoric impairment, or a fundamental disturbance of movement. What features of movement are necessary for normal speech? Darley, et al. (1975) suggest that adequate strength, speed, range, accuracy, steadiness, and muscular tone are necessary.

This chain of events can be appreciated by viewing Figure 12.3.

Against the backdrop of these requisites of movement, the speech production process can be thought of as a chain of events originating in the brain, where the movement plan is conceived, which ends in the formation of acoustic signals that result in sequences of speech sounds (Netsell, 1973). As you can see in Figure 12.3, the genesis of this sequence is in the brain, where the plans of movement are formulated and programmed. Nerve impulses are then generated in the motoric sections of the brain and transmitted along the pathways of the nervous system to the muscles and structures of the speech system. Movements of these muscles and structures (lungs, vocal folds, soft palate, tongue, lips, jaw) create air flows and air pressure that result in the acoustic events we perceive as speech.

These processes were detailed in chapter 4.

These basic concepts of motor speech production have been developed further (Netsell & Daniel, 1979) to focus on some of the control variables that influence aspects of movements of speech. Aspects of muscle strength, muscular tone, and the timing and synchronization of muscular contraction are three of the variables that can have a strong influence on movement patterns. If one or more of these "control variables" is defective, movements can be impaired in range (resulting in either an underexcursion or overexcursion), in velocity, or in direction (resulting in missing the mark or the target of an intended movement). Let us look at each of these variables a little more closely.

FIGURE 12.3
Levels in the Motor Speech Production Process.

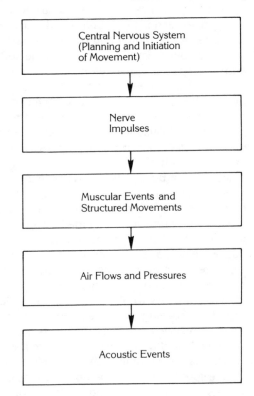

Strength is a concept that is fairly well understood. All of us have experienced or observed differences in strength among individuals. Varying abilities in weight lifting and the experience of having to relinquish the stubborn pickle jar to a person with greater hand strength are reminders of these differences.

Tone refers to the relatively constant background state of muscular contraction that is characteristic of normal muscle. Normal posture is partly dependent on adequate muscle tone. Tone may be decreased or increased (rigid), may wax and wane, or vary rhythmically (cogwheel rigidity).

Timing refers to the accuracy of onset and termination of muscular contraction. It also can refer to the duration of contraction or the complex coordination required for groups of muscles to work in synchrony.

A further concept that is related to the organization and execution of movements is that of programming or planning. The completion of complex skilled movements requires a preplan or program of the order, duration, and other details of movement sequences. Disturbances at this higher level of the organization of movement, when related to speech, may result in apraxia of speech.

It should be understood, and no doubt has been experienced by most of us, that certain other factors can influence the functioning of the motor speech system. Fatigue, motivation, excitement, and stark fear can have important influences on speech. For instance, most of us have experienced the tongue-slipping, voice-cracking effects of anxiety while speaking in front of large groups.

Components of the Motor Speech System

If you wish, review chapter 4 on the physiology of speech.

A simpified view of the functional components of the speech production system might conceive of it as a small decision-making computer that plans and initiates actions (the brain) and transmits these orders along pathways (portions of the central and peripheral nervous system) to the muscles and structures of two large bags of air connected to a series of pipes open at one end (the speech apparatus of the respiratory, laryngeal, and upper airway system). Within the system of air containers and pipes are a series of valves that can be opened and closed to varying degrees to regulate the air pressure or flow that is generated or pumped by the lungs.

Figure 12.4 illustrates the functional components of the speech apparatus when this system is viewed as a pump (the respiratory system) and a series of valves. Each of the seven numbered components is a structure or combination of structures that serve to either generate or valve the speech air stream. Number 1 includes the pump of the system, the muscles and structures of respiration. Included at this level are the abdomen and diaphragm, the muscles and cartilage of the rib cage, and the lungs. Number 2 refers to the structures and muscles of the larynx, and number 3 includes the soft palate (velum) and the muscles in the velopharyngeal area that can move to separate the oral and nasal cavities. Number 4 refers to the blade of the tongue, while number 5 refers to the muscles that regulate the tongue tip. Number 6 refers to all of the facial muscles responsible for lip spreading, rounding, opening, and closing. Number 7 refers to the muscles and structures of the jaw. These basic concepts are important for more than academic reasons. Not only can they provide the framework for a model that will allow a better understanding of the complexities of motor speech, but importantly for the speech-language pathologist, they can offer valuable guidance for the

The use of the point-place system in

processes of diagnosis and treatment of people who suffer motor speech dysfunction. Perceptual signs, the interpretation the listener gives to the sound

FIGURE 12.4

The Functional Components of the Motor Speech System. (Adapted from J. C. Rosenbeck and L. L. LaPointe, "The Dysarthrias: Description, Diagnosis and Treatment." In D. L. Johns (ed.), *Clinical Management of Neurogenic Communicative Disorders.* Boston: Little, Brown, copyright © 1978. Used by permission.)

Point-Place System
(Valves Along the Nile)

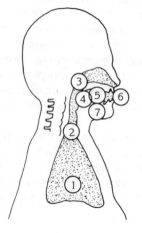

1. Muscles and Structures of Respiration

2. Larynx

3. Soft Palate

4. Tongue Blade

5. Tongue Tip

6. Lips

7. Mandible

of a person's speech, are still important. But, as we will see subsequently, attention to the structures and valves of the speech system can help explain perceptual signs and aid in the planning and execution of treatment. This view is a simplified version of that developed and elaborated upon by Netsell (1973) and also modified by Rosenbek and LaPointe (1978). *assessment is described in detail below.*

CAUSES OF NEUROGENIC SPEECH DISORDERS

Neurological and communication disorders affect 50,000,000 Americans (one out of every five persons), and the dollar cost to the country is $65 billion a year (NIH Publication, 1979). What are the causes of these disturbances? What can go wrong with the nervous system to cause these dehumanizing conditions and erode the capacity of a person to enjoy life and interact with other people?

Many conditions can attack the well-being of the brain and create a web of problems for a person, including movement problems related to the production of speech. Stroke is by far the leading cause of neurogenic speech disorders. It is the number three killer in America; and nearly 500,000 Americans are hospitalized with it every year, one out of every 500 people. Stroke killed Franklin Roosevelt, Winston Churchill, Joseph Stalin, and my grandmother. When it doesn't kill, it leaves ⅔ of its survivors impaired in speech, movement, or feeling.

Trauma is another major cause of nervous system damage and, as we have seen, has plagued man since the invention of the rock. Over 420,000 new cases of head injury occur every year. Automobile and motorcycle accidents account for about 80% of the traumatic head injury in this country, while injuries from recreational activities (diving, skiing, javelin, and so on), power equipment, weapons, blows by objects or persons, and self-inflicted injuries account for the remainder. The young are particularly vulnerable to nervous system trauma. More than ⅔ of the head and spinal injuries occur in the below-35 age group, typically in far more males than females.

Trauma also can affect the peripheral nervous system, and occasionally this can lead to speech disturbance if portions of the PNS that control the structures and muscles of speech production are injured. Cuts, burns, crush injuries, and penetrating wounds can cause these underlying injuries.

Another form of trauma the brain can experience is caused by a variety of toxins (poisons). Mercury, pesticides, lead poisoning, and carbon monoxide poisoning are environmental threats to people, but the most prevalent cause of neurotoxicity is alcohol and drug abuse. Other dramatic neural poisons, even if less frequently encountered, are insect, spider, and snake venoms. Our conditioned reaction of avoiding recreational activities with diamondback rattlers and blackwidow spiders is well-founded.

Brain tumors (neoplasms) are another source of neuropathology. At any one time there are approximately 61,000 people in this country with tumors of the nervous system, many of which can affect the speech system. Damage can occur from the robbing of nutritional requirements from surrounding healthy tissue or the pressing and impinging of a growing mass of cells on surrounding tissue. Some tumors are benign and their growth is self-limited, while others are malignant and can grow and spread their virulent influence to remote regions of the body.

Infections are not the threat to the nervous system they once were, but antibiotics and miracle drugs have not eradicated the problem by any means. Conditions such as bacterial meningitis and viral infections and chronic fungal infections are often treated successfully or prevented by immunization in this generation, though certain neural infections remain a serious problem.

Finally, inherited or acquired diseases can affect the nervous system. In many the disease process is one of slow, painful degeneration which progressively involves areas that regulate speech production. Myasthenia gravis, multiple sclerosis, amyotrophic lateral sclerosis (ALS), Parkinsons's disease, and Huntington's disease are but some of the debilitating progressive conditions that can rob speech, sense, and stability. Lou Gehrig, the baseball player, Woodie Guthrie, the folk balladeer, and a childhood neighbor lady named Mabel suffered the ravages of these degenerative diseases.

Active research continues on the understanding, prevention, or amelioration of these neuropathologies, but until fundamental answers are found, we have no course but to treat their outcomes vigorously to the best of our ability.

CHARACTERISTICS AND TYPES

What does it sound like when someone is unfortunate enough to suffer damage that results in a motor speech disorder? The ear of the beholder is the final arbiter, and a speech difference can only make a difference if listeners perceive it as being unusual or tainted in communicative effectiveness.

The speech sample provided with this chapter gives you an idea of motor disorders of speech, but you should also know that the disorders can vary widely in type or quality. The severity can range from a disturbance that is barely noticeable to one that shackles communication by rendering the speaker completely unintelligible. Type and severity of the disorder are related primarily to the location and extent of the nervous system damage. Generally speaking, large brain lesions result in the most damage; but small areas of destruction, if located in critical brain areas, can produce devastating and severe impairment.

Dysarthria

Clinical research at the Mayo Clinic by Darley and his associates (1975) has contributed a great deal to our understanding of motor speech disorders. One of the most potent contributions of these researchers was to bring into focus some of the deviant speech dimensions heard in the dysarthrias and to associate specific clusters of deviant speech with certain neurologic disorders. We have used the work of Darley and his colleagues to organize our listening skills and perhaps improve our perceptual analysis of dysarthric speakers. The variety of speech features that can go awry in dysarthria sometimes can appear overwhelming to the ear if several parameters of the speech production system are involved. The pattern of signs and symptoms that affect voice, articulation, respiration, and prosody sometimes appear so interwoven as to make individual features unidentifiable. If you know what to expect, though, because of a model of motor speech based on a firm understanding of both process and function, the perceptual onslaught can be less confusing. If the parameters of each speech process are attended to systematically, you can discern patterns of behavior and impose order on the seeming chaos.

In our clinic we use the deviant speech categories presented by the Mayo Clinic research and have adapted them into a checklist to aid us in both sharpening our perceptual skills and pinpointing what is wrong with each patient's speech. This checklist is presented in Table 12.4. What can dysarthric speech sound like? As the checklist shows, the voice may be abnormal along several dimensions.

Pitch level may be too high, too low, monotonous, or may break or squeak. Loudness may be inappropriate. It may decay to inaudible levels, may show rapid and disconcerting changes, or may be too loud or too soft most of the time. Voice quality may reflect too much nasal resonance, breathy or harsh quality, or the strained-strangled quality characteristic of excessive muscular contraction. Respiration may be audible when it should be silent, too shallow (resulting in not enough breath to finish utterances), or irregular. Articulation may be characterized by distorted and imprecisely formed consonant sounds, repeated sounds, abnormally prolonged vowels and consonants, or irregular breakdown in sound production. Finally, prosody (rate, stress, and melodic line) may be too fast, too slow, inappropriate to sentence meaning, or equalized and reduced without regard for normal syllable or word stress.

Overall, the speech pattern of the dysarthric speaker may be affected along two general dimensions, intelligibility and bizarreness. Speech can be perfectly

TABLE 12.4

Checklist of Deviant Speech Dimensions (From Audiology & Speech Pathology Service, Veterans Administration Medical Center, Gainesville, Florida. Adapted from F. L. Darley, A. Aronson, and J. Brown, *Motor Speech Disorders.* Philadelphia: W. B. Saunders, 1975). Used by permission.

VOICE

Pitch characteristics

_____ Pitch level overall	_____ Pitch breaks
_____ Monopitch	_____ Voice tremor

Loudness characteristics

_____ Loudness level overall	_____ Monoloudness
_____ Alternating loudness	_____ Loudness decay
_____ Excess loudness variation	

Quality characteristics

_____ Harsh voice	_____ Breathy voice (transient)
_____ Breath voice (continuous)	_____ Voice stoppages
_____ Strained-strangled voice	_____ Hyponasality
_____ Nasal emission	_____ Hypernasality

RESPIRATION

_____ Forced expiration-inspiration	_____ Audible inspiration
_____ Grunt at end of expiration	

PROSODY

_____ Rate overall	_____ Short phrases
_____ Increased rate overall	_____ Increased rate in segments
_____ Variable rate	_____ Reduced stress
_____ Intervals prolonged	_____ Inappropriate silences
_____ Short rushes of speech	_____ Excess and equal stress

ARTICULATION

_____ Imprecise consonants	_____ Phonemes prolonged
_____ Phonemes repeated	_____ Vowels distorted

INTELLIGIBILITY   1, 2, 3, 4, 5, 6, 7   **BIZARRENESS**   1, 2, 3, 4, 5, 6, 7

intelligible and yet be so bizarre that the listener judges it as abnormal. For example, in some of the neurologic diseases that affect control of muscular contraction of the vocal folds, speech may be relatively clearly articulated and easy to understand, but may be characterized by wildly fluctuating pitch or loudness. This can be disconcerting to listen to, and may call undue attention to the speaker along with judgments of a strange or abnormal speech pattern.

Clusters of Deviant Speech Dimensions

See Rosenbek and LaPointe (1979) for a summary of distinctive characteristics of the various dysarthria types based on this research. This summary associates each type with its underlying neurologic condition, location of neural damage, deficit in neuromuscular tone or movement, cluster of deviant speech dimension, and most distinctive or characteristic speech deviation.

Darley, Aronson, and Brown (1975) attempted not only to refine our perceptual skills by directing our attention to precisely defined behavioral aspects of deviant speech, but also to establish ways to distinguish among the varieties of dysarthria by identifying clusters of deviant speech dimensions associated with specific neurologic disorders. Analysis of these clusters led to deductions about the underlying neuromuscular mechanism that was responsible and led further to the application of an appropriate name for each type of dysarthria. Four distinct types of dysarthria were outlined: (a) flaccid dysarthria (in bulbar palsy or brainstem disorders), (b) spastic dysarthria (in pseudobulbar palsy), (c) ataxic dysarthria (in cerebellar disorders), and (d) hypokinetic dysarthria (in dystonia and chorea). In addition, they describe mixed dysarthrias that result from disorders of multiple motor systems and are associated with the ravaging diseases of ALS, multiple sclerosis, Wilson's disease, and a variety of other conditions. Though the work on motor speech at the Mayo Clinic has done much to highlight differences among the dysarthrias, in clinical practice these distinctions are rarely clear-cut. In our clinic, many of our evaluations result in judgments of "mixed" dysarthria.

Apraxia of Speech

In fact, some authorities consider apraxia to be an integral feature of Broca's aphasia, which is discussed in detail in chapter 14.

"I know what it is but I can't say it." Anyone who has worked with people with apraxia has heard this affirmation frequently. Patients will report that they have a clear idea of what they intend, but cannot get the speech sequence started or keep it rolling once it is started. There is little doubt that, in many instances, they know well what they intend to say since they can write it, describe it, or give salient features of it. What does the resulting speech attempt sound like? From the definition, we expect the signs to be impaired volitional production of articulation and prosody. These articulation and prosodic disturbances do not result from muscular weakness or slowness, nor do they result from the linguistic disturbances in word meaning or impaired use of grammatical rules that we see in aphasia. This is not to say that apraxia of speech cannot coexist with other disorders. The same brain lesion that disturbs programming of speech movements can impinge on areas that affect language or range of motion of the tongue. Frequently these disorders *do* coexist, thus complicating the sorting-out process and making the speech-language pathologist's judgmental skills all the more important in the decisions as to which aspects of deficient speech are the most detrimental to communication, and which ones are amenable to treatment.

A variety of both speech and nonspeech behaviors have been suggested as being characteristic of apraxia of speech. A small explosion of clinical research interest took place in the 1960s and '70s, resulting in many attempts to describe and highlight the salient features of the condition. An excellent synthesis of the articulatory, nonspeech, and prosodic characteristics of apraxia of speech is presented by Wertz (1978). From this summary, we can see that the person with speech apraxia frequently pauses inordinately, gropes for articulatory position, restarts words and sentences, substitutes speech sounds (sometimes adding complicated clusters of sounds for the intended single sound target), and makes prepositioning or postpositioning errors (just as we sometimes do on the typewriter). Amid all this searching and speech sound groping, he slows down his rate and appears to "tip-toe" through speech in the apparent anticipation of problems in stringing sequences together. Remarkable variability on repeated attempts at the same target are often produced.

Johns and LaPointe (1976) trace this development in their chapter on neurogenic disorders of output processing.

An example of some of these features can be seen in the transcribed dialogue below, as one of our speech-language pathologists elicited words from a patient seen in our clinic. This man was a 48-year-old carpenter from Crystal River, Florida, who suffered a left hemisphere stroke about 2 months before the interview.

Speech-Language Pathologist: All right, say these things after me: pen, knife, hospital.

Patient: Pen, knife, hopay, hop, ah, . . . pos, . . . pester, as . . . I can't get all that.

Speech-Language Pathologist: Try it again, hospital.

Patient: Hospin-a . . .

Speech-Language Pathologist: I may go fishing on Sunday.

Patient: I may go fishing on Sunday.

Speech-Language Pathologist: Australia is a small continent.

Patient: Uh . . . Arsale-a is a . . nah, ah, coneh . . . ah, I can't get that.

Speech-Language Pathologist: Try it again, Australia is a small continent.

Patient: A las eh . . . I can't get that.

Speech-Language Pathologist: O.K., we'll go on. You're anxious to get out, huh?

Patient: I gotta get out.

Speech-Language Pathologist: Are you going to go back to work?

Patient: I sure am. Yessir. Soon as I can.

Speech-Language Pathologist: What type of work do you do?

Patient: Construction.

Speech-Language Pathologist: Are you working on a job right now?

Patient: I was, yah. Over in ah, Clivem, ah, ah . . .

Speech-Language Pathologist: What job?

Patient: A church over in Cri . . . Crystal Riv . . .

Speech-Language Pathologist: Over where?

Patient: Critchal, ah, Critchal . . . Ril . . . Ril . . . yah.

Speech-Language Pathologist: Crystal?

Patient: Right. Riddin . . . R-R-Ridden . . .

Speech-Language Pathologist: That's right, Crystal.

Patient: Criden, criden, Crystal . . . River.

Speech-Language Pathologist: What kind of work do you do?

Patient: I'm a coffiney . . . eh. A coffiney. ahhh. Carpenter.

This sample illustrates several aspects of speech apraxia. Dozens of features have been catalogued as characteristic of the disorder, but we feel that there are three cardinal behavioral features.

(1) *Many sound substitutions and transpositions,* frequently including additive substitutions of more complex consonant clusters for a single sound target. For example, asked to repeat the word *bicycle,* the person may say "tise, tise, sicycle, licycle, sprykle, sprickle, . . . spicyle."

(2) *Initiation difficulty,* characterized by stops, restarts, phoneme, syllable, and whole word repetitions, audible groping for articulatory position, and silent searching and posturing of the articulators. When asked "Where do you live?" one person responded, "[pause] Coneve . . . Goneve . . Jah . . . Jah . . . Jake. [silent visible tongue movements] . . . L . . Lakel . . LLLake Geneva . . . Whew."

(3) *Variability of production pattern* on immediate repeated trials of the same target, including changes in type of error and performance varying on and off target. In imitating the word *refrigerator,* one patient said, "Refrig . . . ridgerator, ridgefrigerator, frigerator, frefridgerator, refrigerator, regrigerator, ridgerator."

Recently, speculation has arisen that types of speech apraxia may exist. Clinical observation seems to confirm the impression that the phonologic impairment in persons with lesions more toward the back portions of the brain is less likely to present the halting, groping, initiation difficulty that seems to characterize patients with brain damage that is more towards the front. This is a rich area for future research and description. Severity of apraxia of speech certainly varies; and sometimes the disorder is so severe that the patient is practically speechless and the features that are usually used to define the disorder are not apparent. With these severely impaired individuals, we can only infer from the nature of their speech attempts whether or not the disorder seems to resemble one of disturbed programming of neuromuscular sequences.

Much remains to be learned about the precise nature and the underlying mechanisms of all the motor speech disorders. Much also needs to be learned about what to do to correct them. The work of Netsell, Durango, Kent, Wertz, Rosenbek, and a growing number of others, who are bridging the gap from the speech science laboratory to the rehabilitation clinic, gives us reason to be hopeful.

ASSESSMENT

For the speech-language pathologist who works in a hospital or rehabilitation clinic, the usual request for services arrives in the form of a single sheet of paper, often called a "Request for Consultation Services." This form frequently comes from a physician or a team of health care providers. It includes a summary of the patient's medical diagnosis along with a brief statement of the person's medical history. A typical request might read, "This is a 54-year-old man who suffered a left hemisphere CVA 2 weeks ago that left him hemiplegic and without speech. Please evaluate his communicative status and recommend a course of treatment, if appropriate."

CVA stands for cerebro-vascular accident, or stroke.

This request or any other type of referral then serves as the springboard for setting in motion the assessment or evaluation of the individual's communication.

Purposes of Evaluation

Why do you undertake the assessment process? The evaluation serves to answer a number of crucial questions and has several purposes.

First of all, the evaluator must decide whether or not a significant problem exists. Occasionally a person is referred who has a dialect of English or a foreign accent that is a long-standing speech pattern, and the person neither requires nor desires intervention. On rare occasions the referred patient may have a temporary problem easily corrected at bedside, as in the case of a patient referred to me at a Denver hospital with the diagnosis of "muffled speech . . . hard to understand." Upon bedside interview, the patient spoke with imprecise articulation and minimal jaw excursions during conversational speech. Deft questioning and examination of the intraoral cavity revealed the presence of a wad of chewing tobacco the size of a small cornish hen. Upon removal of the tobacco, this man's speech cleared considerably. The patient revealed that he had a long-standing habit of chewing tobacco and said he wasn't about to stop just because he was hospitalized, even if the doctors had trouble understanding him. In this case, it was determined that no sustaining communication problem existed.

A second purpose is to determine the nature of the impairment. If a disorder exists, it is important to determine if it is classifiable by type and to judge the relative prominence of the deviant speech signs with an eye to determining those that contribute most to the communication handicap.

The next question is how handicapping the condition is. Compared to others with similar problems, is the disorder mild, moderate, or severe? The evaluation will attempt to shed light on these questions of relative severity. Also considered will be the effect of the disorder on functional communication needs for daily living as well as on any specific vocational or life-style peculiarities of the individual.

The establishment of a prognosis is another purpose of the assessment. Information gained from the evaluation will be incorporated with a variety of other variables such as age, time since onset, presence of other medical complications, motivation, and family support. As we have seen, accurate prediction is not a hard science in many areas of speech-language pathology, and here again the speech-language pathologist must be cautious in treading the fine line between dampening hope and igniting unrealistic and unattainable dreams of recovery. Prognosis for what? This is always an important question to answer after assessment is completed, when goals are being established.

Another important function of the evaluation is to find out which functions are intact and which are impaired and to determine baselines of communication performance. Qualitative and quantitative measurements of performance on clearly defined speech tasks can serve as standards of reference to gauge any future change.

Next, the speech-language pathologist will have to begin somewhere if remediation is attempted. The information gained from the evaluation, along with judgments of the relative severity of components of the speech production system and their relative contribution to effective communication, will be invaluable in deciding on the focus and direction of treatment. This may be one of the single most important reasons for assessment—to answer the questions "What's wrong?" and "What should I attempt to correct?"

Finally, questions about the nature, severity, and outcome of the condition will be asked by family, friends, related medical personnel, and the patient, as well as by the source of the referral. Thus another function of evaluation is to provide information. It will be comforting to all to be informed that the condition is known, has a label, has been seen before, and intervention and amelioration can be tried and may well work.

Evaluation Strategies

No standardized measurement batteries are available for the evaluation of motor speech disorders (unlike aphasia, for which there is a wide choice of commercially available tests). Most of the methods for the assessment of speech apraxia and dysarthria have grown out of the clinical experience of the examiner or out of principles based on findings in the speech science laboratories. In recent years a more systematized approach to evaluation has been developing. This approach combines the principles of perceptual evaluation of the speech processes along with analysis of function of the components of the speech production system. This strategy is an amalgamation of ideas developed and refined by a host of researchers and clinicians, including some at the University of Iowa, the Mayo Clinic, the Speech Motor Control Laboratory of the University of Wisconsin, The Boystown Institute for Communicative Disorders, and Veterans Administration Medical Centers in Madison, Memphis, Martinez, Gainesville, and elsewhere.

The fundamentals of the assessment process are similar to those in other speech-language pathologies. These include arriving at conclusions and decisions by piecing together bits of information from four areas:

(1) Personal history (medical, social, educational)
(2) Nonspeech function of the structures of speech
(3) Conversational and social interactive speech
(4) Special speech tasks.

Berry and LaPointe (1974) recommend using a standard recording protocol for this evaluation process. This has been supplemented in recent years by evaluation of performance on a series of special tasks, based on suggestions by Hardy (1967), Hixon (1975), Wertz (1978), Netsell (1973), Darley, et al. (1975), and Rosenbek and LaPointe (1978).

Nonspeech Movement

Nonspeech function of the structures of speech can be evaluated by requesting a series of movements of the articulators. Careful observation of the symmetry, color, configuration, and general appearance of the lips, tongue, soft palate, teeth, and jaw provides the first clues to judgments of normal structure. A series of systematic tasks designed to test the movement of these structures also can reveal gross abnormalities. For instance, the simple request to "pucker the lips" may uncover a fundamental problem.

Not all structures are equally important to speech. It is of little value, for example, to evaluate the status of the "hangey down thing at the back of the throat," or uvula, because it has little role in speech production and we can talk quite well without it.

The Point-Place System

The point-place model for assessment of the functional components of the motor speech system is a useful strategy for evaluating the integrity of each of the valves in the speech production system. Returning to Figure 12.4, we usually start at the bottom of the system and move sequentially through the numbers. This may be crudely analogous to stopping at evaluative checkpoints along a river that moves from south to north, like the Nile River. Thus the caption "valves along the Nile" reminds us of the direction and sequence of the assessment process of the functional components of speech.

Respiration (Number 1)   Hixon (1973) has contributed a good deal to our understanding of the normal respiratory process and how to evaluate it. This is the pump or the energy source for speech; if it is impaired, speech can be weak, with reduced loudness, frequent and abnormal inhalation, decreased syllables per breath, short phrases, and reduced duration of phonation.

Tasks   Tasks specifically designed to evaluate the muscles and structures of respiration include connected, spontaneous speech and the demonstration of rapid control of the system by the ability to rapidly sniff air up the nose, to pant, to demonstrate abrupt changes in loudness, to imitate patterns of loudness change, and to blow into a manometer to observe air pressure matching ability.

Recall the description of a manometer in chapter 4.

Criteria for Normal Performance   On all of these tasks, we need a good deal more research to determine ranges of normal performance, since they are the standards by which performance is measured. In addition to our perceptual impression of whether or not performance falls with our experience of what constitutes normal limits, we have some rather embryonic guidelines for normalcy on some of these special tasks. At the respiratory level, these include the judgment of adequate conversational loudness (including the ability to muster a shout or to talk over noise); enough sustained respiration for speech to produce 10 to 20 syllables on a single breath; the ability to manipulate loudness so that adequate stress for changes in meaning can be produced; and, on the pressure manometer, the ability to generate 5 cm of water pressure for a period of 5 seconds (Netsell & Hixon, 1978); and vowel prolongation for a period of 10 to 20 seconds.

Phonation (Number 2)   The precise control of the laryngeal system for the process of phonation is vital to speech production and is mutually interrelated with the process of respiration. It is somewhat artificial to evaluate them segmentally, as it is for all of the individual components of the system; but for convenience and ease of understanding, focus on specific phonatory tasks can be instructive.

Impaired range, velocity, or direction of movement within the laryngeal system can result in decreased pitch range, slow pitch change, abnormal voiced-voiceless contrasts, slowed voice onset or offset time, breathiness, strained-strangled voice quality, pitch or loudness bursts, or increased habitual pitch use.

Tasks   Evaluation of the laryngeal valve begins with judgments of the normalcy of voice quality during conversational speech. Other parameters of phonation can be assessed by measuring duration of phonation, the ability of attempts to start and stop phonation, steadiness of loudness and vowel production, ability to abruptly change pitch, ability to gradually phonate the unphonated air stream, and production of voiced-voiceless speech sound contrasts (*sip-zip, pen-ben, at-add,* etc.).

You may wish to check back in chapter 6 for further discussion.

Criteria for Normal Performance   Normal phonation requires the judgment of pitch and quality that are appropriate to the sex and age of the individual. Sometimes these judgments, particularly of voice quality, are very subjective and can vary from culture to culture. Though a wide range exists, normal fundamental frequency levels are approximately 130 Hz (about C_3 on a piano keyboard) for males and about an octave higher, 260 Hz (C_4 on the piano), for females. The normal rate of change of frequency is 50 Hz per 100 millisec. This can be determined with the assistance of instruments for voice frequency analysis. Voiced-voiceless consonant distinctions must be judged as being within normal limits, as must intonation and stress changes for meaning.

Resonance (Number 3)   The principle feature of resonance that is evaluated at valve number 3 is that of oral-nasal resonance balance. As we have seen, only a few sounds in English (/m, n, ŋ/) require nasal resonance for their production. The production of all other English speech sounds necessitates a closure or nearly complete closure of the velopharyngeal valve, and several muscle groups are responsible for the adequate functioning of this valve. Inadequate movement of this valve is fairly easy to recognize perceptually.

You may wish to review these techniques, which were presented in chapter 11.

Tasks   Careful listening to conversation is one of the best strategies for detecting either resonance imbalance or the inappropriate emission of a nasal air stream. Some of the instrumental analysis techniques developed for use with people with cleft palates can be used to trace the velar movement in patients with neurogenic damage as well. These include oral-nasal pressure manometers, high speed motion picture X-rays (cineradiography), and a simple device that is plugged into the nostrils and activates a colorful piece of styrofoam within a sealed tube if excesive nasal air escapes during speech.

Another way of determining resonance imbalance is by the cul-de-sac resonance test. For this task the speaker is requested to sustain vowel sounds or repeatedly produce nonnasal consonant-vowel-consonant combinations (for example, *pop, pop, pop*). The examiner then gently pinches and releases the speaker's nose so as to close and open the nostrils. If resonance is normal on these nonnasal samples of speech, no difference should be heard in acoustic quality during the pinched and nonpinched conditions. However, if sound is being inadequately resonated through the nasal cavity, a noticeable change will be heard between the pinched and opened conditions. Another way of checking timing and agility of velar movement is to require the production of alternating nasal and nonnasal consonant-vowel combinations (*ma-ba, ma-ba, ma-ba, . . .*).

Test sentences that have no /m, n, ŋ/ sounds can also be used to judge the presence or absence of nasality. The following sentences should be produced with no nasal resonance.

These rather poetic examples are adapted from some presented by Moncur and Brackett (1974).

(1) Love is a powerful force for good.
(2) Prayers were offered to the Great Spirit of the Sioux.
(3) Raspberry parfait was the featured dessert at the Blue Fox.
(4) Fried foods irritate the gallbladder.
(5) Blue violets hugged the shady slopes of the Ford River.

Conversely, the movements of the velar area must be timed properly for the lowering of the velum to allow normal nasal resonance on words that contain /m, n, ŋ/ sounds. If these movements are mistimed, the result can be inadequate nasal resonance (hyponasality). This is the effect we sometimes hear when the nasal respiratory passages are inflamed or clogged when a person complains "I have a cold id by doze."

To test for inadequate nasal resonance, test words and sentences should be loaded with /m, n, ŋ/ sounds, such as:

(1) John will ring no more.
(2) Monday it was loaned to me for a month.

(3) Many of them are fine with me.
(4) Make me a Hong Kong cookie.
(5) I am reminded of my pants.
(6) Many a young man learned something in Channing.

Criteria for Normal Performance   The objective acoustic correlates of normal nasal balance are unclear, and acceptable levels will vary culturally and from dialect to dialect. Judgments of appropriateness always should be made with community and dialectal standards in mind. The practiced ear is still the final judge as to appropriateness of resonance balance, and when connected speech, the cul-de-sac test, and resonance balance on vowels is deemed adequate and resonance balance is judged to be normal, there is no need for an intervention plan on this particular aspect of speech.

Articulation (Numbers 4, 5, 6, 7)   For many years, the concept of dysarthria was intimately tied to deficient articulation. Deficient range, velocity, or direction of movement with the tongue, lips, and jaw can result in imprecise production of consonant and vowel sounds, and this deficiency can be one of the most noticeable and dramatic barriers to clear speech.

If these structures and valves are affected, we might notice omitted tongue tip consonant sounds /t, d, n, l/, poor vowel differentiation, distorted plosive sounds caused by weakened or light articulatory contacts, slowed transition between articulatory contact points, prolonged vowels or consonants resulting in slowed articulation time, consonant distortions caused by hitting a nonintended point of articulation, or simplification of complex sound clusters (*stop* sounds like *sop*), as well as many other patterns.

Tasks   As with all of the other functional components of the speech production system, the integrity of the valves of the upper airway is best tested by careful observation of their use in connected speech. Another useful measure is a sentence or single word test of articulation. This should be organized *See chapter 5.* so that it systematically elicits all of the sounds of American English in the positions where they are likely to occur. Sometimes a more detailed Sound by Position task, such as that presented by Rosenbek (1978), can shed information on the contextual influences of phonetic errors. A careful inventory of vowel differentiation should be included in these tasks.

Other tasks that reveal slowness, timing, or coordination problems at valves 4, 5, 6, and 7 include measures of Sequential Movement Rate (SMR) and Alternating Movement Rate (AMR). This can be measured by rating the quality as well as the number of times per second an individual can produce the sounds "kuh, kuh, kuh . . ." (valve 4), "tuh, tuh, tuh . . ." (valve 5), "puh, puh, puh . . ."(valve 6), and "puh, tuh, kuh . . ." (valves 6, 5, 4). In order to test the independence of tongue and jaw (valve 7) movement, these SMR and AMR tasks should be done with and without a bite block, which is a small acrylic block or wedge (a small plastic ball point pen will do in a pinch) that is clenched between the back teeth during performance of the "puh, tuh, kuh" tasks. Use of the bite block allows judgments of the quality of independent functioning of the tongue and jaw.

Prosody   As we have seen, *prosody* refers to the aspects of language that convey meaning and melody to the speech act. The meaning conveyed by prosody is in addition to that already conveyed by the semantic aspects of the words. If prosodic variables are impaired, both the intelligibility and perception of normalcy of the speaker can be affected. Fine adjustments at all seven levels can alter rate, stress, or speech melody, and the speech evaluation must consider the contribution of each.

Tasks   Intonation for meaning, or speech melody, can be simply evaluated by carefully listening to a person's ability to contrast declarative statements versus questions. Very different meanings are transmitted by slight variations in pause or melodic inflection. For instance, "What's that in the road ahead?" means something somewhat different from "What's that in the road? A head?" Therefore, having a person imitate and contrast declarative and interrogative sentences often will reveal inability to make these fine adjustments.

> "He ran five miles." "He ran five miles?"
> "She went home." "She went home?"
> "Her name is Joan." "Her name is Joan?"

Sentences such as these can be used to judge ability to change intonation for meaning. Ability to change stress or emphasis can be checked in several ways. Contrastive stress sentences or pairs of words can be used. As pointed out by Rosenbek (1978), the crow would be miffed if he thought we considered all black birds to be blackbirds. The following words illustrate how changes in syllable or word stress can affect meaning.

Black	Bird	Blackbird
Green	House	Greenhouse
Copper	Head	Copperhead
Break	Down	Breakdown
Cross	Word	Crossword
Light	House	Lighthouse
Sail	Boats	Sailboats

Speech rate can be measured by asking the person to read standard passages that can be used to determine numbers of words per minute. Careful listening to spontaneous conversational speech is another efficient method of making judgments of the normal relationship between speaking time and pause time.

Criteria for Normal Performance   Again, much of the burden for judging normal prosody rests on the ear of the listener. Intelligibility can be measured by number of errors on an inventory of articulation or by the percentage of recognizable words or sentences by listeners unfamiliar with the patient's speech pattern. The amount of attention the speech calls to itself, or bizarreness of speech production, depends on the subjective evaluation of the evaluator, though rating scales can be developed to measure degrees of both bizarreness and intelligibility. For example, a listener might be asked to listen to a tape-recorded sample of speech and rate bizarreness on a scale from 1 (normal speech) to 7 (one of the most abnormal patterns I have ever heard).

Judgments of intact intonation and stress for meaning can be made from the contrastive words and sentences presented above. If appropriate meaning is conveyed, this aspect of prosody can be judged as unaffected. A normal oral reading rate is about 150 to 180 words per minute, and inadequate speech rate can be measured against that standard.

Many of the measures used to determine the presence and severity of dysarthria can be used to evaluate apraxia of speech. Spontaneous speech and a variety of automatic and imitative utterances can be used to judge the nature of the disturbance, keeping in mind the definitional characteristics that highlight the speech apraxic patient.

Special tasks, many of which have been described earlier, can contribute information on the integrity of both articulation and prosody. These tasks include:

(1) Repetition of "puh," "tuh," "kuh," and "puh-tuh-kuh"
(2) Imitation of single syllable words
(3) Imitation of longer words (three syllables and greater)
(4) Sentence imitation
(5) Reading aloud standard passages
(6) Spontaneous speech.

The evaluation of oral, nonverbal movements also may shed light on volitional movement disturbance in the apraxic patient, but the relationship of impaired nonverbal movement ("pucker your lips," "blow," "wiggle your tongue," "pretend you are licking a stamp") to impaired speech remains unclear.

After articulation, prosody, and nonverbal skills have been evaluated, the speech-language pathologist has the basis for deciding whether or not the patient's performance meets the definitional requirements of speech apraxia.

Instrumental Evaluation

Not all clinics are equipped with the sophisticated instrumentation of the speech science laboratory, and often the speech-language pathologist in the field must depend primarily on a practical ability to listen carefully. However, in recent years, a variety of biofeedback devices, air flow and air pressure manometers, lip and tongue force transducers, spectrographic (voice print) analysis devices, and other helpful instruments have been adapted to the assessment of motor speech disorders. Some of these strategies are summarized in Rosenbek and LaPointe (1978). In addition, methods presented by Netsell and Daniel (1979) can be instructive for understanding instrumental analysis of the speech signal.

Interpretation of Findings

After all the tests and special tasks have been administered and a stockpile of performance data has accumulated, the speech-language pathologist has the responsibility of making sense of it. Reducing, culling, and organizing the data is no easy job, but it is a crucial one. This is the point when judgments of relative importance of deviant dimensions must be made. The evaluator must decide which deviant aspects of speech contribute most to the nonintelligible or bizarre speech. This is also the time when you can organize hierarchies and priorities of treatment focus. "Relief from the greatest evil" is a good guide for organizing a list of priorities. When the lifeboat springs a leak, you do not worry about how soon it can be given a fresh coat of paint. Similarly, we do not begin dysarthria treatment by polishing the precision of word endings if an impaired respiratory system renders the speech signal barely audible.

Making sense of the assessment data also includes an attempt to find dimensions that are most easily modified, perhaps by postural adjustment,

Chapter 13 discusses some of the ways posture can affect speech.

manipulation of speech rate, or some such change which may have a dramatic effect on speech.

Finally, the treatment plan can be organized by establishing and sometimes writing out precise objectives of treatment. These should be behaviorally and operationally stated so there is little ambiguity as to the specific goal. ("To improve the intelligibility of the patient's speech" would be an unclear and poorly stated treatment objective. "To attain intelligible production of 80% of single syllable words in a 100-word list for three consecutive sessions" would be a little more precise and much easier to measure.)

Though interpretation of findings can be thought of as the final step in the evaluation process, it is easy to conceive of it as interwoven with the treatment process. In fact, it may well be thought of as the first step in the treatment process. It is to the process of intervention that we now turn.

TREATMENT

Early attempts at treating people with motor speech disorders ranged from witchcraft to abandonment. Even in relatively recent times, some writers in speech pathology have expressed the view that little can be done to improve the lot of those afflicted with neurologic speech disorders. The tide has turned in the last few years, though. Not only are people with motor speech disorders no longer neglected, but some exciting advances in clinical management have emerged.

A number of avenues to treatment exist. Some of these are listed in Table 12.5. Most of the time the intervention program chosen by the speech-language pathologist will be behavioral or palliative, or involve the implementation of an alternative communication system. Sometimes, though, we must work in cooperation with the family physican, a surgeon, or a specialist in the construction and fitting of prosthedontic devices to implement the best mode of management.

TABLE 12.5
Possible Avenues of Treatment.

Medical	Alleviate cause
	Pharmaceutic
Surgical	Pharyngeal flap operation
Prosthetic	Construct lift for denervated soft palate
Behavioral	Modify, neuromuscular, aerodynamic events
Palliative	"Hold the line"
	Lessen effect by acceptance
Alternative Mode	Gesture
	Communication aid

As Darley and colleagues (1975) have outlined, there are some basic principles that undergird our treatment of motor speech. These include:

(1) *Developing compensatory strategies*—This includes not only "working around" the physical limitations imposed but also making maximum use of those strengths that remain.
(2) *Automatic to volitional shift*—An inescapable direction to be followed in treatment is that more purposeful control over behaviors that were once automatic and overlearned must be fostered.

(3) _Monitoring behavior and change_—Skills in patient self-monitoring must be an integral part of treatment. Tape-recordings and progress charting are also vital to judgments of change.

(4) _Get an early start_—Many an indecorous habit can be avoided by early attention to more efficient communication.

(5) _Foster motivation_—Treatment must include providing information, concern, support, and warm interaction if the patient's motivation for change is to be influenced.

These basic principles provide a firm foundation for any attempt to manipulate communication potential.

Rosenbek and LaPointe (1978) reiterate some of these principles and supplement them with a _behavioral context_ for treatment of motor speech disorders. This context is relevant to a variety of communication impairments as well as speech apraxia and the variety of dysarthrias that may be encountered.

The first component is _drill_, a usual mode of behavioral therapy that is useful in the modification of the neuromuscular and aerodynamic events impaired in motor speech disturbance. Drill is systematic practice of specially selected and ordered exercises. _Task continua_, another behavioral technique, refers to the development of progressively more difficult tasks. The direction and flow of progress can be directed by moving closer and closer to those skills that approximate normal speech or at least the most efficient means of speech within the limits of the impaired speech production system.

Knowledge of results is a fundamental aspect of treatment. It can be accomplished by instruments that provide visual or auditory feedback of performance, by the direct remarks of the speech-language pathologist ("Good job!" "Not so hot." "That was almost loud enough, but give it a little more oomph!"), by video or audio tape-recordings made periodically during treatment, or by the careful recording of baseline performance and session-by-session progress on a percentage graph. Finally, the _organization of sessions_ entails decisions on scheduling, such as the length, frequency, and format of each session.

Specific Treatment Goals

As we have seen throughout this book, each plan of therapy must be hand-tailored to fit the peculiar characteristics and desires of the individual. Emphasis and focus of therapy will vary according to the priorities and hierarchies of function and dysfunction established during the interpretation of the evaluation results. Style and specific techniques will vary somewhat from setting to setting, but the underlying principles and the ultimate objectives are fairly constant. We like to use the functional component (point-place) and perceptual speech process approach as a model for our treatment. From this base we have established a series of rather specific treatment goals (Rosenbek & LaPointe, 1978). A wide variety of specific techniques are possible to attain these goals, and a few of them will be explained in this section.

As you read through these goals, keep in mind that, depending on the presence and severity of individual signs and symptoms, one or more of these goals may be irrelevant to any specific person. Also, the order is not necessarily sequential as listed and may be rearranged to fit the individual. Some of these specific treatment goals are applicable to people with either dysarthria or apraxia of speech. For example, goal 1 is appropriate to both. Those goals and strategies that are appropriate to only dysarthria or to apraxia of speech are so indicated.

1. Help the Person Become a Productive Patient (Appropriate for the dysarthrias and apraxia of speech)

The techniques here are related to patient counseling and family education and will be discussed in more detail in a following section. To foster productivity we must be sure that the patient agrees on the necessity and value of treatment. Not everyone wants to return to the maximal levels of speech production, and this should be explored and respected. This was brought to my attention recently, in the case of a 43-year-old former 5th grade teacher who suffered a stroke and was making an excellent recovery of communication skills. We thought that, with an intensive program of therapy and a lot of diligent homework, we might be able to see him gain enough communication recovery to return to the classroom in about 12 to 14 months and live happily ever after. We assumed too much, though, and forgot to explore *his* desires. After about 6 months of rather intensive treatment, he informed us, "Look. I've got a pretty good disability pension now. My wife works and we have no financial worries. We have a 20-acre farm, and I'm really enjoying puttering around on the tractor and running the farm. Plus, I never could stand those kids in the classroom and I have no desire to return to teaching. How long does this have to go on?"

The astute speech-language pathologist tunes into these subtle cues of the specific communicative needs and desires of the person. We discharged this gentleman the following week—not only with our blessings but with a bit of envy.

Becoming a more productive patient means a mutual attention to the creation and *order* of specific behavioral goals. At this point the cooperation of other people who are significant to the person should be enlisted, and they can begin to be educated about the disorder and course of treatment as well.

2. Modification of Posture, Tone, Strength (Applicable for the dysarthrias)

Sometimes braces, slings, girdling, or simple postural adjustments can affect tone and strength and ultimately provide a firmer foundation for the speech production system. Modifying strength, tone, and posture is a task that should be done in conjunction with other health care team members. The physician, physical therapist, or occupational therapist can offer valuable guidance in accomplishing this goal. Certain cautions must be observed, particularly in girdling a patient, since altering the respiratory system can cause pneumonia. This procedure should *always* be done under the supervision of a physician.

3. Modification of Respiration (Appropriate for the dysarthrias)

Attempting to modify the respiratory system requires simultaneous attention to the phonatory, resonatory, and articulatory valves, since they work in finely tuned harmony. Though the old elocution school strategies of "breathing exercises" are now passé, with many people practice and improvement in developing controlled exhalation is an important objective. Respiration for speech requires predictable production of consistent, low-pressure exhalation over time. This can be facilitated by biofeedback (using the water manometer, with a goal of producing 5 cm of water pressure for a duration of 5 sec, or by other devices that allow visualization of a sustained air stream).

Such exotic instruments as the stop watch, the tape recorder, and the ear of the speech-language pathologist are mainstays for achieving many of the following specific goals, For respiration, drill on achieving consistent loudness and appropriate loudness change on isolated speech sounds is a start. Expansion to sounds in series (*f-f-f-f-f-f-f-f*) and eventually to words, phrases, and longer utterances is the desired progression.

4. Modification of Phonation (Appropriate for the dysarthrias)

Specific techniques for modification will vary with the underlying neuromuscular problem and the type of motor speech disturbance. For example, for hyperadduction (too much muscular contraction of the vocal folds), which results in harsh or strained-strangled voice quality, attempts are made to counter the overadduction. Using light, gentle articulation contacts, easy yawn-sigh vocalization, and open mouth speech with exaggerated jaw excursions sometimes lessens the effects of the hyperadduction and improves quality.

For hypoadduction, with decreased loudness and breathy voice quality with air wastage, the opposite approach is taken. Increasing the background of muscular effort by pushing, lifting, and attempting quicker phonatory onset are used, as are drills on exaggerated contrastive stress in words and sentences. Any gains in control are expanded to longer, more complex and more spontaneous speech utterances.

If the phonatory problem results from the abnormal coordination of an ataxic motor problem, the speech will be laced with abnormal pitch and loudness breaks and durational abnormalities, because of imprecise timing of turning phonation on and off. These problems sometimes can be influenced by exploring inhibitory postures, by drilling on durational control or increase, or by what I call Ethel Merman therapy ("I Got Rhythm") of rate manipulation. Rate can be manipulated by rhythmical pacing, tapping, squeezing, or the use of external rhythmical sources such as a metronome or amplifying a colleague's heartbeat.

5. Modification of Resonance (Appropriate for the dysarthrias)

Problems at valve 3, the velopharyngeal port, usually result in hypernasal voice quality and nasal emission of air. The individual can be made more aware of how this valve contributes to speech by using mirrors, models, and demonstrations. Visual feedback by using an instrument that detects air leakage through the nose often aids in highlighting the problem. Contrastive speech drills with nasal-nonnasal words (*meat-Pete*; *my-pie*, etc.) and drill on correct timing of palatal elevation in words, phrases, and sentences can be useful in reducing the problem.

For more detail on dealing with these problems, refer to chapter 11 on cleft palate.

Occasionally, with a paralyzed soft palate, the services of the prosthodontist can be called into play for the design and fitting of a palatal lift. This is a device that is worn in the mouth, attaches to the teeth, and is designed to improve resonance balance by elevating the poorly innervated velum. However, the palatal lift is only useful with certain types of cases. Sometimes problems of inadequate retention, persistent mouth irritation, and expense will preclude its use. Occasionally, surgery can be useful to correct the resonance problems caused by an immobile soft palate.

6. Modification of Articulation (Appropriate for the dysarthrias and apraxia of speech)

Lately there seems to be less primary emphasis on treating articulation in the motor speech disorders. In both apraxia of speech and dysarthrias, attention to the interaction of rate, stress, and durational factors in the accuracy of speech sound production is gaining favor.

We attend to the speech sound environment and coarticulating influences on accuracy and generally treat speech movements in syllables instead of isolated sounds. Our speech targets may be the most involved valves or specific sound manner groups such as plosives or fricatives. An underlying principle in modifying articulation is that it is paramount to analyze the errors and attempt to determine the reason for them. If faulty range, velocity, or direction of movement are implicated, the focus of attention in modifying articulation becomes clearer. The objective derived from this principle, then, is to attempt to change the range, velocity, direction, coordination, timing, or ordering of the speech movements in order to produce more acceptable sounds. This can be accomplished by a number of strategies, such as:

(1) *Integral stimulation*—"Watch me. Listen to me. Do what I do."
(2) *Phonetic derivation*—A speech target may be derived from an intact speech gesture, such as producing /n/ by producing /m/ and simultaneously lifting the tongue to the position of /l/ and then parting the lips.
(3) *Phonetic placement*—Points of articulatory contact can be explained and modeled by demonstration, pictures, molding, and hand postures.

Finally, articulatory task continuua can be constructed in steps, such as:

Step (1) /p/ in final position of vowel-consonant (VC) syllables—"ap"
Step (2) /p/ in final position of CVC syllables—"cap"
Step (3) /p/ in medial position in VCV syllables—"apah"
Step (4) /p/ in initial position, CV—"pay"
Step (5) /p/ in varying positions, words, phrases, sentences, controlled conversation

7. Modification of Prosody *(Appropriate for the dysarthrias and apraxia of speech)*

The three prosodic features of rhythm, stress, and intonation have been neglected too often in the management of neurogenic speech disorders. In both apraxia of speech and dysarthria, attention to varying prosody can have rewarding effects on articulation. We believe that prosody interacts potently with articulation and that prosodic manipulation is a rich and fruitful strategy for altering speech intelligibility. Contrastive stress drills, rate manipulation (stop strategies, metronome, pacing, tapping), delayed auditory feedback, and gestural reorganization (gestures accompanied by speech) can be excellent approaches to treatment of both apraxia of speech and some of the dysarthrias.

Details of these techniques are presented in Wertz (1978) and Rosenbek and LaPointe (1978).

8. Providing an Alternate Communication Mode *(Appropriate for the dysarthrias and apraxia of speech)*

Sometimes, because of the severity of the disorder, the development of speech is out of the question and the decision must be made to provide an alternate mode of communication. Though this is never as desirable as natural speech production, it is much preferred over the alternative of isolation and no communication. A variety of alternatives are becoming available for the nonverbal and nonvocal patient these days, and the state of the art appears to be exploding with technological development. Computers, speech synthesizers, and other sophisticated electronic devices are being adapted to the needs of the speechless.

See Figure 12.5.

Other means, including communication and spelling boards, written communication, and gestural systems such as Amer-Ind (based on American

Indian sign language), are more traditional. No doubt the future will bring a rich growth of techniques and devices that will make the instruments of the 1980s look quaint.

FIGURE 12.5

Computers and Voice Synthesizers Adapted to Aid Nonvocal and Nonverbal Persons. The TRS-80 voice synthesizer is packaged in a silver-gray cabinet with black front grill, slightly resembling a speaker enclosure. There is a volume control and device select indicator on the front panel next to a speaker. A ribbon cable emerges from the back of the cabinet, with a length sufficient to set the cabinet on top of the TRS-80 video display unit.

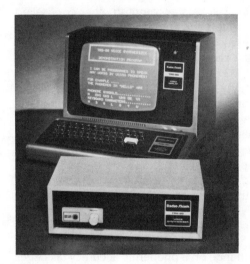

COUNSELING

In the motor speech disorders, as in most of the pathologies of communication, the overall objectives of counseling are threefold: to convey information, to provide reassurance and emotional support, and to improve environmental communication variables. Counseling adults with dysarthria can be viewed as a process of patient and family education (Berry, 1978).

The informational aspect of counseling can be carried out easily and should be accomplished early in the course of management. The most natural questions in the world for anyone afflicted with a health trauma are "What do I have?" "What is it called?" "What caused it?" "Is it serious?" "Does it threaten my life?" "How long will it last?" "Is it common?" "Can you do anything about it?" These are general questions that are almost reflexive to any medical condition. Specific to motor speech disorders, the patient or family might ask "How can I make myself more clearly understood?" "What can we do to help?" "Why are eating and swallowing affected?" "Will medication help?" "Should I slow down or speed up my speech?"

Patient and family counseling also are necessary to establish treatment goals and specific treatment tasks. Good therapy demands that the person with a motor speech disorder know why tasks are selected and the reasons for the employment of particular courses of treatment. The informed patient needs to be counseled on progress as well. The nature of relearning or facilitating speech production tasks must be explained. This means that we must carefully explain the concepts of gradual but consistent change, performance variability as a result of fatigue, illness, or emotional state, and plateauing of behavior.

Berry (1978) suggests that an education or counseling plan be developed, organized around the following questions:

(1) Does the patient/family understand the disorder?
(2) Are the expectations of both patient and family realistic?
(3) Is the environment of the patient and family suitable to facilitate maximal communication?
(4) What other professionals should be part of the educational team?

The informational objectives often will help accomplish other counseling goals, particularly those related to comfort and emotional support. Conveying facts about a disorder will promote understanding, reduce fear, and in most instances increase adjustment to the altered life-style or foster attitudes constructive to rehabilitation.

Throughout the therapy process, the speech-language pathologist should be providing emotional support and reassurance. Thus speech-language therapy is combined with psychotherapy.

The term *psychotherapy* can have a wide range of meanings. At one end of the continuum it refers to structured therapy with people who have suffered psychotic breaks. These are the problems that should be treated only by trained and qualified psychologists, psychiatrists, or professional counselors. Another form of psychotherapy is the emotional support, reinforcement, and encouragement any of us can give whenever a friend or patient needs a "boost" or a positive stroke. This can range from a pat on the arm accompanied by a genuine smile to the more objective approach of indicating "excellent work" by showing an 80% change on a phonemic accuracy task after four sessions of practice.

Since treatment for the neurogenic disorders of speech production relies heavily on structured drill and systematic practice, we must be careful to avoid the suggestion that the therapeutic process is automatized, unswervingly programmed, or rigidly fixed in direction. There is plenty of room in a therapy session for pause, reflection, encouragement, "Way to go!", humor, some small talk, and the warmth of human interaction. Often the planned activities of the session are best set aside so that more pressing emotional or information issues can be discussed. The quality of interaction, after all, is the core of the therapeutic process; without it, little can be expected in the arduous process of mending shattered communication.

CONCLUSION

The past 30 years have seen dramatic and awe-inspiring advances in the development of a sophisticated technology of aerospace, electronic microcircuitry, plastics, and a host of other areas that make life more convenient. Some would argue, though, that the advances in fundamental knowledge of normal function of speech and a clearer understanding of the disruptions which occur in communication disorders are equally as impressive as the emergence of the cordless hedgetrimmer, the hot comb, and frozen yoghurt.

These are exciting times for those who have committed and those who will commit their efforts and talents to the study and remediation of neurogenic speech impairment. Perhaps many of the current ideas we have about the nature and causes of neurologic speech disorders will be regarded as tentative working hypotheses in the future. There is no doubt, however, that we have a firm foundation for continued observation and systematic clinical research that will refine our abilities to help people afflicted with these disorders. The communication barriers created by neurologic disorders can be isolating, dehumanizing, and identity wrenching. Efforts to dissolve these barriers and restore efficient communicative interaction can be one of the noblest contributions to the restoration of human dignity.

SELECTED READINGS

Johns, D., & LaPointe, L. L. Neurogenic disorders of output processing: Apraxia of speech. In H. Avakian-Whitaker & H. A. Whitaker (Eds.), *Current trends in neurolinguistics.* New York: Academic Press, 1976.

LaPointe, L. L. Neurologic abnormalities affecting speech. In D. B. Tower (Ed.), *The nervous system, Vol. 3: Human communication and its disorders.* New York: Raven Press, 1975.

Netsell, R. Speech physiology. In F. D. Minifie, T. J. Hixon, & F. Williams (Eds.), *Normal aspects of speech, hearing, and language.* Englewood Cliffs, N.J.: Prentice-Hall, 1973.

Netsell, R., & Daniel, B. Dysarthria in adults: Physiologic approach to rehabilitation. *Archives of Physical Medicine and Rehabilitation,* 1979, *60,* 502–508.

Rosenbek, J. C. Treating apraxia of speech. In D. F. Johns (Ed.), *Clinical management of neurogenic communicative disorders.* Boston: Little, Brown, 1978.

Rosenbek, J. C., & LaPointe, L. L. The dysarthrias: Description, diagnosis and treatment. In D. F. Johns (Ed.), *Clinical management of neurogenic communicative disorders.* Boston: Little, Brown, 1978.

Wertz, R. T. Neuropathologies of speech and language: An introduction to patient management. In D. F. Johns (Ed.), *Clinical management of neurogenic communicative disorders.* Boston: Little, Brown, 1978.

REFERENCES

Berry, W. R. *Adults with dysarthria: Patient/family education.* Paper presented at Conference on Treatment of Motor Speech Disorders, Mayo Clinic, Rochester, Minnesota, 1978.

Berry, W. R., & LaPointe, L. L. *The adult dysarthric patient: Part I, evaluation.* Video Cassette. Washington, D.C.: Medical Media Service, Veterans Administration, 1974.

Darley, F. L. Lacunae and research approaches to them. IV. In C. Milliken & F. L. Darley (Eds.), *Brain mechanisms underlying speech and language.* New York: Grune & Stratton, 1967.

Darley, F. L., Aronson, A., & Brown, J. *Motor speech disorders.* Philadelphia: W. B. Saunders, 1975.

Hardy, J. C. Suggestions for physiological research in dysarthria. *Cortex,* 1967, *3,* 128–156.

Hixon, T. J. Respiratory function in speech. In F. D. Minifie, T. J. Hixon, & F. Williams (Eds.), *Normal aspects of speech, hearing, and language.* Englewood Cliffs, N.J.: Prentice-Hall, 1973.

Hixon, T. J. *Respiratory-laryngeal evaluation.* Paper presented at Veterans Administration Workshop on Motor Speech Disorders, Madison, Wisconsin, 1975.

Johns, D., & LaPointe, L. L. Neurogenic disorders of output processing: Apraxia of speech. In H. Avakian-Whitaker & H. A. Whitaker (Eds.), *Current trends in neurolinguistics.* New York: Academic Press, 1976.

Kertesz, A. *Aphasia and associated disorders: Taxonomy, localization and recovery.* New York: Grune & Stratton, 1979.

LaPointe, L. L. Neurologic abnormalities affecting speech. In D. B. Tower (Ed.), *The nervous system, Vol 3: Human communication and its disorders.* New York: Raven Press, 1975.

Martin, A. D. Some objections to the term "Apraxia of Speech." *Journal of Speech and Hearing Disorders,* 1974, *39,* 53–64.

Moncur, J., & Brackett, I. *Modifying vocal behavior.* New York: Harper & Row, 1974.

National Institutes of Health. *National research strategy for neurological and communicative disorders.* Washington, D.C.: National Institutes of Health, No. 79-1910, 1979.

Netsell, R. Speech physiology. In F. D. Minifie, T. J. Hixon, & F. Williams (Eds.), *Normal aspects of speech, hearing, and language.* Englewood Cliffs, N.J.: Prentice-Hall, 1973.

Netsell, R., & Daniel, B. Dysarthria in adults: Physiologic approach to rehabilitation. *Archives of Physical Medicine and Rehabilitation,* 1979, *60,* 502–508.

Netsell, R., & Hixon, T. J. Noninvasive method for clinically estimating subglottal air pressure. *Journal of Speech and Hearing Disorders,* 1978, *43,* 326–330.

Rosenbek, J. C. Treating apraxia of speech. In D. F. Johns (Ed.), *Clinical management of neurogenic communicative disorders.* Boston: Little, Brown, 1978.

Rosenbek, J. C., & LaPointe, L. L. The dysarthrias: Description, diagnosis and treatment. In D. F. Johns (Ed.), *Clinical management of neurogenic communicative disorders.* Boston: Little, Brown, 1978.

Wertz, R. T. Neuropathologies of speech and langauge: An introduction to patient management. In D. F. Johns (Ed.), *Clinical management of neurogenic communicative disorders.* Boston: Little, Brown, 1978.

CEREBRAL PALSY 13

Edward D. Mysak

Sally was born in 1975. Her mother suffered from high blood pressure during the pregnancy. Because Sally was in a breech position, she was delivered by Caesarean section. She weighed 5 pounds at birth and was placed in an incubator. She remained in the hospital for about 2 weeks.

Sally's early development was slow. She did not sit alone until she was about 15 months old, did not crawl until she was about 2½ years old, and did not walk until she was almost 4 years old. At 4 years of age, toilet training was still a problem and she had not developed speech. She also had recurring ear infections.

Because of what appeared to be poor muscle tone, Sally returned to the hospital at 6 weeks of age, and at 10 months of age had a muscle biopsy. When Sally was 4 years 5 months old, she was given a complete speech and hearing evaluation at a university speech and hearing center. The impression was that Sally exhibited a severe delay in speech, language, and cognitive abilities apparently related to her neurological involvement. More specifically, eye contact was poor, head rocking was noted, auditory awareness was poor, and vocalization appeared confined to infrequent monosyllabic babbling.

At age 5 a neurologic evaluation confirmed the diagnosis of central nervous system dysfunction reflected by generalized hypotonia and developmental delay, including intellect and language. At 4 years 11 months of age, an educational evaluation stated that Sally was functioning far below expectations in all areas of development. More specifically, she was described as a child who was not toilet trained, did not ask for food, and did not make eye contact. A psychological evaluation estimated that Sally was functioning in the severely retarded range, that her poorest performance was on expressive language tasks, and that she was most advanced in the area of gross motor functioning. A social history report indicated that Sally was attending a normal nursery school and received special occupational and speech therapy. It stated that Sally's mother was very concerned about Sally's educational needs and about obtaining an appropriate school placement for her. The social worker also recommended that the mother receive some supportive help as well.

A total therapy program was recommended. It included facilitation of cognitive development, stabilization of speech postures in the on-elbows, sit, and stand positions, stimulation of listening movements and behavior, and stimulation of imitative vocalization and expressive communication, *including "hands and face talk." A home program involving the mother was also developed.*

After about 1½ years of therapy, modest gains can be reported. There has been a decrease in head rocking. Improvement has been noted in language comprehension. Sally's monosyllabic vocalizations include plosives, nasals, and fricatives. Some multisyllabic utterances marked by intonation, stress, and prosody features have also been heard. One or two true words appear to be emerging.

Although Sally has made some progress, a lot more needs to be done. More family participation in the habilitation program will be requested. Increased emphasis will be placed on the stimulation of listening movements and behavior. Increased emphasis will also be placed on developing compensatory communication along with continuing efforts to stimulate speech communication.

You may now wish to listen to the speech sample accompanying this chapter, found on Audio Disc 2, Side 4 (sample #9).

As Sally has not yet developed an intelligible speech, the speech sample is of a young adult male diagnosed as having a tension athetotic type of cerebral palsy.

Like hearing impairment and cleft palates, cerebral palsy is a physical condition that often causes speech and communication disorders. **Cerebral palsy** is a general term for a brain injury resulting in a display of certain kinds of neurological symptoms. As such, it may be thought of as a neurogenic disorder. It is not a disease; it does not have a single specific cause or lead to specific symptoms. In fact, cerebral palsy can be so slight that it is hard to detect or so severe that the person may never be able to be completely independent of support services. It is usually associated with the period of childhood, is thought of as chronic and crippling, and again, is commonly accompanied by significant speech problems. Many people with cerebral palsy are noticeable because of their motor and postural problems, which also affect their speech. Yet these same people, who may be confined to wheelchairs, may have average or above average intelligence.

The primary and secondary symptoms associated with cerebral palsy may affect most of the important human functions, including the neurosensory, neuromotor, perceptual, cognitive, behavioral, and speech functions. To more fully understand the communication problems associated with cerebral palsy, then, we will first examine the general problem and then follow with a discussion of the speech problem and its management.

CHARACTERISTICS OF CEREBRAL PALSY

See general texts (such as Marks, 1974; Cruickshank, 1976; Connor, Williamson, & Siepp, 1978) for more information on the management of cerebral palsy.

Because of the nature of cerebral palsy, much has been written about the various problems that occur among these children (including medical, intellectual, personality, visual, and dental problems) and about the various types of management they need (including medical, psychological, special educational, occupational, and physical therapy, social work, and vocational guidance). The professional organization devoted to the understanding and care of cerebral palsy is the American Academy for Cerebral Palsy and Developmental Medicine; the official journal of the academy is *Developmental Medicine and Child Neurology.*

Prenatal, infantile, and early childhood brain injury and consequent brain dysfunction have no doubt been a bane of humans from the earliest of times. Descriptions of crippled individuals appear in ancient Hebrew and Greek writings and in the Bible, and there is no reason to believe that some of the people referred to did not have neurological symptoms that today would be called *cerebral palsy*.

During the second half of the 15th century, pediatric textbooks began to describe symptoms of brain dysfunction; however, the classic paper on the connection between abnormal birth histories and childhood brain dysfunctions did not appear until 1861, written by an English physician by the name of Dr. Little (Little, 1861). In the United States, concern for helping these children grew rapidly in the early 1940s. Dr. Winthrop Phelps (1940) organized one of the earliest systematic programs of management for children with cerebral palsy.

Cerebral palsy is an umbrella term for a variety of congenital and early neurological disorders. Cerebral palsy, as we use it here, includes the full range of chronic brain syndromes from isolated articulation problems—which may only be heard and seen during the speech act—to severe and generalized sensorimotor involvement in which the child is unable to walk, stand, sit, or even hold up his head, and where reaching, eating, and speaking movements are severely restricted. Cerebral palsy is usually considered static; that is, the symptoms get neither better nor worse with age.

More specifically, cerebral palsies are complexes that result from damage to various parts of the brain, occur between conception and 2 years of age or so, and appear in various forms and combinations of sensorimotor, perceptual, behavioral, and speech disorders.

Like many other conditions we have looked at, it is hard to pinpoint a specific cause for most cases of cerebral palsy. In general, we can say that the causes may be divided into two categories, familial and environmental.

Certain cranial malformations, degenerative diseases, and static conditions such as familial tremor contribute a relatively small number of cases to the congenital cerebral palsies. Further, cranial malformations and degenerative diseases are usually excluded from the more restrictive definition of childhood cerebral palsy as a chronic and static disease.

Recall that a congenital disorder is present at birth.

Lesions acquired during the period from conception to about 1 month following birth account for the large majority of conditions that are eventually diagnosed as cerebral palsy. Prenatal causes, or all those factors that may contribute to brain injury before birth, include infections in the mother such as mumps, rubella, and influenza; blood incompatibility in the mother, such as the Rh-negative factor; anesthesia, irradiation, and accidents; and placental and cord anomalies and disturbances. Central nervous system (CNS) malformations in the embryo and fetus can also be prenatal causes of cerebral palsy.

Natal factors, or all those factors that may contribute to brain injury during the actual birth period, include precipitate (less than 2 hours) or prolonged (more than 24 hours) deliveries, premature deliveries, breech or caesarean deliveries, irregular implantation of the placenta, and forceps manipulation and trauma. In fact, the number of new cases of cerebral palsy has dramatically decreased as fewer and fewer babies are delivered with forceps.

Postnatal factors, or all those factors that may contribute to brain injury during approximately the first month of life, include infections such as meningitis, encephalitis, roseola, measles, and whooping cough; lead poisoning; trauma; anoxia; and neoplasms or growths of the brain.

This long list of possible environmental causes of cerebral palsy suggests that in any one case more than one factor may be operative. In addition, the many disease processes represented may be related to lesions in different parts of the brain, which helps explain the variety of symptoms found in any one case of cerebral palsy.

Incidence

For a review of studies of incidence, see Cruickshank, 1976, chapter 1.

The true incidence of cerebral palsy is difficult to determine for a number of reasons. Not all specialists agree on the definition of the disorder with respect to the time of occurrence, the location of the lesion, and the type, severity, and predominance of the symptoms. Consistency, or lack of it, in reporting the disorder is another factor. Reported rates of occurrence of cerebral palsy range from 1 to 6 per 1,000.

Types

We recognize a number of types of cerebral palsy. The types are named basically for clinical findings because of the lack of consistency between presenting symptoms and their severity and the location, cause, and size of the lesion. Spasticity, athetosis, ataxia, rigidity, tremor, and atonia are traditional terms currently used to describe various forms of cerebral palsy. Pure forms of tremor or atonia are rare and are more likely to appear as part of other forms of cerebral palsy; on the other hand, mixed types are common, but usually children are classified according to their predominant symptoms. The speech-language pathologist may find it useful to include congenital isolated articulation problems and other manifestations of limited involvement of the brain under the category of subclinical forms of cerebral palsy.

Subclinical

These problems were discussed in depth in chapters 8 and 9.

The term *subclinical* refers to those children who do not show obvious sensorimotor problems, but who nevertheless have central nervous system (CNS) involvement. Children with neurogenic learning disabilities including dyslexia or those with perceptual problems, for example, may be viewed as having minimal brain dysfunction or "subclinical cerebral palsy." These children may display uneven intellectual profiles, hyperactivity, and delayed onset of speech. The potential value of viewing these minimally involved children as having subclinical cerebral palsy is that many may benefit from some of the management techniques developed for children with obvious cerebral palsy.

One condition that may be considered a specific form of subclinical cerebral palsy is congenital suprabulbar paresis (Worster-Drought, 1968). At least two forms of the condition are recognized: the complete syndrome, characterized by paralysis of the lips, tongue, velum, larynx, and swallowing difficulty; and the incomplete syndrome, characterized by an isolated paresis of the velum or tongue.

Movements of children with **spastic** (spasmogenic) cerebral palsy are described as labored, still, or jerky. They show increased muscle tone and consistent limitations in directions and range of movements of body parts. The standing spastic child may demonstrate flexor spasms and inward rotation of the upper limbs or shoulder, elbow, and wrist, and extensor spasms and inward rotation of the lower limbs or thigh, knee, and foot. The walking spastic child may exhibit toe-walking because her lower limbs are hyperextended and "scissors gait" or leg crossover because of the overadduction and inward rotation of the thighs.

When a muscle flexes, it contracts and tightens; when it extends, it stretches.

Traditionally, spastic symptoms are thought to be caused by involvement of the pyramidal tract in the cortical or subcortical areas of the brain and sometimes by lesions in the brainstem and upper spinal cord. The neurodynamics of the condition may be described as a lack of automatic inhibition by the cerebrum of various levels of the CNS from which basic muscle tone is controlled. Neurological signs of this interference with higher center regulation over lower centers include exaggerated stretch reflexes (uncontrolled counteraction to the muscle being stretched), Babinski's reflexes (fanning of toes in response to a stimulus applied to the sole of the foot), and ankle clonus (alternating contraction and relaxation of the foot in response to sudden flexion of the ankle).

These portions of the central nervous system are described in chapter 4.

Figure 13.1 shows a child with a spastic posture.

Movements of children with **athetotic** cerebral palsy are described as involuntary and wormlike or writhing. They are characterized by variability in mus-

Athetosis *means without a fixed base.*

FIGURE 13.1
Two Views of a Child Displaying a Spastic Posture.

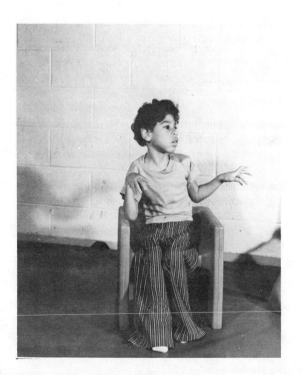 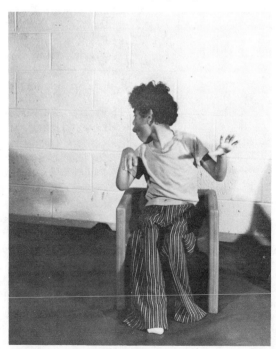

cle tone and by inconsistency in movements in appropriate directions and of appropriate ranges. The child with athetosis who is at rest and relaxed may make few of these involuntary movements; however, when he is required to reach for something or to speak, he may have a burst of involuntary, writhing movements. Attempts at voluntary movements during periods of emotion or excitement usually intensify the problem.

Traditionally, athetotic symptoms are ascribed to involvement of the basal nuclei and their connections or to involvement of the extrapyramidal system. The neurodynamics of the condition may be described in at least two ways: (*a*) interference of the regulating or smoothening influence of the extrapyramidal system over the pyramidal system, or (*b*) a lack of control by the higher, voluntary movement centers of the pyramidal system over the lower, automatic movement centers of the extrapyramidal system. The neurological signs of this impairment in the relationship between pyramidal and extrapyramidal systems are preemptive movements (involuntary movements preceding voluntary ones), writhing movements, and variable muscle tone.

Ataxic

Ataxis *means lack of order.*

Movements of children with **ataxic** cerebral palsy are described as awkward, clumsy, and uncoordinated. They are characterized by reduced muscle tone (hypotonia), and problems in the guidance of movements in appropriate directions. Because of her problems in maintaining balance, the standing ataxic child may display a wide-based stance. When walking she may display a birdlike posture of a forward placed head and backward placed arms in addition to a gait which accelerates involuntarily.

Traditionally, ataxic symptoms are ascribed to involvement of the cerebellum. The neurodynamics of the condition may be described as a failure of the CNS to receive appropriate feedback concerning the progress of movements due to disturbance in general proprioception (muscle, joint, tendon sense) and special proprioception (balance sense from the ears). The cerebellum appears to compare the intended movements of the voluntary motor center with the actual movements, as reflected by the position and movement feedback it receives. If there are discrepancies, the cerebellum automatically relays adjustment signals to the voluntary motor center until there is a match between intended and actual movements. Neurological signs of cerebellar dysfunction include:

(1) Problems in simultaneous coordination of multimuscle groups, as may be used in returning a ping-pong ball, for example (dyssynergia);
(2) Undershooting or overshooting a fork on the table with a reaching hand, for example (dysmetria);
(3) Difficulty in maintaining a serial repetitive movement such as repetitive eyebrow raising, panting, or uttering /pʌ/ rapidly and rhythmically (dysdiadochocinesia);
(4) A tremor that appears only during a voluntary movement; and
(5) Ocular and head **nystagmus** (an involuntary slow movement in one direction followed by a rapid movement in the opposite direction).

Rigidity

Children with cerebral palsy of the rigidity type show extremely limited or almost no movements. They appear stiff and inflexible. In the extreme form, a child with rigidity who is lying on the back may exhibit a "bridging" posture, where his head and feet are in contact with the surface and the rest of his body is arched upward from the surface.

Traditionally, rigidity symptoms are ascribed to widespread involvement of inhibitory centers of the brain. The neurodynamics of the condition are similiar to those of spasticity. In rigidity, the resistance to slow passive motion is greater than that to rapid passive motion, antagonists to antigravity muscles are more involved, and clonus and stretch reflexes are absent.

Figure 13.2 shows a child with a rigidity posture.

FIGURE 13.2

A Child Displaying a Rigidity Posture in Supine Position.

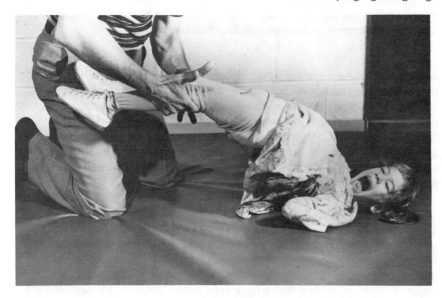

Tremor and Atonia

Pure tremor or atonia types of cerebral palsy are rare and usually appear as part of the symptom complexes of other forms of cerebral palsy. *Tremor* means trembling or shaking; unlike the writhing movements found in athetosis, tremor is characterized by regular and symmetrical movements produced by the alternating contraction of muscles and their antagonists. Tremor appears in two forms: intention or nonintention. Intention tremor, or that tremor triggered by a voluntary movement, is traditionally attributed to cerebellar involvement, while nonintention tremor, or the tremor that appears when the individual is at rest, is traditionally attributed to basal nuclei involvement.

Atonia describes a condition where the muscles are "overrelaxed" or flaccid. The atonic infant may be described as a floppy baby. Traditionally, the condition is attributed to involvement of the cerebellum—the center responsible for maintaining normal muscle tension.

Neurophysiological Age

Before leaving this section of the chapter, we should describe a nontraditional basis for classifying cerebral palsy—the neurophysiological basis—which is growing in use. A number of workers have developed orientations and management approaches to cerebral palsy that are based less on the traditional types and more on what might be called the "neurophysiological age" of the child. I myself take this approach; see Mysak, 1980. As Twitchell (1965) said, "from the neurophysiological view, the separation of patients into various cat-

See, for example, Rood, 1954; Bobath & Bobath, 1967.

egories—such as spasticity, rigidity, athetosis, tremor—is wholly artificial." Regardless of classification, the same physiological substrata for the different cerebral palsies can be demonstrated in all children. "Strict adherence to the various classifications of cerebral palsy are artificial and based on unphysiologic tenets" (Twitchell, 1965).

In short, a classification system based on neurophysiological age entails an analysis of the child's development and functional level. That is, does the child exhibit the reflexes and reactions that allow for head balance, for rolling over, for body support on elbows, and for sitting and standing? This approach also entails neuroanalyses of hand movements, basic speech reflexes, and skilled speech movements. Later in the chapter, we will see the implications of this orientation for speech diagnosis and speech therapy.

Component Problems

Along with the characteristic neuromotor symptoms, cerebral palsy often carries many other components. Among these component problems are convulsions, mental retardation, emotional problems, sensory disturbances, and perceptual problems. There is no clear-cut relationship between the severity of the neuromotor problem and the number or severity of the component problems. That is, a severely spastic child may show normal intelligence, normal vision, and normal hearing, while another with mild athetosis may be moderately retarded and deaf.

Convulsions

Since cerebral palsy results from various types of brain injury and since brain injury predisposes people to seizure disorders, it is not surprising that these children show a higher than normal incidence of convulsive disorders. The incidence of convulsive disorders among cerebral palsied children varies depending on the source; as we have seen before, incidence figures are influenced by the reporter's definitions and by the accuracy of diagnosis of the wide range of possible symptoms. Among athetotics, figures of about 2, 10, and 30% have been reported, while among spastics, figures as high as 50, 60, and 80% have been reported. Almost every possible variety of seizure has been reported. Speech-language pathologists who deal with children with seizure disorders should become familiar with the types of seizures, procedures for handling a seizure, and the medications often prescribed to prevent them.

One good source of information is the Epilepsy Foundation of America, 1828 L Street, N.W., Washington, D.C. 20036.

Mental Retardation

Intellectual development and achievement among children with cerebral palsy varies considerably. Some people with cerebral palsy are profoundly retarded; others are gifted. Primary factors that contribute to this variability include the different locations and sizes of the offending brain lesions and the degrees of specific linguistic involvement. In addition, many children with cerebral palsy have fewer than normal sensory-perceptual experiences, both because their mobility is limited and because of the overprotectiveness of their parents and other caretakers. Cerebral palsy is frequently associated with relatively severe retardation, and these children may have drastically limited communication skills, as well as reduced environmental stimulation and social interactions.

It is difficult to assess the intelligence of these children accurately because of their motor, sensory, perceptual, and communication limitations. Therefore, incidence figures on mental retardation in this population must be interpreted with caution. Figures range from about 30% up to about 70%, with most around 50%.

Emotional Problems

Given the complex of sensorimotor, perceptual, and communication problems of children with cerebral palsy, it is easy to understand how their socioemotional development may be affected. Complicating the situation are not-infrequent parental reactions of guilt, rejection, and overprotection. The reactions of other people to a child who drools, who jerks, who makes facial grimaces, or who walks strangely further compound the problem. Emotional immaturity and instability, introversion, and depression are findings that are likely to appear in psychological studies of these children.

Sensory-Perceptual Problems

Because the motor problems of children with cerebral palsy are so obvious, their many sensory-perceptual involvements may go relatively unnoticed. Adding to the problem of undetected or unnoticed sensory problems is the difficulty in testing the various senses, especially when the child's ability to communicate is limited or nonexistent.

Sensory problems found among these children include problems in tactile sensation, two-point discrimination, position sense, and pain and temperature sense. Visual acuity problems have been observed in over 50% of these children and visual field defects in about 25%. To further complicate matters, many people with cerebral palsy are hearing impaired.

Tactile, auditory, and visual perception problems may also be found among children with cerebral palsy. Difficulty in perceiving objects grasped or placed in their hands, such as small toys, figures, or coins, and in perceiving plastic forms representing various shapes placed in their mouths may be observed. Hearing the difference between certain sounds, synthesizing combinations of sounds, and memory span for sounds may also be a problem. Problems in seeing the whole pattern of a letter, the word pattern of a group of letters, or discriminating a visual figure on a background of other visual stimuli are also found. Complicating these visual perceptual problems are problems of binocular balance **(strabismus)** and ocular nystagmus. Oculomotor imbalances have been observed in over half of these children.

SPEECH AND LANGUAGE DISORDERS

It should be clear by now that cerebral palsy is an extremely complex "disorder." All or any one of the component problems we have just discussed—convulsions, mental retardation, emotional problems, sensory-perceptual problems—can contribute to an individual's speech and language difficulties. The speech-language pathologist should expect to find a large variety of factors underlying any one communication disorder and a large variety of patterns of communication disorders. One child may have no speech at all; another may show little (if any) difference from children without cerebral palsy. But the reported incidence of communication problems among people with cerebral palsy ranges from 70% (Wolfe, 1950) to 86% (Achilles, 1955).

An important concept is postural readiness for speech. Sometime after the age of 10 months, a normal child reaches neurophysiological readiness for true speech. This readiness is reflected in the development of the erect pos-

This concept is a complicated one and is beyond the scope of this chapter; for more information on this topic and other issues dealing with treatment of cerebral palsy, see Mysak, 1980.

ture, or of at least head and trunk balance, the use of a preferred hand, and the maturation of certain infantile oral reflexes, which shows up when the child stops nursing and eats solid food. Before the speech mechanism can be properly used, it must be appropriately supported in an upright and balanced framework or "speech chasis." Adding to the problems of the infant with cerebral palsy, he may not have full head or trunk balance when he is on his back, on his elbows, or sitting; hence, his auditory, articulatory, resonatory, and phonatory mechanisms (which reside within the head and neck) and the respiratory mechanism (which resides within the trunk) may not be able to function properly for speech.

At least two types of symptoms may be found in developmental cerebral palsies: those of immaturity and those of paralysis or pathology. Whenever a brain lesion develops before birth or in infancy, it may contribute to general delay, retardation, or arrest of certain functions (immaturity); depending on the location of the lesion, it may cause some specific defect of function

See chapter 14.

(paralysis or pathology symptom). For example, a lesion in the frontal lobe of the brain may contribute to general symptoms of immaturity in a child, such as persisting infantile feeding reflexes; but because it is near the primary motor area that supplies muscles of the tongue, the child may also show specific difficulty in raising the tongue tip.

Characteristics of Communication Deficits

Because the communication disorders in cerebral palsy are so complex, we cannot describe a typical case. A more useful approach is to attempt to identify the possible components of any one case. The job of the speech-language pathologist is to study each child for all the components that appear to be present, as well as to identify the immaturity and paralysis features of each component. Let us now look at several types of communication disorders associated with cerebral palsy: disorders of posture, listening, breathing, voice, articulation, and language. As we discuss each one, we will also discuss diagnostic considerations. In addition, you may wish to refer to the section on assessment in the chapters relating to each specific type of disorder.

Speech Posture Disorders

An important feature of the progression of motor control in the human being is that postural control of a part of the body always precedes movement control of that part. The concept of the importance of the relationship between postural control and movement control has not been well developed in clinical speech-language pathology, but we do have some information available. To listen for speech, a child should be able to assume trunk and head positions

Chapter 10 shows development sequences in listening.

that facilitate the reception of the speech signal. In other words, if a child is able to quickly orient his upper trunk and head toward the source of speech signals, listening for speech is facilitated. In speaking, coordinated movements of respiratory, phonatory, resonatory, and articulatory mechanisms depend to a meaningful degree on postural control of the trunk, neck, and head. This postural control may be observed when a child speaks while lying on his back, lying on his elbows, sitting in various positions, and standing.

Since problems in trunk, neck, and head balance and control are a common part of cerebral palsy, their possible role in a presenting speech disorder should be appreciated and assessed. Figure 13.3 shows a person who has difficulty in assuming and maintaining sit and stand speech postures.

FIGURE 13.3
A Child Who Has Problems in Sit and Stand Speech Postures.

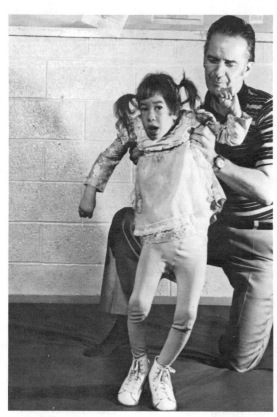 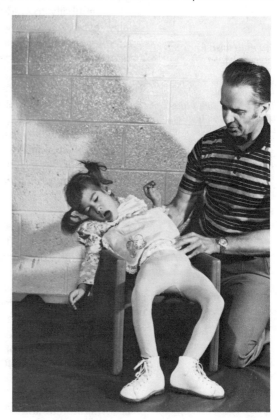

Listening Disorders

We use the word *listening* rather than *hearing* to describe the auditory disorders that may be found in children with cerebral palsy. Here, listening denotes not only hearing for speech, but also that body position and preparation designed to facilitate hearing.

Immaturity

Symptoms of listening immaturity in the cerebral palsied child may include the inability of the child to automatically assume the head and trunk positions that facilitate hearing speech and the persistence of the auditory Moro and cry reflexes in response to sound. Underdeveloped postural control and persistent startle reflexes are likely to interfere with processing speech signals. Also, the child may show a delay or retardation in the ability to localize speech, for example, the localization of the primary caretaker's voice (which normally appears around age 6 months).

*A **Moro reflex** is an extensor startle pattern in response to sound.*

Pathology

Almost every type of hearing loss, including conductive, sensorineural, and central types, has been found among people with cerebral palsy. Defects have been found in the external, middle, and inner ears and in the central auditory tracts and cortices. Estimates of the incidence of hearing loss among people with cerebral palsy range from 6% to 41%, but in general the incidence appears to be about 20% (Nober, 1976).

Susceptibility to middle ear disease has also been observed in cerebral palsy, especially among spastics. Sources of inner ear problems include hereditary deafness, viral infections, and toxemia. Some athetotics have been suspected of showing central deafness.

You may wish to review chapter 10.

Diagnosis

The special difficulties of audiometric testing with the multiply handicapped were discussed in chapter 10.

Among the factors that a speech-language pathologist must keep in mind when evaluating the listening behavior of the cerebral palsied person are the high rate of involvement, the wide range in types of involvement, and the difficulty of audiometric testing and interpreting findings. These factors all suggest that testing by a trained audiologist is essential. Differentiating between symptoms of immaturity and pathology is also important.

Breathing Disorders

As we have seen, there are at least two forms of breathing: vegetative breathing and speech breathing. To recap, vegetative breathing is characterized by nasal breathing with approximately even inspiratory and expiratory phases; speech breathing is characterized by oral breathing with a rapid inspiratory phase followed by a long expiratory phase. Automatic and rapid shifting from vegetative breathing (vb) to speech breathing (sb) is a prerequisite of efficient speech. This automatic vb-sb shifting requires intact central mechanisms for respiratory regulation, and these are unfortunately frequently involved in cerebral palsy. Reported breathing problems among the different types of cerebral palsy range from 40% to 80%.

Immaturity

All sorts of breathing differences among cerebral palsied children have been reported by researchers and clinicians. Most of these differences appear related to immaturity of the CNS centers involved with the regulation of breathing.

Some children may show a delay in the vb-sb shift, while others may not be able to effect the shift at all. Breaths per minute may remain high, and the depth of the breathing cycle may remain shallow. Also, some people show simultaneous inspiratory and expiratory movements or "oppositional breathing."

Paralysis

Some of the breathing problems among people with cerebral palsy appear to be related to irregular innervation of the muscles that are directly or indirectly involved with respiration rather than to immaturity of neuroregulatory centers. Among the paralytic symptoms may be weak thoracic and abdominal muscles, respiration accompanied by retracted abdominal muscles and little movement of the diaphragm, and air stream obstruction due to irregular movements of the vocal folds.

Diagnosis

When evaluating the breathing mechanisms, the speech-language pathologist must again be alert to the high rate of involvement and the wide range in types of involvement. When attempting to relate breathing dysfunctions to possible speech symptoms, the following possible relationships should be considered: (*a*) problems in vb-sb shifting and delay in voluntary phonation, producing only one or two syllables per expiration, and slow and irregular rate; (*b*) poor thoracic-abdominal muscle coordination (including fixation of muscles) and weak voice, forced voice, difficulty in sustaining voice, interrupted voice, and inspiratory voice; (*c*) poor respiratory-laryngeal coordination and inspiratory voice, forced voice, sudden arrest of voice, and uncontrolled loudness; (*d*) shallow breathing cycles and weak voices; and (*e*) high rates of breaths per minute and reduced voicing time and irregular rate.

Voice Disorders

Efficient voicing (including resonation) results from the coordination of inspiratory and expiratory movements with laryngeal and velopharyngeal movements and from primary monitoring of the consequent phonation by the ear. Given the high rate of hearing and breathing disorders alone, voice problems among people with cerebral palsy are not surprising.

Immaturity

Voicing inefficiency may be related to the immaturity of various reflexes. The glottic-opening reflex, which allows for inspiration, the glottic-closing reflex, which allows for build-up of intrathoracic pressure, and crying, for example, may be unregulated and be the cause of phonatory problems. The velar opening reflex, which allows nasal inspiration, and the velar closing reflex, which allows for the creation of negative or positive oral pressure, may also be unregulated and cause problems in speech resonance.

These problems may be similar to those caused by cleft palates and related disorders. See chapter 6 and 11.

Paralysis

In addition to unregulated glottic and velar reflexes influencing voicing and resonation, voice problems may also stem from difficulties with the voluntary use of laryngeal muscles. Possible reflections of this difficulty are flaccid or weak vocal folds, as well as spasms and arhythmic activity of the folds.

Diagnosis

To properly diagnose voice problems among the cerebral palsied, the speech-language pathologist should be concerned about differentiating symptoms of immaturity from paralysis and should also attempt to identify whether the source of the problem is respiratory, laryngeal, or the coordination of the two.

More specifically, the following possible relationships should be considered: (*a*) involuntary open-close activity of the glottis (unregulated glottic reflexes) and inspiratory voice, sudden loss of voice, intermittent voice, uncontrolled loudness, and forced voice; (*b*) involuntary open-close activity of the velum (unregulated velar reflexes) and reduced nasality, increased nasality, and mixed and intermittent imbalance in nasality; (*c*) flaccid paralysis of the folds and breathy voice; and (*d*) hypertonic vocal folds and difficulty in initiating voice and hoarseness.

Articulation Disorders

Also see chapter 12 for an indepth discussion of dysarthria and apraxia.

Problems with articulation are usually the most obvious component of the communication disorder. In the context of cerebral palsy, these disorders are referred to as *developmental dysarthrias*. We have already seen that articulation is related to and dependent on respiration and phonation and hence is influenced by problems of breathing and voicing. In some cases of cerebral palsy, the dysarthria may be the major observable symptom; articulation may be almost normal in a child with major symptoms in other areas; or it may appear in severe form with only minor symptoms in other areas. Reports of the incidence of some degree of articulation disorder among the cerebral palsied range as high as 80% and higher.

Immaturity

Some of the articulation problems in cerebral palsy may be attributed to the persistence, exaggeration, and irregular appearance of feeding reflexes such as rooting, lip, mouth-opening, biting, and suckling reflexes. These conditions affect speech only when particular speech efforts also elicit certain reflexive movements; for example, when movement for tongue-tip sounds stimulates the suckle reflex and the tongue moves too far forward and into an interdental position; when efforts at producing /r/ or /l/ sounds stimulate the lip reflex and there is simultaneous lip rounding accompanying the tongue-tip elevation; or when efforts at producing an open-mouth sound like /a/ stimulate the mouth-opening reflex and there is an exaggeration of the open-mouth posture.

Indirect causes of articulatory immaturity may be hearing loss and mental retardation.

Paralysis

Various forms of paralytic involvement of the articulators complicate articulation disorders among people with cerebral palsy. The paralytic involvement may be spastic, athetotic, ataxic, or apraxic.

In spasticity, the articulators may move in a labored fashion and be either hypertonic or flaccid. In addition, the child may have pathological stretch reflexes. In athetosis, the articulators may move involuntarily before the voluntary speech movement is attempted. The movements may be slow and irregular. Movements of the articulators in ataxia may be slow, clumsy, and inaccurate. Finally, in apraxia, the person may have no difficulty in moving the articulators spontaneously, but great difficulty in moving them voluntarily in order to speak.

Diagnosis

In evaluating cerebral palsy articulation disorders, the speech-language pathologist must first assess the possible roles of listening disorders and of mental retardation. Separating out immaturity symptoms from paralytic symptoms should also be attempted.

More specifically, the following possible relationships should be considered: (a) speech-elicited rooting reflex and lateralization of sibilants, lip reflex and bilabialized /r/ and /l/, mouth-opening reflex and vowel distortion, and suckle reflex and forward placed tongue-tip sounds; (b) slow, clumsy movements characterized by consistent limitations in directions and range of movements and spastic dysarthria (especially with tongue-tip sounds); (c) involuntary movements characterized by inconsistency in moving in appropriate directions with appropriate ranges and athetotic dysarthria (all sounds may be involved during athetotic episodes); (d) clumsy, uncoordinated movements characterized by uncertainty and inconsistency in the direction and range of movements and ataxic dysarthria; and (e) difficulty in voluntarily reproducing certain movements that can be made spontaneously and apraxic dysarthria.

Language Disorders

We have seen that children develop language as they develop other cognitive skills. In particular, spoken language develops as a function of general motor maturation up to standing, which allows the child to move around and experience the world; perceptual maturation, which allows the child to develop perceptual representations of things in the world; and central speech mechanism maturation, which allows the child to learn and associate oral symbols with their referents. Since children with cerebral palsy may show involvement with all these aspects of spoken language development, many of them also are delayed in developing language.

Immaturity

Oral language immaturity is reflected in delay in the onset of speech as well as in the development of vocabulary and grammar. The oral language of some children with cerebral palsy is characterized by a predominance of social gesture speech, such as "hi" and "bye," memorized speech, such as counting and nursery rhymes, and emotional utterances. The child may communicate only to express his wants or needs. Frequently, conversation and narration forms of speech are minimal or nonexistent. In short, the form and function of speech is infantile and could be called simple language retardation.

Indirect causes of retardation of speech development include substantial hearing loss, mental retardation, perceptual dysfunction, socioemotional problems, and limited stimulation and experience.

Pathology

Complicating language disorders among people with cerebral palsy may be symptoms that appear more directly related to involvement of the central neural mechanisms devoted to the function of spoken language. Symptoms may be observed that are similar to those found among otherwise normal children and adults who have language disorders due to some form of brain lesion. Among these symptoms may be perseveration, echolalia, confusion between similar-sounding words, syllable reversals, grammatical confusions, word-finding difficulty, and telegraphic speech.

Diagnosis

In the analysis of the child with a language disorder, the speech-language pathologist needs to determine the relative influence of factors such as listening disorder, speech mechanism paralysis, mental retardation, and reduction in general mobility and sensory-perceptual stimulation. Differentiating simple language retardation from specific language pathology is another important task.

SPEECH THERAPY

How well a speech therapy program for any particular child with cerebral palsy may work depends on many factors, including how accurately the speech-langauge pathologist has identified the components of the child's problem and formulated an individualized therapy regimen. Because the disorder in any given case may have begun at birth or before, may have various causes, and may present itself in various forms, we must take a wide-spectrum approach to management.

Incorporated within the concept of a wide-spectrum approach are the principles of holistic and early intervention. By holistic intervention, we mean that the speech-language pathologist must not only be concerned with the child's speech development, but also with how that development relates to and depends upon the child's overall motor, perceptual, cognitive, and socio-emotional development. By early intervention we mean the earliest possible intervention after the diagnosis of cerebral palsy has been made. Early intervention should help minimize secondary communication problems. Wide-spectrum management includes the consideration of primary and secondary preventive measures as well as causal, symptom, compensatory, and supportive therapies. Because the area of speech therapy for the cerebral palsied is so large and complex, we will present only a philosophy of therapy and some basic principles and methods.

If you have a special interest in therapy, you might wish to read further; see for example Lencione, 1976; Mysak, 1980.

Primary Preventive Measures

It is said that *the* goal of every clinical field is to put itself out of business. Prevention then should be a password in every profession, and we should spend major amounts of energy and resources on it. Alas, as in many other fields, the field of speech-language pathology and audiology has not done too well in this area. With respect to communication problems in cerebral palsy, the best way to prevent them is to prevent cerebral palsy. And one important way to help prevent cerebral palsy is through public education conducted by all concerned agencies and specialists.

Cerebral Palsy

Whenever possible, speech specialists should be directly or indirectly involved in premarital counseling with respect to speech and hearing problems. Young couples should be reminded of any familial tendencies for degenerative diseases such as progressive spastic paraplegia and for static conditions such as familial athetosis, paraplegia, and tremor.

Mothers-to-be should also be informed that various infections and conditions within them may cause cerebral palsy and should be guarded against. These prenatal causal factors include mumps, rubella, influenza, Rh-negative factor, and toxemia. Similary, mothers should guard their infants against infections such as meningitis, encephalitis, and measles, as well as against trauma and lead poisoning.

Communication

In those cases of existing cerebral palsy where speech and hearing mechanisms seem to be intact, certain primary preventive measures may also be carried out. Certainly, parents must obtain immediate medical attention for any ear infections in their child. Frequent audiometric screening is also recommended to identify and treat undetected problems so as to ensure against the development of future speech problems.

Facilitating the development of normal speech and hearing processes may also be viewed as a primary preventive measure. Parents may be advised to keep their child near talkative children and adults, to speak a lot when the child is experiencing good feelings (for instance, during feeding, bathing, playing), to expand and enrich the child's social and perceptual spheres by exposure to speakers and places outside the home, and to reward all efforts on the part of the child to perceive and produce speech. These measures would also be helpful in dealing with children with other physical disabilities, such as cleft palate, which may affect communication. The imaginative specialist may think of more ways to have parents facilitate the speech and hearing development of their child.

The aim of secondary preventive measures for the cerebral palsied child is to ensure that the child's personal reaction to his problems and the reactions of those around him do not add to his communication problems. A number of helpful suggestions may be given to parents by the speech-language pathologist.

The parents should be informed that, in general, a therapeutic environment is one in which the child is regularly exposed to situations where carefully measured challenge always exceeds carefully measured assistance. Accordingly, he should be allowed to spend as much time as possible in positions in which he can support himself; for example, on elbows or in various floor-sit positions (tailor position, side-sit, or long-sit positions). He should be given *every* opportunity to move from point to point using whatever mode of body progression is available to him. The child should be allowed to nurse and be exposed to solid foods as soon as possible (depending on circumstances, supplementary feeding may also be necessary). Whether it be supporting a particular body posture (perhaps sitting), moving through space, or eating, the child must be encouraged and allowed to try to do as much as possible for himself and to begin doing whatever he can for others. This may mean that everything the child needs to do will take a little longer to accomplish, but for the child it is time well spent.

The parents should also use the ideas we mentioned above to facilitate the development of normal speech and hearing processes. In general, the parents should be sure to provide an atmosphere rich with adult and child speakers, create situations that require the child to communicate orally, and reward all attempts to communicate and any growth in communication skills.

Causal Therapy

Causal therapy includes all those techniques aimed at what the speech-language pathologist thinks is directly responsible for the presenting speech problem. Techniques designed to counteract disorders of speech posture, listening, breathing-voicing, and articulation are described here.

Speech Posture Techniques

Postural control of the trunk, neck, and head contributes substantially to movement control of the speech mechanism. Helping the child with cerebral palsy to develop balance in a back-pattern speech posture, an on-elbows speech posture, or a sit-pattern speech posture is, therefore, an important goal of speech therapy. Physicians, physical therapists, occupational therapists, and parents all share this goal, and hence their efforts can contribute to reaching it. In order to apply specific techniques for developing speech postures, a good deal of background information is required that cannot be given here. In many cases, the speech-language pathologist will want to work closely with a physical therapist to choose and develop postures that facilitate speech and inhibit normal reflexes.

Listening Techniques

Developing head balance and control in speech postures also serves the listening function of allowing the child to orient her hearing mechanism toward the source of speech signals. Early use of amplification and the stimulation of auditory localizing and perception are also listening goals.

Whenever a hearing loss is detected, appropriate listening enhancement techniques should be applied as early as possible. This includes fitting a personal hearing aid, decreasing the distance between the child and speakers, having speakers raise their loudness level, and making sure that the child is in a position to see the speaker's face.

Localizing exercises involving speech and nonspeech stimuli should be done with the child in back-pattern, elbow-pattern, and sit-pattern speech postures whenever possible. Head localization should be stimulated, first to the right and then the left and first upward and then downward. Interesting, novel, and changing stimuli should be used inside and outside the home. Distances from the stimuli should be progressively increased and loudness levels progressively decreased. When the child does not spontaneously move her head, a therapy partner should initiate and guide these movements until the child develops some degree of independent localization.

Perceptual exercises include the abundant use of pleasant voice by family and friends, especially during feeding, bathing, and play periods. Localizing the voices of various family members should also be stimulated; these movements may be facilitated by having the different individuals vary the pitch, loudness, quality, and time dimensions of their voices. Span is developed, for example, by having the child point or eye-localize a progressively increasing number of things named by the adult; discrimination is developed, for example, by having the child signal whether pairs of syllables, words, or phrases are the same or different; and sequencing is developed, for example, by having the child execute a progressively longer series of simple instructions and in the right order.

More on hearing and auditory disorders in general is found in chapter 10 of this book.

Breathing-Voicing Techniques

Improving vegetative breathing and speech breathing are each important goals, and of course, breathing is also essential to voicing. Goals in vegetative breathing are to deepen breathing cycles, normalize breaths per minute, and stimulate thoracic participation. The goal in speech breathing is to effect a rapid vb-sb shift, which includes a shift from nasal to oral inspiration and from a ratio of 40% time spent in the inspiratory phase as compared to the expiratory phase of breathing to one of about 15%. There are many maneuvers available for facilitating inspiration, and we will describe two of them here.

The "leg-roll technique" is done with the child lying on a mat, for example, with the speech-language pathologist at the child's feet or at his side. The clinician grasps the child's shins, flexes and abducts the legs, and presses them toward the child's armpits, thereby displacing the internal organs upward, stretching the diaphragm, and facilitating expiration. Following the expiratory phase, the speech-language pathologist quickly extends and brings the legs downward, returning them to their original position and facilitating inspiration.

The "butterfly technique" is done with the child on a stool and with the speech-language pathologist behind the child. The clinician places the child's clasped hands on the back of the child's head, abducts the child's elbows, and extends his head and dorsal spine, thus facilitating inspiration. Following the inspiratory phase, the clinician quickly abducts the elbows, flexes the child's head and spine, and brings the head, arms, and shoulders down between abducted knees, facilitating expiration.

In applying both techniques, a rhythm similar to normal vegetative breathing should be imposed first. Next, the expiratory phase is lengthened and the

FIGURE 13.4
Inspiratory Facilitation Maneuvers: Leg-Roll (top row) and Butterfly (bottom row) Techniques.

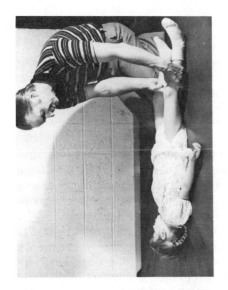
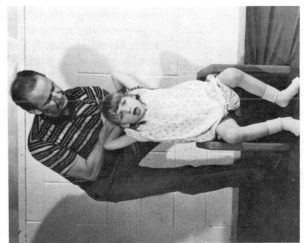
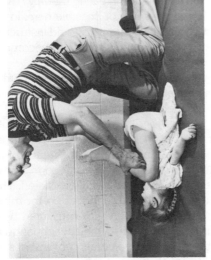
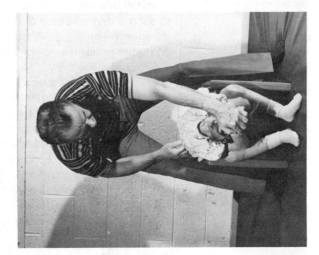
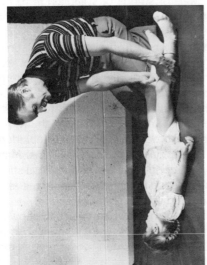
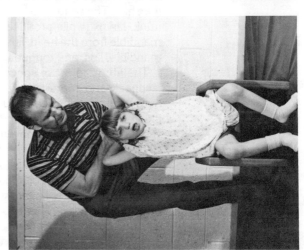

speech-language pathologist stimulates voicing, either sustained vowels or syllable strings, during the maneuver. At the same time, the inspiratory phase is quickened so that it lasts for approximately 10% to 15% of the entire breathing cycle. Examples of the maneuvers are shown in Figure 13.4.

Articulation Techniques

The major goals of articulation techniques are to increase the kinds, range, accuracy, and speed of movements of the mandible, lips, and tongue and to coordinate those movements with the breathing-voicing mechanism. Work on vegetative movements of the articulators as well as direct work on speech movements and their coordination should serve these goals.

Many experts believe that improvement of early eating movements like suckling, chewing, and swallowing contribute to the development of articulatory movements. Among the early advocates of eating therapy to improve speech movements were Meader (1940), Palmer (1947), and Westlake (1951); there has been a continued interest and development of this therapy by many new workers. Methods and techniques in eating therapy have grown to such a degree that a discussion of them is not possible here. In general, the speech-language pathologist or physical therapist should instruct parents and other family members in eating therapy and should not become a main provider of it.

See, for example, Mueller, 1972; Davis, 1978.

Causal therapy for speech movements and their coordination includes work in moving a body part in isolation from other body parts, in performing specific movements, and in performing speeded movements.

The first goal here is for the child to be able to move one articulator in isolation from other articulators and from all other body parts. It is done through a technique appropriately called an *isolation maneuver.* First, the speech-language pathologist holds or stablilizes all body parts, sometimes with the aid of an assistant, except for the part to be differentiated. The child is then asked to move the isolated part. If the child cannot do so, the movement of the part is assisted by the professional. Progress is measured by the reduction in the amount of stabilization imposed by the speech-language pathologist and by the increase in the amount of voluntary movement shown by the child. The sequence in the differentiation process is as follows: head from trunk, larynx (while producing vowels or strings of syllables) from the head, mandible from the head, lips from the head, tongue from the head, and finally mandible, lips, and tongue from the head and from each other.

The ability to move specific articulators is improved through stimulating-feedback and movement-facilitation maneuvers and movement exercises. Stimulating-feedback maneuvers impose particular articulatory patterns upon the child's mechanism, with the expectation that the imposed feedback will encourage the target movement to develop. Therapeutic feedback is provided, therefore, by bringing the child's articulators through the movements and points of contact associated with production of bilabial, labiodental, linguadental, lingua-alveolar, and linguavelar articulatory patterns. Maneuvers should be carried out along with appropriately timed audio-visual stimulation from the speech-language pathologist so that the child receives all the important sensory information associated with a particular sound.

Because these techniques require some background information and knowledge of

Movement-facilitation maneuvers are used when the child shows certain limitations in direction and range of articulatory movements. Among the maneuvers that could be used are the resisted-movement, associated-movement, countermovement, reversed-movement, and reflex-movement maneuvers.

Movement exercises are used to ensure the full use of movement potential that is developed through the stimulating-feedback and movement-facilitation techniques. Among the exercises that the child may perform are serial production of discrete on-off voicing, of nasal-nonnasal sound distinctions (for example, /mʌ-bʌ/), and of the production of various sets of two-syllable, three-syllable, and four-syllable combinations. An example of a typical two-syllable set is /bʌ-vʌ, bʌ-tʌ, bʌ-dʌ, bʌ-nʌ, bʌ-lʌ, bʌ-dʒʌ, bʌ-rʌ, bʌ-gʌ/. Sounds that the child has difficulty producing are excluded from the exercise sets. As progress is made with the production of the syllable sets, the element of speed is added.

neurofacilitatory techniques, they cannot be discussed in detail here. See Mysak, 1980.

Symptom Therapy

Symptom therapy is aimed directly at improving the child's use of oral language and speech production skills. Its goal is to capitalize on all the potential for speech production that emerges from the effort spent in secondary preventive measures and causal therapy. There are at least two reasons why any one child may not be speaking at maximum potential: the child learned sounds at a time when his articulatory system was not as efficient as it may now be, and the child did not automatically make use of any new potential resulting from preventive and causal therapy.

Articulation

If a particular child is not articulating certain sounds, either because she learned the sounds prior to her being able to make certain articulatory movements, or because she has not put to use new movements that have resulted from causal therapy, various traditional approaches to articulation therapy may be applied.

For information on these approaches, look back at chapter 5.

Language

Information on language symptom work is found in chapters 8 and 9.

Some general principles for language stimulation may be applied by all those individuals who come into contact with the child. Basic goals are to provide large amounts of speech stimulation when the child is experiencing pleasant sensations, to reward the child for all listening attitudes and efforts at communication, to ask the child to name first silently and then aloud whatever his eyes fix upon in the environment, and to ask the child to accompany his activities with a running description of them. Also, those around the child may describe aloud the child's activities or objects in the child's visual field whenever the child is not speaking. They can also describe aloud (simply and appropriately) their own activities whenever the child is nearby, watching and listening.

Sociocommunication situations that require various functional uses of speech and various role-playing activities also provide good language stimulation. For example, to develop intrapersonal communication skills, you can ask the child to imagine that he is about to say something very important to someone and that he should first rehearse what he wants to say in his mind. Skills for communicating can be developed by telling the child that you will pretend to be different people seeking various kinds of information that he is to provide. A control situation can be developed by telling the child that you will pretend to be his father, for example, and that he must talk you into doing something for him. To encourage the child to express emotions, you could ask her to pretend that she is happy, angry, or frightened about something and tell her that she should express that emotion. Finally, to teach the child identification skills, you could tell the child that you will pretend to be a stranger and that he should tell you all about yourself.

Compensatory Therapy

Compensatory therapy techniques are used to facilitate the development of spoken language and to supplement or replace spoken language when its development is proceeding slowly, is limited, or there is little hope of achieving it. Both modified speech forms and nonspeech forms are available.

Modified Speech

Forms of modified speech include spell and topic talk, electronically treated speech, and synthethic speech.

Spell and topic talk are ways to improve communication in instances of questionable intelligibility. Children should be willing and ready to spell aloud words which they believe listeners are having trouble understanding and should identify the topic of what they intend to talk about before they begin to communicate.

Electronically treated speech requires the child to wear a device that is designed to increase understandability. Two such devices have been developed: the electronic speaking aid (National Institute for Rehabilitation Engineering, Pompton Lakes, New Jersey) and the Auditory Feedback Mechanism, or AFM (Berko, 1965). The electronic speaking aid basically amplifies and filters the child's speech and transmits the treated signal into a loudspeaker. The AFM also amplifies and filters the child's speech, but then the treated speech is fed back to a headset worn by the child.

Synthetic speech may also be viewed as a form of modified speech. Portable models of speech synthesizers that can "speak" for the child are now commercially available (Phonic Mirror, H. C. Electronics, Inc.). High cost and a particular child's physical and mental abilities limit the use of these synthesizers.

Nonvocal communication

Nonspeech/nonvocal forms of compensatory therapy include the use of signals and code, symbols, and communication boards. These modes of communication are used with more severely involved children, often those who are severely retarded. Mental abilities, motivation, and voluntary movements available to the child are considerations in the selection of an alternate mode of communication. Also important is the cooperation of the child's parents, family, friends, teachers, and therapists. It is important to note that the use of nonspeech communication should not preclude speech therapy, since a number of studies have shown that an increase in speech attempts and intelligibility accompany their use.

See, for example, McDonald and Schultz, 1973; Beukelman and Yorkston, 1977.

Signal and code forms of communication include the use of a simple yes-no system, audio-signalling, and Morse code. Yes or no signals may be given by the child via some sort of hand, head, face, or eye movement. A portable audio-oscillator that emits a loud tone has been used to teach cerebral palsied children four simple signals: I need help; Yes; No; See the list (Hagen, Porter,

& Brink, 1973). Morse code has also been used as a means of communication for severely involved children (Clement, 1961).

Symbol forms of communication involve the use of special symbols that represent sounds or words. Two symbol systems have been frequently used with cerebral palsied children. First, Blissymbol communication has been effectively used with certain severely involved children with cerebral palsy (Vanderheiden & Harris-Vanderheiden, 1976). Blissymbols represent concepts rather than specific words. Depending on the child's ability, Blissymbol vocabularies of up to 400 items may be learned. Second, an electronic conversation board called the "Expressor" was designed to facilitate the use of the Initial Teaching Alphabet (ITA) (Shane, 1972). In this system, one symbol represents one sound; if the child learns the 44 symbols, he would be capable of producing any English word.

A final compensatory system is the use of communication boards, which may be nonelectronic or electronic. Nonelectronic boards have been used with the cerebral palsied for some time (McDonald & Chance, 1961; Westlake & Rutherford, 1964). Boards should be developed on an individual basis in accordance with each child's needs and physical and intellectual abilities. More organized forms of communication boards have recently been developed (McDonald & Schultz, 1973). These boards may display numbers, letters, words, pictures, and sentences. They may also display Blissymbols, the ITA, or other symbol systems. The vocabulary should reflect the child's own priorities and interests. An electronic communication board called the Auto-Monitoring Communication Board or Auto-Com has also been used with a severely involved cerebral palsied child (Bullock, Dalrymple, & Danca, 1975). Some of the features of the Auto-Com include a capacity to print out letters, words, phrases, and sentences; a television read-out component; and interfacing with a typewriter.

Supportive Therapy

In certain cases of cerebral palsy, the speech-language pathologist may find that there is little hope for any kind of progress in verbal or nonverbal communication. Such cases are, unfortunately, appearing with increasing frequency in the caseload of the speech-language pathologist who now, more than in the past, may be working in state developmental centers.

In such cases, the clinician has at least two goals: (a) to ensure that parents and others who relate with the child comprehend any body, hands, facial, or sound communication that the child may be able to use, and (b) to help the parents and others who relate with the child to understand and accept the child's severe limitations in the use of any form of verbal or nonverbal communication.

CONCLUSION

After reading this chapter, there should be little doubt that the analysis of the communication problem in cerebral palsy, the formulation of an individualized therapy plan, and the effective execution of that plan should be regarded as some of the greatest challenges to the clinical speech-language pathologist. Some of the greatest rewards await those who accept and meet those challenges.

SELECTED READINGS

Connor, F. P., Williamson, G. G., & Siepp, J. M. (Eds.). *Program guide for infants and toddlers with neuromotor and other developmental disabilities.* New York: Teachers College Press, Teachers College, Columbia University, 1978.

Cruickshank, W. M. (Ed.). *Cerebral palsy: Its individual and community problems.* Syracuse: Syracuse University Press, 1976.

Lencione, R. M. The development of communication skills. In W. J. Cruickshank (Ed.), *Cerebral palsy: A developmental disability.* Syracuse: Syracuse University Press, 1976.

McDonald, E. T., & Schultz, A. Communication boards for cerebral palsied children. *Journal of Speech and Hearing Disorders,* 1973, *38,* 73–88.

Mueller, H. Facilitating feeding and prespeech. In P. H. Pearson & C. E. Williams (Eds.), *Physical therapy services in the developmental disabilities.* Springfield, Ill.: Charles C Thomas, 1972.

Nober, E. H. Auditory processing. In W. J. Cruickshank (Ed.), *Cerebral palsy: A developmental disability.* Syracuse: Syracuse University Press, 1976.

Westlake, H., & Rutherford, D. *Speech therapy for the cerebral palsied.* Chicago: National Society for Crippled Children and Adults, 1964.

REFERENCES

Achilles, R. F. Communicative anomalies of individuals with cerebral palsy: I. Analysis of communicative processes in 151 cases of cerebral palsy. *Cerebral Palsy Review,* 1955, *16,* 15–24.

Berko, F. *Amelioration of athetoid speech by manipulation of auditory feedback.* Unpublished doctoral dissertation, Cornell University, 1965.

Beukelman, D., & Yorkston, K. A communication system for the severely dysarthric speaker with an intact language system. *Journal of Speech and Hearing Disorders,* 1977, *42,* 265–270.

Bobath, K., & Bobath, B. The neuro-developmental treatment of cerebral palsy. *Journal of American Physical Therapy Association,* 1967, *47,* 1039–1041.

Bullock, A., Dalrymple, G. F., & Danca, J. M. Communication and the nonverbal, multihandicapped child. *American Journal of Occupational Therapy,* 1975, *29,* 150–152.

Clement, M. Morse code method of communication for the severely handicapped cerebral palsied child. *Cerebral Palsy Review,* 1961, *22,* 15–16.

Connor, F. P., Williamson, G. G., & Siepp, J. M. (Eds.). *Program guide for infants and toddlers with neuromotor and other developmental disabilities.* New York: Teachers College Press, Teachers College, Columbia University, 1978.

Cruickshank, W. M. (Ed.). *Cerebral palsy: Its individual and community problems.* Syracuse: Syracuse University Press, 1976.

Davis, L. F. Pre-speech. In F. P. Connor, G. F. Williamson, & J. M. Siepp (Eds.), *Program guide for infants and toddlers with neuromotor and other developmental disabilities.* New York: Teachers College Press, Teachers College, Columbia University, 1978.

Hagen, C., Porter, W., & Brink, J. Nonverbal communication: An alternative mode of communication of the child with severe cerebral palsy. *Journal of Speech and Hearing Disorders,* 1973, *38,* 448–455.

Lencione, R. M. The development of communication skills. In W. J. Cruickshank (Ed.), *Cerebral palsy: A developmental disability.* Syracuse: Syracuse University Press, 1976.

Little, W. J. On the influence of abnormal parturition, difficult labor, premature birth, and asphyxia neonatorum in the mental and physical condition of the child, especially in relation to deformities. *Transcripts of the Obstetrical Society of London,* 1861, *3,* 293.

Marks, N. C. *Cerebral palsied and learning disabled children.* Springfield, Ill.: Charles C Thomas, 1974.

McDonald, E. T., & Chance, B. *Cerebral palsy.* Englewood Cliffs, N. J.: Prentice-Hall, 1964.

McDonald, E. T., & Schultz, A. Communication boards for cerebral palsied children. *Journal of Speech and Hearing Disorders,* 1973, *38,* 73–88.

Meader, M. H. The effect of disturbances in the developmental processes upon emergent specificity of function. *Journal of Speech Disorders,* 1940, *5,* 211–219.

Mueller, H. Facilitating feeding and prespeech. In P. H. Pearson & C. E. Williams (Eds.), *Physical therapy services in the developmental disabilities.* Springfield, Ill.: Charles C Thomas, 1972.

Mysak, E. D. *Neurospeech therapy for the cerebral palsied.* New York: Teachers College Press, Teachers College, Columbia University, 1980.

Nober, E. H. Auditory processing. In W. J. Cruickshank (Ed.), *Cerebral palsy: A developmental disability.* Syracuse: Syracuse University Press, 1976.

Palmer, M. Studies in clinical techniques II: Normalization of chewing, sucking and swallowing reflexes in cerebral palsy: A home program. *Journal of Speech and Hearing Disorders,* 1947, *12,* 415–418.

Phelps, W. M. The treatment of cerebral palsies. *Journal of Bone Joint Surgery,* 1940, *22,* 1004–1012.

Rood, M. S. Neurophysiological reactions as a basis for physical therapy. *Physical Therapy Review,* 1954, *34,* 444–448.

Shane, H. *A device and program for aphonic communication.* Unpublished master's thesis, University of Massachusetts, 1972.

Twitchell, T. E. Variations and abnormalities of motor development. *Journal of American Physical Therapy Association,* 1965, *45,* 424–430.

Vanderheiden, G., & Harris-Vanderheiden, D. Communication techniques and aids. In L. Lloyd (Ed.), *Communication assessment and intervention strategies.* Baltimore: University Park Press, 1976.

Westlake, H. Muscle training for cerebral palsied speech cases. *Journal of Speech and Hearing Disorders,* 1951, *16,* 103–109.

Westlake, H., & Rutherford, D. *Speech therapy for the cerebral palsied.* Chicago: National Society for Crippled Children and Adults, 1964.

Wolfe, W. G. A comprehensive evaluation of fifty cases of cerebral palsy. *Journal of Speech and Hearing Disorders,* 1950, *15,* 234–251.

Worster-Drought, C. Speech disorders in children. *Developmental Medicine and Neurology,* 1968, *10,* 427–440.

14 APHASIA IN ADULTS

Audrey L. Holland
O. M. Reinmuth

Janice, age 46, suffered a stroke involving the left middle cerebral artery. As a result, she developed moderate aphasia. One month after her stroke, her verbal output was limited in quantity and she had marked word-finding problems. Characteristically she spoke in short phrases, and some grammatical problems were evident. Her auditory comprehension was considerably better than her speech, although she had some problems comprehending complex instructions and messages. Janice's reading was minimally affected, and her writing was similar to her speech, although complicated by a mild residual muscle weakness which presented mechanical difficulties with writing.

Before her stroke, Janice had led an active life, working in the public relations department of the Pittsburgh Steelers, raising two teen-age children, and managing her household with no help beside her husband, a chemical engineer. Janice was an avid potter, and her other interests included professional sports, scuba diving, and reading.

One month after her stroke, having been transferred from acute care to a rehabilitation center, Janice was engaged in a full-scale rehabilitation program including physical therapy, where she had already received instruction in walking with the aid of a short leg brace; occupational therapy, which was centered primarily on regaining use of her weak arm; and speech-language therapy directed primarily at increasing her functional communication and at decreasing her anxiety about her presently faltering speech and language skills. Her formal evaluation at that time indicated a mild to moderate mixed aphasia, with disproportionate word-finding difficulty. Psychologically, Janice was mildly depressed, but the gains she had already made in physical therapy had begun to lift her spirits and she was working with determination in speech-language therapy. Janice's family visited her every other day, and her husband had begun to attend the family group sessions run once a week by the Rehabilitation Center to prepare families for patients' return home. Both the social worker and the staff psychologist had been alerted to Janice's depression and had initiated brief counseling sessions. The social worker had centered his activities on realistic appraisal of potential for return to work; the psychologist had centered hers in exploring Janice's self-concept in relation to her problems.

Janice was dismissed after 6 weeks at the Rehabilitation Center. She was walking with the aid of a cane at that point and had made enough gains in use of her arm to be able to perform most of the activities of daily living, including being able to perform the manual activities necessary for cooking.

Many gains in language abilities had also been made, particularly in auditory comprehension, which had been restored to normal. Persisting, however, were the word-finding problem and difficulty with both reading and writing. It was decided that speech-language therapy should be continued on an outpatient basis, and arrangements were made with the local University Clinic for that treatment.

Janice came to the University Clinic for both individual and group treatment 2 times a week during the ensuing year. Consistent but slow progress was maintained for approximately 10 months, with no apparent progress after that time. She was discharged from treatment at the end of that year.

At the time of her discharge from treatment, Janice evidenced minimal speech-language problems when rested and comfortable; however, pressure on her often created some difficulty in speech. During her time in the Clinic, a number of family decisions had been made that had impact on her case. First, Janice altered her rehabilitation goals. While initially she was highly concerned about returning to work and determined to do so, she decided against this, citing her remaining language difficulty and her reticence at returning in any capacity less demanding and fulfilling than her job before her stroke. She had not, however, retired from life; in addition to returning to her major managerial role at home, she had decided to forgo household help and was totally responsible for maintaining her home. In addition, she undertook a responsible role in her local stroke club. At the time of her discharge, she had become responsible for developing a visitation program for stroke patients by stroke patients. This program had as its primary goal informing recent stroke victims of the helping services available in the community and inspiring them to become involved to the maximum in their own recovery.

Janice's family was presently functioning well with the less than total status of her recovery. Her teenaged children, almost ready for college, felt that they had had both a significant learning experience brought about by their altered family structure and roles in the last few years. They were impressed with their mother's courage and the strength she demonstrated in pursuing her recovery. Janice's husband, who felt the major financial burden and some of the major effects of his wife's stroke, was optimistic about what their future holds. "We've learned a lot. We've learned to handle adversity. We've learned what we're made of. I'm terribly sorry it happened. But we've survived it—and survived it well."

"Boy, I'm sweating, I'm awful nervous, you know once in a while I get caught up. I can't mention the tarripoi, a month ago, quite a little, I've done a lot well, I impose a lot, while, on the other hand, you know what I mean, I have to run around, look it over, trebbin and all that sort of stuff."

Wernicke aphasic patient quoted by
Gardner (1975, p. 68) in response to question,
"What brings you to the hospital?"

Q. What happened to make you lose your speech?
A. Head, fall, Jesus Christ, me no good, str, str . . . oh, Jesus . . . stroke.
Q. I see. Could you tell me what you've been doing in the hospital?
A. Yes, sure, me go er uh P.T. nine o'cot, speech two times . . . read . . .
    wr . . . ripe, er, rike, er write . . . practice . . . get-ting better.

Question and answer sequence,
Howard Gardner and Broca aphasic patient
(Gardner, 1975, p. 61)

By this time in your life, when you are old enough to be interested in reading this chapter, whether or not you have (or had) most of the other problems described in this book is a matter of record. This chapter, along with the adult disorders described in chapter 12, deals with an exception to that statement. This chapter is about a communication disorder called *aphasia,* which is usually acquired in adulthood. Aphasia is not simply a speech disturbance; in addition to wreaking havoc on speech and verbal output, it also produces disturbances in comprehending the speech of others, in reading, and in writing. The examples above demonstrate two extremes of aphasic difficulty. Aphasia is actually a general term used to describe a number of related but separable syndromes, as we shall see later. It refers to a breakdown in the ability to formulate, or to retrieve, and to decode the arbitrary symbols of *language.* Aphasia's onset is most often abrupt, occurring without warning to people who have had no history of speech or language problems. Although injury to the head, brain tumors, and some other neurologic diseases may produce aphasia, it occurs most often in the wake of a stroke. Because strokes most commonly occur in older people, it is not likely that you may have one in the near future. However, aphasia is the most prevalent of adult language problems, due to the frequency of stroke in this society; and most of us know an older relative, neighbor, or relative of a friend who has experienced its disastrous consequences. Thus, aphasia is a language problem with which you are likely to have direct personal experience.

This contrasts to disorders of speech production, which were covered in chapter 12.

The purpose of this chapter is to acquaint you with the mechanisms that produce aphasia, with the various forms the disorder takes, and with treatment for the problem. In addition, we will consider the profound effects of aphasia on the previously normal speaker and his family and introduce you to some aphasic persons through brief case histories.

Aphasia is a fascinating topic, not only to speech-language pathologists but to neurologists, linguists, and neuropsychologists, to name a few. This is because aphasia affords a unique opportunity to study some of our most perplexing questions about ourselves. These include the nature of brain-behavior interaction, the relationship of thought to language, and the neurologic substrata of cognitive activities. As a result, there is a large, often highly contradictory and controversial body of information regarding aphasia that has been accumulating for more than a century since its formal study was begun. We will merely scratch the surface in what follows. We hope that, in the process, you will catch enough of the excitement that can be generated by studying aphasia and working with aphasic adults to read more of its vast literature.

APHASIA AND THE BRAIN

Basic Neuroanatomic Considerations

Although damage to many different parts of the brain can cause some sort of speech problem, the cortex, or covering, of the cerebrum is of most interest to aphasiologists. This is because this wrinkled and crumpled grey surface appears to be the body's major integrative network, allowing for implementing and conducting our most complex cognitive activities. Among these activities are, of course, speaking, writing, and comprehending others' speech and reading. Predictably then, damage to the cortex (and *cortical* as opposed to *subcortical* brain damage) is most likely to produce aphasia.

Brain damage can also cause the neurogenic speech disorders covered in chapter 12; recall that these disorders can coexist with aphasia.

But this statement is too simple; damage just anywhere to the cortex is not sufficient to produce aphasia. Although controversy still exists over just what particular site of damage produces just what form of language problem, and no one yet has but the vaguest understanding of just how the damage extracts its toll, some principles of neurologic function allow us to be more specific about cortical damage and aphasia.

To explain, we must become a bit more familiar with the cerebral hemispheres. Like some other organs of the body (the kidneys, for example), the cortex-covered cerebrum appears actually to be a pair of organs. It consists of two halves, called *hemispheres,* which are roughly similar in size and shape. Most perfectly normal brain functioning requires both halves to be operating properly. However, the function of each half of the brain is not reduplicative, each half doing sometimes subtly different and often grossly different things. We must discuss three broad types of cortical activities—motor, sensory, and cognitive—in terms of their hemispheric control in order to understand a few of the very basics of brain-language relationships.

You may wish to review the description of the brain in chapter 4.

Movement

Our only means of affecting our environment is through movement. Even our thoughts are inaccessible to the world around us, except as we can move our speech musculature to put our thoughts into their active forms as words or move our bodies to communicate them nonverbally. Movement seems the most obvious of our abilities, yet how movement is accomplished, how the brain controls the body's muscles, remains at the scientific frontier. The enormous complexity of neuromotor control is yet to be satisfactorily explained.

Among the knowns, however, is that for highly skilled motor behavior, nature plays an interesting trick. The left half of the brain (left cerebral hemisphere) controls movement of the right side of the body, and the right half (right cerebral hemisphere) controls the left side of the body. Thus, if cortical brain damage results in some motor impairment (and it frequently does), we can often observe a paralysis of only one side of the body. This condition, called **hemiplegia** or **hemiparesis,** allows us to predict which side of the brain was damaged. If a left hemiplegia is noted, we can infer right cortical brain damage; if a right hemiplegia is noted, we can infer damage to the left hemisphere.

Sensory Systems

We perceive the world around us by hearing, seeing, touching, smelling, and tasting it. Our remarks will be limited to describing the two sensory systems that are most important to language: vision and audition. Let us first consider vision. Indeed, in organisms with monocular vision, such as pigeons, vision in the left eye is in the province of the right hemisphere, and vice versa. But human beings (and some other animals as well) have binocular, rather than monocular, vision; and in humans the visual pathways are partially (as opposed to totally) crossed. The partial crossing can be described by a do-it-yourself example. Direct both of your eyes to a point in front of you, perhaps an object directly above the upper edge of this book. Note that both eyes participate in seeing the object. All visual information to the right of that point (the right visual field) is fed by each eye to the left hemisphere; and information to the left of that point (the left visual field), to the right hemisphere. This crossing of the optic nerve fibers (optic tract) occurs in the optic chiasm, not very far behind the eyeballs. Beyond this crossing point, damage either to the optic tract or to the area of the cortex which receives visual impulses causes a loss of vision of one half of what is being viewed. This loss is called **hemi-anopsia.** An interruption of the left optic tract or occipital lobe therefore causes loss of the right half of the visual space before each eye. The loss of the *same* visual half field is identified by the term *homonymous* loss—hence, right homonymous hemianopsia.

As with vision, there is also a peculiarity about auditory information and its cortical reception, although the difficulty is much harder to demonstrate. This difficulty is due both to the nature of sound waves themselves and to the fact that auditory information is quite generously distributed to both hemispheres. While roughly 70% of the auditory fibers from each ear cross to the opposite hemisphere, the remaining fibers do not. Few, if any, effects on hearing sensitivity are caused by purely cortical damage. Deafness in one or the other ear occurs as a result of damage to the ear itself or the sensory pathways much below the level of the cortex. The role of the cortex in audition is rather the *interpretation* of auditory signals and messages, that is, making sense out of the signals received by the ear.

Recall the discussion in chapter 10.

In the case of visual and auditory information, it appears that nature has been careful to protect these two major sources for apprehending the world around us. First, by giving us two eyes and ears, nature has arranged things so that if one member of either pair is damaged, we are not totally cut out of its sensory contributions to our understanding. Nature has also protected us by arranging for each member of the pair to have access to both cortical hemispheres. This further assures access to visual and auditory information, this time by protecting sensory mechanisms against unilateral brain damage.

Cognitive Function: Left vs. Right Hemisphere

We have seen how sensory input from the eyes and ears is differentially received by the left and right hemispheres. We have also been alerted to the manner in which motor output is differentially controlled by the hemispheres. What about the *cognitive* functions of these two halves of the brain? Is there a difference in the hemispheres' respective roles in integrating, in processing information, in thinking?

It has been recognized for a long time that aphasia usually occurs with damage to the left hemisphere, and that people with brain damage limited to the right hemisphere usually escape language disorders. Thus, language appears to be a function of the left hemisphere. (If the brain-damaged person's lesion also involves the cortical motor areas, you can also predict, from what you have just read about motor control, that he will have difficulty using the right side of his body and a right hemiplegia as well. Similarly, if he has an associated visual problem it will be with his right visual field; he will have a right homonymous hemianopsia.) And indeed language sets the tone for the sorts of cognitive activities the left hemisphere appears to perform—the logical, sequential aspects of thinking and mental operations.

For many years, because language had already been localized to the left hemisphere and because language was so prominent in Western society's beliefs about thinking, the left hemisphere was referred to as the "dominant" hemisphere, with the added implication that the right hemisphere was a sort of spare part, to be called into thinking only when and if the left was damaged in some way. It was further believed that in left-handed people this situation was reversed, with the right hemisphere having dominance, and the left being a cognitive spare part.

Recent advances in neuropsychology have begun to change that view. Far from being the subservient hemisphere, the right hemisphere is increasingly being demonstrated to make its own distinctive contributions to our thinking skills. Briefly, the right hemisphere is presently thought to have major responsibility for nonverbal aspects of thinking, such as visuo-spatial problem solving and artistic and creative mental activities. It appears particularly sensitive to music and its appreciation, as another example. If the cognitive operations of the left hemisphere can be characterized as logical, the cognitive operations of the right are by contrast probably more intuitive. Further, this dichotomy of function is no longer thought to be totally related to handedness, but to be probably true of most people's cognitive organization. That is, the left hemisphere for most of us probably has a subtly different role than does the right; neither hemisphere is "dominant." They are, rather, different; and perhaps each dominates in different types of cognitive activity.

Persons who have damaged right hemispheres have a characteristic set of disturbed behaviors which is beyond the purpose of this chapter to detail. We therefore return to the left hemisphere, where one major way that the consequences of brain damage may be manifested is in the symptoms of aphasia.

It is important to give you a warning at this point. Most of what we know about how the brain functions in normal cognitive activities comes from two sources: both animal and human investigations under two broad sorts of unnatural conditions—surgical removal or destruction and direct cortical stimulation. Each of these two techniques may yield misinformation. When animals serve as subjects in either stimulation or surgical experiments, a further error source is added; due to differences in brain structure, the value of animal analogues to human brain function may be limited.

In studies of humans, cortical stimulation is perhaps most easily exemplified by the considerable contributions of Penfield and his associates (Penfield & Roberts, 1959), who mapped cortical function by direct electrical stimulation of the cortices of patients who were undergoing surgery to correct brain diseases. There is no doubt that this work is invaluable. Yet it is important to remind ourselves that direct cortical stimulation by an experimental electrode is an unusual circumstance; and further, that since Penfield's patients came to be experimental subjects *because* of neurologic problems, the results may not be generalizable to normal function without some caution.

Finally, a third case—what happens to behavior when parts are destroyed—is the most fruitful of information, and frankly also the most open to suspicion. Over 100 years ago, Hughlings Jackson warned us that localization of a symptom is not the same as localization of a function. What he meant was that interrupting an area of the normally working cortex, with its complex, interconnected circuitry, disrupts the integrity of the whole system. Only if the cortex actually physically maps psychological events, that is, if there is a tiny spot in the cortex that controls nouns or verbs or speech sounds or sentences (fill in whatever units you wish), can the correlation between damage and behavioral consequences be totally justified or can we use this information to explain normal cognitive behavior fully. If the brain works in a more complex way, if the cognitive psychological event itself is a product of the brain's activity, then the correlation of damage and consequence cannot be totally justified. For the same reasons, it is even less justifiable to assume that a particular cognitive function resides in a given area if we see a disruption of that function following damage to the given area. What we observe in the cognitive behavior of the brain-damaged person is generally a matter of how the brain adapts to damage, how it uses its remaining tissue, in addition to being a manifestation of the damage itself. Because language is a psychological, cognitive event, as are functions like making music and reading maps, Jackson's argument must always be kept in mind.

The Left Cerebral Hemisphere and Aphasia

You might wish to review Figure 4.30, which shows the functions of various areas in the brain.

Figure 14.1 shows a lateral (side) view of the left hemisphere. Note that the brain lobes are named after the bones of the skull under which the areas lie, with separation between them only partly related to anatomic features of the brain itself. Although the anatomy of the right hemisphere is almost identical to that of the left, its contribution to cognitive function differs in important ways (such as its apparent minimal role in speech), of which we understand much less.

By and large, the regions of the cortex posterior to the fissure of Rolando and above the Sylvian fissure are responsible for the primary analysis of sensation. The occipital lobe is specialized for vision, the parietal for somatic sensory analysis, and the temporal lobe for audition. The area directly anterior to the fissure of Rolando has an intimate relationship to the initiation of movement. Farther forward in the frontal lobe the nature of the function is more subtle and harder to describe. The frontal lobes play an executive role in initiating, planning, and integrating the whole spectrum of behavior so essential for directing the individual in affecting the environment.

FIGURE 14.1
The Human Brain.

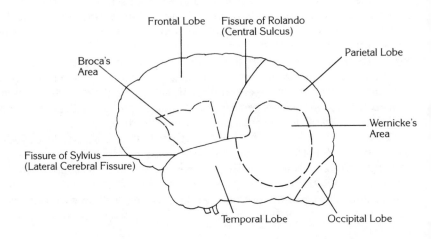

Frontal Lobe   Fissure of Rolando (Central Sulcus)

Broca's Area

Parietal Lobe

Wernicke's Area

Fissure of Sylvius (Lateral Cerebral Fissure)

Temporal Lobe   Occipital Lobe

Notice on Figure 14.1 two darkened areas, one adjacent and anterior to the motor cortex in the frontal lobe, the other primarily in the temporal, but extending up into the parietal lobe. These two areas are thought to be primarily responsible for speech and language functions. The frontal area is called *Broca's area,* and the temporo-parietal area is termed *Wernicke's area.* Each has been named for the 19th century researcher who first began to delimit the area's special roles in language function: in the first instance, the French physician Paul Broca, and in the second, the German neurologist Carl Wernicke. These areas are, in fact, idealized approximations, but destruction in these general areas of the left hemisphere significantly affects speech and language performance and brings about aphasia. That this differentiation of the language areas is merely approximate can most succinctly be summarized by a remark made by Joseph Bogen, an eminent neurosurgeon, addressing the Academy of Aphasia: "We know where Broca's area is, we are merely uncertain about what it does. And we know what Wernicke's area does, we are merely uncertain about where it is"(1977). With that warning in mind, we will talk about each in turn, beginning with Wernicke's area.

Wernicke's Area   Remember that the posterior cortex is concerned with reception and analysis of stimuli from the outside world. Note that Wernicke's area lies in the temporal lobe (with its responsibility for hearing), and extends back toward the occipital lobe (where visual stimuli are received) and upward into the parietal area (where somatic sensation is integrated). Accepting the statement that some language difficulty results from damage to Wernicke's area, it would make logical sense that damage to these regions produces difficulty with the input or stimulus side of language—that is, with understanding language. And, indeed, this is the case. Damage to the *posterior* parts of the language area produces difficulties with comprehending speech, and in many instances difficulty with reading as well. Since the posterior part of Wernicke's area can be thought of as the meeting place for the different types of language, it is easy to see that major difficulties *across* the language modalities can occur with damage here. Finally, although no damage has occurred to the motor speech center itself (Broca's area), it should be obvious that, if your ability to comprehend speech or to read is compromised, there should be some rather profound effects on speech itself. And, in fact, the aphasic patient with damage to Wernicke's area is not in much better shape for comprehending his own speech than he is the speech of others. While fluent, and often even grammatically and phonologically correct, the speech of a patient with Wernicke's aphasia contains many semantic errors and, like the example presented at the beginning of this chapter, is often almost incomprehensible to the listener.

We shall talk in more detail about this later in the chapter.

Thus, in one classification system Wernicke's aphasia is called receptive aphasia.

Broca's Area   We have indicated the frontal lobe as responsible for movement (behavior) and its initiation. Its speech area, thus, can be responsible for output, for speaking. Damage here does much less to affect the comprehension of the speech of others, but instead takes its major toll on fluent, well-articulated, initiative speech. The speech of a person with Broca aphasia is slow and labored, lacking the prosody and flow of normal speech. Lying adjacent to the motor areas, damage to Broca's area often results in articulatory problems as well, and produces motor programming deficits as well as difficulty in finding the words one wishes to say, either for speaking or for writing (where hemiplegia can also affect the mechanics of writing).

Broca's aphasia is also called expressive aphasia.

SYNDROMES OF APHASIA

Principles of Typing

Between the poles of fluent Wernicke aphasic speech, with its major disruptions of auditory comprehension, and nonfluent Broca aphasic speech, with intact auditory comprehension, a notable array of variations occur. These variations are often discrete enough to be referred to as syndromes. The aphasia syndromes are related not only to the site of lesion, but to the extent of damage, to the idiosyncracies of a person's individual cortical structures, and to some degree, to the general health condition and life circumstances at the time the aphasia-producing damage is incurred. After setting some of the ground rules, we will briefly describe the most common of these syndromes.

Here are the ground rules, the things to keep in the back of your head as you read about the syndromes (or types) of aphasia.

First, aphasic symptoms are not bizarre and mysterious. They are actually extreme variants of everyday occurrences. For example, all of us have misspelled a word we know well; all of us have experienced difficulty in remembering a name or a word, or have heard or read something, even in our own language, which we simply couldn't understand. It is quite useful to keep those experiences in mind when you explore the world of aphasia.

We hope this chapter is not one of your examples.

Second, regardless of the cardinal symptoms, the bottom line is that people who have aphasia have some basic underlying problems (perhaps only brought to light through sophisticated testing) with two aspects of language—comprehension and word retrieval. You should be alert to the fact that some authorities emphasize the features that are common to most aphasic patients, while others approach the analysis by distinguishing patients by how they differ. Each approach may serve a useful function in the attempt to find rules and patterns of organization that help further our imperfect understanding of the mechanisms. These differing approaches may also suggest new ways to test patients as well as new ways to approach corrective therapy.

A major proponent of the view that what aphasic patients have in common is more important than the ways in which they differ was Hildred Schuell, a distinguished speech-language pathologist. She viewed aphasia, thus, as a disturbance of language. Her work, which emphasizes the role of auditory comprehension in aphasia, is of enormous rehabilitative significance, and will be discussed later. While acknowledging the impact and importance of this point of view, we must also acknowledge our preference for a multidimensional view of aphasia. That is, we prefer differentiating symptom complexes as specifically as possible. You need to know, however, that other, perfectly viable and useful viewpoints exist in this frontier field of neural behavior. It will be a useful exercise, in what follows and as examples are given, to look for the common factors in the behavioral descriptions, as well as the differences, which are emphasized.

To confound the issue more, even within the group of scientists who are interested in differentiating types of aphasia, the same patients may be described differently. Similar syndromes may be differently named. Rather than discourage you by this terminology swamp so early in your study of aphasia, we wish only to alert you to the problem. We use the terminology of Geschwind, Benson, and their coworkers because it appears to be presently in widest currency in the United States and is widely used by the many students of language in several different disciplines.

See, for instance, Benson and Geschwind, 1976.

Since aphasia is a language disorder, rather than a speech disorder, it is appropriate to describe details about other language modalities in addition to speech. In what follows, therefore, relevant details of speaking, comprehending, reading, writing, and repeating are included.

Some of the syndromes we will describe are inherently more devastating to langue than are others. Within each syndrome, there is a continuum of severity as well. Thus, you will often find qualifying terms, such as *mild, moderate,* or *severe,* used to describe the conditions and their effects upon language.

Finally, as we have seen, lesions involving the posterior portions of the left hemisphere (temporal-parietal-occipital lobes) produce fluent aphasia; we have used Wernicke aphasia as an example. Lesions involving the anterior portion (the frontal lobe) produce nonfluent aphasia. (Here we have discussed Broca aphasia.) However, this relationship can vary. Some people escape aphasia altogether, even if their damage is to these regions. Others show minor language difficulty in the presence of vast areas of damage. Although we have stated that the left hemisphere is usually afflicted when aphasia occurs, even in left-handers, right hemispheric lesions can produce aphasia in left-handers and, even more rarely, in right-handers. Finally, aphasias have been documented to occur with subcortical, rather than cortical, brain damage as well. Lesions to the left thalamus, for example, have been shown to produce transitory aphasic behavior.

With all of those ground rules in mind, the following major patterns of syndromes can be described.

Table 14.1 summarizes the features of the types of aphasia in terms of a few of the language modalities we discuss.

TABLE 14.1

Basic Language Characteristics of Some Major Syndromes of Aphasia.

Language Form	Wernicke	Anomic	Conduction	Transcortical Sensory	Broca	Transcortical Motor	Global
Conversational speech	Fluent, paraphasic	Fluent, empty	Fluent, paraphasic	Fluent, paraphasic, echolalic	Nonfluent	Nonfluent	Nonfluent
Comprehension of speech	Below normal to poor	Relatively good	Relatively good	Poor to extremely poor	Relatively good	Relatively good	Poor
Repetition	Predictable from comprehension	Good	Not predictable from comprehension, poor	Not predictable from comprehension, good to excellent	Predictable from comprehension, good	Predictable from comprehension, good to excellent	Predictable from comprehension, poor
Confrontation naming	Defective to poor	Defective	Usually defective	Poor	Defective to poor	Defective	Poor
Reading comprehension	Defective to poor	Usually moderately good	Usually good	Defective to poor	Not predictable	Not predictable	Poor
Writing	Poor	Moderately good; abnormal in substantive word finding	Moderately impaired	Poor	Moderately impaired	Moderately impaired	Poor

Fluent Aphasias

Wernicke Aphasia

This type has also been called sensory, syntactic, *and* receptive *aphasia.*

Jargon *here refers to new words composed for the most part of phonologically correct syllables but without apparent meaning and delivered in fluent profusion.*

Although we have already described this syndrome, we need to add further details here. The patient with Wernicke aphasia speaks fairly fluently and often with excessive volubility, referred to by some as "press of speech." The speech of such a patient often lacks clear content and direction; in most severe cases, speech consists almost entirely of neologistic jargon. The uninitiated listener often initially mistakes the hyperfluent output of the Wernicke patient for normal speech; for even in patients whose speech is totally jargon, the prosodic features of the aphasic patient's native language are maintained, and the speaker's jargon observes the sound-combining rules of his native language. He shows reduced ability to comprehend not only the speech of others, but often his own speech as well. In most of the more common types of aphasia, reading and writing abilities are similar to the auditory comprehension and speech patterns upon which they are built. The Wernicke aphasic patient is a good example. Reading is poor, and writing is similar to speech. Handwriting itself is minimally affected, emphasizing that hemiplegia is usually absent in this type of aphasia; however, the writing has no comprehensible content. Its pattern mirrors the patient's speech. Repetition, as you will see below, is often a sensitive diagnostic sign regarding the nature of the aphasic syndrome a given patient is manifesting. In the case of the Wernicke patient, his repetition skills are impaired due to the impairment of auditory comprehension. In fact, the ability to repeat is an interesting first approximation of the extent of the comprehension deficit.

Refer to the first example at the beginning of this chapter to refresh your understanding of Wernicke aphasic speech.

Anomic Aphasia

Anomic aphasia has also been called nominal, semantic, *and* amnesic *aphasia.*

Another of the fluent aphasias is *anomic aphasia.* The anomic aphasic patient's otherwise almost normal language is marred by word-finding difficulties. Auditory comprehension is usually near normal in anomic aphasia, as is reading, but the groping inability to produce substantive words extends to these patients' writing. When the word she is searching for is furnished to the anomic patient, she usually recognizes it immediately. Thus, her repetition can be expected to be better than her spontaneously produced speech. Word retrieval problems that typify anomic aphasia are common to all aphasias, but only in these patients do they contribute the salient symptom. Word-retrieval problems allow speculation about the role of memory in the generation of aphasic problems. While aphasia can hardly be explained as a language-specific memory loss, memory certainly plays a role in aphasia and short-term memory difficulties often coexist with it.

Here is an example of a patient with anomic aphasia. He is describing a busy scene from the stimulus pictures of the Boston Diagnostic Aphasia Examination (Goodglass & Kaplan, 1972), in which a little boy and girl are stealing cookies. The stool they are standing on is about to topple. And their mother serenely washes dishes, oblivious both to the cookie theft and to the fact that her sink is running over.

> This is a boy an that's a . . . thing! (Laughs) An' this is goin' off pretty soon (points to toppling stool). This is a . . . a place that is mostly in (Examiner: "Could you name the room . . . a bathroom?") No . . . kitchen . . . kitchen. An' this is a girl . . . an' that something that they're running an' they've got the water going down here. . . . (Goodglass & Kaplan, 1972, p. 65)

Conduction aphasia is still another fluent aphasia syndrome. Here, comprehension of language is good, but speech is frequently marred by inappropriate words. (These are called *verbal* or *semantic paraphasias*.) Another type of speech error, caused by substituting an incorrect sound in a word, is also found. (These are called *literal* or *phonemic paraphasias*.) In the rare patient with severe conduction aphasia, these errors occur frequently enough to cause the speech to be unintelligible. More typically, since the conduction aphasic patient has good comprehension, his speech is moderately good; but because of his awareness of his own words it is often marked by unsuccessful self-corrective attempts. The hallmark of the conduction aphasic patient is his disproportionate inability to repeat or to make use of verbal cues supplied by others, even though he is quick to recognize the correct word when it is said by another person. In this way, he differs markedly from the anomic patient. Reading and writing are usually somewhat better preserved. The damage responsible for conduction aphasia is generally assumed to be in the subcortical fiber tracts connecting auditory association areas in the temporal lobe to Broca's area frontally. The arcuate fasciculus is the tract most researchers hold responsible.

Here is an example from a conduction aphasic speech. Again, the cookie theft picture is being described.

> Well, this um . . . somebody's . . . a mather is takin the . . . washin' the dayshes an' the water. . . . the water is falling . . . is flowing all over the place, an' the kids sneakin' out in back behind her, takin' the cookies in the . . . out of the top in the . . . what do you call that? (Examiner: "Shelf?") Yes . . . and there's a . . . then the girl . . . not the girl . . . the boy who's getting the cookies is on this ah . . . strool an' startin' to fall off. That's about all I see. (Goodglass & Kaplan, 1972, p. 69)

Transcortical sensory aphasia is the last fluent aphasia we will describe here. It is a rare syndrome, and it usually results from a lesion that isolates the function of the speech areas from input and control from other areas of the cortex. It is much more likely to result from more generalized neurologic diseases than from stroke, and therefore there is some question as to whether it should be included among the aphasias. Transcortical sensory aphasia most closely resembles Wernicke aphasia, except that repetition is intact, even echolalic.

Broca aphasia is by far the most common of the nonfluent aphasias. To recap, it is characterized by scarcity of speech, difficulties in word retrieval, labored and slow rate of speech, and often omission of small, grammatically important words such as *the, is, on*. Comprehension of spoken and written language is much better than speaking. Repetition is marred by the difficulty in talking with fluency, and writing mirrors the speech output. The mechanics of writing also are impaired since most of these patients also have right arm and hand paralysis. Often they must learn to use their left hands for writing.

You might want to reread the second example at the beginning of this chapter to emphasize this important aphasia type.

Sidebar

Conduction Aphasia

This type of aphasia has also been called central *or* afferent motor *aphasia.*

Transcortical Sensory Aphasia

Since the speech is so similar to Wernicke speech, no example is provided.

Nonfluent Aphasias

Broca Aphasia

Broca aphasia is also known as *expressive,* motor, *and* verbal *aphasia.*

This condition is called agrammatism.

Transcortical Motor Aphasia

This type is also referred to as dynamic *aphasia.*

The remaining nonfluent syndrome is *transcortical motor aphasia.* Like its fluent transcortical counterpart, it is probably the result of some form of isolation of the speech areas from surrounding cortex, it is very rare, and it has as its hallmark intact repetition. In this case, however, the excellent repetition is embedded in Broca-like symptoms. Repetition has been documented to be the *only* surviving speaking skill in the extreme case. It also occurs in general damage more frequently than in focal lesions and, as such, is questionably included in aphasia *per se.*

Since the speech is Broca-like, no example is given here.

Mixed and Global Aphasia

It is not unusual for the aphasia-producing lesion to encompass both the anterior and posterior speech areas. The result is likely to be a mixed or global aphasia. The distinction between mixed and global aphasia is a practical one, typically made on the basis of the severity of the presenting problem. Mixed aphasia usually refers to patients whose problems involve both comprehension and production, but are less severe; global aphasic patients are the more severely impaired. Global aphasia produces the scarcity of speech typical of nonfluent aphasia and the difficulties with comprehension typical of the Wernicke patient. Often, globally aphasic patients have only a few utterances available to them, which are both appropriately and inappropriately used. These are called *stereotypys,* but if they are an often-repeated nonsense word, they are sometimes called *neologisms.* We know a global aphasic person whose entire verbal repertoire was "weema-jeema." Both reading and writing are seriously compromised, and repetition capability is poor. Global aphasia is generally considered to be the most severely debilitating of the common aphasic syndromes. Unfortunately, it is also the most common.

MECHANISMS OF APHASIA

Let us turn now to the manner in which a person might become aphasic. We have been using the term *lesion* frequently in this chapter. A lesion here is an injury that leaves an area of cortical tissue incapable of functioning in its normal way. Tissues may be destroyed directly, as in the case of a wound by a penetrating missile such as a bullet. They may be rendered incapable of functioning because other tissues push upon them and distort them in some way, as when a tumor grows into or displaces the brain. And tissue may die as the result of an infectious process, or of being denied the nourishment necessary to its healthy function, usually by interruption of the blood supply.

We mentioned earlier that stroke is by far the most common cause of aphasia. *Stroke* is the term used by physicians to describe the abnormal neurologic function that occurs when a brain artery is blocked and the area of brain it nourished is destroyed. Figure 14.2 shows the arteries that feed the left cerebral hemisphere. Note especially the area supplied by the middle cerebral artery. Because its territory encompasses the speech areas we have been talking about, it is easy to see that problems with this artery are frequently responsible for aphasia-producing strokes.

This condition is called arteriosclerosis, *or hardening of the arteries.*

Strokes are of three basic types: (*a*) thrombotic, (*b*) embolic, and (*c*) hemorrhagic. In thrombotic strokes, a build-up of plaque blocks a vessel, which then thromboses (clots). An embolic stroke results when a clot or thrombosis forms elsewhere, as in the heart or the great vessels of the chest or neck, and

FIGURE 14.2
Vascular System of the Brain.

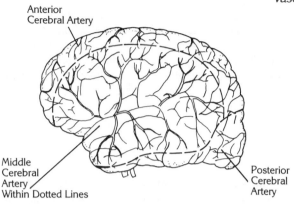

breaks off to become an embolus that may then be carried to a brain artery. Such an embolus often arises from a location in the carotid artery in the neck—a site predisposed to blockage and embolus formation. Since the basic processes are the same, the term *thromboembolic stroke* is sometimes used to describe these two types. Hemorrhages are different. Arterial walls, weakened by the effects of high blood pressure or losing elasticity due to aging, occasionally burst under pressure. The blood rips into the brain tissue, dissecting it and causing intense inflammation and swelling.

Another cause for hemorrhage that is less common but that may occur in young adults as well as in older individuals is the rupture of saccular ("berry") aneurysms. These are blister-like balloonings of arteries occurring at vessel branch points. They develop through early adult life. When aneurysms rupture, they often bleed into the fluid-filled subarachnoid space surrounding the surfaces of the brain. Although bleeding into this space may damage the brain or even cause death, it is only when the bleeding is directly into the brain tissue itself that characteristic stroke syndromes like aphasia are likely. A well-publicized example of this disorder is the illness suffered by the movie actress Patricia Neal. Even less common, but noteworthy because of the ability to produce hemorrhagic stroke, is bleeding into the brain from abnormal arterial and venous tangles of vessels occasionally present from birth—called an *arteriovenous malformation.*

You may well ask why localized rather than more general damage to the brain occurs in the stroke process. Shouldn't the whole cortex, beyond the point of disruption, be affected by arterial occlusion? You can answer this question by referring again to Figure 14.2. Note the rich intertwining of the vascular tree and the possibilities it affords for developing secondary vascular pathways. The complexity of the vascular network also helps to explain the differences in both extent and severity of damage and the variability of symptoms we find in aphasic patients. Part of this variability is due to the effectiveness with which alternative routes are found for supplying an individual's cortex with its blood supply.

At the beginning of this section, we mentioned other causes for aphasia, including trauma to the head and tumors. While damage to the speech areas by injury can certainly occur, and tumors can grow in such a way as to put pressure directly on the speech areas, it is quite likely in these cases that other cortical areas are also damaged. In the cases of progressive neurologic disorders and infectious disease, more generalized cortical involvement is the most typical result. Thus, while aphasic symptoms frequently are found in these conditions, many other changes in cortical function are almost always present as well. Describing the head-injured or postencephalitic person as "aphasic" is often likely to be rather inaccurate; disturbances in language complicated by generalized brain damage often produce far more encompassing and difficult clinical problems than does aphasia occurring as the result of a focal brain lesion.

THE APHASIC PERSON

We are roughly halfway through this chapter and only now are we in a position to begin to discuss the person who has aphasia. This illustrates a problem in the larger aphasia literature as well. Because there is so much to be learned about language by describing its breakdown, and so many provocative aspects of the relationships between brain and cognition that can be productively studied by the study of aphasia itself, the literature dealing with the person who becomes aphasic and the effects of it upon his and his family's life is sparse by comparison. The result is that we know a great deal more about aphasia than we do about aphasic people.

At the beginning of our courses in aphasia, it has been our practice to ask students to describe the way they would feel if injury or illness rendered them aphasic tomorrow. Frequently, the students attempt to displace the problem in time to some future date, to when they are older. This rather straightforwardly suggests that our students (like their teachers) have some fear of the problem, and some real difficulty accepting the premises of the classroom exercise. Sent back to the task, the expected descriptions begin to emerge. Commonly listed words include *afraid, frustrated, angry, anxious, depressed, crazy, stupid, useless.* The list goes on, but almost totally in the same vein, never cheerier than perhaps the wistful word *challenged.*

We believe the students do a good job both in their initial reticence and in their final listings of describing the ways aphasic patients themselves feel in the aftermath of stroke. Once they have discovered their own survival, the devastating effects of aphasia begin to emerge and to be experienced.

Our most precious skill, often unappreciated and simply taken for granted, is our ability to communicate our needs and wants to others, our power to affect our world with words, which are our major avenue for presenting ourselves to others. When these skills are suddenly withdrawn or limited to some degree, not only does a person become powerless in his own terms, but his very self-concept is threatened and/or seriously compromised. It is important to understand these reactions to the language problem. Even though they may, in fact often do, lessen to some degree as time passes and adjustments are made, and as gains are made toward reaching normal function again, they are a formidable part of the aphasic profile and must be dealt with in therapeutic encounters.

In addition to the patient's reaction to the language loss, there are other factors to contend with in the aftermath of stroke. We have already mentioned the likelihood of sensory and motor problems, hemianopsia and hemiplegia, respectively. Particularly in the case of hemiplegia, a patient's loss of mobility may pose a huge deterrent to a return to normal life. Even the patient who escapes aphasia, but must learn to contend with living in a wheelchair, or using a cane and leg brace, or finding himself only able to awkwardly use his left hand for eating, dressing, or writing faces some amount of depression and fear.

Brain damage itself often subtly changes some aspects of a person's cognition, regardless of the presence of aphasia. Included in these changes are some tendencies to think more concretely—that is, more literally—than previously (reflecting a subtle loss of abstract thinking skills), to engage in perseverative behaviors, to be more sensitive to emotional events than previously, to lose some initiative, and at the same time to be less inhibited. Among other brain-damage effects are the possibility that the asphasic patient may exhibit some **agnosia,** or loss of ability to perceive and integrate incoming stimuli, or to demonstrate **apraxia,** a loss of ability in programming, planning, sequencing, and initiating motor behaviors.

A special difficulty is apraxia of speech, which was described in detail in chapter 12.

There is much speculation but little hard information concerning the overall effects of aphasia on a person's personality. It has been our experience that aphasia does not produce basic personality changes. Rather, the effect of the disorder is to emphasize, to heighten a person's cognitive and social style. Perhaps this is due to the previously mentioned loss of inhibition. Whatever the explanation, there are few deficits of human function in which the full display of differences of personality and of coping mechanisms are so clearly seen in aphasic patients.

We have increasingly been learning to view aphasia as a family's, rather than just an individual's, problem. The adjectives used to describe the person's reaction may well apply to the family as well. Aphasia takes its toll not only on the patient himself, but on those around him, primarily because it seriously upsets the family's sense of balance and requires a restructuring of familiar family roles. Financial changes and role reassignments may be the most obvious, but other social roles are affected as well. Webster and Larkins (1979) report four family problems to be paramount. They are: (*a*) the nonaphasic spouse has no time alone, (*b*) finances, (*c*) getting used to the new roles that aphasia creates for both spouses, and finally (*d*) finding ways to deal with the issue of dependence/independence for the aphasic spouse. In addition, guilt for the striken member's becoming aphasic is the most frequently asserted reaction by family members. A crucial aspect of rehabilitation involves helping the family not only to work through their feelings about the problem, but mobilizing other members of the helping community to help the family in the restructuring and role changes that may be required in the wake of aphasia.

Finally, for both the aphasic patient and the family, it is important to remember that aphasia does not occur only to previously well-adjusted people and families. It occurs to people who have the same chances as the rest of us for having unresolved personal, financial, social, and family problems (to name a few). And aphasia cures none of them. It merely adds another solemn dimension to them.

We have, to this point, been almost inadvertently stressing the darker side of aphasia. There is a brighter side as well. We find work with aphasic patients and their families is among the most rewarding of clinical speech-language pathology activities. In these encounters you have an almost constant awareness of the indomitability of the human spirit. Aphasic patients, if their earliest reactions are worked through successfully, often have a tenacity for solving their problems that exposes the clinician to the basic strength and ability to rise to challenge that dignifies us all.

Perhaps the best summary of this can be found in the words of the husband of a remarkable aphasic woman.

> When she first got her problem, we (the family) were really scared and we all helped out too much. Then we got angry at her because she needed the help. We finally worked all of that out, due to her. I really didn't know who I was married to until E. became aphasic. I thought I had a nice, passive, typical housewife on my hands. Instead, I have this tough, gutsy, talented, independent woman. It's not at all bad.

Seven years after her stroke, this woman is still experiencing a moderate degree of Broca aphasia. Her right hand is useless. She has only recently been able to walk without a leg brace, and she still uses a cane. But she is a mover in the local stroke club, she has learned to paint with her left hand, and she has had numerous, critically successful, one-woman shows. Her social life is active, and she runs her three-child household as well as ever. Her rehabilitation is a success story, brought about not only by her, but by her family's frontal attack on aphasia.

THE NATURAL RECOVERY PROCESS IN APHASIA

Immediately following the event which produces the aphasia, the aphasic person's language, along with other neurological dysfunction, is at its worst. Of course, this is related to the severity of the event and to the extent of the cortical damage it has produced. Within a few days, however, the natural recovery process gets underway. Swelling begins to reduce, and some injured cells begin to function more normally again, although damaged brain cells never completely recover. A clearer picture of the residual damage begins to emerge. Nonetheless, in the early few weeks after damage, it is difficult to predict the course and the degree of a given patient's recovery.

The natural recovery is influenced by a number of factors, including age, the extent of damage, the location of the damage, general physical condition, and to some extent the quality of care a patient receives. In spite of these uncertainties, we may be sure that a repair process continues no less than 3 to 6 months, sometimes even longer, and with it the expectation of improvement of the aphasic deficit. This naturally occurring improvement is called *spontaneous recovery*. It is most rapid soon after onset of brain damage, and as time progresses the rate of change slows down. It occurs not only for speech and language, but for motor impairment as well.

During the period of spontaneous recovery, the greatest gains are usually seen in auditory comprehension (Kertesz & McCabe, 1977). The whole presenting syndrome, however, may evolve into another, usually milder, form. The most likely expectation of evolution is with global aphasia, which may evolve into any of the other types.

Although there is some controversy over just how long the period of spontaneous recovery may continue, it is generally agreed that the greatest change occurs in the first 3 months. The degree to which it continues for a longer period of time is likely to depend on a variety of individual factors.

There is also controversy over the optimal time to begin intervention. This particular concern impinges upon the matter of the efficacy of treatment. Because in most cases aphasia is the most resistant of the patient's problems to improvement, it is difficult to determine whether improvement is the result of the intervention or of spontaneous recovery alone. At the least, it is problematical to attack the question of just how much of the gains are related either to the natural process or treatment. Some authorities argue that, until we know more about the so-called contaminating effects of spontaneous recovery, intervention should wait for a period of time. In that way, we could separate the contributing effects and make clearer statements about both unaided and aided recovery.

Other authorities, bowing to the complexity of the problem, suggest that the greatest therapeutic gains can be accomplished when the patient is improving anyway and that the question of efficacy of treatment must be answered by other means. Therefore, they suggest early intervention. We have no clear scientific evidence to suggest whether early intervention is preferred or whether it should be deferred until after spontaneous recovery has occurred. It seems logical that a patient's individual condition should determine when to initiate direct treatment. Patients who are responsive to their environments are probably good candidates for treatment. However, counseling of both patient and family by trained counselors concerning some of the psychosocial effects we have just looked at should probably be undertaken as soon as possible following onset.

The bulk of our direct intervention strategies have been designed for working with the *chronically* aphasic patient, that is, the patient whose spontaneous recovery process has reached a plateau. We shall discuss therapy for these patients next.

THE ASSISTED RECOVERY PROCESS IN APHASIA

Successful rehabilitation of the aphasic patient is essentially an interdisciplinary endeavor, requiring cooperative effort between a number of medical and paramedical specialists. The optimal team includes a neurologist, a psychiatrist, a physiatrist, physical and occupational therapists, a neuropsychologist, a social worker, and a speech-language pathologist. Although what follows describes langauge evaluation and treatment, the context for aphasia rehabilitation is one of interdisciplinary interaction.

A physiatrist is a physician who specializes in rehabilitation by prescribing physical therapy.

Evaluation

Before undertaking treatment, the speech-language pathologist should conduct a detailed evaluation. Some aphasic patients, notably those with severe global aphasias or whose aphasias coexist with other problems such as severe confusion or serious medical problems, are not good candidates for rehabilitation. The first goal of evaluation, therefore, is to determine if clinical intervention is feasible. The case history is one of the most important features of the evaluation, but more direct assessment of language is also critical. This direct assessment includes detailed analysis of the aphasic patient's language performance, aimed at defining and describing the type of aphasia the patient has and measuring the extent of auditory comprehension and/or motor programming deficits. It also includes identification of other disorders, such as apraxia of speech, that can appear along with aphasia.

See chapter 12.

The formality of the initial evaluation will be directly related to how long after brain damage the evaluation is made. Early evaluation tends to be less structured, and often assessment is unobtrusive and heavily reliant upon observation. After the aphasic patient's condition has become stabilized, observation is supplemented with formal tests of language ability, comprehension of speech, reading, and writing. Among the tests most widely used today by speech-language pathologists are the *Porch Index of Communicative Ability* (PICA) (Porch, 1967), the *Boston Diagnostic Aphasia Examination* (BDAE) (Goodglass & Kaplan, 1972), and the *Minnesota Test of Differential Diagnosis of Aphasia* (MTDDA) (Schuell, 1965), although many other tests are available. Darley (1979), for example, has included reviews of 15 tests in his handbook of tests.

These tests share a number of features. All sample a range of language behaviors, including reading and writing. All attempt, either by the nature of the stimuli or by the way a response is to be scored or interpreted, to disentangle what might be causing a particular patient to have difficulty with a given language task. For example, from the syndromes we have described earlier, you can tell that it is important to know if a patient does not supply the appropriate label for a fork because he is unable to retrieve it or because he does not comprehend the question he has been asked. And this is only the smallest of examples.

Different tests also measure language somewhat differently, and often carry with them a bias about many of the controversies we have discussed earlier. The BDAE, for example, is used not only to gain a detailed description of language behavior, but to profile the various syndromes. Neither the PICA nor the MTDDA makes distinctions as to type of aphasia. The PICA, further, attempts to quantify prediction for recovery, a matter addressed by no other test. Finally, some measures, like the measure of *Communicative Ability in Daily Living* (CADL) (Holland, 1980) and the *Functional Communication Profile* (FCP) (Sarno, 1969), are not really interested in language behavior at all, but in how a patient gets along communicatively in his daily life. Whatever tests a speech-language pathologist might decide to use, therefore, not only reflect his or her beliefs about what aspects of the problem are worth describing but, to some degree, direct the course of treatment. While many of the decisions involved in appropriate disposition of the treatment depend on the evaluation, it is important to point out that the supportive counseling we have been talking about should be initiated at the time of first evaluation.

Treatment

Treatment for aphasic patients, as it is presently practiced in the United States, had its real beginning during World War II, and is thus a relatively new field. The impetus, of course, was the large number of head-injured military survivors of that war. One of the most important books about aided recovery, still extremely influential in terms of present treatment procedures, is Wepman's (1951) careful description of that intensive rehabilitation process and his scientific evaluation of it. Wepman's, as well as others', early efforts developed for American aphasiology a model of treatment and evaluation which has continued to typify rehabilitation efforts in aphasia.

All of the evaluation information is brought into play in determining the exact nature of clinical intervention, as well as its goals. Dictated in large measure by the extent of the deficit uncovered by formal evaluation, other aspects of the patient's life-style, motivation, medical needs, and so on are also important in planning rehabilitation. It should be clear that both techniques and goals for treatment will differ for a global aphasic patient and for a patient whose residual language deficits are very minimal. However, in even those extreme cases, the goals and plans will be influenced by the nonlanguage factors. In the ideal case, goals are made clear, set, and mutually agreed upon by the aphasic patient, his family, and the speech-language pathologist.

There are many approaches to rehabilitating the aphasic adult. Most are outgrowths of the speech-language pathologist's theoretical position regarding how best to effect recovery. One class of techniques stresses that the patient is best served by concentrating clinical activities on underlying processes such as memory or auditory comprehension skills. The techniques for improving memory generally reflect Luria's beliefs about rehabilitation following brain damage (1970), and those for auditory skills come from Schuell's beliefs that auditory skills are the foundation upon which aphasia rehabilitation should rest. No one can tell what actually happens to the brain as it begins to use language again. Nonetheless, Luria hypothesized that to regain function it is necessary to lead the cortex into reorganizing itself, to develop new pathways for receiving and acting upon stimuli. One way to reorganize the cortex is through practice with a number of cross-modal activities, for example, involving tactile sensation in reading by having the patient trace letters in sand or other rough material. Schuell hypothesized that "reauditorization"—building sound organization internally—was a key deficit in aphasia, and consistently invoked the auditory modality in clinical activities to retrain the ability to reauditorize. "Deblocking"—that is, using the patient's most intact language modality to trigger his use of others (Weigl, 1970)—is still another example of attempting to reorganize the cortex.

This approach is an application of the developmental or process approaches we have seen used to deal with other disorders.

Still in this vein of dealing with the underlying process, some clinical techniques have been devised to involve the right hemisphere in the language activities we have previously ascribed to the left hemisphere. Melodic intonation therapy (Sparks, Helm, & Albert, 1974) is an excellent example. In this approach, the aphasic patient's usually unimpaired ability to sing or to intone is capitalized upon. The patient, usually one with Broca aphasia, is taught first to intone words and phrases systematically. The intonation is then gradually faded and supplanted by nonintoned word and phrase production; finally, these words are incorporated into contextual speech. Another right hemispheric technique is the use of visual imagery and training in its application to word finding.

It is worth repeating that we do not know how the brain capitalizes on the activities provided to the patient. A different school of thought regarding that issue is that the damaged brain, still capable of learning, must be taught again what has been lost. The principles of learning are thus applied to the process of aphasia therapy. The language act is dissected into its component parts and then hierarchically arranged. Systematic practice, using appropriate contingencies of reinforcement, is invoked to retrain areas of deficit. Simultaneously, components of language left relatively intact by aphasia are sought for, and their use is reinforced.

This is, of course, the application of the learning theory approaches.

LaPointe (1978) provides many examples of how different components of language behavior are shaped in conjunction with the use of behavioral management principles. By using a carefully constructed record-keeping system, which he calls *Base-10 programming,* he charts the target behaviors, stimuli used to evoke those behaviors, the reinforcement contingency, and the patient's responses to the stimuli on repeated presentations. Thus, he provides both patient and speech-language pathologist with an on-going record of progress. Illustrative tasks include writing to dictation, generating sentences, reading printed commands, and verbal responses to functional questions. In all these cases, positive changes over time are also reported.

Review chapter 13 for more on nonspeech systems.

A third major approach contains within it the bias that brain damage, by and large, remains invariant. Solutions to communication problems, therefore, must involve reliance upon alternative strategies and still-intact cerebral mechanisms. Particularly where speech itself is most seriously compromised, nonspeech communication systems, such as communication boards of AMERIND (American Indian) sign, may be used. Patients are often taught systematically to use alternative communication strategies. In this approach, whatever helps the patient to comprehend (for example, repeats of messages) or to communicate expressively (for example, combining speech attempts with gesture) is sought. Once found, they are explained to the patient, who is then required by the speech-language pathologist to use them. PACE (an acronym for *Promoting Aphasic Communication Effectiveness*) (Wilcox & Davis, in press) is yet another of these functional approaches. Using a situation which is a controlled analogue to the give-and-take of natural communication, in which previously unknown requests and responses are exchanged, the aphasic patient is required to test out the effectiveness of a variety of his communicative attempts, from gesture to writing. Effectiveness in PACE is meant to be getting a message across, not necessarily talking. The patient is then trained to use the most effective of his communication strategies.

The thoroughly trained and sensitive speech-language pathologist knows a variety of these techniques, and often applies more than one to the effective treatment of a given aphasic patient. In the ideal case, direct treatment is always used in conjunction with patient and family counseling. One important goal of the counseling, in addition to its psychosocial adjustment goals, is to help the family communicate with the patient and to further the advances made in the clinic by involving the family in daily practice outside the treatment room.

No one really knows the best schedule for direct aphasia treatment, nor really how long it should continue. We believe that the patient's overall condition, his progress in therapy, and his communicated feelings about the usefulness of therapy should all contribute to individual decisions in these matters. We also believe that intensive treatment, that is, frequent clinical sessions, is probably more useful than even the same number of sessions spread over a longer period of time.

In addition to individual sessions, the ideal treatment plan should include group sessions as well. Sometimes these groups sessions are used to practice and gain experience with some of the skills developed in individual sessions. These sessions also give the aphasic patient an opportunity to exchange his feelings with other people who are experiencing similar problems, and to provide an opportunity to help other people in the group with their difficulties—not a small benefit to all the patients' rehabilitation. In a similar vein, we have found family groups to be an extremely effective way for working through many of the family adjustment problems we have described earlier.

We have briefly summarized some of the ways speech-language pathologists assist aphasic patients to maximize their potential for language recovery. In the process, it is possible that you might be concluding that it is a relatively clear-cut and simple matter for the aphasic patient to regain her former language proficiency. This could not be farther from the truth. The treatment of aphasia is, indeed, often successful in helping the aphasic patient to improve her language abilities, but total recovery of language function is a rarity. Moreover, it is difficult and often highly emotional work for both professional and patient. With all these strikes against it, it may surprise you to read that we believe it to be the most satisfying of clinical work in the discipline. This is because it is always surprising, constantly challenging, and an unwavering reminder of human resiliency.

Arthur Kopit, in the preface to his remarkable play *Wings* (1978), which explores what the inner world of the aphasic patient might contain, eloquently describes it:

> I had met the older woman while accompanying my father one afternoon on his rounds. When he went down for speech therapy, she was one of the three other patients in the room. I had never observed a speech therapy session before and was nervous. The day, I recall vividly, was warm, humid. The windows of the room were open. A scent of flowers suffused the air. To get the session started, the therapist asked the older woman if she could name the seasons of the year. With much effort, she did, though not in proper order. She seemed annoyed with herself for having any difficulty at all with such a task. The therapist then asked her which of these seasons corresponded to the present. The woman turned at once to the window. She could see the garden, the flowers. Her eyes were clear, alert; there was no question but that she understood what was wanted. I cannot remember having ever witnessed such an intense struggle. At first, she did nothing but sit calmly and wait for the word to arrive on its own. When it didn't, she tried to force the word out by herself, through thinking; as if to assist what clearly was a process of expulsion, she scrunched her face up, squeezed her eyelids shut. But no word emerged. Physically drained, her face drenched with sweat, she tried another trick; she cocked her head and listened to the birds, whose sound was incessant. When this too led to nothing, she sniffed the air. When nothing came of this strategy either, she turned her attention to what she was wearing, a light cotton dress; she even touched the fabric. Finally, something connected. Her lips began to form a word. She shut her eyes. Waited. The word emerged. WINTER.
>
> When informed that it was summer she seemed astonished, how was it possible? . . . a mistake like that . . . obviously she knew what season it was, anyone with eyes could tell at once what season it was! . . . and yet . . She looked over at where I sat and shook her head in dismay, then laughed and said, "This is really nuts, isn't it!"
>
> I sat there, stunned. I could not believe that anyone making a mistake of such gross proportions and with such catastrophic implications could laugh at it.
>
> So there would be no misunderstanding, the therapist quickly pointed out that this mistake was stemmed completely from her stroke; in no way was she demented. The woman smiled (she knew all that) and turned away, stared back out the window at the garden. This is really nuts, isn't it!—I could not get her phrase from my mind. In its intonation, it had conveyed no feeling of anger, resignation, or despair. Rather it conveyed amazement, and in that amazement, a trace (incredible as it seemed) of delight. This is not to suggest that anyone witnessing this incident could, even for an instant, have imagined that she was in any sense pleased with her condition. The amazement, and its concomitant delight, seemed to me to reflect only an acknowledgement that her condition was extraordinary, and in no way denied or obviated the terror or the horror that were at its core. By some (I supposed) nourishing spring of inner strength and light, of whose source I had no idea, she had come to a station in her life from which she could perceive in what was happening something that bore the aspect of adventure, and it was through this perhaps innate capacity to perceive and appreciate adventure, and perhaps in this sense only, that she found some remaining modicum of delight, which I suspect kept her going. (pp. ix-xi)

Efficacy of Treatment

We have briefly touched upon the issue of the value of aphasia therapy. Perhaps because of the interdisciplinary context in which treatment is conducted, as well as the frequency with which third-party payment is used to finance treatment, the speech-language pathologist who works with aphasic people must take the matter of efficacy of treatment very seriously. As a result, the discipline has developed a stronger literature related to the issue of accountability than we find with most speech problems. It seems worth summarizing here.

The problem inherent in developing a single, thorough, adequately controlled study of the effectiveness of aphasia rehabilitiation are great, possibly even insurmountable. They involve statistical issues, such as adequate sample size; ethical questions, such as the justification for withholding treatment; and problems with controlling the multitude of variables presumed to influence recovery from aphasia. These include age, initial severity of the aphasia, the role of spontaneous recovery, and type and frequency of treatment. A *Lancet* editorial recently discussed these problems in assessing recovery from aphasia and concluded that, until more is known about aphasia itself, investigations of treatment should concentrate on small, well-defined studies comparing one mode with another (1977). Of the more than 20 presently available studies regarding the effectiveness of treatment, the clear majority conclude that treatment has a positive effect on recovery from aphasia (Darley, 1972, 1975).

The most impressive evidence for the effectiveness of treatment, however, comes from two recent studies, that of Wertz et al. (1978) and that of Basso, Capitani, and Vignolo (1979). Wertz' well-designed and tightly controlled study compares the effectiveness of 1 year of individual versus group treatment for a large number of aphasic patients carefully screened to approximate the normal distribution of poststroke aphasias at five VA hospitals. The results of that study showed patients receiving either of the two types of treatment to have made significant gains in language ability as measured by *Porch Index of Communicative Ability* (Porch, 1967). The few significant differences between treatment groups that did occur all favored individual over group treatment.

The Basso study involved 271 patients, roughly divided among those treated and not treated. Treated patients made significantly more gains, as measured by a series of tests for aphasia, than did the untreated group. This study, however, illustrates some of the difficulties in control alluded to above. Control patients in this Italian study were self-selected. That is, patients who comprised the control group were patients who were offered treatment but could not or would not take advantage of the offer. Thus, the possibility of bias in group assignment remains. D. Frank Benson, in reviewing the Basso, et al. study, concludes.:

> The findings of this Italian study . . . strongly suggest that therapy does affect recovery from aphasia. How much of the improvement stems from the psychic support offered by the therapy program and how much is due to actual language training techniques remains unknown. While this study may have technical deficiencies (for the epidemiologist/statistician), it is so large, has sufficiently definite results and would be so difficult to improve upon that it commands respect. It would appear more fruitful to focus future efforts on improving therapy techniques rather than on additional statistical refinements of the treatment:no-treatment comparison. (1979, p. 182)

ACQUIRED APHASIA IN CHILDREN

Other chapters in this book address the matter of developmental language disorders in children. And to this point, we have dealt here only with adults. Children who have developed and who are in the process of developing language normally also can acquire aphasia. If the term *aphasia* is applied to children, it is almost invariably preceded by a modifier such as *childhood* or *developmental*. As we describe children below, we will also modify the term. This time the modifier is *acquired*. Thus, children who *become* aphasic, rather than fail to develop language, have a condition referred to as *acquired aphasia*.

See chapter 8 also.

Acquired aphasia results from the same causes as does aphasia in adults, although by far the most common cause is head injury, rather than stroke. Stroke is exceedingly rare in children; however, Black children who suffer sickle cell disease contribute a disproportionate percentage to the child stroke population. In children, head injury induced aphasia, as well as aphasia resulting from neurologic diseases such as encephalitis, potentially can produce the same types of generalized defects in memory and cognition that we have cautioned against in regard to adults. Psychiatric disorders often follow as well.

However, there are some striking differences between acquired aphasia in children and in adults. Two of these differences, symptom pattern and recovery pattern, are of particular significance and will be covered next.

Symptom Pattern

Rather than showing the wide variation in type of language deficits we have described earlier, it appears that some smaller numbers of patterns predominate in children. Typically, once children have recovered consciousness, their former level of ability to comprehend language returns rather rapidly, with their ability to speak lagging far behind. It is not uncommon for a child to remain mute for some time, after comprehension of speech appropriate to his or her age has begun to be re-established. If the child was a reader before the trauma, level-appropriate reading may also begin to return before speech. Often initial speech attempts are apractic; as this evolves, word-finding difficulties are apparent. Therefore, the patterns we have earlier described as Broca aphasia and anomic aphasia are typical of the problems encountered by children who become aphasic.

Recovery

The second major difference has to do with recovery rate. Children appear to recover language both more rapidly and more extensively than do adults. Obviously this is affected by the severity of the initial injury, but if it were possible to compare recovery in two identical injuries, one occurring in a child and the other in an adult, it would be a safe prediction that the child would show the greatest speed and extent of recovery.

The reasons for this difference are not entirely clear, but most authorities believe that the child's brain is more plastic than the adult's. That is, children's brains are less "set in their ways" than are adults' brains; they are more capable of developing alternative routes for transmission of neural messages.

We must emphasize that actually very little is known about acquired aphasias in children, and that like everything else in this chapter, we have more questions than answers. Even the two generalizations above have enough exceptions to make them tentative. For example, some children, particularly those with seizure disorders which only become apparent after the onset of language, often have profound and unremitting disorders of auditory comprehension. For another example, even though some children appear to recover language fully, subtle learning deficits, particularly as they relate to language-based skills such as reading, plague these children when they return to school.

Diagnosis and Treatment

The diagnosis and treatment of acquired aphasia in children presents one of the strongest examples of cooperative effort in speech-language pathology. The medical and paramedical specialists we have already listed as part of the interdisciplinary team retain their importance in diagnosis and treatment of the child who has acquired aphasia. But some additional disciplines must be involved, including educational specialists and child developmentalists. More striking is the fact that diagnosing and treating children with acquired aphasia requires the *intradisciplinary* cooperation of the specialist in adult language disorders with those fellow professionals who specialize in language acquisition in children. To determine if a child's language "errors" are manifestations of his level of syntactic and lexical development (that is, age-appropriate) or if they represent deviations from the normal brought on by brain damage, you must know a great deal about processes and stages in normal language acquisitions. Only a few adult language specialists remain expert enough in child language to accomplish this diagnostic process alone; similarly, only an occasional child language specialist is well-enough trained in the effects of brain damage occurring after birth to accomplish the same end. Thus, both child and adult language specialists cooperate in diagnosis of acquired aphasia in children.

Their work has been described in chapters 8 and 9.

Because many aphasic children recover quite rapidly, often the speech-language pathologist's role is minimal. For children who recover well enough to return to school, the treatment required can usually be handled adequately by speech professionals who work in the schools. Often the learning disability specialist is part of this public school team.

For the unfortunate minority of head-injured children who have extensive residual problems, intensive and integrated interdisciplinary rehabilitation centers or special schools become the appropriate placement. In such settings restitution of linguistic, cognitive, and physical skills is the primary goal.

CONCLUSION

In this chapter we have tried to introduce you to the problem of aphasia in both its academic and practical aspects. No attempt has been made to gloss over how very much is unknown about aphasia. We hope that, in the process, you might be challenged by the mysteries and complexities of aphasia, as well as becoming more sensitive to people who risk losing some part of themselves in losing some part of their language.

SELECTED READINGS

Darley, F. L. *Evaluation of appraisal techniques in spech and language pathology.* Reading, Mass.: Addison-Wesley, 1979.

Gardner, H. *The shattered mind.* New York: Knopf, 1975.

LaPointe, L. L. Aphasia therapy: Some principles and strategies for treatment. In D. Johns (Ed.), *Clinical management of neurogenic communicative disorders.* Boston: Little, Brown, 1978.

Wepman, J. M. *Recovery from aphasia.* New York: Ronald Press, 1951.

Wertz, R., et al. *Language rehabilitation in aphasia: An examination of the process and its effects.* Final report, Veterans Administration Cooperative Study, 1978.

REFERENCES

Basso, A., Capitani, E., & Vignolo, L. Influence of rehabilitation on language skills in aphasic patients. *Archives of Neurology,* 1979, *36,* 190–196.

Benson, D. F. *Aphasia, alexia, apraxia.* New York: Churchill Livingstone, 1979.

Benson, D. F., & Geschwind, N. The aphasias and related disturbances. In A. B. Baker & L. H. Baker (Eds.), *Clinical neurology* (Vol. 1). Hagerstown, Md.: Harper & Row, 1976.

Bogen, J. Unpublished address, Academy of Aphasia, 1977.

Darley, F. Efficacy of language rehabilitation in aphasia. *Journal of Speech and Hearing Disorders,* 1972, *37,* 3–21.

Darley, F. Treatment of acquired aphasia. In W. Friedlander (Ed.), *Advances in neurology, Vol 6: Current review of higher nervous system dysfunction.* New York: Raven Press, 1975.

Darley, F. L. *Evaluation of appraisal techniques in speech and language pathology.* Reading, Mass.: Addison-Wesley, 1979.

Editorial: Prognosis in aphasia. *Lancet,* 1977, *2,* 24.

Gardner, H. *The shattered mind.* New York: Knopf, 1975.

Goodglass, H., & Kaplan, E. *Boston Diagnostic Aphasia Examination.* Philadelphia: Lea & Febiger, 1972.

Holland, A. *Communicative Abilities in Daily Living: A Test of Functional Communication for Aphasic Adults.* Baltimore: University Park Press, 1980.

Kertesz, A., & McCabe, P. Recovery patterns and prognosis in aphasia. *Archives of Neurology,* 1977, *34,* 590–601.

Kopit, A. *Wings.* New York: Hill & Wang, 1978.

LaPointe, L. L. Aphasia therapy: Some principles and strategies for treatment. In D. Johns (Ed.), *Clinical management of neurogenic communicative disorders.* Boston: Little, Brown, 1978.

Luria, A. *Traumatic aphasia.* The Hague: Mouton, 1970.

Penfield, W., & Roberts, L. *Speech and brain mechanisms.* Princeton, N.J.: Princeton University Press, 1959.

Porch, B. E. *Porch Index of Communicative Ability.* Palo Alto, Calif.: Consulting Psychologists Press, 1967.

Sarno, M. T. *The Functional Communication Profile.* New York: New York University Medical Center, Institute of Rehabilitation Medicine, 1969.

Schuell, H. M. *The Minnesota Test for Differential Diagnosis of Aphasia.* Minneapolis: University of Minnesota Press, 1965.

Sparks, R., Helm, N., & Albert, M. Aphasia rehabilitation resulting from melodic intonation therapy. *Cortex,* 1974, *10,* 303–310.

Webster, E., & Larkins, P. *Counseling aphasic families.* Videotape lecture, 1979.

Weigl, E. Neuropsychological studies of structure and dynamics of semantic fields with the deblocking methods. In A. T. Greimes et al. (Eds.), *Sign, language, culture.* The Hague: Mouton, 1970.

Wepman, J. M. *Recovery from aphasia.* New York: Ronald Press, 1951.

Wertz, R., et al. *Language rehabilitation in aphasia: An examination of the process and its effects.* Final report, Veterans Administration Cooperative Study, 1978.

Wilcox, M. J. & Davis, G. A. Promoting aphasics' communicative effectiveness (PACE): A treatment program. *Journal of Speech & Hearing Disorders,* in press.

THE CLINICAL PROCESS AND THE SPEECH-LANGUAGE PATHOLOGIST

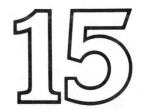

Albert T. Murphy

During several days before I began this chapter, I became increasingly aware of my feelings about the subject, the clinical process in speech-language pathology and audiology. I finally recognized a feeling of celebration for the life of the speech-language pathologist in clinical practice. I was momentarily, though pleasantly, surprised. I could not deny the feeling of wanting to salute speech-language pathologists because of the tasks they perform, tasks as caring individuals committed to helping people communicate. As we have stressed throughout this book, there are few more important human adventures.

The need for self-expression may not be as fundamental as the need for water, air, food, and sex, but it could be called the fifth need. Communicating with others helps us find the differences between us and understand ourselves. We are the talking and writing animals. The impulse to communicate is so strong that it can help people conquer even combined deafness and blindness—witness Helen Keller and Laura Bridgeman.

To live and grow, we must be able to convey our thoughts and feelings to others so that they are clearly understood and to clearly understand the experiences expressed by others. Speech-language pathologists strike directly to the heart of this ideal. The chance to help others to live fully is a remarkable opportunity. What makes it even greater is that, in order to help others to communicate effectively, we must constantly seek to improve our own ability to communicate. In the world of work, it is seldom that devotion to *self-*improvement has such direct benefit to your work relationships.

We could say that life's primary task is to grow or to create oneself continually as a communicative system. In no small way, our work is a search for ways to help persons with speech, language, and hearing problems to grow through widened experience and personal relationships.

Speech-language pathologists confront this reality all the time: the recent stroke patient who has lost the human connection with old friends because he cannot talk; the cerebral palsied adolescent who yearns to declare her independence from her parents; the deaf child bewildered by rejection from his classmates; the child made fun of because of infantile speech. Their struggles are not only efforts to improve some specific communication skill; they are a search for an existence with greater meaning and happiness. And they remind us that there can be a large gulf between our learning and analysis of communication behavior and our understanding of it.

In one sense, this chapter celebrates life. The effort to help the other person may deepen the professional's self-knowledge. These efforts, though having a common base professionally, are unique for each speech-language pathologist. They require personal strengths and even felicitous idiosyncracies.

It is now time to come full circle in this book—to take a slightly different view of the various roles the speech-language pathologist can take. But before we turn to that task, we need to make clear some assumptions about human interactions.

BASIC ASSUMPTIONS

(1) Each person has a natural urge to grow and an interest in the world beyond the self, an interest that reaches out beyond mere existence or simple survival.

> There are times when maintaining this belief is difficult for both the professional and the person in therapy, especially in situations of severe impairment such as brain damage or severe retardation.

(2) Each person has natural tendencies toward higher levels of independent functioning and relating to others.

> Individuals may resist progress in treatments, or even appear to punish themselves. The faith of the professional, the client, and often the family may be severely tested.

(3) We see others not so much as they are, but as we are.

> The reality each of us has within us is, for each of us, the only reality we know. Some speech-language pathologists never allow their true selves to speak. While revealing yourself carries risks, it is a vital part of the clinical relationship—of all relationships.

(4) Creation and revision are better than fixation of beliefs and techniques.

> Time and again we cling to the things we have been taught or care for. This could be wise professional fidelity, but sometimes it is only inertia. We are still looking for causes, theories, and treatments that are more effective—and more rapid—than those we are using now.

(5) While knowledge of scientific fact and method are important, where clinical relationships are concerned, the personal relationship with the patient is more important than facts, even scientifically respectable ones.

> The speech-language pathologist *has* a relationship with each client, and improvement in the clinical condition is influenced by all the clinician's attitudes.

(6) The live wire of human sympathy is more valuable than clinical technique, but it needs to be well-grounded in professional knowledge and experience.

(7) There are many ways (some apparently strange) of struggling to be more human; many an expression of frustration, anger, or despair over one's communication ability is a disguised cry for understanding and a human touch, the desire to feel oneself a person of worth.

> Certainly I have had this belief challenged severely. There was one father who punished his deaf son with cigarette burns on the child's arms, and other parents who dehumanized their children and themselves in even more horrifying ways. It is hard to keep from rejecting the person while abhorring the behavior. Yet, given the opportunity to know such individuals better, I developed an appreciation of their

confusion, and with it the ability to move into a more productive relationship with them.

(8) Therapy is most likely to succeed when it is in accord with the goals of those receiving it.

The sources of these deeper well-springs of human action often lie beyond the surface manifestations of speech, language, or hearing behavior.

(9) Any communication misfortune—language loss, sensory deprivation, speech dysfluency or distortion— can be transformed into an experience of value.

It is not always easy to believe in Shakespeare's words "Sweet are the uses of adversity," but the belief in the ability to overcome can help create the fact.

(10) In human communication, part-functions are always functions of the system as a whole.

We need to understand and to modify the separate components of the act of communication, but we can understand the significance of the parts—the phonemes, the sound discrimination ability, the intonations—only by seeing how they integrate with the whole person. In real life we regard others in their totality; that is how they normally behave and want to be regarded. Causes and effects of disorders are seldom unidimensional; they are generally complex. There is no such thing, for example, as good speech in itself; speech is "good" when it is an expression of authentic human experience and understandable as such.

(11) People with speech, language, or hearing disorders—even unmotivated, uncooperative, or defiant ones—are, in any final reckoning, on your side.

COMMUNICATION PROCESSES: LEVELS AND RELATIONSHIPS

Let's now look again at the word *communication,* this time from a clinically functional perspective. We will discuss a few typical premises or uses of terms at the outset.

The most frequent conception of *communication* refers to all of those processes by which one mind may influence another. In the broadest sense, this includes verbal and nonverbal—in fact, all—human behavior. Let us simply say that *communicate* is a verb; and, whatever each of us is, we are always changing. In the best of clinical sessions, the professional grows as the client is growing.

We can spell out the functions of communication more precisely. In the simplest sense, communication serves to affect others, the environment, or ourselves. We wish to produce a response or achieve some purpose. We may wish to inform, share, persuade, control, or entertain, to express feelings. Any speech-language pathologist who has seen both a child who is totally unconcerned about his speech misarticulations and his mother who is terribly anxious about them recognizes that the assignment of meanings is highly personalized.

Transactions and Communication

The proper study of persons with communication disorders should always occur in terms of relationships between individuals. In relationship, communication is never simply linear or one-way. We do not communicate to or at other people, we communicate *with* them. When a lisping child speaks to you, both you and the child are affected. The communicator, in fact, may be more affected than the listener.

Intrapersonal Communication

As we have seen, *intrapersonal communication* refers to conscious or unconscious communication within the self or individual person. This is the level of individual neurophysiology or neuropsychology. It includes the processes of thinking, feeling, self-observation, self-regard, self-talk, and introspection. It can also refer to the degree of harmony between thought and feeling, between feeling and action, or between action and thought. I am reminded of this sentence from *The Upanishads:* "May my speech be one with my mind, and my mind be one with my speech."

For communication with the outer world to be successful, communication within the individual's inner world must be. To integrate harmoniously with others, our own personal functions must be integrated. My skill in communicating with myself is the same skill I use in communicating with those I help as a speech-language pathologist.

Clinical situations provide many examples of intrapersonal communication disorder: the stroke patient who has lost the ability to associate the appropriate meaning or name with a body part or function, to evoke within himself an emotion appropriate to his thought; the stutterer whose self-image is destructive to clear thinking; the autistic child whose verbal outpourings appear to have no connection with her general behavior or feelings; the language-learning disabled child who struggles to analyze and integrate his own learning patterns.

Interpersonal Communication

Again, this is the term used to refer to person-to-person communication, the basic human relationship. Obviously, *intrapersonal* dynamics permeate interpersonal ones. We might say that a *transaction* occurs between the intra- and interpersonal processes, each affecting and being affected by the other. The client-clinician meeting is a transaction which functions as prototype for relationships with others.

Interprofessional Communication

This refers to a subset of interpersonal communication, one which has not received the attention it deserves. Delivery of service to persons with communication disorders varies according to the degree to which workers communicate efficiently with each other—within or between professions. Communication disorders can be complex; for this reason they constitute an area of multidisciplinary interest. While the American Speech-Language-Hearing Association constitutes the central professional axis for the field of communication disorders, many other professional groups are involved. However, there is no significant movement toward cohesive action among the groups. Each has its own special organization, its special nomenclature, its own territorial imperatives.

See Figure 15.1.

This lack of communication, in company with other factors, can sometimes lead to feelings of alienation not only between professional groups but between individuals within a profession, and occasionally to rifts between individuals and the professional association of which they are members. I believe

FIGURE 15.1

Professions Related to Human Communications Disorders.

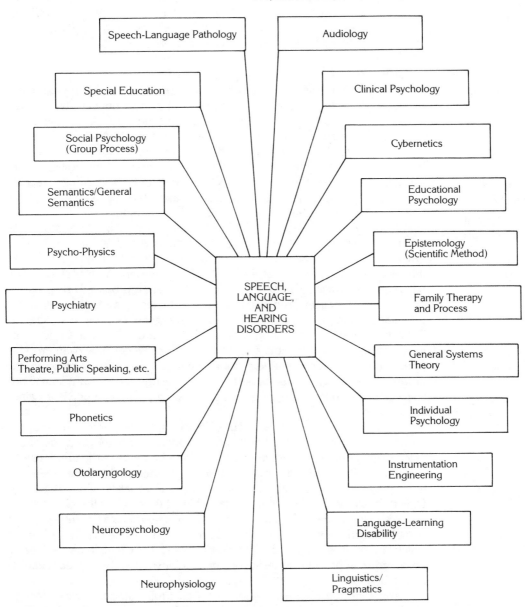

that the attitudes of speech-language pathologists toward clients are in part a function of the soundness of their relationship with their own profession or organization. In addition, attitudes of alienation with your own professional group are revealed by and shape your attitudes toward members of other professions having similar or related roles. The stronger and more openly communicative the professional and the primary professional affiliation, the better are the chances for successful relationships with allied workers and professional groups.

It requires dedication and effort for professionals to communicate well. The necessary ingredients are those found to be necessary in all human experiences if healthy communication is to occur: openness to others, security in knowledge and acceptance of oneself, and the desire to share knowledge and process in a caring relationship. It is not only an ideal to believe that different fields, theories, and practices should coexist as mutually supportive enterprises—they often do and ideally must coexist as such.

Clinician-Supervisor Communication

Because of the impor-tance of clinician-supervisor relation-ships, you may wish to read further on this topic. See, among others, Cogan, 1973; Gerstman, 1977; Gold-hammer, 1969; Miner, Prather, Kunz, Brown, and Haller, 1967; Pannbacker, 1975; Van Riper, 1979; Villereal, 1964; Ward and Webster, 1965.

The relationship between the speech-language pathologist and the supervisor is critical not only as you work to improve your professional ability; it is also, in many respects, representative of what happens in the clinician-client relationship. The purposes of supervision are to translate theory and knowledge into practice, to develop skills, and to learn to relate productively to persons having a variety of communication disorders. While your training experience should be fruitful, some stress is practically unavoidable. As a new speech-language pathologist, your success in this relationship can deeply affect your entire outlook and self-concept as a professional person.

In the beginning, trainees typically have faith in their ability and often an enormous enthusiasm. Vital as these ingredients are, they are not enough. While most trainees have mixed emotions when meeting their first clients, they do feel initial pleasure and anticipatory excitement. In later stages, perhaps when the phase of spontaneous improvement has passed and progress slows, when the client's motivation wanes and support systems weaken, the new speech-language pathologist naturally experiences some frustration. They may have feelings of hopelessness, anger, and self-doubt. Under more trying circumstances, doubts about the choice of career may even crop up. Sometimes without expressing it, trainees develop critical feelings toward the program, theory, methods, or staff. These feelings are not unusual. Their successful resolution depends greatly on the strength of the supervisor-trainee relationship.

Many factors affect this relationship. For example, the participants may not share the same experimental or theoretical background; they may differ significantly in their emphasis on or comfort with biological or learning factors compared with psychodynamic ones. Your manner and attitude when with the supervisor may be quite different compared to your behavior with a client. Direct observation of the trainee is desirable, of course, but the observations by the supervisor cannot match your actual experience as a speech-language pathologist on the spot, nor can the supervisor experience the subtle feelings which you may sense only in close proximity with the client. In general, being observed may provoke anxiety; you may feel insecure, threatened, subordinate, vulnerable.

Competent and concerned supervisors take full account of these factors. They not only bring the stabilizing leavening of more experience to the setting, but they are warmly supportive and accepting, objective but flexible. Their role is a challenging one. It is the supervisor's responsibility to point out gaps and strengths in your knowledge, techniques, and interpersonal relationships—sometimes to be critical.

Most trainees, at any level of training, do not accept criticism well, even when it is constructive; they find it painful to admit failure, error, or even obvious stupidity. It can be painful to confront yourself. These traits are not unique to trainees; many experienced professionals have similar reactions. Some speech-language pathologists reveal professional near-sightedness by worshipping their own approaches, which, in severe cases, can solidify into a kind of cultism. This behavior constitutes a kind of "psychic hearing impairment" of others' views, brought about by chronic adoration of one's own clichés. It is behavior to be avoided. As we have seen in almost every chapter in Parts II and III, there are more than one valid approach to most problems. As a new professional, you should try to remain open to your supervisor's suggestions.

If the supervisor has the basic responsibility for the therapy outcome, you must comply with the supervisor's directions. The supervisor also has responsibility to the client, his or her family, the school or clinic, and even in some cases to a research design. If the channels of communication between supervisor and trainee are open, your experience is enriched because you are exposed to these realities.

Of course it is necessary to develop a mutual understanding of language and concepts in order to share a common frame of reference. But rigid adherence to procedure or specialized terminology serves as a barrier to effective liaison. In the healthiest of trainee-supervisor partnerships, both parties in the transaction have opportunities to learn about themselves, not just about each other. Neither is likely to grow significantly where extreme views are held or where strict allegiance is required. For example, in a written report to her campus-based supervisor, one student who had requested a clinical practicum in a residential institution for mentally retarded persons revealed her unhappiness with that work setting. She pointed out that the institution seemed to exist primarily to control and not to rehabilitate the patients. She was a very creative woman, but her novel ideas were regarded only as troublesome in a setting geared to conformity. Unfortunately, creative learning produces some instability. When institutions or supervisors require conformity and control, trainees and clients suffer.

Mature and growing supervisor-trainee relationships include options for selecting alternate procedures while the basic repertoire of necessary skills is being developed. The superior supervisor is able to send clear messages and to behave unambiguously, yet withstand the ambiguity of others. As a trainee, you should be able to examine your own behaviors—your attitudes, language usage, clinical skills, and appearance as a professional person.

Professional Communications and Ethics

The supervisor-trainee relationship may also be a beginning model not only in terms of subsequent contacts with children and adults who need assistance, but also in terms of relationships with colleagues both within and beyond your professional discipline. Because of the nature of communication disorders, professionals from a wide range of disciplines may be involved, or may wish to be involved, in treatment. This can create a sensitive situation. For example, some clients may need, or think they need, psychotherapy. And in fact, emotional disturbance in clients will show up from time to time. The speech-language pathologist's participation in therapy for the emotional causes or results of communication disorders depends on many factors; no simple rule of conduct is possible. Training and experience vary, even within a profession. Many individuals certified as speech-language pathologists are also physicians, clinical psychologists, or educational specialists.

However, most speech-language pathologists are not qualified to practice as psychotherapists, and states vary greatly in their certification and practice boundaries. Most speech-language pathologists, nevertheless, should and do have courses in abnormal and personality psychology and learning theory, the ability to recognize psychotic or chronic neurotic behaviors, and knowledge about how to refer to appropriate personnel.

Inclinations to refer depend on many factors. Obviously, your self-regard as a speech-language pathologist is critical, as are your evaluations of your clients. Referrals will also vary according to work setting. A public school clinician may be operating under an administrative requirement which makes referral impossible; a hospital clinician may be working as a member of a team of specialists which includes a psychiatrist or psychiatric social worker. The types of communication disorders also will affect referral rate. It will be higher, for instance, in relation to autistic children, some stuttering individuals, or certain voice disorders.

You will usually be able to serve the great majority of communication-connected emotional disturbances in the clients you encounter. Most clients profit and are well served, not only by gains in communication competency, but by a supportive atmosphere and perhaps occasional opportunities for the unmonitored release of feelings. That you have the capacity to feel deeply is necessary. Plunges into the shadows of the client's mind are usually not.

As we saw as early as chapter 1 of this book, another arena of possible conflict is the public school. You may feel strongly that a particular child needs your individualized services in therapy, yet the administrative structure of the school (or its budget) might make that impossible. You must then develop skills as a teacher trainer and consultant, perhaps providing direct services only in initial diagnosis and periodic reassessment.

Much of what happens in these interprofessional "twilight zones" depends on how comfortable you feel in the relationship and with the particular behaviors. Of course, it is vital that you be realistic in your own self-evaluation. I have at times counseled clinicians stuck in a therapeutic dilemma to "give yourself what you need." But this assumes that the clinician is a well-adjusted person.

It is impossible for the speech-language pathologist to avoid some emotional involvement. You soon learn this in sitting repeatedly at the hospital bedside of a stroke patient; in administering speech therapy to a young lady who has recently been jailed "for being drunk" when, in reality, her difficulty walking was caused by her cerebral palsy; in speaking with the high-school stutterer whose depression seems almost overwhelming; in helping the language-disordered child deal with his parents' unrealistic expectations and his own; in looking at the repeated drawings of faces with twisted, hostile mouths by a child with severe articulation errors. You cannot refuse to be responsive in such instances. Many speech-language pathologists have learned that they must do as much as possible, for they are frequently the only specialist the person ever sees, ever can see.

See Appendix B.

Fortunately, problems in ethics seldom occur. The majority, in fact, are caused not so much by behavior outrightly deviating from ASHA's Code of Ethics as by repetitively immature or careless behavior which may be observed by colleagues, and perhaps more seriously, by members of other professions. A few speech-language pathologists do not recognize their proper limits. They refuse to admit that no one can be equally competent with every variety of problem; that no matter what their background or training, they will be better equipped to deal with some persons than with others. Some fear criticism if they do not "accept every case" (their fears may be well-grounded, depending on the administration in the work setting). It takes courage to say, "I cannot work equally well with everyone. It would be better to assign me someone else." We would hope that such courage could elicit a responsive chord from colleagues. But we must recognize that risk may be involved.

ROLES OF SPEECH-LANGUAGE PATHOLOGISTS

First and foremost, the speech-language pathologist must be able to communicate creatively. By modifying some criteria developed by Satir (1967, 1972), we can say that communicatively creative persons (clients *or* speech-language pathologists):

(1) Reveal themselves clearly to others
(2) Are in touch with their own feelings
(3) Have a realistic picture of themselves
(4) Regard each person as unique
(5) Treat differentness as an opportunity to learn something rather than as a threat or signal for conflict
(6) Deal with persons according to their *contexts* and in terms of how they really are rather than how they might wish them to be
(7) Accept responsibility for how they speak, perceive, and relate without denying any of it or unreasonably attributing negative influences to others
(8) Have the ability to achieve and clarify meaning between themselves and others.

Creative speech-language pathologists, in addition, regard themselves as reasonably secure and capable in their professional functions. They are able to function in a variety of professional roles.

The Clinician as Observer

Each participant in a relationship, including the clinical one, is an observer both of the other and of the self. The properties of the observer must be made explicit. Let us assume that we wish to observe a young man who stutters. As Ruesch and Bateson (1968) have pointed out, in determining the unique position of the observer, we must identify:

(1) The position of the observer—What we observe differs if we are in the client's public-speaking class, his home during mealtime, and with him while he converses with his best friend or in a group discussion
(2) The theoretical system of the observer (consciously or implicitly held)
(3) The methods and instruments of the observer ("editorial" implements)
(4) The purpose of the observer
(5) The biases of the observer.

Speech-language pathologists of more orthodox scientific bent claim that, the more successful we are in isolating the behaviors we observe, the more precise will be the data obtained. But if they concentrate too much on details, they learn less about the *relationship* of these events to larger perspectives. On the other hand, the broader view of the observers, the more information they gather about connections; but they lose information concerning details which may be critical. In speech-language pathology, we move constantly between these two poles, especially if we work with a large variety of disorders or procedures. Most of us avoid either extreme. But whatever your view, it is wise to remain aware of your position as an observer in the clinical encounter.

Clinicians and Linguistic Relativity

Eugene O'Neill, in his play *Strange Interlude* (1959), wrote, "How we poor monkeys hide from ourselves behind the sounds called words." Even the language we use as speech-language pathologists sensitizes us to some phenomena and blinds us to others, depending on how we employ it.

As we saw in chapter 2, the Whorf-Sapir hypothesis states in brief that language structures reality; one's manner of viewing, responding to, and thinking about the world is seen as a function of one's lexicon and, more importantly, one's grammar. In this view, languages are thought-systems bonding syntax and semantics, form and meaning, in an inseparable fusion. Language thus not only transmits thought, it shapes it. Our linguistic behaviors shape the way in which we perceive and regard reality.

At the level of common sense, it occurs to us that language has structure. If individual and cultural behavior is conditioned by language, we can assume there is some relationship between the two—the structure of language and the structure of our behaviors. If we apply this thought to clinical encounters, we can see some provocative possibilities.

If, for example, groups having different linguistic systems think and perceive differently and have different views of the world, are there implications for speech-language pathologists who speak from widely different theoretical, methodological, or terminological perspectives? No one is able to describe clinical process with absolute impartiality; we are constrained by individual style of interpretation which functions by way of "method," "technique," or "approach."

Consider a group of mentally retarded or autistic children in a residential setting. Could their linguistic systems be significantly different from ours? If so, how are we to arrive at their view of the world (assuming we wish to), unless we can better match our linguistic characters? How can we identify with them so as to be in better communication and relationship? If we do not understand their linguistic systems, how can we understand their minds?

The Clinician as Assessor

Some authorities (Perkins, 1978) use the term *diagnosis* for medical assessment and the term *assessment* for the speech-language pathologist's functions. Many communication disorders specialists employ both terms, often interchangeably. As we have explained earlier, most agree that the fundamental purpose of assessment is to ascertain the nature and severity of the disorder and most try to estimate prognosis. Not all are interested in determining etiology, either because they view the determination of causes as beyond the realm of their professional competence, or else because they maintain that initial causes cannot be altered or are identified only on a conjectural rather than a factual basis. And anyway, they maintain, even were causes (of a neurophysiological kind, for example) identified, coping procedures (such as surgery or drugs) lie beyond their range of professional competency or certification. For such reasons, only publicly observable behavior may be focused upon.

Because of the broad array of communication-disordered people who pass through our doors, flexibility in assessment procedures is a must. An actual disorder may turn out to be far more complex than the referring complaint might have suggested. Thus, a quick review of your notes (mental or otherwise) for articulation assessment, for instance, is not sufficient; you must be prepared to follow where the data take you. With growing experience, speech-language pathologists feel more secure in varying from fixed routines. Individual clinical styles differ, some leaning toward a formal and objective "battery" of instruments and procedures, while others prefer a more informal and pliable approach. Probably neither extreme is helpful.

In initial meetings, it is not uncommon to have the participants spend much of the time trying to clarify what the meeting is about. Role assignation and mutual explorations occur, and at least tentative agreements are reached. In regard to "role," for example, Ruesch and Bateson (1968) state that the term refers wholly to the code which is used to interpret the flow of messages. For instance, the statements of a father concerning his son, who stutters, might be interpreted very differently when it dawns upon you that the father also stutters and refers to himself as a stutterer, while letting his wife do most of the talking. The father has, in effect, announced a rule he would like to follow: his wife is to do the majority of the talking. If you regularly return to the father for a response, you give notice of a clinic rule: we find it necessary to hear from both parents.

If, at the initial interview, a child is whisked off to a separate assessment room with barely a word being spoken to his parents, a rule is declared concerning the parents' role. An interview in which you do little more than ask parents printed questions of a factual nature reveals another rule. The channels of communication are prescribed, the sequence of messages regulated. Even though clinicians are highly aware of the "rules" by which they set up communications, we need to be mindful of these more subtle elements. Rules are not intrinsically bad, but increasing our awareness of how we employ them, often in barely noticeable ways, pays clinical dividends.

Clinical Styles and Split Decisions

It is observable in the world at large, and sometimes dramatically in the professional world, that many people appear to be almost entirely intuitive and others entirely logical. Not infrequently those at one extreme derogate the others, usually out of defensiveness or because they have very little awareness of the value of these two kinds of functioning. The two perspectives should exist as complementary modes of communication. Frequently, however, they are poorly integrated.

The situation is analogous to the two modes of thinking shown to be localized in the cerebral cortex, as evidenced in recent studies of brain lesions or alterations, most notable in terms of "split-brain" patients (Sagan, 1977). The evidence suggests that functions we typically describe as "rational" reside mainly in the right brain. From such explorations into cortical functioning, we can surmise that a particular child might be able to solve a problem employing verbal symbols more easily than visual-spatial ones; for another child, the opposite might hold true. Education or therapy which forces each child into the inappropriate mode could produce great frustration regarding self, teacher, or learning process.

Recall that this relates also to people with aphasia caused by strokes.

In one view of speech-language pathologists, their functioning "styles" can be seen as inclined toward one side or the other of the rational-intuitive continuum. Clinical style will reflect and shape your perspectives as an observer, your interpretive bent, your theoretical or methodological underpinnings, your descriptive/analytical biases and therapy choices.

Behavioristic-rationalistic speech-language pathologists who set up what they do after the model of physics, mathematics, and the scientific analysis of behavior identify, describe, and analyze publicly observable behaviors. They try to use communication styles which fit the observable facts. Those who are more personalistic and phenomenological also try to identify problem behavior; in addition, they emphasize the importance of understanding the behavior from the client's perspective and then taking into account how they themselves personally affect the client and the interaction. While we may tend to lean toward one orientation or the other, most of us use a blend. There are places for the variety of orientations in dealing with disorder. In this sense, you "work both hemispheres"—as scientist in a humane pursuit of broadly applicable knowledge and technique and as artist in imagining the possibilities in a human relationship.

The Speech-Language Pathologist's Personality

The impact of the speech-language pathologist's personality on the clinical process has been suggested throughout, but several additional observations are in order. Try as we might to be "completely objective," clients will skillfully engage us—stimulate, frustrate, and elate us—and each of us will react differently. Two similarly qualified professionals, even two with the same training history, will manage similar communication disorders differently.

All of us inevitably form our own approaches which are composites of training, experience, personal likes and dislikes, needs, successes, and failures. I have worked with some who, though trained with a psychodynamic or client-centered emphasis, were inclined by nature to be directive and even authoritarian. They suffered as they attempted to allow clients to set their own targets and improvement rates. The tension interfered with their normal modes of functioning. Under pliable training conditions or in independent practice later, those individuals may learn to function more in keeping with their natures.

Clients are more responsive to professionals who appear natural. The abandonment of artificiality and the subsequent reinforcement from clients encourages us even more to be ourselves. In a psychological sense, we have a continuing responsibility to try to match our procedures with our own individual personalities, beyond that degree which naturally might occur. The large majority of workers reveal no chronically disabling personality features, and cases brought before ethics committees are relatively few in number. A therapeutic ideal would be to be able to selectively risk deeply felt emotional investments which, while being related primarily to the client's needs, would stem from and reinforce mature motives in the speech-language pathologist.

Speech-Language Pathologists as "Optimal Systems"

Knowledge, techniques, theories, or practices do not spring to life or grow in the abstract. They are products of living organisms in various social contexts. Modern "systems theory," which veteran speech-language pathologists see reflected in the work of Gestalt psychologists, points up the complex interdependability of persons and setting (Buckley, 1968). Systems thinking is now in the forefront of a shift from statics, structure, and single-source casuality to process, transformation, and feedback patterns.

See Table 15.1 for some contrasts between open and closed systems.

All living systems are open systems, but they differ greatly in their degrees of openness. Common sense about ourselves as clinicians and our clients tells us so. There is the nonverbal child who "cannot be reached"; the parents who seem unable to consider professional advice; workers who operate according to fixed beliefs. These persons are relatively closed, and human

TABLE 15.1
Characteristics of "Closed-System" and "Open-System" Clinicians.

Closed-System	Open-System
Need to reduce uncertainty	Admits and accepts uncertainty
Cautionary communicative style	Spontaneous communicative mode
Predictable	Unpredictable
Resistant to new information	Accessible to new information (even occasional dissonance)
Stereotyped behavior	Adaptable behavior
Solutions assumed known	Solutions assumed improvable
Steady goals	Variable, evolving goals
Resistance to change	Changeable
Rigid, static	Pliable, dynamic

systems which are closed are unhealthy to themselves and, eventually, less helpful to others.

In an organismic or holistic sense, we know our clients as dynamic systems—their speech and hearing behaviors, their linguistic patterns, their relationships—but also their cognitive styles, their attitudes and motives, their strengths. But we are still deficient if we do not take into account their life situations and backgrounds.

A helpful blending of the systems concept with a communication model has been made by the distinguished family therapist, Virginia Satir (1967). In her efforts to teach families to communicate more effectively, she developed a number of communication games. I have found one of her games particularly useful with adolescents or adults and their family members, usually in instances of stuttering, aphasia, cerebral palsy, or laryngectomy. Satir observed that people seem to find it almost impossible to express discordant or angry messages if they have steady eye or skin contact with the other person. An example follows as it has occurred in a clinic setting.

> The dysphasic adult and his wife are placed standing back to back and asked to talk about anything. Then they are requested to face each other and "eyeball" each other without talking or touching. Next, they are asked to "eyeball" and touch without talking. They are then asked to hold hands, eyes closed. They then "eyeball" and talk without touching. Finally, the couple is asked to talk, touch, and "eyeball" and try to argue with each other. It's usually impossible. They usually end up enjoying the experience. (Adapted from Satir, 1967, p. 188)

Here we see an example of trying to open up two people who had begun to close out each other. We could have been discussing a high-school stutterer and his parents or a learning-disabled adolescent and a perfectionistic father. I have also found the technique useful in seminars on interprofessional communication.

Open-system speech-language pathologists are more likely to have open minds. To remain healthy, professional disciplines also must be open. Workers must remain to some degree in a state of creative insecurity, open to alternatives to change in philosophy or method, and to the possibility of weakness, even of insignificance, in one's way of functioning. It is impossible to believe, given the vast range and variability found in persons with communication disorders, with all of their possible etiologies, accompanying personal factors,

For more on open versus closed systems, see Allport, 1961.

and living situations, that a single philosophy or method could automatically be considered as appropriate for any large cluster of such patterns.

The Speech-Language Pathologist as Technician

If the professions devoted to communication disorders can claim any area of abundance, it must be the veritable mountain of techniques which exist. By *technique* we mean any routine or complex standardized means for obtaining a predetermined result. Its goal is maximum efficiency of communication performance. As I have tried to make clear, a danger arises when formulas and procedures, once established, do not vary; as though, indeed, the speech-language pathologist considered them inviolable magic. As Ellul (1964) says:

> Strict adherence to form is one of the characteristics of magic: forms and rituals, masks which never vary, the same kinds of prayer wheels, the same ingredients for divination, and so on. All these became set and were passed on: the slightest variation in word or gesture would alter the magical equilibrium. (p. 24)

It may sometimes seem easier to focus on more specific, more manipulatable behavior over which we can feel a sense of control and perhaps comfort. But it is not necessarily wiser. Sometimes this may be represented, as Alfred North Whitehead might have said, as a "fallacy of misplaced concreteness." Creative pliability, on the other hand, I think of as the "validity of well-placed abstractness."

The most effective speech-language pathologist can use a number of techniques, posit an appropriate rationale for their use, place them in a context of total-person function, and be ready to modify or even to abandon them. Some learn a limited number of techniques and tend to apply them repeatedly, regardless of disorder or unsuitability. Most of us are limited in some degree by our character structures so as to be inclined toward some techniques rather than others. No one can efficiently manage all the available techniques. But even those techniques we *do* know are insignificant, unless they are used with conviction and faith. Techniques are dead things until, working with a child or adult with a communication problem, you breathe a life into them. Techniques are powerful in a positive sense when used with balance and perspective; they may be powerful in a negative sense in the hands of professionals snared in an ecstatic technical vertigo.

Nonverbal Communication

Long before the current fashion, communication disorder specialists were deeply interested in understanding the significance of body language, especially those nonverbal characteristics connected with speech and listening—vocal pitch, loudness, quality, range, pattern, rate, and fluency. There has always been interest in these metalinguistic elements in determining and enhancing the flow of the client-clinician relationship:

(1) As indicators of the client's attitude toward professional, self, and setting
(2) As indicators of a client's perception of *verbal* behaviors in the transaction
(3) As an auxiliary mode, such as music therapy, in treatment programs.

The study of nonverbal behaviors by our profession has been modest. An article by

Of course, speech-language pathologists have worked directly with many of these behaviors—not simply as indicators of "hidden significances," but as primary focus, as things in themselves to be dealt with directly. For our purposes here, however, we wish to note only that clinical sensitivity to nonverbal communications assists us in comprehending the fuller picture of the persons we meet in clinical work. A wealth of this material is presented to us. For example, below are some notes I made during one day of observation of workers in a speech and hearing training clinic.

(1) The speech-language pathologist, when escorting the parents into the interview area, said, "I'd appreciate it if you didn't smoke." Ten minutes after the interview began, the father lighted a cigar.

(2) The same man said little, but when he did speak his voice was hardly audible. Upon their leaving, his voice was heard to be loud and resonant.

(3) At one point, the mother said, "I want to be completely honest with you." At the same moment, she pushed her chair back slightly from the desk, clasped her hands on her knees, and went silent.

(4) The speech-language pathologist asked Larry, who stuttered, to walk out once again into the corridor and ask a stranger for the corrct time. Larry replied pleasantly, "O.K.," but as the clinician turned away, Larry rolled his eyes toward the ceiling and bit his lip before finally shuffling off to the task.

(5) I shook hands with a young trainee who had only several moments before been informed that I would be observing him working with a child. His palm was sweaty and his pupils were dilated.

(6) In the discussion practice of the young adult cerebral palsy group, the speech-language pathologist directed her gaze three times as often to one person (the most verbal) as to the average for all others. She did not look directly at one of the group members at all. At the outset she had stated, "I want you to think of me as just one of the group." However, upon speaking these words, she stood and remained standing at the head of the conference table.

(7) The learning disabled 10-year-old was a very active handful for all concerned. The mother, upon leaving, commented ruefully, "Sometimes I think I should sell him," but she immediately hugged the lad, and left the clinic with her hand around his waist.

(8) The autistic child kept rocking silently; but whenever the cookies were visible, he'd stop rocking unitl he got one.

(9) The professor lectured to the trainees, several of whom dozed while one read a paperback novel.

(10) Though it was during a heat-wave, during an initial interview the obviously anxious mother of a retarded child wore a heavy coat buttoned from the neck down. As she began to relax, she unbuttoned her coat, one button at a time, over a 45-minute period. As she opened up, the coat did, too.

(11) As a young man arrived for his appointment, his speech-language pathologist commented, "Late as usual. He hasn't been on time once."

(12) Of the five professors with offices in the clinic, the desks of two stood between their chairs and the chairs of visitors. The desks of the other three were positioned so that nothing separated the sitting positions.

Egolf and Chester (1973) provides an excellent brief introduction. A substantial, more detailed survey and bibliography have been prepared by Harrison (1974), in a book containing an extra dividend, a helpful discussion on systems, mentioned earlier. A particularly valuable chapter on nonverbal behaviors related to language and learning disability in adolescence is found in a text by Wiig and Semel (1976).

One of the remarkable characteristics of this profession is that it contributes to and participates in such a wide variety of knowledge and skill areas. Of course, just as it is impossible to utter the sound for the letter *b* without uttering two phonemes, it is impossible, as has been frequently observed, *not* to communicate. In speaking, we always communicate on several levels of discourse.

The Clinician as Listener

As several authors in this book have stressed, speech, language, and hearing specialists should know how to listen to the language that is spoken. The auditory channel is our primary assessment modality. It is also the pathway serving as basis for our emphathic responses. Most speech-language pathologists, to be good clinicians, do not need to have perfect hearing. But you do need to know how to listen well with the hearing you do have. While it is important to be able to discriminate /s/ from /ʃ/ sounds, it is also important to be able to discriminate any child from all others, to hear his special-ness. To be effective, we must see clients as unique individuals, not only as "speech cases."

Each of us, when we listen, listens selectively, depending on our experiences, beliefs, interests, and biases. We "shape" what we hear. Selective perception is unavoidable; the total lack of self-awareness of *how* we listen *is* avoidable.

There can be a danger in selective listening which is too circumscribed and rigidly maintained. If, for example, you listen to a stroke patient only in terms of analyzing the grammar or syntax or of recording utterances according to a set, pre-arranged schema, the larger significance of the behavior may be missed. Dissection may be necessary for analysis but may be detrimental to understanding the *person* in a more practical sense. It is not enough that we hear the notes; we must also listen for the melody.

You should try to listen on several planes: (a) *silent listening,* perhaps with nonverbal reinforcement to the client; (b) *active listening,* such as restating in order to clarify a message or to signal comprehension; (c) *vector listening,* such as to phonemes, syllable rate, voice quality, or feeling tone; (d) *intrapersonal listening,* or self-monitoring; and (e) *interpersonal listening,* listening for the meaning of the total behavior or relationship. To listen with scientific accuracy takes skill, but to listen with understanding takes human concern. We must not listen so narrowly that what the person is "saying" never gets heard.

The Speech-Language Pathologist as Scientist

Specialists in communication disorders range in function from researchers in vocal physiology and cortical functioning to practitioners in reinforcement and programming procedures to those conducting traditional speech and language training and play therapy. While the professional knowledge for all specialists should be solidly grounded in experience, some workers aspire more pointedly to the role or status of scientist in the sense of physical or natural science. For most speech-language pathologists, however, dealing as they usually do directly with complex and rapidly changing behaviors, rapidly made decisions cannot always await scientific proof.

The speech, language, and hearing profession is basically an applied behavioral discipline, but there is a place in it for the "harder" science. This is especially true if we broaden the definition of natural science and scientific method somewhat. When clinicians work, there is often science in their method, be it acknowledged as such or not. Let me illustrate.

Speech-language pathologists collect the "facts" concerning their clients (evidence). These facts are inspected in order to ascertain the shape they make (patterns). Missing facts are dug for through observation and experiment (investigation) and continuing effort (trial and error). The variance of the facts or behaviors is inspected as a function of the situation (context). Alterations in perspective, hypothesis, and procedure are made (adaptation).

Beyond these steps, a design may be drawn to allow for generalization beyond the particular case—a scheme of the empirical world including basic premises and concepts (modeling process and theory). Estimates are made as to what behaviors will ensue, given the facts and variables (prediction). This is essentially, of course, the scientific method, and speech-language clinicians operate by it daily.

Again, however, even this "objective" method has its "subjective" elements. Superficiality, unthinking conventionality, and rigid adherence to a single point of view are well-known thorns in the sides of empirical science. Instances in which *method* intractably determines the nature of the data debase genuine scientific inquiry. The significance of patterns of behavior may be ascertained by mechanical or statistical procedures or frequency counts, but most of us do better to arrive at meaningful connections through judicious reflection. Methods have value, but methods are mere dry bones until workers breathe a spark into them.

One occasionally encounters scientifically oriented speech-language pathologists who routinely turn to their use of "operational definitions" as validation of their work as worthy. An operational definition is one that attaches meaning to a construct or variable by specifying the activities or "operations" required to measure the construct or variable. For example, let us suppose that we wish to measure the self-concepts of stutterers. We have no *direct* measure of self-concept. But we may assume that we can draw inferences about the concept from figure-drawings stutterers make. Self-concept then would be defined in terms of certain, selected behaviors in the drawing. Obviously this procedure would not yield a complete picture of the individual's self-concept. A fuller picture could be attained only by studying the self-concept as it was experienced in the clinic, school, home, or at play.

The communication disorder specialist as scientist is primarily a behavioral scientist, one interested not only in behavior but in people. Capable in scientific structure and procedure, the speech-language pathologist is also grounded in the flesh and bones of everyday living.

Speech-Language Pathologists As Students of the Self

A recurrent theme throughout this chapter is that our persons are more important than our methods or techniques and that awareness of ourselves is advantageous. In their small but winning book, Zunin and Zunin (1972) have made some suggestions for self-study for individuals interested in improving their abilities in social relationships. I have adopted some of their materials and applied them to the teaching of student speech-language pathologists. Trainees keep a personal diary which includes responses to the items shown in Figure 15.2. The trainee has the option of sharing the diary with the supervisor or of keeping it, in whole or in part, confidential. This material has served as an important resource in individual or group trainee conferences.

Along the professional way, perhaps as trainee but more often as fully qualified speech-language pathologists, we become aware of the many roles that become part of the clinical life. Again this is not surprising, given a profession which deals with a remarkably broad range of human behaviors. Depending upon the client's needs and our own individual qualifications, we are at different times:

(1) *Teacher* in the traditional sense—Imparting information, instructing in skill-development, drawing out latent capacities

FIGURE 15.2
Trainee Self-Study Work Sheet.

(1) What three characteristics do your friends like about you?

(2) What three characteristics could you improve or acquire to make you a better person or friend?

(3) What are your three outstanding strengths as a clinician? Weaknesses?

(4) List three incidents in your life that contributed importantly to your character. Explain how they exhibit themselves or influence your behavior today.

(5) List one or more consequential situations you have experienced in working with people. How have they influenced your behavior or self-image?

(6) Name a critical incident in your life which, though difficult at the time, proved eventually to be a strengthening experience for you.

(7) What are the illusions you have about yourself? Your appearance? Weight? Speaking ability? Voice quality? Intelligence? Do you pretend to be more secure and independent or happier than you are? (If you answer, "None," is that an illusion?) What are the implications for working as a clinician?

(8) List several of your worst habits and describe approaches you could institute to modify or eliminate them.

(9) What are your basic professional goals? Are you pushed toward or pulled to them?

(10) What in clinical or social relationships makes you feel important? Happy? Strong? Uncomfortable? Weak? Depressed? Angry?

(11) Do you tend to elicit positive, negative, or neutral responses from co-workers? What are the work implications of your response?

(12) List three issues in your training program which trouble you (philosophy of staff, interpersonal frictions, confidence in skills, etc.).

(13) Are you able to show warmth and caring in your voice and general manner without being unduly anxious?

(14) Does your life have balance and perspective? Can you handle both success and failure?

(15) How do you think others in the program regard you?

(16) How do you regard yourself in relation to other persons in the program?

---

(2) *Counselor*—Supporting, encouraging, perhaps enhancing the client's knowledge of self

(3) *Role-model*—Serving as a kind of reference point against whom clients may elect to evaluate or compare themselves, be it for specific speech behavior or a more general communicative or interpersonal style

(4) *Reinforcer*—Strengthening through careful responses the desirable behaviors and weakening those less desirable

(5) *Interpreter*—Pointing out or comparing the possible meanings and effects of communication acts and

(6) *Confronter*—Helping clients to face issues and self more realistically.

The list of roles we play is a long and ever-changing one.

Fully Functioning Speech-Language Pathologists

The important features of the perhaps ideal speech-language pathologists have been suggested throughout this chapter. Now it is time for a direct thrust at describing this ideal.

Outstanding clinicians are not a rare breed in the speech, language, and hearing fields—there are many. I suspect this has some correlation with whatever interests in language, communication, or speech processes brings them into the profession in the first place. You are not apt to be interested in human communication without being interested in humans. Similarly, in working to enlarge your own capacity as a communicator, you are likely to improve proportionately in enhancing related interpersonal skills. Many efforts have been made to describe "the good clinican," including not a few of my own.

Fully functioning speech-language pathologists are devoted to the process of person transaction, not simply to isolated acts. They are accepting of and honest with themselves and others. They are able to be directive when the situation warrants, permissive at other times. They are attentive without being overbearing, sociable without being unduly familiar, professionally committed but personally involved. They have love and caring in them, but have no abiding need for the client's love. They are task-oriented and willing messengers of realistic limitation, but also of hope. They are able to express themselves so as to be widely understood. They view target behaviors in their contexts, not only in isolation. As they study their field and clients, they study themselves. They seem to regard communication disorders not merely as challenging but frequently as fascinating. They possess, though not absolutely, a pervasive optimism about their work, and yet they are grounded in reality. They recognize and are wary of glib explanations and extreme points of view. They can be relatively spontaneous and improvisational. They have an ability to accept the apparent absurdity that is, from time to time, part of life and work as a speech-language pathologist. They appear to be tolerant of their own inner impulses and accepting of the range of emotions others reveal.

You may pale at such a long list of characteristics as unreachable ideals. Perhaps, in their total, we should regard them as we do stars, not fully touchable but serving as guides on our journey.

See for example, Murphy, 1954; 1964; 1969; 1977a, 1977b, 1977c; 1980.

RELATIONSHIP AND COMMUNICATION: THE SYMBIOTIC AFFINITY

In professions serving handicapped children, the word "symbiotic" is typically used in a negative sense. For example, if a parent and child are emotionally immature, inseparable, and feed on each other's infantile behaviors, their relationship is said to be symbiotic. The relationship is reciprocally destructive. But an interpersonal connection may also be mutually developmental— symbiotic in a positive sense.

There is no relationship without communication, and communication both suggests and exists for relationship. Their affinity, however, can be creative or destructive. Growth in relationships tends to improve communicative behavior; thus, my use of the phrase "symbiotic affinity."

While the need for human relationship is basic, some clients appear to resist it (Murphy, 1974). The beauty of stepping forward into relationship is that it may enhance life; the beast about it is that, if you do not have a healthy sense of self, a relationship may be seen as a threat to your identity. Threat is experienced, paradoxically, as the danger of being understood, of being heard, even of being loved.

Trust and Relationship

Not only in extreme but in all clinical relationships, trust must be present if the encounter is to be successful. Trusting the other person is to let go; it includes an element of risk and perhaps a leap into the unknown, both of which require courage. Speech-language pathologists and parents sometimes unknowingly declare a lack of trust by trying to force a child into a certain mold or even perhaps by caring too much and overprotecting. The parent who makes all the stuttering son's telephone calls for him and the speech-language pathologist who makes all of the decisions for a learning disabled client may be serving primarily their own needs.

A speech-language pathologist's trust could also be based on a belief in the client's ability to take responsibility and to grow. It could include the assumption that the client (and professional) can learn from mistakes. Such trust cannot be faked. It is not simply a technique. You can act trustingly only to the degree you actually are. As one stroke patient said, "My wife says every day I will get better. Then she goes and does everything. I can do things but I don't get a chance." He was missing opportunities to improve independent functioning and to develop trust in himself. Among life's building blocks, self-trust is one of the most necessary.

Faith and Relationship

Faith is the twin of trust. Without faith by the speech-language pathologist in the approach taken, by the client in the professional, or by both in the appropriateness of their relationship, improvement is not as likely to occur. Faith and trust are scarcely to be found as topics in the professional literature; yet without them, progress may be impossible. It really is quite remarkable, in a person who has failed a thousand times to utter a particular sound fluently, or to spell a given sound-blend correctly, or to speak with less nasal voice quality, to see him try again. This kind of perseverance shows faith in the possibility for change.

Love and Relationship

Occasionally we encounter speech-language pathologists or parents who behave as though "love for the children" alone will carry them through to success with the child. Love goes a long way, but it alone cannot cure all ills. The parents of a 16-year-old cerebral palsied lad could not bear to give him the independence he pleaded for because they were so painfully intent on "making him happy," rather than on understanding him. To love someone in the most valid sense is to want that person to live fully in relationship or independently, when appropriate. Nor does this mean that anger or disagreement must never occur. They do occur, but our reactions are to the disagreeable behavior, not the whole person.

In such ways as these, in its auxiliary sense, love *may* be enough (Murphy, 1969). But love alone cannot guarantee clinical success any more than the ability to appreciate Beethoven guarantees us the ability to compose like him.

Relation and Dialogue

The essential purpose of speech, language, and hearing programs is to satisfy the basic hunger people have for a sense of community. This hunger for identification and growth through authentic dialogue or relationship is the impulse behind all creative efforts, including clinical ones.

FINALE

Our professional lives run the gamut of the human experience. We see this depicted beautifully in the partial autobiography of a remarkable odyssey, *A Career in Speech Pathology* by Charles Van Riper (1979), which should be required reading for all students of speech-language pathology. In this gem of a book, representing more than seven decades of involvement with communication disorders, we see clearly that to communicate well is to live well, and that living well contributes to communication. The personalized coverage of basic concepts and roles in speech and language disorders by Perkins (1978) is also a noteworthy and readable insight into the lives of clinicians.

Most speech-language pathologists and parents eventually conclude that the purpose of life is not to be forever happy, but to matter, to have an impact, to be in a significant relationship with at least one other person. Happiness in this noblest sense comes in large measure through helping relationships with others, stretching our professional resources and the resources of the mind and heart. Every now and then something in our deeper selves enables us to realize that what truly counts in life is not a matter of what is in you or what is in me but of what occurs between us. That divine spark of relationship may be the most fundamental life-force of all.

SELECTED READINGS

Carr, J. B. *Communicating and relating.* Menlo Park, Calif.: Benjamin Cummings Publishers, 1979.

Chinn, P. C., Winn, J., & Walters, R. H. *Two-way talking with parents of special children.* St. Louis: C. V. Mosby, 1978.

Johnson, W. *People in quandaries.* New York: Harper, 1946.

Perkins, W. H. *Human perspectives in speech and language disorders* St. Louis: C. V. Mosby, 1978.

Rogers, C. R. *On becoming a person.* Boston: Houghton-Miffllin, 1961.

Ruesch, J. *Therapeutic communication.* New York: W. W. Norton, 1961.

Van Riper, C. *A career in speech pathology.* Englewood Cliffs, N.J.: Prentice-Hall, 1979.

REFERENCES

Allport, G. W. The open system in personality theory. *Journal of Abnormal and Social Psychology,* 1961, *61,* 301–310.

Buckley, W. (Ed.). *Modern systems research for the behavioral scientist: A sourcebook.* Chicago: Aldine, 1968.

Cogan, M. L. *Clinical supervision.* Boston: Houghton Mifflin, 1973.

Egolf, D. B., & Chester, S. Nonverbal communication and the disorders of speech and language. *Asha,* 1973, *15,* 511–518.

Ellul, J. *The technological society.* (J. Wilkinson, Trans.). New York: Random House, 1964.

Gerstman, H. L. Supervisory relationships: Experiences in dynamic communication. *Asha,* 1977, *19,* 527–529.

Goldhammer, R. *Clinical supervision: Special methods for the supervision of teachers.* New York: Holt, Rinehart & Winston, 1969.

Harrison, R. P. *Beyond words.* Englewood Cliffs, N.J.: Prentice-Hall, 1974.

Miner, A., Prather, E., Kunz, L., Brown, E., & Haller, R. A symposium: Improving supervision of clinical practicum. *Asha,* 1967, *9,* 471–481.

Murphy, A.T. Personal relations in a profession. *The Volta Review,* 1954, *56,* 261–262.

Murphy, A.T. *Functional voice disorders*. Englewood Cliffs, N.J.: Prentice-Hall, 1964.

Murphy, A.T. Love may be enough: The passionate investments of clinicians. *Seminars in Psychiatry*, 1969, *1*(3).

Murphy, A.T. The quiet hyena: Two monologues in search of a dialogue. In L. L. Emerick & S. B. Hood (Eds.), *The client-clinician relationship*. Springfield, Ill.: Charles C Thomas, 1974.

Murphy, A.T. Authenticity and creativity in stuttering theory and therapy. In R. W. Rieber (Ed.), *The problem of stuttering: Theory and therapy*. Amsterdam: Elsevier North-Holland, 1977. (a)

Murphy, A.T. Counseling ways: Lessons parents have taught me. *The Volta Review*, 1977, 145–152. (b)

Murphy, A.T. Parent counseling and exceptionality: From creative insecurity to increased humanness. In E. Webster (Ed.), *New approaches in counseling parents of handicapped children*. Springfield, Ill.: Charles C Thomas, 1977. (c)

Murphy, A.T. *Special children, special parents: Personal issues in families with handicapped children*. Englewood Cliffs, N.J.: Prentice-Hall, 1980.

Pannbacker, M. Bibliography for supervision. *Asha*, 1975, *17*, 105–106.

Perkins, W. H. *Human perspectives in speech and language disorders*. St. Louis: C. V. Mosby, 1978.

Ruesch, J., & Bateson, G. *Communication: The social matrix of psychiatry*. New York: W. W. Norton, 1968.

Sagan, C. *The dragons of Eden: Speculations on the evolution of human intelligence*. New York: Random House, 1977.

Satir, V. *Conjoint family therapy* (Rev. ed.). Palo Alto, Calif.: Science and Behavior Books, 1967.

Satir, V. *People-making*. Palo Alto, Calif.: Science and Behavior Books, 1972.

Van Riper, C. Supervision of clinical practice. *Asha*, 1965, *7*, 75–77.

Van Riper, C. *A career in speech pathology*. Englewood Cliffs, N.J.: Prentice-Hall, 1979.

Villereal, J. (Ed.). *Seminar on guidelines for supervision of clinical practicum*. Washington, D.C.: American Speech, Language and Hearing Association, 1964.

Ward, L. M., & Webster, E. J, The training of clinical personnel: II. A concept of clinical preparation. *Asha*, 1965, *7*, 103–107.

Wiig, E. H., & Semel, E. S. *Language disabilities in children and adolescents*. Columbus, Ohio: Charles E. Merrill, 1976.

Zunin, L., & Zunin, N. *Contact: The first four minutes*. Los Angeles: Nash, 1972.

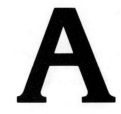

appendix

Requirements for the Certificates of Clinical Competence

(Revised January 1, 1981)

The American Speech-Language-Hearing Association issues Certificates of Clinical Competence to individuals who present satisfactory evidence of their ability to provide independent clinical services to persons who have disorders of communication (speech, language, and/or hearing). An individual who meets these requirements may be awarded a Certificate in Speech-Language Pathology or in Audiology, depending upon the emphasis of preparation; a person who meets the requirements in both professional areas may be awarded both Certificates.

I. STANDARDS

The individual who is awarded either, or both of the Certificates of Clinical Competence must hold a master's degree or equivalent with major emphasis in speech-language pathology, audiology, or speech-language and hearing science. The individual must also meet the following qualifications:

I,A. General Background Education
As stipulated below, applicants for a certificate should have completed specialized academic training and preparatory professional experience that provides an in-depth knowledge of normal communication processes, development and disorders thereof, evaluation procedures to assess the bases of such disorders, and clinical techniques that have been shown to improve or eradicate them. It is expected that the applicant will have obtained a broad general education to serve as a background prior to such study and experience. The specific content of this general background education is left to the discretion of the applicant and to the training program attended. However, it is highly desirable that it include study in the areas of human psychology, sociology, psychological and physical development, the physical sciences (especially those that pertain to acoustic and biological phenomena) and human anatomy and physiology, including neuroanatomy and neurophysiology.

Equivalent is defined as holding a bachelor's degree from an accredited college or university, and at least 42 post baccalaureate semester hours acceptable toward a master's degree, of which at least 30 semester hours must be in the areas of speech-language pathology, audiology, or speech-language and hearing science. At least 21 of these 42 semester hours must be obtained from a single college or university, none may have been completed more than 10 years prior to the date of application and no more than six semester hours may be credit offered for clinical practicum.

I,B. Required Education

In evaluation of credits, one quarter hour will be considered the equivalent of two-thirds of a semester hour. Transcripts that do not report credit in terms of semester or quarter hours should be submitted for special evaluation.

A total of 60 semester hours of academic credit must have been accumulated from accredited colleges or universities that demonstrate that the applicant has obtained a well-integrated program of course study dealing with the normal aspects of human communication, development thereof, disorders thereof, and clinical techniques for evaluation and management of such disorders.

Twelve (12) of these 60 semester hours must be obtained in courses that provide information that pertains to normal development and use of speech, language, and hearing.

Thirty (30) of these 60 semester hours must be in courses that provide (1) information relative to communication disorders, and (2) information about and training in evaluation and management of speech, language and hearing disorders. At least 24 of these 30 semester hours must be in courses in the professional area (speech-language pathology or audiology) for which the certificate is requested, and no less than (6) semester hours may be in audiology for the certificate in speech-language pathology or in speech-language pathology for the certificate in audiology. Moreover, no more than six (6) semester hours may be in courses that provide credit for clinical practice obtained during academic training.

Credit for study of information pertaining to related fields that augment the work of the clinical practitioner of speech-language pathology and/or audiology may also apply toward the total 60 semester hours.

This requirement may be met by courses completed as an undergraduate providing the college or university in which they are taken specifies that these courses would be acceptable toward a graduate degree if they were taken at the graduate level.

Thirty (30) of the total 60 semester hours that are required for a certificate must be in courses that are acceptable toward a graduate degree by the college or university in which they are taken. Moreover, 21 of those 30 semester hours must be within the 24 semester hours required in the professional area (speech-language pathology or audiology) for which the certificate is requested or within the six (6) semester hours required in the other area.

I,C. Academic Clinical Practicum

The applicant must have completed a minimum of 300 clock hours of supervised clinical experience with individuals who present a variety of communication disorders, and this experience must have been obtained within the training institution or in one of its cooperating programs.

I,D. The Clinical Fellowship Year

The applicant must have obtained the equivalent of nine (9) months of full-time professional experience (the Clinical Fellowship Year) in which bona fide clinical work has been accomplished in the major professional area (speech-language pathology or audiology) in which the certificate is being sought. The Clinical Fellowship Year must have begun after completion of the academic and clinical practicum experiences specified in Standards I,A., I,B., and I,C. above.

I,E. The National Examinations in Speech-Language-Pathology and Audiology

The applicant must have passed one of the National Examinations in Speech-Language-Pathology and Audiology, either the National Examination in Speech-Language-Pathology or the National Examination in Audiology.

II. EXPLANATORY NOTES

II,A. General Background Education

While the broadest possible general educational background for the future clinical practitioner of speech-language pathology and/or audiology is encouraged, the nature of the clinician's professional endeavors suggests the necessity for some emphasis in general education. For example, elementary courses in general psychology and sociology are desirable as are studies in mathematics, general physics, zoology, as well as human anatomy and physiology. Those areas of introductory study that do not deal specifically with communication processes are not to be credited to the minimum 60 semester hours of education specified in Standard I,B.

II,B. Required Education

II,B,1. Basic Communication Processes Area

The 12 semester hours in courses that provide information applicable to the normal development and use of speech, language, and hearing should be selected with emphasis on the normal aspects of human communication in order that the applicant has a wide exposure to the diverse kinds of information suggested by the content areas given under the three broad categories that follow: (1) anatomic and physiologic bases for the normal development and use of speech, language, and hearing, such as anatomy, neurology, and physiology of speech, language, and hearing mechanisms; (2) physical bases and processes of the production and perception of speech, language and hearing, such as (a) acoustics or physics of sound, (b) phonology, (c) physiologic and acoustic phonetics, (d) perceptual processes, and (e) psychoacoustics; and (3) linguistic and psycholinguistic variables related to normal development and use of speech, language, and hearing, such as (a) linguistics (historical, descriptive, sociolinguistics, urban language), (b) psychology of language, (c) psycholinguistics, (d) language and speech acquisition, and (e) verbal learning or verbal behavior.

It is emphasized that the three broad categories of required education given above, and the examples of areas of study within these classifications, are not meant to be analogous with, or imply, specific course titles. Neither are the examples of areas of study within these categories meant to be exhaustive.

At least two (2) semester hours of credit must be earned in each of the three categories.

Obviously, some of these 12 semester hours may be obtained in courses that are taught in departments other than those offering speech-language pathology and audiology programs. Courses designed to improve the speaking and writing ability of the student will not be credited.

II,B,2. Major Professional Area, Certificate in Speech-Language-Pathology

The 24 semester hours of professional education required for the Certificate of Clinical Competence in Speech-Language-Pathology should include mastery of information pertaining to speech and language disorders as follows: (1) understanding of speech and language disorders, such as (a) various types of disorders of communication, (b) their manifestations, and (c) their classifications and causes; (2) evaluation skills, such as procedures, techniques, and instrumentation used to assess (a) the speech and language status of children and adults, and (b) the bases of disorders of speech and language, and (3) management procedures, such as principles in remedial methods used in habilitation and rehabilitation for children and adults with various disorders of communication.

Within these categories at least six (6) semester hours must deal with speech disorders and at least six (6) hours must deal with language disorders.

II,B,3. Minor Professional Area, Certificate in Speech-Language-Pathology

For the individual to obtain the Certificate in Speech-Language Pathology, no less than six (6) semester hours of academic credit in audiology is required. Where only this minimum requirement of six (6) semester hours is met, three (3) semester hours must be in habilitative/rehabilitative procedures with speech and language problems associated with hearing impairment, and three (3) semester hours must be in study of the pathologies of the auditory system and assessment of auditory disorders. However, when more than the minimum six (6) semester hours is met, study of habilitative/rehabilitative procedures may be counted in the Major Professional Area for the Certificate in Speech-Language-Pathology (see Section II,B,8).

II,B,4. Major Professional Area, Certificate in Audiology

The 24 semester hours of professional education required for the Certificate of Clinical Competence in Audiology should be in the broad, but not necessarily exclusive, categories of study as follows: (1) auditory disorders, such as (a) pathologies of the auditory system, and (b) assessment of auditory disorders and their effect on communication; (2) habilitative/rehabilitative procedures, such as (a) selection and use of appropriate amplification instrumentation for the hearing impaired, both wearable and group, (b) evaluation of speech and language problems of the hearing impaired, and (c) management procedures for speech and language habilitation and/or rehabilitation of the hearing impaired (that may include manual communication); (3) conservation of hearing, such as (a) environmental noise control, and (b) identification audiometry (school, military, industry); and (4) instrumentation, such as (a) electronics, (b) calibration techniques, and (c) characteristics of amplifying systems.

Not less than six (6) semester hours must be in the auditory pathology category, and not less than six (6) semester hours must be in the habilitation/rehabilitation category.

II,B,5. Minor Professional Area, Certificate in Audiology

For the individual to obtain the Certificate in Audiology, not less than six (6) semester hours must be obtained in the areas of speech and language pathology, of these three (3) hours must be in the area of speech pathology and three (3) hours in the area of language pathology. It is suggested that where only this minimum requirement of six (6) semester hours is met, such study be in the areas of evaluation procedures and management of speech and language problems that are not associated with hearing impairment.

II,B,6. Related Areas

In addition to the 12 semester hours of course study in the Basic Communication Processes Area, the 24 semester hours in the Major Professional Area and the six (6) semester hours in the Minor Professional Area, the applicant may receive credit toward the minimum requirement of 60 semester hours of required education through advanced study in a variety of related areas. Such study should pertain to the understanding of human behavior, both normal and abnormal, as well as services available from related professions, and in general should augment the background for a professional career. Examples of such areas of study are as follows: (a) theories of learning and behavior, (b) services available from related professions that also deal with persons who have disorders of communication, and (c) information from these professions about the sensory, physical, emotional, social, and/or intellectual status of a child or an adult.

Academic credit that is obtained for practice teaching or practicum work in other professions will not be counted toward the minimum requirements.

In order that the future applicant for one of the certificates will be capable of critically reviewing scientific matters dealing with clinical issues relative to speech-language pathology and audiology, credit for study in the area of statistics, beyond an introductory course, will be allowed to a maximum of three (3) semester hours. Academic study of the administrative organization of speech-language pathology and audiology programs also may be applied to a maximum of three (3) semester hours.

II,B,7. Education Applicable to All Areas

Certain types of course work may be acceptable among more than one of the areas of study specified above, depending upon the emphasis. For example, courses that provide an overview of research, e.g., introduction to graduate study or introduction to research, that consist primarily of a critical review of research in communication sciences, disorders, or management thereof, and/or a more general presentation of research procedures and techniques that will permit the clinician to read and evaluate literature critically will be acceptable to a maximum of three (3) semester hours. Such courses may be credited to the Basic Communication Processes Area, or one of the Professional Areas or the Related Area, if substantive content of the course(s) covers material in those areas. Academic credit for a thesis or dissertation may be acceptable to a maximum of three (3) semester hours in the appropriate area. An abstract of the study must be submitted with the application if such credit is requested. In order to be acceptable, the thesis or dissertation must have been an experimental or descriptive investigation in the areas of speech, language and hearing science, speech-language pathology or audiology; that is, credit will not be allowed if the project was a survey of opinions, a study of professional issues, an annotated bibliography, biography, or a study of curricular design.

As implied by the above, the academic credit hours obtained for one course or one enrollment, may, and should, be in some instances divided among the Basic Communication Processes Area, one of the Professional Areas, and/or the Related Area. In such cases, a description of the content of that course should accompany the application. This description should be extensive enough to provide the Clinical Certification Board with information necessary to evaluate the validity of the request to apply the content to more than one of the areas.

II,B,8. Major Professional Education Applicable to Both Certificates

Study in the area of understanding, evaluation, and management of speech and language disorders associated with hearing impairment may apply to the 24 semester hours of Major Professional Area required for either certificate (speech-language pathology or audiology). However, no more than six (6) semester hours of that study will be allowed in that manner for the certificate in speech-language pathology.

II,C. Academic Clinical Practicum

It is highly desirable that students who anticipate applying for one of the Certificates of Clinical Competence have the opportunity, relatively early in their training program, to observe the various procedures involved in a clinical program in speech-language pathology and audiology, but this passive participation is not to be construed as direct clinical practicum during academic training. The student should participate in supervised, direct clinical experience during that training only after the student has had sufficient course work to qualify for work as a student clinician and only after the student has sufficient background to undertake clinical practice under direct supervision. A minimum of 150 clock hours of the supervised clinical experience must be obtained during graduate study. Once this experience is undertaken, a substantial period of time may be spent in writing reports, in preparation for clinical sessions, in conferences with supervisors, and in class attendance to discuss clinical procedures and experiences; such time may not be credited toward the 300 minimum clock hours of supervised clinical experience required.

All student clinicians are expected to obtain direct clinical experience with both children and adults, and it is recommended that some of their direct clinical experience be conducted with groups. Although the student clinician should have experience with both speech-language and hearing disorders, at least 200 clock hours of this supervised experience must be obtained in the major professional area (speech-language pathology or audiology) in which certification is sought, and not less than 35 clock hours must be obtained in the minor area. A minimum of 50 supervised clock hours of the required 300 hours of clinical experience must be obtained in each of two distinctly different clinical settings. (The two separate clinical settings may be within the organizational structure of the same institution and may include the academic program's clinic and affliliated medical facilities, community clinics, public schools, etc.)

For certification in speech-language pathology, the student clinician is expected to have experience in both the evaluation and management of a variety of speech and language problems. The student must have no less than 50 clock hours of experience in evaluation of speech and language problems. The applicant must also have no less than 75 clock hours of experience in management of language disorders of children and adults, and no less than 25 clock hours each of experience in management of children and adults with whom disorders of (1) voice, (2) artic-ulation, and (3) fluency are significant aspects of the communication handicap.

Work with multiple problems may be credited among these types of disorders. For example, a child with an articulation prob-lem may also have a voice disorder. The clock hours of work with that child may be credited to experience with either articula-tion or voice disorders, whichever is most appropriate.

Where only the minimum 35 clock hours of clinical practicum in audiology is met that is required for the persons seeking certification in speech-language pathol-ogy, that practicum must include 15 clock hours in assessment and/or manage-ment of speech and language problems associated with hearing impairment, and 15 clock hours must be in assessment of auditory disorders. However, where more than this minimum requirement is met, clinical practicum in assessment and/or management of speech and language problems associated with hearing impair-ment may be counted toward the minimum clock hours obtained with language and/or speech disorders.

For the student clinician who is preparing for certification in audiology, 50 clock hours of direct supervised experience must be obtained in identification and eval-uation of hearing impairment, and 50 clock hours must be obtained in habilitation or rehabilitation of the communication handicaps of the hearing impaired. It is suggested that the 35 clock hours of clinical practicum in speech-language pathol-ogy required for certification in audiology be in evelution and management of speech and language problems that are not related to a hearing impairment.

An applicant whose application has been rejected may reapply if changes in the requirements make his application acceptable as a result of such changes. However, if the Clini-cal Fellowship Year is not initiated within two years of the time academic and practi-cum requirements are completed, the appli-cant must meet aca-demic and practicum requirements that are current when the Clin-ical Fellowship Year is begun.

Supervisors of clinical practicum must be competent professional workers who hold a Certificate of Clinical Competence in the professional area (speech-language pathology or audiology) in which supervision is provided. This supervision must entail the personal and direct involvement of the supervisor in any and all ways that will permit the supervisor to attest to the adequacy of the student's performance in the clinical training experience. At least 25% of the therapy sessions conducted by a student clinician must be directly supervised, with such supervision being appro-priately scheduled throughout the training period. (Direct supervision is defined as on-site observation or closed-circuit TV monitoring of the student clinician.) At least one-half of each diagnostic evaluation conducted by a student clinician must be directly supervised. (The amount of direct supervision beyond these minima should be adjusted upward depending on the student's level of competence.) The first 25 hours of a student's clinical practicum must be supervised by a qualified clinical supervisor who is a member of the program's professional staff (i.e., a primary employee of the training program). In addition to the required direct supervision, supervisors may use a variety of other ways to obtain knowledge of the student's clinical work such as conferences, audio- and videotape recordings, written reports, staffings, and discussions with other persons who have participated in the student's clinical training.

II,D. The Clinical Fellowship Year

Upon completion of professional and clinical practicum education, the applicant must complete a Clinical Fellowship Year under the supervision of one who holds the Certificate of Clinical Competence in the professional area (speech-language pathology or audiology) in which that applicant is working (and seeking certifi-cation).

Professional experience is construed to mean direct clinical work with patients, consultations, record keeping, or any other duties relevant to a bona fide program of clinical work. It is expected, however, that a significant amount of clinical expe-rience will be in direct clinical contact with persons who have communication handicaps. Time spent in supervision of students, academic teaching, and research, as well as administrative activity that does not deal directly with management programs of specific patients or clients will not be counted as professional experience in this context.

The Clinical Fellowship Year is defined as no less than nine months of full-time professional employment with full-time employment defined as a mimimum of 30 clock hours of work a week. This requirement also may be fulfilled by part-time employment as follows: (1) work of 15-19 hours per week over 18 months; (2) work of 20-24 hours per week over 15 months; or, (3) work of 25-29 hours per week over 12 months. In the event that part-time employment is used to fulfill a part of the Clinical Fellowship Year, 100% of the minimum hours of the part-time work per week requirement must be spent in direct professional experience as defined above. The Clinical Fellowship Year must be completed within a maximum period of 36 consecutive months. Professional employment of less than 15 hours per week will not fulfull any part of this requirement. If the CFY is not initiated within two years of the date the academic and practicum education is completed, the applicant must meet the academic and practicum requirements current when the CFY is begun. Whether or not the Clinical Fellow (CF) is a member of ASHA, the CF must understand and abide by the ASHA Code of Ethics.

CFY supervision must entail the personal and direct involvement of the supervisor in any and all ways that will permit the CFY supervisor to monitor, improve, and evaluate the CF's performance in professional clinical employment. The supervision must include on-site observations of the CF. Other monitoring activities such as conferences with the CF, evaluation of written reports, evaluations by professional colleagues, and so on may be executed by correspondence. The CFY supervisor must base the total evaluation on no less than 36 occasions of monitoring activities (a minimum of four hours each month). The monitoring activities must include at least 18 on-site observations (a minimum of two hours each month). Should any supervisor suspect that at any time during the Clinical Fellowship Year that the CF under supervision will not meet requirements, the CFY supervisor must counsel the CF both orally and in writing and maintain careful written records of all contacts and conferences in the ensuing months.

Further requirements for the Clinical Fellowship Year are available, and, moreover, such requirements are provided with application material for certification.

II,E. The National Examinations in Speech-Language-Pathology and Audiology

The National Examinations in Speech-Language-Pathology and Audiology are designed to assess, in a comprehensive fashion, the applicant's mastery of professional concepts as outlined above to which the applicant has been exposed throughout professional education and clinical practicum. The applicant must pass the National Examination, in either Speech-Language Pathology or Audiology that is appropriate to the certificate being sought. An applicant will be declared eligible for the National Examination on notification of the acceptable completion of the educational and clinical practicum requirements. The Examination must be passed within three years after the first administration for which an applicant is notified of eligibility.

In the event the applicant fails the examination, it may be retaken. If the examination is not successfully completed within the above mentioned three years, the person's application for certification will lapse. If the examination is passed at a later date, the person may reapply for clinical certification.

Upon such reapplication, the individual's application will be reviewed and current requirements will be applied. Appropriate fees will be charged for this review.

III. Procedures for Obtaining the Certificates

III,A.

The applicant must submit to the Clinical Certification Board, a description of professional education and academic clinical practicum on forms provided for that

Application material for certification, including a schedule of fees, may be obtained by writing to Information Services Section, American Speech-Language-Hearing Association, 10801 Rockville Pike, Rockville, Maryland 20852.

purpose. The applicant should recognize that it is highly desirable to list upon this application form the entire professional education and academic clinical practicum training.

No credit may be allowed for courses listed on the application unless satisfactory completion is verified by an official transcript. *Satisfactory completion* is defined as the applicant's having received academic credit (i.e., semester hours, quarter hours, or other unit of credit) with a passing grade as defined by the training institution. If the majority of an applicant's professional training is received at a program accredited by the Education and Training Board (ETB) of the American Speech-Language-Hearing Association (ASHA), approval of educational and academic clinical practicum requirements will be automatic.

The applicant must request that the director of the training program where the majority of graduate training was obtained sign the application. In the case where that training program is not accredited by the ETB of ASHA, that director, by signature, (1) certifies that the application is correct, and (2) recommends that the applicant receive the certificate upon completion of all the requirements. In the case where the training program is accredited by the ETB of ASHA, that director (1) certifies that the applicant has met the educational and clinical practicum requirements, and (2) recommends that the applicant receive the certificate upon completion of all the requirements.

In the event that the applicant cannot obtain the recommendation of the director of the training program, the applicant should send with the application a letter giving in detail the reasons for the inability to do so. In such an instance letters of recommendation from other faculty members may be submitted.

Application for approval of educational requirements and academic clinical practicum experiences should be made (1) as soon as possible after completion of these experiences, and (2) either before or shortly after the Clinical Fellowship Year is begun.

III,B

Upon completion of educational and academic clinical practicum training, the applicant should proceed to obtain professional employment and a supervisor for the Clinical Fellowship Year. Although the filing of a CFY Plan is not required, applicants may submit such a plan to the Clinical Certification Board (CCB) if they wish prior approval of the planned professional experience. Within one month following completion of the Clinical Fellowship Year, the CF and the CFY supervisor must submit a CFY Report to the Clinical Certification Board.

III,C

Upon notification by the Clinical Certification Board of approval of the academic course work and clinical practicum requirements the applicant will be sent registration material for the National Examinations in Speech-Language-Pathology and Audiology. Upon approval of the Clincal Fellowship Year, achieving a passing score on the National Examination, and payment of all fees the applicant will become certified.

III,D

As mentioned in Footnote 8, a schedule of fees for certification may be obtained, and payment of these fees is requisite for the various steps involved in obtaining a certificate. Checks should be made payable to the American Speech-Language-Hearing Association.

IV. APPEALS

In the event that at any stage the Clinical Certification Board informs the applicant that the application has been rejected, the applicant has the right of formal appeal.

In order to initiate such an appeal, the applicant must write to the Chairman of the Clinical Certification Board and specifically request a formal review of the application. If that review results, again, in rejection, the applicant has the right to request a review of the case by the Council on Professional Standards in Speech-Language Pathology and Audiology (COPS) by writing to the Chairman of the COPS at the National Office of the American Speech-Language-Hearing Association. The decision of the COPS will be final.

B

Code of Ethics of the
American Speech-Language-Hearing Association

(Revised January 1, 1979)

PREAMBLE

The preservation of the highest standards of integrity and ethical principles is vital to the successful discharge of the professional responsibilities of all speech-language pathologists and audiologists. The Code of Ethics has been promulgated by the Association in an effort to stress the fundamental rules considered essential to this basic purpose. Any action that is in violation of the spirit and purpose of this Code shall be considered unethical. Failure to specify any particular responsibility or practice in this Code of Ethics should not be construed as denial of the existence of other responsibilities or practices.

The fundamental rules of ethical conduct are described in three categories: Principles of Ethics, Ethical Proscriptions, Matters of Professional Propriety.

1. *Principles of Ethics.* Six principles serve as a basis for the ethical evaluation of professional conduct and form the underlying moral basis for the Code of Ethics. Individuals subscribing to this Code shall observe these principles as affirmative obligations under all conditions of professional activity.

2. *Ethical Proscriptions.* Ethical Proscriptions are formal statements of prohibitions that are derived from the Principles of Ethics.

3. *Matters of Professional Propriety.* Matters of Professional Propriety represent guidelines of conduct designed to promote the public interest and thereby better inform the public and particularly the persons in need of speech-language pathology and audiology services as to the availability and the rules regarding the delivery of those services.

PRINCIPLE OF ETHICS I

Individuals shall hold paramount the welfare of persons served professionally.

A. Individuals shall use every resource available, including referral to other specialists as needed, to provide the best service possible.

B. Individuals shall fully inform persons served of the nature and possible effects of the services.

C. Individuals shall fully inform subjects participating in research or teaching activities of the nature and possible effects of these activities.

D. Individuals' fees shall be commensurate with services rendered.

E. Individuals shall provide appropriate access to records of persons served professionally.

F. Individuals shall take all reasonable precautions to avoid injuring persons in the delivery of professional services.

G. Individuals shall evaluate services rendered to determine effectiveness.

Ethical Proscriptions

1. Individuals must not exploit persons in the delivery of professional services, including accepting persons for treatment when benefit cannot reasonably be expected or continuing treatment unnecessarily.

2. Individuals must not guarantee the results of any therapeutic procedures, directly or by implication. A reasonable statement of prognosis may be made, but caution must be exercised not to mislead persons served professionally to expect results that cannot be predicted from sound evidence.

3. Individuals must not use persons for teaching or research in a manner that constitutes invasion of privacy or fails to afford informed free choice to participate.

4. Individuals must not evaluate or treat speech, language, or hearing disorders except in a professional relationship. They must not evaluate or treat solely by correspondence. This does not preclude follow-up correspondence with persons previously seen, nor providing them with general information of an educational nature.

5. Individuals must not reveal to unauthorized persons any professional or personal information obtained from the person served professionally, unless required by law or unless necessary to protect the welfare of the person or the community.

6. Individuals must not discriminate in the delivery of professional services on any basis that is unjustifiable or irrelevent to the need for and potential benefit from such services, such as race, sex, or religion.

7. Individuals must not charge for services not rendered.

PRINCIPLE OF ETHICS II

Individuals shall maintain high standards of professional competence.

A. Individuals engaging in clinical practice shall possess appropriate qualifications which are provided by the Association's program for certification of clinical competence.

B. Individuals shall continue their professional development throughout their careers.

C. Individuals shall identify competent, dependable referral sources for persons served professionally.

D. Individuals shall maintain adequate records of professional services rendered.

Ethical Proscriptions

1. Individuals must neither provide services nor supervision of services for which they have not been properly prepared, not permit services to be provided by any of their staff who are not properly prepared.

2. Individuals must not provide clinical services by prescription of anyone who does not hold the Certificate of Clinical Competence.

3. Individuals must not delegate any service requiring the professional competence of a certified clinician to anyone unqualified.

4. Individuals must not offer clinical services by supportive personnel for whom they do not provide appropriate supervision and assume full responsibility.

5. Individuals must not require anyone under their supervision to engage in any practice that is a violation of the Code of Ethics.

PRINCIPLE OF ETHICS III

Individuals' statements to persons served professionally and to the public shall provide accurate information about the nature and management of communicative disorders, and about the profession and services rendered by its practitioners.

1. Individuals must not misrepresent their training or competence.

2. Individuals' public statements providing information about professional services and products must not contain representations or claims that are false, deceptive, or misleading.

3. Individuals must not use professional or commercial affiliations in any way that would mislead or limit services to persons served professionally.

Matters of Professional Propriety

1. Individuals should announce services in a manner consonant with highest professional standards in the community.

PRINCIPLES OF ETHICS IV

Individuals shall maintain objectivity in all matters concerning the welfare of persons served professionally.

A. Individuals who dispense products to persons served professionally shall observe the following standards:

(1) Products associated with professional practice must be dispensed to the person served as a part of a program of comprehensive habilitative care.

(2) Fees established for the professional services must be independent of whether a product is dispensed.

(3) Persons served must be provided freedom of choice for the source of services and products.

(4) Price information about professional services rendered and products dispensed must be disclosed by providing to or posting for persons served a complete schedule of fees and charges in advance of rendering services, which schedule differentiates between fees for professional services and charges for products dispensed.

(5) Products dispensed to the person served must be evaluated to determine effectiveness.

Ethical Proscriptions

1. Individuals must not participate in activities that constitute a conflict of professional interest.

Matters of Professional Propriety

1. Individuals should not accept compensation for supervision or sponsorship from the clinician being supervised or sponsored.

2. Individuals should present products they have developed to their colleagues in a manner consonant with highest professional standards.

PRINCIPLE OF ETHICS V

Individuals shall honor their responsibilities to the public, their profession, and their relationships with colleagues and members of allied professions.

Matters of Professional Propriety

1. Individuals should seek to provide and expand services to persons with speech, language, and hearing handicaps as well as to assist in establishing high professional standards for such programs.

2. Individuals should educate the public about speech, language and hearing processes, speech, language and hearing problems, and matters related to professional competence.

3. Individuals should strive to increase knowledge within the profession and share research with colleagues.

4. Individuals should establish harmonious relations with colleagues and members of other professions, and endeavor to inform members of related professions of services provided by speech-language pathologists and audiologists, as well as seek information from them.

5. Individuals should assign credit to those who have contributed to a publication in proportion to their contribution.

PRINCIPLES OF ETHICS VI

Individuals shall uphold the dignity of the profession and freely accept the profession's self-imposed standards.

A. Individuals shall inform the Ethical Practice Board of violations of this Code of Ethics.

B. Individuals shall cooperate fully with the Ethical Practice Board inquiries into matters of professional conduct related to this Code of Ethics.

Sources of
Additional Information

JOURNALS

American Journal of Mental Deficiency

Published by the American Association on Mental Deficiency (AAMD). Issued bi-monthly. Designed to present discussions and research of behavioral and biological aspects of mental retardation.

Education and Training of the Mentally Retarded

Published by the Council for Exceptional Children (CEC), Division on Mental Retardation. Issued four times during the school year. Designed to present investigations and discussions of the education of the mentally retarded.

Exceptional Children

Published by the Council for Exceptional Children (CEC). Issued eight times each year. Designed to assist special educators and other professionals and specialists who serve exceptional children.

Journal of Learning Disabilities

Published by Professional Press. Issued ten times a year. Designed to present research and theoretical discussions relating to learning disabilities.

Journal of Speech and Hearing Disorders

Published by the American Speech-Language-Hearing Association (ASHA). Issued quarterly. Designed to present applied research and critical discussions relating to the nature, assessment, and treatment of communication disorders.

Journal of Speech and Hearing Research

Published by the American Speech-Language-Hearing Association (ASHA). Issued quarterly. Designed to feature theoretical and technical research in communication sciences and disorders.

Language, Speech, and Hearing Services in the Schools

Published by the American Speech-Language-Hearing Association (ASHA). Issued quarterly. Designed to address the application of theories and research to the assessment and treatment of communication disorders in educational settings.

Learning Disability Quarterly

Published by the Council for Exceptional Children (CEC), Division for Children with Learning Disabilities. Issued four times each year. Designed to present applied research, theory, and practices in the area of learning disabilities.

Mental Retardation

Published by the American Assocation on Mental Deficiency (AAMD). Issued bi-monthly. Designed to present new approaches to methods, critical discussions, and applied research in mental retardation.

ORGANIZATIONS

American Association of Mental Deficiency (AAMD)

5201 Connecticut Avenue, N.W., Washington, DC 20015
An organization of researchers, teacher educators, and psychologists associated with the field of mental retardation.

American Speech-Language-Hearing Association (ASHA)

10801 Rockville Pike, Rockville, MD 20852
The major professional organization for individuals involved in the study of communication sciences and in serving individuals with communication disorders.

Association for Children with Learning Disabilities (ACLD)

5255 Grace Street, Pittsburgh, PA 15236
An organization of parents and professionals devoted to advocacy for learning disabled children and youth.

Division for Children with Communication Disorders (DCCD)

Council for Exceptional Children
1920 Association Drive, Reston, VA 22091
An organizational unit of speech, language, and hearing clinicians and other specialists working with children with disorders of communication.

Division for Children with Learning Disabilities (DCLD)

Council for Exceptional Children
1920 Association Drive, Reston, VA 22091
An organizational unit of teachers, special educators, and other specialists working with learning disabled children and youth.

Division on Mental Retardation (DMR)

Council for Exceptional Children
1920 Association Drive, Reston, VA 22091
An organizational unit of teachers, teacher educators, and other members of CEC working with the mentally retarded.

Glossary

Abdomen	That portion of the body lying between the thorax and pelvis.
Abduct	To draw away from the midline.
Adduct	To move toward the midline.
Agnosia	Loss of ability to perceive, integrate, and attach meaning to sensory stimuli.
Alexia	Acquired inability to perform some or all of the tasks involved in reading; caused by brain damage.
Allophone	A speech sound that is accepted as a variant of a phoneme but is not used to differentiate two words in a language.
Alveolus	A small hollow or pit.
Ambiguous	Word or other linguistic unit with multiple meanings.
Anacusis	Total hearing loss.
Ankylosis	Impairment of arytenoid movement resulting from stiffness or fixation of the cricoarytenoid joint.
Anomia	Acquired word-finding difficulty, caused by brain damage.
Anoxia	Lack of oxygen.
Antagonist	Muscle which acts in opposition to another muscle.
Antecedent Event	Event which occurs before target response.
Anterior	Toward the front; away from the back.
Aphasia	Acquired language disorder caused by brain damage, resulting in partial or complete impairment of language comprehension, formulation, and use for communication.
Aphonia	Complex loss of voice.
Apraxia	Neurologic, phonologic disorder resulting from sensorimotor impairment of the capacity to select, program, or execute, in coordinated and normally timed sequences, the positioning of the speech muscles for the volitional production of speech sounds; involuntary movements remain intact. Sometimes considered a form of aphasia.
Arbitrary	Word which derives meaning from a random choice rather than from a similarity, logical reason, resemblance, or need.
Articulation	(1) A joint or point of juncture of bones; (2) movement of and placement of body structures known as *articulators* during speech production.
Articulators	Those structures responsible for modification of the vocal tract; i.e., tongue, lips, soft and hard palates, and teeth.
Ataxia	(1) Lack of order; (2) Type of cerebral palsy characterized by poor sense of body position and balance and lack of coordination of voluntary muscles.
Athetosis	(1) Without a fixed base; (2) Type of cerebral palsy characterized by large, irregular, uncontrollable twisting actions; muscles may have too much or too little tone.
Auditory Training	Program to teach hearing impaired to make maximum use of residual hearing.

Autonomous Phonemic	Traditional study of the sounds of a language, independent of changes which may occur between or within words.
Baseline	The pretreatment level of a target behavior, which, when quantified, can be used as a basis against which to measure progress.
Behavior Modification	Systematic application of behavioral learning principles in order to increase or decrease a target response.
Biopsy	Surgical removal of a small sample of tissue that is then examined microscopically.
Black English	The collective varieties of English spoken by people of African descent throughout the world, including American Black English (the collective varieties of English spoken by Blacks in the United States).
Black English Vernacular	The varieties of Black English spoken by people of African descent in formal situations throughout the world, including American Black English Vernacular.
Block	An instance of stuttering usually characterized by a complete or partial interruption of the smooth flow of speech.
Bronch-, Broncho-	Referring to the windpipe.
Bronchiole	The smallest division of the bronchial tree.
Cartilage	A nonvascular connective tissue, softer and more flexible than bone.
Cerebral Palsy	A group of irreversible, nondeteriorating disorders caused by an irregularity in the central nervous system, primarily at motor control centers; damage may be caused at any time before muscular coordination is attained. Characteristics may include too much or too little muscle tone, abnormal positioning, and general lack of coordination. Intellect, speech, hearing, vision, and emotional control may be affected.
Circumlocution	The substitution of a word or phrase for a more direct expression; talking around the point.
Classical Conditioning	Process in which two stimuli are repeatedly paired in order to give one (the conditioned stimulus) the power to elicit the unconditioned response (reflex) already elicited by the other (unconditioned) stimulus.
Cluttering	Very rapid, often unintelligible speech; characterized by omission of speech sounds or entire words.
Coarticulation	Influence of one speech sound upon another.
Code Switching	The act of shifting from one language or one dialect of a language to another, usually under the control of the social situation or context.
Cognates	Pair of consonant phonemes with the same place and manner of articulation, differing only in voicing.
Communication Competence	Knowledge which users of a language must have in order to understand and produce an infinite number of acceptable grammatical structures.
Concha	A shell-like organ or structure; pronounced *khongka.*
Conductive Hearing Loss	Loss caused by a breakdown or obstruction to the mechanical conductors of sound; contrasts with *sensorineural hearing loss.*
Congenital	Present at birth.
Consequence	Contingent event following a response that functions to increase or decrease the probability that the response will occur again.
Creole	A language formed on the basis of the phonology and grammar of a dominant language, but using the vocabulary of a nondominant language.
Criterion-Referenced	Test which compares an individual's scores to a standard for mastery (rather than to scores of other subjects).
Deaf	Person with a hearing loss of at least 70 dB HL, which precludes comprehending speech aurally.
Decibel (dB)	Arbitrary unit of loudness that expresses the ratio of a measured power or pressure to a reference value.
Deciduous	Temporary; falling off and shedding at maturity.

Decoding	Process of deducing a thought or message from oral or written language.
Derivation	Process of adding an ending to a base word form to change its grammatical class and allow the new (derived) word to function differently (e.g., *teach-teacher*).
Dialect	A variety within a specific language.
Diaphragm	(1) A partition separating two cavities; (2) Muscle which separates thorax from abdomen.
Diphthong	Speech sound within a syllable produced by movement from the articulatory position of one phoneme to that of another.
Disfluencies	Properties in speech that interrupt the smooth, forward flow of an utterance; usually refers to pauses, hesitations, interjections, prolongations, and repetitions.
Distortion	Articulation error type in which phoneme is present but produced incorrectly.
Distributed	Practice session which are separated by rest period.
Down's Syndrome	Specific syndrome caused by chromosomal abnormality, occurring in approximately 1 in 700 births; often characterized by wide-set, Oriental-looking eyes; mild to moderate mental retardation; a Simian or single crease across the palm; and a wide range of other birth defects.
Dysarthria	A group of motor speech disorders caused by nervous system damage; may involve respiration, articulation, phonation, or prosody deviations, because of inability either to initiate or to control muscular movements.
Dyslexia	Failure to master reading at expected age level in the absence of a major debilitating disorder.
Dysnomia	Developmental word-finding difficulty which interferes with accuracy in finding intended words.
Dysphemia	Theory of causation of stuttering which posits stuttering to be a biological breakdown which occurs under emotional or physical stress. Related to biochemical theory, which states that the breakdown is specifically biochemical.
Dysphonia	Poor or unpleasant voice quality.
Edematous	Filled with fluid; swollen.
Encoding	Translating a thought or message into written or oral language.
Erythema	Abnormal redness.
Etiology	Cause or causes of a problem.
Extinguish	To irradicate an undesirable behavior completely.
Extrinsic	Originating outside the part.
Fissure	A cleft or split.
Formant (Bonds)	Regions of prominent energy distribution in a speech sound.
Functional	Having no known physical cause.
Glottal Fry	A grating or popping sound that occurs most often toward the end of sentences or phrases, where the pitch and breath pressure customarily drop.
Glottal Stop	A plosive sound produced when air held beneath the glottis is suddenly released.
Glottal Tone	The tone generated by the vibrating vocal folds, to be distinguished from the tone produced by the oscillation or ringing of the vocal tract.
Glottis	The space betwen the vocal folds.
Gyrus	A fold in the cerebral cortex; a convolution.
Hard-of-Hearing	A person with a hearing loss of 35 to 69 dB HL, which makes comprehension of speech by hearing alone difficult, but not impossible.
Hearing Impaired	Suffering from any degree of hearing loss.
Hematoma	A tumor filled with blood, such as a blood blister.
Hemianopsia (Hemianopia)	Defective vision in one-half of the visual field of one eye. Homonymous hemianopsia indicates a corresponding visual field loss in both eyes.
Hemiparesis	Weakness of one lateral half of the body.

Hemiplegia	Paralysis of one lateral half of the body.
Hertz (Hz)	Measurement of wave frequency in cycles per second.
High Self-Reinforcer	Person who has a tendency to provide his own reinforcers as a means of regulating his own behavior.
Homonymous	Having the same meaning.
Hypernasal	Speech which is too greatly resonated in the nasal cavities.
Hyponasal	Speech which varies from the norm in having very little or no nasal resonance.
Iconic	Word which bears a resemblance to its reference, as a picture, gesture, or sound.
Ideation	Organization of ideas into concepts which can be communicated.
Inflection	(1) The rising and falling of the voice during speech; (2) Grammatical change of a word to fit different grammatical functions, such as number or tense, by adding a word ending (e.g., *boy, boys*; *walk, walked*).
Intelligibility	How readily a person's speech can be understood by listeners.
Intrinsic	Rising from the nature or constitution of a thing; inherent, situated within.
Kinesics	The study of bodily movement, particularly in relation to communication.
Kinesthetic Feedback	Knowledge of location of muscles and body parts or whether they are moving, derived from sensory end-organs in the muscles, tendons, joints, and sometimes inner ears.
Language	A system of oral or written symbols used by a group of people with marked consistency in order to communicate.
Language-Learning Disability	The developmental language disability associated with a diagnosed learning disability.
Language Retardation	Developmental delay in language acquisition associated with mental retardation.
Laryngectomy	Surgical removal of the larynx.
Larynx	Anatomical structure located above the trachea and below the hyoid bone and tongue root; consists of cartilage and muscle and, due to its vocal folds, is the primary organ of phonation.
Lexicon	Vocabulary.
Ligament	A band of fibrous tissue which connects bones or holds organs in place.
Low Self-Reinforcer	A person who has a tendency to require reinforcement from others in regulating his behavior.
Mainstreaming	Process of placing children with handicaps in regular classroom setting or in the most nearly normal setting in which the child can succeed.
Mandible	Lower jaw.
Manometer	Instrument for measuring the pressure of liquids or gases.
Marked Word	Word in an antonym pair with negative, nonpreferred, or unusual reference, e.g., *hate (love)*.
Masking	Process of presenting a sound to the nontest ear to remove it from an audiological test procedure.
Massed	Continuous practice sessions which are not separated by rest periods.
Maxilla	Upper jaw.
Meatus	An opening to a passageway in the body.
Medial	Toward the axis; near the midline.
Membrane	A thin layer of tissue that binds structures, divides spaces or organs, and lines cavities.
Metacommunication	Nonverbal aspects of communication.
Middle Ear Effusion	Accumulation of fluid behind the tympanic membrane.
Mongolism	Vernacular term for Down's syndrome.
Moro Reflex	Extensor startle pattern in response to sound, exhibited by most newborns.

Morpheme	The smallest unit of meaning in a language; can be a root word, prefix, infix, or suffix.
Morphology	The study of the arrangement of sounds into words or other units which carry meaning.
Myasthenia	Overall condition of muscular weakness.
Narrow-Band Noise	Filtered noise presented in certain frequencies at near-equal intensities.
Neurogenic	Arising from the nervous system.
Noise	Any complex sound composed of irregular vibrations to which a pure pitch cannot be assigned.
Nonverbal Communication	Reciprocal interaction between two or more individuals without the use of oral or written symbols.
Norm-Referenced	Test in which an individual's score is compared to the test scores of a large number of subjects who have previously taken the test.
Normative Data	Information derived from study of large groups of subjects performing a particular behavior.
Nystagmus	An involuntary slow movement in one direction followed by a rapid movement in the opposite direction.
Omission	Articulation error type in which phoneme is totally omitted.
Operant Conditioning	Systematic arrangement of antecedent and consequent events to increase or decrease a target behavior.
Organic	Having a physical cause or source.
Origin	The place of attachment of a muscle, remaining relatively fixed during contraction.
Otitis Media	Inflammation of the middle ear.
Paralanguage	The study of prosodic variation; sounds produced in speech that are not part of the phonetic code.
Pharynx	The membranous-muscular tube connecting the mouth and posterior nares with the esophagus and larynx.
Phonation	The production of sound by the vibration of the vocal folds.
Phone	Any speech sound.
Phoneme	Smallest unit of sound in a language which can be distinguished and which serves to differentiate two words.
Phonological Conditioning	Process by which the choice of inflectional word ending is governed by the sound immediately preceding it.
Phonology	The study of the linguistic rules for combining sound segments into larger units.
Pitch	Quality of sound caused by its frequency; perceived on a scale from low to high.
Pleura	The serous membranes lining the thoracic cavity and investing the surfaces of the lungs.
Posterior	Toward the back; away from the front.
Postlingual Hearing Loss	Loss acquired after the person has developed language.
Pragmatics	The branch of linguistics dealing with the relations between language and context.
Prelingual Hearing Loss	Loss which occurs before a child develops language.
Prognosis	Indication of how rapidly recovery from a disorder will occur and how complete recovery will be.
Prosodic	Referring to the stress pattern—voice, pitch, loudness, duration—of an utterance.
Proxemics	The study of bodily position and spatial relations, in particular in relation to communication.
Pseudoglottis	An artificial glottis.
Punishment	Process of presenting a consequence to decrease the frequency of the behavior it follows.

Reauditorization	Process of reconstructing or rehearsing digits, words, phrases, or sentences you have heard to yourself, "in your head."
Referent	The event or object to which a symbol refers.
Reflex	An involuntary, relatively invariable, adaptive response to a stimulus.
Register	Range of word, phrase, sentence, and utterance choices and language styles available to a speaker to meet the needs or expectations of a given listener.
Reinforcement	Consequent event which increases the probability that the behavior it follows will occur again.
Relaxation Pressure	Intrapulmonic pressure due to tissue elasticity, torque, and gravity, which tends to expel air from the lungs.
Residual Hearing	Amount of hearing present along with some loss.
Residual Volume	Quantity of air that cannot be expelled from the lungs; usually expressed in cm^3.
Resonant Frequency	The rate at which any given object can most easily be made to vibrate.
Respiration	The interchange of gases between living organisms and their environment.
Respiratory Tract	The nares, nasal cavities, pharynx, oral cavity, larynx, trachea, and bronchial tubes.
Screening	Any assessment given to large numbers of subjects in order to identify those who are "at-risk" of having difficulty and who thus need more indepth assessment.
Segmentation	Process of dividing a stream of speech into discrete sounds, words, and sentences.
Semantics	The study of meaning in language.
Semivowels	Sounds that are neither completely vowel nor consonant, but fall between them in articulation and perception.
Sensorineural Hearing Loss	The inability to hear caused by failure of nerves to transmit sound impulses; contrasts with *conductive hearing loss*.
Shaping	Process of using antecedent and consequent events to change behavior through gradually closer approximations of target.
Sociolinguistic Variables	Nonlinguistic factors which may change an act of communication; e.g., audience, topic, or setting.
Sociolinguistics	The study of social and cultural influences on language and its use within speech communities.
Sonogram	Graph of a sound or sounds produced by a special electromechanical device.
Southern White Non-standard English	Dialect of American English spoken by working-class Southern Whites.
Spastic	(1) Characterized by muscle contractions which are involuntary and jerky; (2) A type of cerebral palsy characterized by spastic movements and too much muscle tone.
Speech Community	A group of individuals sharing a common set of linguistic and communication rules, values, and experiences.
Spirometer	An instrument for measuring vital capacity or volume of inspired and exhaled air.
Standard Black English	Varieties of English spoken by formerly educated people of African descent throughout the world; used especially in formal situations.
Standard Dialect	The primary language spoken by groups within a society with the highest social, economic, political, or educational prestige and power.
Stimulability	Ability to produce a misarticulated sound in response to a model of the correct production of the sound.
Stoma	An opening.
Strabismus	Inability to focus the eyes caused by unbalanced muscular strength or control in one eye.
Strider	Membranous partition, extending usually from one vocal fold to the other; a laryngeal web.
Structural Ambiguity	Characteristics of sentence structure that allows it to be interpreted in more than one way.

Substitution	Articulation error type in which one phoneme is used in place of the correct phoneme.
Sulcus	Furrow or groove, especially in the brain.
Suprasegmental	Characteristics greater than segments; relating to junctural or prosodic features.
Symbol	Oral or written expression used to represent an object, event, or idea.
Syndrome	Group of symptoms or characteristics which, when taken together, constitute an identifiable condition or disease.
Syntax	Branch of language dealing with structure; i.e., relation of word order to meaning.
Systematic Phonemic	A system of the study of sounds which tries to classify and explain changes in sounds as words are used in different ways.
Tendon	A nonelastic band of connective tissue that attaches a muscle to bone or cartilage.
Tetrahedral	Having the form of a tetrahedron, which is a solid contained by four triangular plane faces (a triangular pyramid).
Thoraco-	Pertaining to the chest.
Tidal Volume	The quantity of air exchanged during a cycle of quiet, normal breathing; usually expressed in cm^3.
Trachea	The tube extending from the larynx to the bronchi.
Transformation	Operation in which elements in the base structure of an utterance are substituted, deleted, or rearranged into an appropriate surface structure.
Tympanometry	Method of measuring the resistance of acoustical energy flow at different pressure changes at the tympanic membrane.
Unmarked Word	Word in an antonym pair with positive, preferred, or usual reference, e.g., *love* (*hate*).
Unvoiced	Consonant sound produced with no vibration of the larynx.
Velum	Thin, veil-like structure; the muscular portion of the soft palate.
Vernacular	Common mode of expression in a speech community, especially used for informal exchanges among members of that community.
Vital Capacity	The maximum amount of air that can be exhaled after a maximum inhalation.
Voiced	Sound produced with vibration of the vocal folds; includes some consonants and all vowels.

Name Index

Subject Index

Contributors

George H. Shames, Professor in Speech and Psychology and Chairman of the Graduate Training Program in Speech Pathology and Audiology at the University of Pittsburgh, has had a dual interest in stuttering and in training of speech-language pathologists for many years. He has been guest lecturer at universities and colleges throughout the United States and in Australia, in addition to presenting many miniseminars, short courses, and workshops on the management of stuttering. A member of the American Speech-Hearing-Language Association, American Cleft Palate Association, American Psychological Association, and American Association for the Advancement of Science, Shames holds a CCC in Speech and is a Licensed Clinical Psychologist. He is an active leader of ASHA and ACPA and has served as a site visitor for and on the Educational and Training Board of the American Board of Examiners in Speech Pathology and Audiology. He has been a consultant in research, training, and curriculum developments, as well as at a variety of clinical sites. A long list of research grants and a wide range of clinical experiences have produced an even longer list of papers, articles, international presentations, and books, including *Stutter-Free Speech: A Goal for Therapy* (with C. L. Florance).

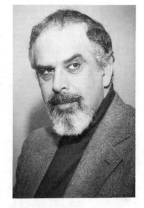

A native of Denmark, where she received her B.S., **Elisabeth H. Wiig** completed her professional schooling in the United States with a Ph.D. from Case Western Reserve University. She is currently a Professor in the Department of Speech Pathology and Audiology at Boston University. In addition to holding the CCC in Audiology and the CCC in Speech Pathology, Wiig is a member of the American Association of Mental Deficiency, the International Neuropsychology Society, the Academy of Aphasia, the American Speech-Language-Hearing Association, and the Massachusetts Speech and Hearing Association, of which she was president in 1976–77. She has published more than 25 articles and made numerous conference presentations dealing primarily with aphasia and with learning disabilities. Her current research focus on the language problems of learning disabled children and adolescents is reflected in her most recent text, *Language Assessment and Intervention for the Learning Disabled,* and a program of screening tests and a diagnostic battery, *CELF: Clinical Evaluation of Language Functions* (both with E.M. Semel).

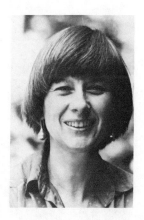

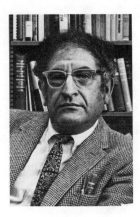

Jack Matthews, who is Professor and Chairman, Speech and Theatre Arts Department, University of Pittsburgh, has been a leader in the fields of speech pathology and psychology for more than 20 years. A past president of the Pennsylvania Speech Association, American Cleft Palate Association, and American Speech and Hearing Association, he has also served as assistant editor or on the editorial board of many of the fields' most highly respected journals. He has been and continues to act as a consultant for many private and governmental agencies, including the National Advisory Committee on Handicapped Children, the National Institutes of Health, United Cerebral Palsy, and the Departments of Health, Education and Welfare and of Defense. His many interests range from teaching speech skills to special students to teaching machine concepts.

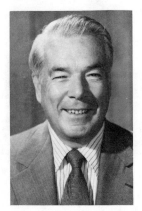

John Valeur Irwin has also had a distinguished career in speech pathology. He has taught at the Universities of Minnesota, where he was Director of the Voice Science Laboratory; Wisconsin, where he was also Director of the Speech and Hearing Clinics; and Kansas where he was Roy A. Roberts Professor of Speech. In 1970 he was designated the Pope M. Farrington Professor of Speech Pathology at Memphis State University, a position he held until his retirement in 1980. He currently serves as Distinguished Lecturer and Consultant at Eastern Kentucky University. A member of Phi Beta Kappa, Omicron Delta Kappa, and Phi Kappa Phi, and a fellow of The American Speech-Language-Hearing Association, Irwin was awarded The Honors of the Association in 1970. He has also served as president of ASHA and on many panels, site teams, and committees for both the Office of Education and the National Institutes of Health. A former editor of *Acta Symbolica,* Irwin has contributed both to textbooks and to many professional journals.

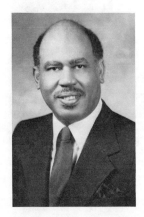

Orlando L. Taylor is now a Graduate Research Professor at Howard University's Department of Communication Arts and Sciences, after heading that department for 5 years. He is also Adjunct Professor at the University of Pittsburgh. His graduate degrees focus on speech pathology, psychology, linguistics, sociology, and reading. He has directed urban language research at the University of the District of Columbia, directed language programs and taught at many universities, both in the United States and abroad, and directed a clinic at Indiana's Fort Wayne State Hospital. His professional credits include work as a speech clinician; membership in numerous professional organizations; consulting for *Sesame Street,* the public schools, and government projects; and authoring articles and books on aphasia, testing, and Black English. For his outstanding work developing the Afro-American Program at Indiana University, he won the Leather Medal.

A Professor of Speech and Hearing Science and School of Basic Medical Sciences at the University of Illinois, **Willard R. Zemlin** has had a career-long interest in the anatomy and physiology of speech and hearing. He is a member of the American Speech-Language-Hearing Association (of which he is a Fellow), the Acoustic Society of America, and the American Association of Phonetic Sciences. Zemlin has written numerous books and articles and presented dozens of papers on speech and hearing science and the related physiological mechanisms in humans and animals (from dalmations to guinea pigs). He is also actively involved in directing graduate student research. His many honors include winning the 1972–73 Swedish Medical Research Council Fellowship.

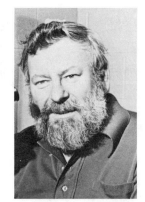

Leija V. McReynolds is a Professor of Hearing and Speech at the University of Kansas Medical Center and a Research Associate at the Bureau of Child Research Laboratory and at the Kansas Center for Mental Retardation and Human Development. A member of several professional organizations, she has also served in editorial functions for the *Journal of Speech and Hearing Disorders,* the *Journal of Applied Behavior Analysis,* and *Analysis and Intervention in Developmental Disabilities.* McReynolds' interest in the application of behavior modification techniques to language impairments, especially articulation disorders, has been demonstrated in numerous articles, chapters in books, journal reviews, and workshops presented from coast-to-coast. Her current interests focus on articulation disorders and normal phonological development from the point of view of linguistics.

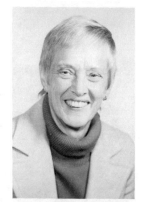

G. Paul Moore has been a recognized leader in the study of the voice and laryngeal function for more than 30 years. His career was capped by his appointment as Distinguished Service Professor at the University of Florida in 1977, where the Annual Symposium on the Care of the Professional Voice is named the G. Paul Moore Lecture. A former president of the American Speech and Hearing Association, the American Speech and Hearing Foundation, and the Central States Speech Association, he has also been a member of several professional organizations, editorial boards, and government advisory committees. His many writings on voice, the singing voice, and the larynx have appeared in professional journals in the United States, Europe, and Australia. He has also authored or coauthored nine films on voice or the larynx.

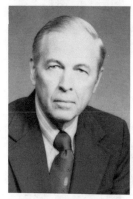

Cheri L. Florance is Director of the Communication Disorders Institute at St. Anthony Hospital in Columbus, Ohio. Certified as CCC in Speech, she received her Ph.D. in Speech and Hearing Science from The Ohio State University. Her extensive clinical experience includes work in hospitals, a rehabilitation center, community speech and hearing clinics, and university clinics. Florance has given many workshops and research presentations at conferences, and has written numerous articles dealing with apraxia of speech, early language development, and language training of handicapped children, as well as stuttering. She is coauthor (with George Shames) of *Stutter-Free Speech: A Goal for Therapy.*

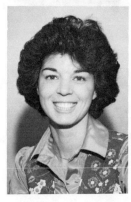

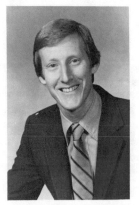

Laurence B. Leonard is a Professor in the Department of Audiology and Speech Sciences at Purdue University. Leonard received his B.A. degree in psychology and M.S. degree in speech-language pathology from the University of South Florida. Prior to receiving his Ph.D. in speech-language pathology from the University of Pittsburgh, he was employed as a speech-language pathologist and, later, as a clinical supervisor. His primary interests center on language development and language disorders in children. Leonard's work on this subject appears in a number of professional journals and textbooks.

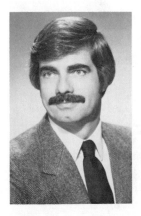

Jerry L. Northern is Professor of Otolaryngology, Associate Professor of Pediatrics, and Head, Audiology Division, Department of Otolaryngology at the University of Colorado Health Sciences Center. Before joining the University of Colorado, he had held positions as Assistant Director of the Army Audiology and Speech Center at Walter Reed Hospital and as Chief of Audiology at Brooke General Hospital, Ft. Sam Houston, Texas. He has also had a private practice in audiology. He has presented papers in nearly 200 professional meetings throughout his career, and has presented in South Vietnam, the Republic of China, and several Central and South American countries. He has written or edited seven books and contributed many chapters, book reviews, and articles in professional journals. His special interests include audiological assessments of hearing impaired and other handicapped children.

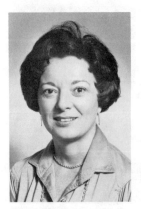

Margaret L. Lemme has more than 13 years experience in speech-language pathology and education, most recently as Associate Professor at the University of Denver, and Clinical Associate Professor of Physical Medicine and Rehabilitation, Colorado Health Sciences Center. Previous to these current assignments, she taught in the Department of Communication Disorders and Speech Sciences, University of Colorado, at Gallaudet College for the Deaf, and in the public schools of Fort Knox, Kentucky. Lemme earned a master's degree in Communication Disorders from Oklahoma Health Sciences Center, Oklahoma City, and a doctorate in Speech-Language Pathology and Audiology from the University of Colorado. She has been active in the American Speech-Language-Hearing Association, serving as Colorado Legislative Counselor, as chairman of Speech Disorders III and IV for the Program Committee, and as Instructor for Communication Problems and Behaviors of the Older American. She serves as Treasurer of Clinical Aphasiology and is active in the Colorado Speech-Language-Hearing Association. Lemme has published articles in *JSHD, LSHSS,* and *CAC Proceedings* in the areas of neurogenic communication disorders and auditory processing. Her most recent interest deals with models of auditory linguistic processing.

The distinguished career of **Betty Jane McWilliams** has been committed to individuals with cleft palate and related disorders. A past president of the American Cleft Palate Association and current editor of the *Cleft Palate Journal,* she is Director of the Cleft Palate Center and Professor of Audiology and Speech Patholgoy at the University of Pittsburgh. She continues to be active in her community and at the university, along with writing numerous books, chapters, and articles focusing on both the technical and the interpersonal management of cleft palate. McWilliams has been honored as a Fellow of both the American Speech and Hearing Association and the American College of Dentists and with the Service Award of the American Cleft Palate Association (1975) and the Herbert Cooper Memorial Award (1979).

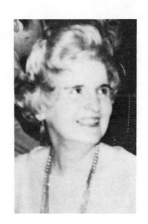

Leonard L. (Chick) LaPointe (L^3) began his professional career as an itinerant speech-language clinician in 10 schools in Menasha, Wisconsin. During his graduate studies at the University of Colorado at Boulder, he acquired his on-going interest in brain function and communication by serving traineeships and internships at Rose Memorial Hospital, the Denver Veterans Administration Hospital, the University of Colorado Medical School, and Fitzsimons Army Hospital. He is now Coordinator of Instruction in Audiology and Speech Pathology at the Veterans Administration Medical Center in Gainesville, Florida, while holding adjunct positions in the Department of Speech and the Department of Communicative Disorders at the University of Florida. LaPointe has authored or coauthored one book, seven book chapters, two films, a reading test for aphasia, over 25 scientific articles, and more than 100 papers, invited lectures, and workshops. His other interests include the crafts and culture of American Indians, humor and nonsense, and the cultivation of optimism.

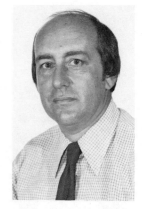

A Professor of Speech Pathology and Chairman of the Department of Speech Pathology and Audiology at Teachers College, Columbia University, **Edward D. Mysak** teaches and does research on stuttering, cleft palate, and diagnostic methods a well as on cerebral palsy. He has been a leader in ASHA for many years and holds both the CCC in Speech Pathology and the CCC in Audiology. Mysak has written five textbooks dealing with speech or cerebral palsy, along with numerous articles, chapters, and films. Since 1960, he has presented over 100 talks and short courses at conventions, colleges and universities, hospitals, and special schools, on a wide range of topics, including language development and disorders, vocal aging, stuttering, cerebral palsy, feedback theory, cleft palate, articulation, dysarthria, and speech systems theory.

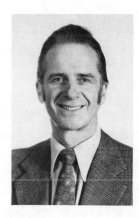

Audrey L. Holland is Professor of Speech and Research Assistant Professor of Psychiatry at the University of Pittsburgh, where she received her undergraduate and graduate training. An active member of her university community, she is also a leader in both the American Speech-Language-Hearing Association and the Academy of Aphasia. She has served in editorial roles for the *Journal of Speech and Hearing Disorders, Behavioral Sciences and Allied Health,* and *Journal of Speech and Hearing Research.* Holland has written many articles, reviews, and textbook chapters, as well as *Communicative Abilities in Daily Living: An Assessment Procedure for Aphasic Adults.* Her career is marked by a two-fold interest in applied research and in clinical management, most particularly dealing with aphasia, neurogenic speech-language disorders, and neurolinguistics.

O. M. Reinmuth, M.D., completed his undergraduate education at the University of Texas. He obtained his M.D. degree from Duke University, where he also completed his internship. This was followed by residencies in Internal Medicine at Yale University and in Neurology at Harvard University (Boston City Hospital) and at Queen's Square Hospital, London, England. He served as Professor of Neurology at the University of Miami Medical School before becoming Professor and Chairman, Department of Neurology, University of Pittsburgh, a position he has held for the past 4 years. He is a Fellow of the American Academy of Neurology and the American College of Physicians, a member and past officer of the American Neurological Association, and is currently serving as Chairman of the Stroke Council of the American Heart Association.

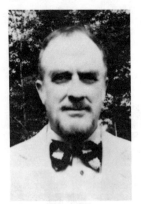

Albert T. Murphy is Professor of Special Education, Communicative Disorders, and Rehabilitation Medicine at Boston University, where he has been Director of the Psycho-Educational Clinic, the Speech and Hearing Clinic, and Chairman of the Division of Special and Counselor Education. He is also a Licensed Clinical Psychologist. Murphy is a consultant to a number of government agencies, including the U.S. Office of Special Education and the U.S. Overseas Dependency Schools. In the last several years, he has helped put P.L. 94-142 in place for U.S. citizens in Europe and the Orient. Murphy is the author of 65 publications dealing with handicapping conditions, including books on the families of handicapped children, psychological voice disorders, and hearing impaired children; and he has coauthored several books on stuttering. In recent years he has been an editorial board member of such journals as *Mental Retardation, The Exceptional Parent* and *The Volta Review.* His most recent publication is *Special Parents, Special Children: Personal Issues with Handicapped Children.*